MW01284435

Manual of Canine and Feline Cardiology

Fourth Edition

Manual of Canine and Feline Cardiology

Fourth Edition

Larry P. Tilley, DVM
Diplomate, American College of Veterinary
Internal Medicine (Internal Medicine)
President, VetMed Consultants, Inc.
Consultant, New Mexico Veterinary Specialty Referral Center
Santa Fe, New Mexico

Francis W. K. Smith, Jr., DVM
Diplomate, American College of Veterinary
Internal Medicine (Internal Medicine & Cardiology)
Vice President, VetMed Consultants, Inc.
Lexington, Massachusetts;
Clinical Assistant Professor, Department of Medicine
Cummings School of Veterinary Medicine, Tufts University
North Grafton, Massachusetts

Mark A. Oyama, DVM
Diplomate, American College of Veterinary
Internal Medicine (Cardiology)
Associate Professor
Department of Clinical Studies
School of Veterinary Medicine
University of Pennsylvania
Philadelphia, Pennsylvania

Meg M. Sleeper, VMD
Diplomate, American College of Veterinary
Internal Medicine (Cardiology)
Assistant Professor and Section Chief, Cardiology
Department of Clinical Studies
School of Veterinary Medicine
University of Pennsylvania
Philadelphia, Pennsylvania

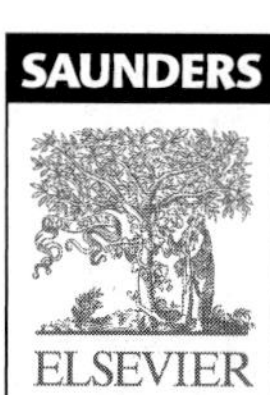

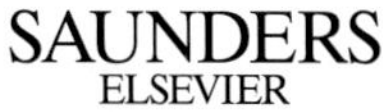

11830 Westline Industrial Drive
St. Louis, Missouri 63146

MANUAL OF CANINE AND FELINE CARDIOLOGY
FOURTH EDITION

ISBN: 978-1-4160-2398-2

Notice

Knowledge and best practice in this field are constantly changing. As new research and experience broaden our knowledge, changes in practice, treatment and drug therapy may become necessary or appropriate. Readers are advised to check the most current information provided (i) on procedures featured or (ii) by the manufacturer of each product to be administered, to verify the recommended dose or formula, the method and duration of administration, and contraindications. It is the responsibility of the practitioner, relying on their own experience and knowledge of the patient, to make diagnoses, to determine dosages and the best treatment for each individual patient, and to take all appropriate safety precautions. To the fullest extent of the law, neither the Publisher nor the Editors assume any liability for any injury and/or damage to persons or property arising out of or related to any use of the material contained in this book.

The Publisher

Previous editions copyrighted 2001, 1995, 1985.

Library of Congress Control Number: 2007928036

ISBN: 978-1-4160-2398-2

Vice President and Publisher: Linda Duncan
Senior Acquisitions Editor: Anthony Winkel
Developmental Editor: Shelly Stringer
Publishing Services Manager: Pat Joiner-Myers
Senior Project Manager: Gena Magouirk
Design Direction: Karen O'Keefe Owens

Printed in Canada

Last digit is the print number: 9 8 7 6 5 4 3 2

To my wife, Jeri, my son, Kyle, mother, Dorothy
In honor of that secret correspondence and love within our hearts

Larry P. Tilley

To the ever-popular Ben Smith and his charming sister Jade,
thanks for keeping life fun. You are the best! To my wife May,
who warms my heart every day, thanks for always being there.

Francis W. K. Smith, Jr.

To my parents, who made this all possible.
To Emi, K.A., Miya, and Audrey, who keep the kid in me alive.

Mark A. Oyama

To Dave, whose support enables my dreams; and my father, who inspired them.

Meg M. Sleeper

Contributors

Jonathan A. Abbott, DVM, DACVIM (Cardiology)
Associate Professor
Department of Small Animal Clinical Sciences
Virginia-Maryland Regional College of Veterinary Medicine
Virginia Polytechnic Institute and State University
Blacksburg, Virginia
Acquired Valvular Disease

Janice McIntosh Bright, BSN, MS, DVM, DACVIM (Cardiology and Internal Medicine)
Professor of Cardiology
Department of Clinical Sciences
College of Veterinary Medicine and
Biomedical Sciences
Colorado State University
Fort Collins, Colorado
Pacemaker Therapy

Scott A. Brown, VMD, PhD, DACVIM (Internal Medicine)
Josiah Meigs Distinguished Professor
Associate Dean for Academic Affairs
Department of Physiology and Pharmacology
University of Georgia
College of Veterinary Medicine
Athens, Georgia
Systemic Hypertension

Clay A. Calvert, DVM, DACVIM (Internal Medicine)
Professor
Small Animal Medicine and Surgery
College of Veterinary Medicine
The University of Georgia
Athens, Georgia
Heartworm Disease

Kathleen E. Cavanagh, BSc, DVM
Haskell Valley Veterinary Hospital
Orleans, New York;
Niagara Veterinary Emergency Clinic
St. Catharines, Ontario, Canada
Appendix 1: Canine Breed Predilections for Heart Disease

Steven G. Cole, DVM, DACVECC, DACVIM (Cardiology)
Section of Critical Care
Department of Clinical Studies – Philadelphia
School of Veterinary Medicine
University of Pennsylvania
Philadelphia, Pennsylvania
Cardiopulmonary Resuscitation
Emergency Management and Critical Care

Thomas K. Day, DVM, MS, DACVA, DACVECC
Owner, Emergency and Critical Care Veterinarian, Anesthesiologist
Louisville Veterinary Specialty and Emergency Services
Louisville, Kentucky
Anesthesia of the Cardiac Patient

Kenneth J. Drobatz, DVM, MSCE, DACVIM (Internal Medicine), DACVECC
Professor, Section of Critical Care
Department of Clinical Studies – Philadelphia
School of Veterinary Medicine
University of Pennsylvania;
Director, Emergency Service
Ryan Veterinary Hospital of the University of Pennsylvania
Philadelphia, Pennsylvania
Cardiopulmonary Resuscitation
Emergency Management and Critical Care

Virginia Luis Fuentes, MA, VETMB, PhD, CertVR, DVC, DACVIM (Cardiology), DECVIM-CA (Cardiology), MRCVS
Senior Lecturer in Small Animal Medicine
Veterinary Clinical Sciences
Royal Veterinary College
Hatfield, United Kingdom
Echocardiography and Doppler Ultrasound

Anna R. M. Gelzer, Dr.med.vet., DACVIM (Cardiology)
Assistant Professor
Department of Clinical Sciences
College of Veterinary Medicine
Cornell University
Ithaca, New York
Treatment of Cardiac Arrhythmias and Conduction Disturbances

Rebecca E. Gompf, DVM, MS, DACVIM (Cardiology)
Associate Professor of Cardiology
Department of Small Animal Clinical Sciences
University of Tennessee
College of Veterinary Medicine
Knoxville, Tennessee
The History and Physical Examination

Rosemary A. Henik, DVM, MS, DACVIM (Internal Medicine)
Clinical Associate Professor
Department of Medical Sciences
University of Wisconsin – Madison
Madison, Wisconsin
Systemic Hypertension

Lynelle R. Johnson, DVM, PhD, DACVIM (Internal Medicine)
Assistant Professor
Department of Veterinary Medicine and Epidemiology
College of Veterinary Medicine
University of California–Davis
Davis, California
Cor Pulmonale and Pulmonary Thromboembolism

Richard D. Kienle, DVM, DACVIM (Cardiology)
Staff Cardiologist
Bay Area Veterinary Specialists
San Leandro, California;
Owner
Mission Valley Veterinary Cardiology
Gilroy, California
Feline Cardiomyopathy

Marc S. Kraus, DVM, DACVIM (Cardiology and Internal Medicine)
Lecturer
Department of Clinical Sciences
College of Veterinary Medicine
Cornell University
Ithaca, New York
Treatment of Cardiac Arrhythmias and Conduction Disturbances

Elizabeth A. McNiel, DVM, PhD, DACVIM (Oncology), ACVR (Radiation Oncology)
Assistant Professor
Department of Veterinary Clinical Sciences
College of Veterinary Medicine
University of Minnesota
St. Paul, Minnesota
Pericardial Disorders and Cardiac Tumors

Sydney Moise, DVM, MS, DACVIM (Cardiology and Internal Medicine)
Professor of Medicine, Section Chief Cardiology
Department of Clinical Sciences
College of Veterinary Medicine
Cornell University
Ithaca, New York
Treatment of Cardiac Arrhythmias and Conduction Disturbances

E. Christopher Orton, DVM, PhD, DACVS
Professor
Department of Clinical Sciences
Veterinary Medical Center
Colorado State University
Fort Collins, Colorado
Cardiac Surgery

Mark A. Oyama, DVM, DACVIM (Cardiology)
Associate Professor
Department of Clinical Studies
School of Veterinary Medicine
University of Pennsylvania
Philadelphia, Pennsylvania
Canine Cardiomyopathy
Appendix 2: Common Cardiovascular Drugs

Brian A. Poteet, MS, DVM, DACVR, ABSVM
Director,
Gulf Coast Veterinary Diagnostic Imaging
Gulf Coast Veterinary Specialists
Houston, Texas
Radiology of the Heart

Carl D. Sammarco, BVSc, DACVIM (Cardiology)
Senior Cardiologist
Department of Cardiology
Red Bank Veterinary Hospital
Tinton Falls, New Jersey
Cardiovascular Effects of Systemic Diseases

Donald P. Schrope, DVM, DACVIM (Cardiology)
Oradell Animal Hospital
Department of Cardiology
Paramus, New Jersey
Cardiovascular Effects of Systemic Diseases

Meg M. Sleeper, VMD, DACVIM (Cardiology)
Assistant Professor and Section Chief, Cardiology
Department of Clinical Studies
School of Veterinary Medicine
University of Pennsylvania
Philadelphia, Pennsylvania
Special Diagnostic Techniques for Evaluation of Cardiac Disease
Appendix 2: Common Cardiovascular Drugs

Francis W. K. Smith, Jr., DVM, DACVIM (Internal Medicine and Cardiology)
Vice President
VetMed Consultants, Inc.
Lexington, Massachusetts;
Clinical Assistant Professor
Department of Medicine
Cummings School of Veterinary Medicine
Tufts University
North Grafton, Massachusetts
Electrocardiography
Cardiovascular Effects of Systemic Diseases
Appendix 1: Canine Breed Predilections for Heart Disease
Appendix 2: Common Cardiovascular Drugs

Keith N. Strickland, DVM, DACVIM (Cardiology)
Clinical Associate Professor of Veterinary Cardiology
Department of Veterinary Clinical Sciences
School of Veterinary Medicine
Louisiana State University
Baton Rouge, Louisiana
Congenital Heart Disease
Pathophysiology and Therapy of Heart Failure

Justin David Thomason, DVM, DACVIM (Internal Medicine)
Assistant Professor
Department of Veterinary Clinical Science
Center for Veterinary Health Sciences
Oklahoma State University
Stillwater, Oklahoma
Heartworm Disease

Larry P. Tilley, DVM, DAVCIM (Internal Medicine)
President, VetMed Consultants, Inc.
Consultant, New Mexico
Veterinary Specialty Referral Center
Santa Fe, New Mexico
Electrocardiography
Appendix 2: Common Cardiovascular Drugs

Anthony H. Tobias, BVSc, PhD, DACVIM (Cardiology)
Associate Professor
Department of Clinical Sciences
College of Veterinary Medicine
University of Minnesota
St. Paul, Minnesota
Pericardial Disorders and Cardiac Tumors

Preface

In the last 5 years there have been a number of excellent textbook chapters and journal articles describing new findings in the field of canine and feline cardiology. However, for the practicing veterinarian and veterinary student, the amount of information is overwhelming. Many veterinarians and students have stated, in past surveys, the difficulty in keeping up with cardiovascular advances in the most time-effective way. The *Manual of Canine and Feline Cardiology,* now in its fourth edition, has been updated to continue to meet the need for a current textbook that can provide useful and practical information on cardiac disease in the dog and cat. We have worked hard to make this book a most reliable source for practicing cardiovascular medicine in the dog and cat. For the new edition, we have expanded the number of contributors, with each chapter written by an expert. We have also worked to conserve reading time by using an easy-to-use format. The *Manual of Canine and Feline Cardiology,* Fourth Edition, is unique as a quick reference with consistency of presentation. The new edition now also has generous use of figures and charts, with many in color.

This practical approach to the diagnosis and therapy of cardiac disease will be useful to a wide audience, from the veterinary student to the fully trained cardiologist. The approach is largely clinical and includes the practical as well as the most sophisticated methods for diagnosis and therapy.

Cardiovascular disorders in the dog and cat represent a substantial portion of diseases seen in the average veterinary practice. It is important for veterinary students and practitioners to understand the principles of diagnosis and treatment of the numerous cardiovascular disorders. New chapters that have been added include cardiac surgery, cor pulmonale, pulmonary thromboembolism, and pacemaker therapy. A table of canine breed predilections for heart disease has been added to the appendixes.

Since the third edition of this textbook was published, there has been tremendous growth in the field of canine and feline cardiology. The fourth edition has been carefully revised, edited, and updated to reflect the latest technologies and approaches to cardiac care.

The methods of diagnosis of heart diseases in the dog and the cat are described in Section I The first five chapters follow the sequence that the veterinarian uses in approaching the patient. Chapter 1 covers the history and physical examination; Chapter 2, radiology of the heart; Chapter 3, electrocardiography; Chapter 4, echocardiography and Doppler ultrasound; and Chapter 5, special diagnostic techniques for evaluation of cardiac disease.

Section II presents in a step-by-step fashion a description of the various cardiac disorders that occur in the dog and cat, starting in each chapter with general considerations (e.g., definitions, incidence, pathophysiology, etiology), history, physical examination, electrocardiography, thoracic radiography, special diagnostic techniques, differential diagnosis, and finally, the therapeutic approach.

Section III includes chapters describing the treatment of cardiac failure, treatment of arrhythmias and conduction disturbances, and two separate chapters on cardiopulmonary arrest and resuscitation and on emergency management and critical care in cardiology. Chapters on anesthesia of the cardiac patient, cardiac surgery, and pacemaker therapy complete this section.

Appendix 1, Canine Breed Predilections for Heart Disease, represents the most current listing of breed-associated cardiac disorders.

Appendix 2 is a cardiopulmonary drug formulary that contains extensive cardiopulmonary drug tables with indications, dosages, side effects, contraindications, and drug interactions. An extraordinary array of new cardiovascular drugs has become available, and both students and veterinarians have difficulty deciding which drugs from various drug classes should be prescribed.

Appendix 3, Echocardiographic Normals, is an easy-to-refer-to list of normal values by body weight and breed.

The *Manual of Canine and Feline Cardiology,* Fourth Edition, will help to eliminate the aura of mystery that surrounds the diagnostic and therapeutic principles of veterinary cardiology. The teaching principles that are presented will allow even the novice to make an intelligent assessment of a cardiac case. This manual will be useful to a wide audience, but comprehensive enough to serve as a reference for the advanced student and the veterinarian with expertise in cardiology.

LARRY P. TILLEY
FRANCIS W. K. SMITH, JR.
MARK A. OYAMA
MEG M. SLEEPER

Acknowledgments

The completion of this manual provides a welcome opportunity to recognize in writing the many individuals who have helped along the way. All authors have board certification and are uniquely qualified to give an update or review of their respective disciplines.

In addition to thanking veterinarians who have referred cases to us, we would like to express our gratitude to each of the veterinary students, interns, and residents whom we have had the pleasure of teaching. Their curiosity and intellectual stimulation have enabled us to grow and prompted us to undertake the task of writing this manual.

The last edition was co-edited by John Karl Goodwin, and since then he has unfortunately passed away. John's teaching principles in veterinary medicine were clearly drawn from clinical experience, and this edition continues to maintain that focus. I will always remember what John had posted on a wall at his office: "No one cares how much you know until they know how much you care." That saying was John's philosophy and one that all of us should follow.

Finally, a special thank you goes to Tony Winkel, Editor, Elsevier, whose vision and support were critical for this fourth edition. The unique format and use of numerous images demonstrates the educational vision he had. For this edition, we would also like to thank Shelly Stringer, Developmental Editor and the rest of the Elsevier staff, including everyone in the Production Department. They are all meticulous workers and kind people who made the final stages of preparing this book both inspiring and fun.

LARRY P. TILLEY
FRANCIS W. K. SMITH, JR.
MARK A. OYAMA
MEG M. SLEEPER

Contents

Appendixes

Manual of
Canine and Feline Cardiology

Fourth Edition

SECTION I

Diagnosis of Heart Disease

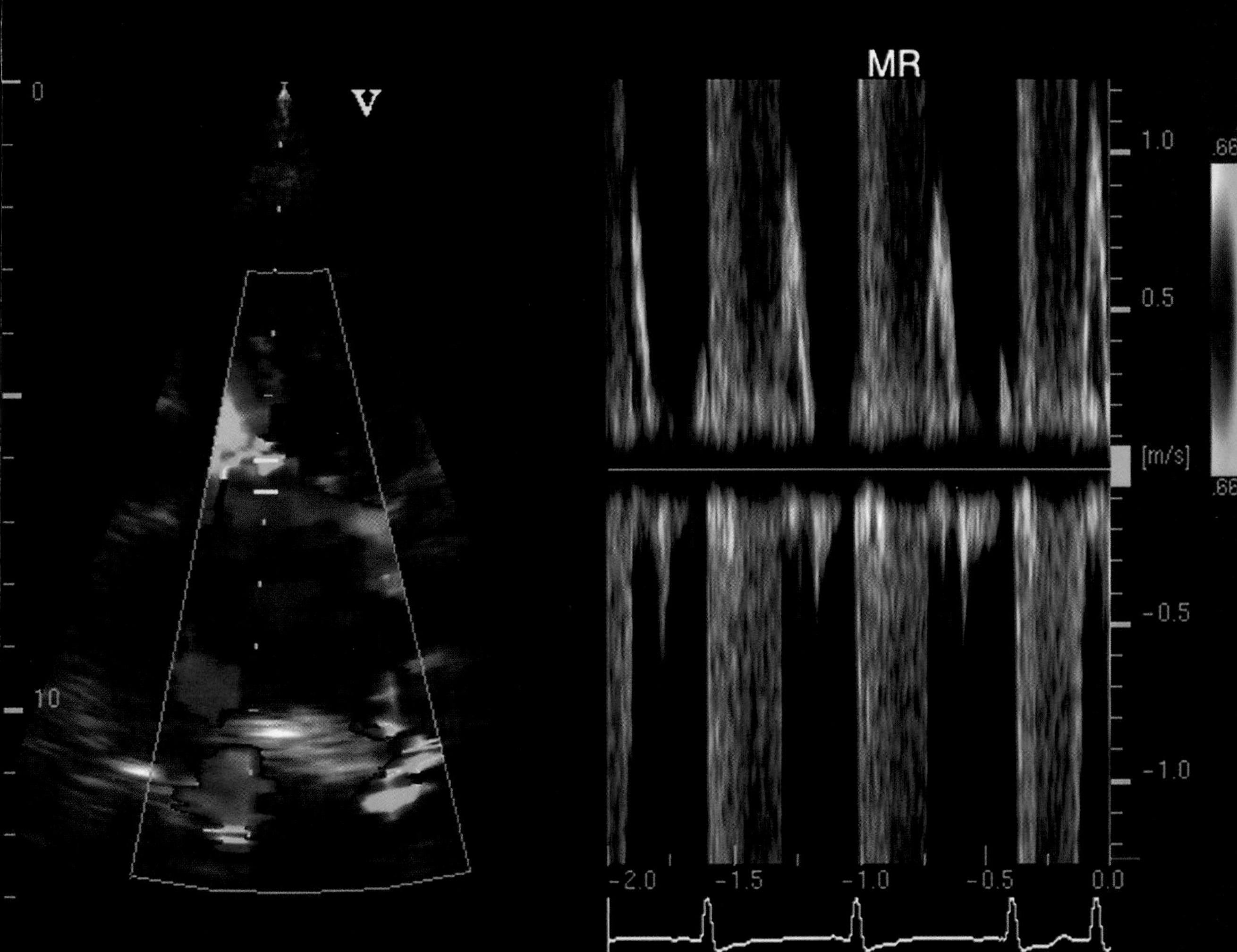

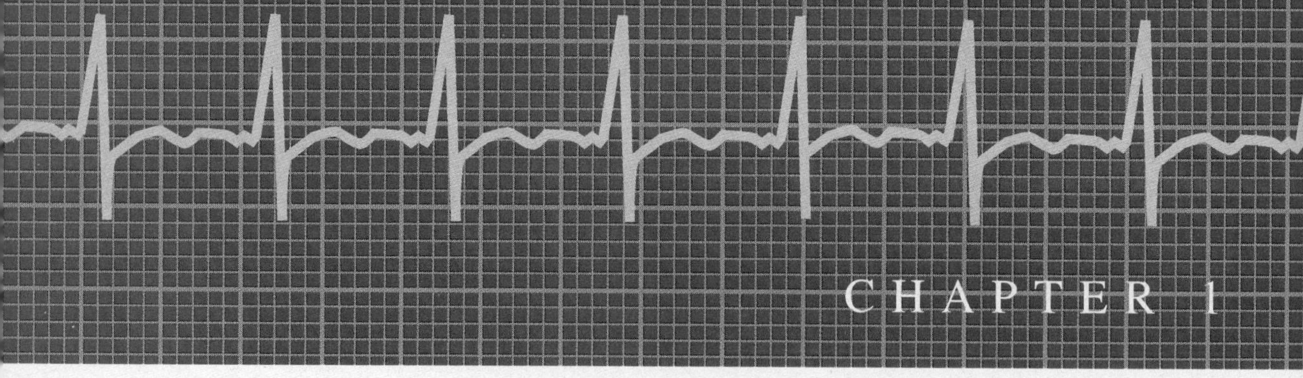

CHAPTER 1

The History and Physical Examination

Rebecca E. Gompf

INTRODUCTION

Despite the technical nature of many cardiovascular diagnostics, such as electrocardiography and echocardiography, the history and physical examination remain the most crucial steps in establishing the correct diagnosis. Findings from a careful history and physical examination prompt the clinician to the probability or presence of heart disease. Results of the cardiovascular physical examination will usually allow the clinician to make a tentative diagnosis or formulate a specific differential diagnosis. The history and physical examination also provide important information regarding the stage of heart disease present, which may significantly impact therapy.

- A good history and physical exam are invaluable in making a diagnosis of heart disease and helping to differentiate heart disease from pulmonary disease.
- Besides helping to make the diagnosis, a good history and physical exam help to tell the extent of the problem, how well the animal is responding to previous therapy, if the owner is able to medicate the animal consistently, and if other medical problems are present.

KEY POINT

Clinicians should do a thorough history and physical exam in order to properly diagnose and treat an animal with heart disease.

MEDICAL HISTORY

Signalment

Age

Young animals usually present with congenital diseases (e.g., patent ductus arteriosus [PDA]), whereas older animals usually present with acquired diseases, such as degenerative diseases (e.g., mitral and tricuspid regurgitations) or neoplastic diseases (e.g., heart base tumor). Exceptions can occur because cardiomyopathies can occur in young dogs and cats (aged 6 months or younger), and older dogs can have congenital heart defects that were not diagnosed when they were young (e.g., PDA, atrial septal defect). Also, cardiac disease in older animals can be modified or affected by other concurrent disease processes (e.g., collapsing trachea, renal or liver disease).

Breed

Certain cardiac defects are more common in some breeds of animals; however there can be a regional difference in the rate of occurrence of cardiac problems. See Appendix for a summary of some of the cardiac defects found in certain breeds of dogs and cats.

Sex

Males are more susceptible to certain cardiac diseases (e.g., male cocker spaniels to endocardiosis of the mitral valve, and large-breed males to dilated cardiomyopathy). However, sick sinus syndrome occurs in the female miniature schnauzer and PDA is more common in females than in males.

Weight

The animal's weight influences several aspects of treatment including the dose of cardiac medication to use, evaluation of the response to diuretic medication, and the monitoring of cardiac cachexia. A Pickwickian syndrome (characterized by severe obesity, somnolence, and hypoventilation) can occur in an animal that is so obese that its ability to breathe is restricted.

Utilization of the Animal

It is important to know how an animal is going to be used when giving a long term prognosis for a cardiac disease. For example, hunting dogs with severe heartworm disease may not be able to hunt again after treatment. Also, some animals with congenital heart defects may have normal life spans and may make good pets; however, they should not be used for breeding purposes, because the defect could be perpetuated.

KEY POINT

The age, breed, and sex of the animal may help the clinician to make an accurate diagnosis; however, there are always exceptions to every rule, so a clinician should not ignore the fact that an animal could have an atypical problem for its age, breed, or sex.

History

- A good history will establish the presence of a cardiac problem, help to differentiate between cardiac and respiratory problems, and help to monitor the course of the disease and the response to therapy. It must be done carefully to prevent an owner from giving a misleading history.
- It includes several key questions such as the reason the animal is being presented, the problems noted by the owner, the onset and duration of the problem(s), the progression of the disease, any known exposure to infectious diseases, vaccination history, any current medications the animal is receiving, the animal's response to any medications that have been given, and the owner's ability to give the medication(s).
- It will also define the animal's attitude and behavior by asking if the animal is listless and depressed or alert and playful. Does the animal tire easily with exercise?
- It covers the family history of the siblings and parents, especially if congenital disease is present in the patient.
- It will ask about the health of other pets in the household.
- It includes the results of previous tests done on the patient.
- It covers other relevant information that may help to identify the patient's problem(s), such as what and how much is being fed and the patient's appetite and water consumption. How frequently is the animal urinating, and does it have any diarrhea? Does the patient have any vomiting or regurgitation? Has the patient had any seizures or syncopal episodes? What is the patient's reproductive status? Does the patient have any lameness or paresis? Is the patient coughing, sneezing, or having difficulty breathing? Has the patient had any previous trauma? Where is the animal housed (e.g., indoors, outdoors, fenced-in yard)?
- It includes information about other diseases such as hyperthyroidism, chronic renal disease, respiratory diseases, or other diseases that can also affect the heart or can affect how the animal's heart disease is treated.
- Once a problem is identified, more specific questions can be asked such as the character of a cough, when the cough occurs, and stimuli evoking the cough.
- Common presenting complaints for cardiac disease include dyspnea or tachypnea, coughing, exercise intolerance, syncope, abdominal swelling, cyanosis, anorexia or decreased appetite, and poor growth or performance.
- Other symptoms can be associated with cardiovascular disease. Polydipsia and polyuria are common in animals on diuretics or that have a concurrent disease (e.g., renal disease), whereas oliguria occurs with severe left-heart failure. Hemoglobinuria is found with the postcaval syndrome of heartworm disease.
- Cardiac drugs such as digitalis, quinidine, and procainamide can cause vomiting and diarrhea. Regurgitation occurs with congenital vascular ring anomalies. Right-heart failure can cause intestinal edema and a protein-losing enteropathy resulting in diarrhea. Cats with cardiomyopathy can develop hemorrhagic enteritis secondary to thromboembolism of the gastric or mesenteric arteries.

KEY POINT

A good history will uncover all of the animal's symptoms and problems whether they are due to a cardiac problem or to another concurrent problem. Also, by the end of a good history, an astute clinician will have a good idea as to the potential causes of the animal's problems.

SPECIFIC SYMPTOMS

Coughing

- Coughing is the most common complaint in dogs with significant heart disease, but cats rarely cough even when they have an enlarged left atrium.
- Coughing is a sudden, forced expiration and is a normal defense mechanism to clear debris from the tracheobronchial tree. It can originate from many different areas such as the pharynx, trachea, bronchi, bronchioli, pleura, pericardium, and diaphragm.
- A cardiac cough can be difficult to differentiate from a respiratory cough. Table 1-1 lists some of the characteristic coughs and their associated causes.
- Dogs with pulmonary edema often have an acute onset of coughing that progresses rapidly to a severe cough and dyspnea. These coughs are usually soft.
- Dogs with chronic heart disease usually have mild, intermittent coughs. They may also have nocturnal dyspnea, coughing, and restlessness. Their coughs tend to be harsh and lower pitched.
- Dogs with fulminant left-heart failure may have pink foam in their mouth and nose and be dyspneic, but they may or may not be coughing.
- Dogs with a loud, harsh, dry cough of sudden onset followed by a nonproductive gag commonly have tracheobronchitis.
- Dogs with a honking, high-pitched cough often have a collapsing trachea and/or collapsed bronchi.
- Small breeds of dogs with large airway disease will have a chronic, paroxysmal cough that is hard, loud, and honking, and usually occurs with excitement.
- Dogs that cough after drinking may have cardiac disease, collapsing trachea, chronic tracheitis, tracheobronchitis, laryngeal problems, or other causes of dysphagia.
- Dog that cough without an inciting factor may have cardiac, pulmonary, or extrapulmonary disease.
- Dogs that cough after eating have pharyngeal dysphagia, megaesophagus, vascular ring anomalies, esophageal diverticula, esophageal foreign bodies, or esophageal tumors.
- It is unusual for cats to cough with congestive heart failure; however, they will cough with heartworm disease. If the clinician compresses

Table 1-1 Characteristics of Coughs and Their Associated Causes in Dogs and Cats

Type of Cough	Causes
Acute cough	Tonsillitis, pharyngitis, tracheobronchitis, acutebronchitis, pleuritis, acute left heart failure (dogs)
Chronic cough	Right or left heart disease, heartworms, enlarged left atrium compressing the left mainstem bronchus (dog only), pulmonary neoplasia, asthma (cat only), chronic respiratory problem, chronic bronchitis (dog only)
Acute onset, soft that rapidly becomes worse in dogs with dyspnea	Pulmonary edema
Mild, intermittent cough, harsh, low pitched in dogs	Chronic heart disease
Loud, harsh, dry, sudden onset followed by gag in dogs	Tracheobronchitis
Honking, high-pitched in dogs	Collapsing trachea or bronchi
Chronic, paroxysmal, loud, honking with excitement in dogs	Large airway disease
Cough after drinking in dogs	Cardiac disease, collapsing trachea, chronic tracheitis, tracheobronchitis, laryngeal paralysis, dysphagia
Cough after eating in dogs	Pharyngeal dysfunction, megaesophagus, vascular ring anomalies, esophageal diverticula, esophageal foreign bodies, esophageal tumors
Cough without an inciting factor	Cardiac, pulmonary, or extrapulmonary disease

KEY POINT

It is important to distinguish between a cough due to cardiac disease versus one due to respiratory disease. The history can be the first step in differentiating between the two major causes of coughing.

the cat's trachea and the cat has a prolonged bout of coughing, then coughing is likely to be part of the cat's problem.

Dyspnea

- Dyspnea is difficult, labored, or painful breathing. It is usually preceded by tachypnea (an increased rate of breathing), which owners may miss. It is a good idea to have the owner of a cardiac patient learn to count his or her pet's respiratory rate at rest. The respiratory rate should be less than 30 per minute in a dog at rest, and if it goes over 50 per minute, then the dog has tachypnea.
- Dyspnea will occur whenever anything increases the amount of air that must be breathed by the animal. Box 1-1 lists the problems that can cause dyspnea.
- The most common cardiac cause of dyspnea in the dog is left-heart failure causing pulmonary edema. The most common cardiac cause of dyspnea in the cat is right-heart failure causing pleural effusion or left-heart failure causing pulmonary edema.
- Dyspnea can be accompanied in cardiac patients by stridor, which is a harsh, high-pitched respiratory sound. Other sounds include rhonchi, which sound like dry, coarse crackles. Also, dyspnea can be accompanied by wheezing, which is more typical of respiratory problems than cardiac problems.
- Table 1-2 lists the different types of dyspnea and the problems associated with each type.
- Acute dyspnea is usually caused by pulmonary edema (cardiac and noncardiac), severe pneumonia, airway obstruction, pneumothorax, or pulmonary embolism.
- Chronic, progressive dyspnea is caused by right-heart failure with ascites and/or pleural effusion, pericardial diseases, bronchial disease, lung diseases such as emphysema, pleural effusions, progressive anemia, and primary or secondary pulmonary neoplasia.
- Dyspnea at rest occurs with pneumothorax, pulmonary embolism, and severe left- or right-heart failure.
- Exertional dyspnea occurs after or during activity and can be associated with heart diseases, such as dilated cardiomyopathy, when the animal goes into heart failure. It can also be associated with chronic, obstructive lung disease.
- Expiratory dyspnea is prolonged and labored expiration and is due to lower respiratory tract obstruction or disease.
- Inspiratory dyspnea is prolonged and labored inspiration and is due to upper airway obstruction.
- Mixed dyspnea is due to severe pulmonary edema caused by left-heart failure or severe pneumonia.
- Orthopnea means that the dyspnea occurs when the animal lies down but not when it is standing. It is associated with severe pulmonary edema, pleural effusion, pericardial effusion, pneumothorax, diaphragmatic hernia, and severe respiratory problems.
- Paroxysmal dyspnea means that the dyspnea comes and goes. It can be associated with arrhythmias that cause either bradycardia or tachycardia.
- Simple dyspnea, or polypnea, is an increased rate of respiration due to fever, fear, pain, or excitement.
- Cats with severe hyperthyroidism can also be dyspneic.
- Dyspnea that improves when treated with diuretics and angiotensin-converting enzyme inhibitors

Box 1-1 Causes of Dyspnea

Acidosis
Anemia
Central nervous system disorders
Excitement
High altitude
Pain
Pericardial effusions
Pleural effusions
Primary cardiac diseases causing pulmonary edema or pleural effusion
Pulmonary edema
Secondary cardiac diseases
Strenuous exercise
Thoracic wall problems (e.g., fractured ribs)

KEY POINT

Dyspnea is a sign of significant cardiac, respiratory, or other systemic problems. It requires immediate diagnostic tests to identify the cause of the dyspnea so that specific therapy can be started. However, all tests should be done with minimal stress to the animal as these patients are very fragile and could die with stress.

Table 1-2 Types of Dyspnea and Their Associated Diseases or Problems

Type of Dyspnea	Disease or Problem
Acute dyspnea	Pulmonary edema (cardiogenic and noncardiogenic), severe pneumonia, airway obstruction, pneumothorax, pulmonary embolism
Chronic, progressive dyspnea	Right heart failure with ascites and/or pleural effusion, pericardial diseases, bronchial disease, lung diseases (e.g., emphysema), pleural effusions, progressive anemia, primary and secondary neoplasia
Dyspnea at rest	Pneumothorax, pulmonary embolism, severe left or right heart failure
Exertional dyspnea	Heart disease (e.g., dilated cardiomyopathy) or chronic obstructive lung disease
Expiratory dyspnea	Lower respiratory tract obstruction or disease
Inspiratory dyspnea	Upper airway obstruction
Mixed dyspnea	Pulmonary edema due to left heart failure or severe pneumonia
Orthopnea	Severe pulmonary edema, pericardial effusion, pleural effusion, diaphragmatic hernia, pneumothorax, severe pulmonary disease
Paroxysmal dyspnea	Arrhythmias (e.g., bradycardia or tachycardia)
Simple dyspnea	Fever, fear, pain, or excitement

plus or minus digoxin is suggestive of left-heart failure as the cause of the dyspnea.
- Dyspnea that improves when treated with bronchodilators, antibiotics, or steroids is suggestive of respiratory disease as the cause of the dyspnea.

Hemoptysis

- Hemoptysis is coughing up of blood. It is uncommon in animals, as they usually swallow their sputum. It is a sign of very severe pulmonary disease.
- The causes of hemoptysis are listed in Box 1-2.
- Cardiac causes of hemoptysis include severe pulmonary edema (e.g., ruptured chordae tendineae) and severe heartworm disease, usually with pulmonary embolism.

Box 1-2 Causes of Hemoptysis

Acute and chronic bronchitis
Chronic pulmonary granulomas
Clotting disorders
Disseminated intravascular coagulopathy
Lung abscesses
Lung lobe torsions
Oral or other neoplasia
Pulmonary embolism
Pulmonary fungal infections
Pulmonary neoplasia
Respiratory foreign bodies
Severe heartworm disease with pulmonary embolism
Severe pneumonia
Severe pulmonary edema (e.g., from ruptured chordae tendineae)
Trauma with severe pulmonary contusions

KEY POINT

Hemoptysis is a sign of a very serious underlying abnormality in the lungs, which may be caused by either a severe cardiac or respiratory problem.

Syncope

- Syncope is a loss of consciousness due to inadequate cerebral blood flow. It can reoccur and is usually brief.
- Syncope can be hard to differentiate from seizures. Animals usually fall over suddenly, get back up quickly, and are normal before and after the syncopal episode.
- Box 1-3 lists the causes of syncope in dogs and cats.
- In a dog with no other cardiac problems, syncope may be associated with severe bradycardias (e.g., third degree heart block or sick sinus syndrome), or with marked sustained tachycardias (e.g., atrial or ventricular tachycardias), which are usually paroxysmal (i.e., they come and go).
- Small dogs with chronic, severe mitral regurgitation that cough when they get excited can have syncopal episodes.

Box 1-3 Causes of Syncope in Dogs and Cats

Disease with very poor cardiac output (e.g., dilated cardiomyopathy)
Severe bradycardia (e.g., complete heart block, sick sinus syndrome)
Severe sustained tachycardias (e.g., atrial or ventricular tachycardia)
Severe hypertrophic cardiomyopathy in cats
Systemic hypotension including arteriolar dilator therapy
Severe pulmonary hypertension
Severe subaortic stenosis
Severe pulmonic stenosis
Small dogs with severe mitral regurgitation that cough when excited
Tetralogy of Fallot

- Dogs with severe subaortic stenosis, pulmonic stenosis, pulmonary hypertension, or tetralogy of Fallot can have arrhythmias associated with their ventricular hypertrophy and myocardial hypoxia. Syncope can also occur in cats with severe hypertrophic cardiomyopathy.
- Animals with poor cardiac output due to dilated cardiomyopathy can have syncope, especially if they also have arrhythmias such as atrial fibrillation or ventricular premature beats that further reduce their cardiac output.
- Vasodilators, especially arterial dilators, can result in systemic hypotension, which can cause syncope.

KEY POINT

Syncope must be distinguished from seizures by careful history and physical examination. Having the owner videotape an episode can also help the clinician to distinguish between the two. Further tests such as Holter or event monitoring may be necessary to determine if an arrhythmia is causing the syncope.

Weakness and Exercise Intolerance

- Weakness and exercise intolerance are nonspecific signs of heart disease. Many diseases such as severe anemia, systemic diseases, metabolic diseases (e.g., hyperadrenocorticism), drug toxicities, and severe respiratory diseases can cause these signs. See Box 1-4 for causes of weakness and exercise intolerance.
- Because most animals do not exercise very hard, weakness and exercise intolerance are uncommon presenting complaints. Some owners think that their animal is slowing down due to old age and not due to heart disease or other problems.
- Both complaints can be an early sign of decompensated heart failure, as the heart cannot pump enough blood to the muscles due to:
    - Myocardial dysfunction (e.g., dilated cardiomyopathy or advanced mitral valve disease)
    - Obstruction to left ventricular outflow (e.g., subaortic stenosis or hypertrophic obstructive cardiomyopathy)
    - Inadequate ventricular filling (e.g., arrhythmias, pericardial diseases, hypertrophic cardiomyopathy)
    - Decreased arterial oxygen (e.g., pulmonary edema or pleural effusion).

Box 1-4 Causes of Weakness and Exercise Intolerance

Cardiac disease with myocardial dysfunction (e.g., dilated cardiomyopathy)
Cardiac disease with obstruction to left ventricular outflow (e.g., subaortic stenosis, hypertrophic obstructive cardiomyopathy)
Decreased arterial oxygen (e.g., pulmonary edema, pleural effusion or other pulmonary diseases)
Inadequate ventricular filling (e.g., arrhythmias, pericardial diseases)
Drug toxicities
Severe anemia
Severe metabolic disease
Severe respiratory diseases
Severe systemic diseases

KEY POINT

It is important to distinguish between exercise intolerance due to heart disease versus other causes.

Ascites

- Ascites is an accumulation of fluid in the abdomen.
- Ascites caused by cardiac problems is either due to the right heart being unable to pump the blood presented to it or because of pericardial disease, in which the blood cannot get into the right heart. In either case the blood accumulates in the liver and spleen and causes congestion and increased venous pressure. Eventually fluid leaks out of the capsule of the liver causing the ascites.

- Ascites is seen more frequently with right-heart failure in dogs due to acquired diseases (e.g., tricuspid regurgitation due to endocardiosis, advanced heartworm disease, dilated cardiomyopathy, pericardial effusions, restrictive pericarditis) and congenital heart defects (e.g., tricuspid dysplasia, large ventricular septal defect, large atrial septal defect). See Figure 1-1 for an example of ascites and Box 1-5 for a list of causes of ascites in the dog.
- Ascites is less common in cats and is usually due to tricuspid dysplasia but occasionally can be seen with other problems such as dilated cardiomyopathy.
- Large amounts of ascites will put pressure on the diaphragm, resulting in tachypnea or dyspnea.
- Ascites associated with right-heart failure is usually a modified transudate and accumulates slowly.

KEY POINT

Decompensated heart diseases that result in ascites may not have an associated murmur (e.g., pericardial effusion, some dilated cardiomyopathies, heartworm disease). Thus, any time ascites occurs, right-heart failure must be included in the differential diagnosis.

Cyanosis

- Cyanosis is blue-tinged mucous membranes of the gums, tongue, eyes, ears, and so on and is associated most commonly with right-to-left shunting congenital heart defects. Occasionally it is seen with severe left-heart failure or severe respiratory disease. It is rarely seen with abnormal hemoglobin production.

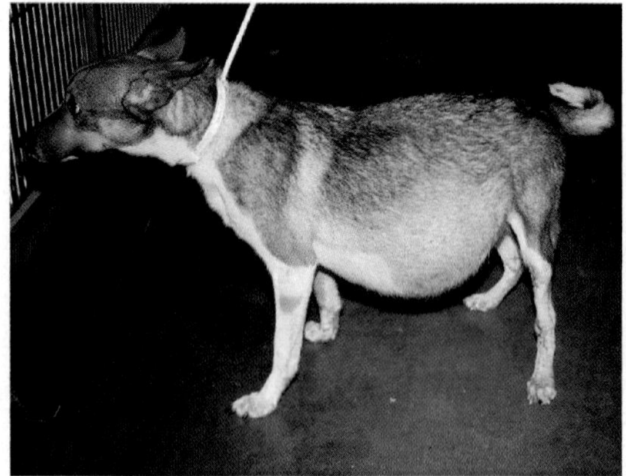

Figure 1-1. Notice the severe ascites in this dog with right-heart failure due to severe pulmonic stenosis and severe tricuspid dysplasia.

Box 1-5 Causes of Ascites in the Dog

Advanced heartworm disease
Dilated cardiomyopathy
Large atrial septal defect
Large ventricular septal defect
Pericardial effusion
Restrictive pericarditis
Tricuspid dysplasia
Tricuspid regurgitation due to endocardiosis

- Cyanosis is a very insensitive way of detecting hypoxemia in dogs and cats because the oxygen saturation has to be very low to cause it and animals have darker mucous membranes, which makes cyanosis harder to detect until it is severe.
- Right-to-left shunting cardiac defects such as tetralogy of Fallot result in low oxygen saturation plus high deoxygenated hemoglobin levels, which make affected animals cyanotic. These patients also have polycythemia, and the increased number of red blood cells has increased amounts of reduced hemoglobin, which contributes to the cyanosis.
- Cyanosis gets worse with exercise because the peripheral vascular resistance will decrease while the pulmonary vascular pressure is unchanged so more deoxygenated venous blood will go systemically.

KEY POINT

Cyanosis is a very late finding in severe cardiac disease, except in right to left shunting congenital heart defects, and so it is an insensitive indicator of membrane oxygenation and cardiac function.

Weight Loss

- Weight loss occurs in dogs with chronic, severe right-heart failure (e.g., severe tricuspid regurgitation, dilated cardiomyopathy, advanced heartworm disease).
- Weight loss in cats is usually associated with hyperthyroidism or infiltrative bowel disease, although cats with chronic right-heart failure can also lose weight.
- Cardiac cachexia is the loss of total body fat and lean body mass, especially skeletal muscle, despite a normal appetite and adequate therapy for the underlying heart disease. It can be a rapid loss of body condition in some dogs with dilated

cardiomyopathy (Figure 1-2). See Box 1-6 for a list of the problems that contribute to cardiac cachexia in dogs.

Weight loss is associated with:

- Ascites. Dogs with ascites may have mild discomfort from the fluid which makes them reluctant to eat. Also, the ascites and congested liver will compress the stomach so that the animal feels full after eating only a small amount of food. The fluid also restricts gastric emptying. Finally, if an unpalatable diet is fed, the animal is even more reluctant to eat and does not consume enough calories to keep from losing weight.

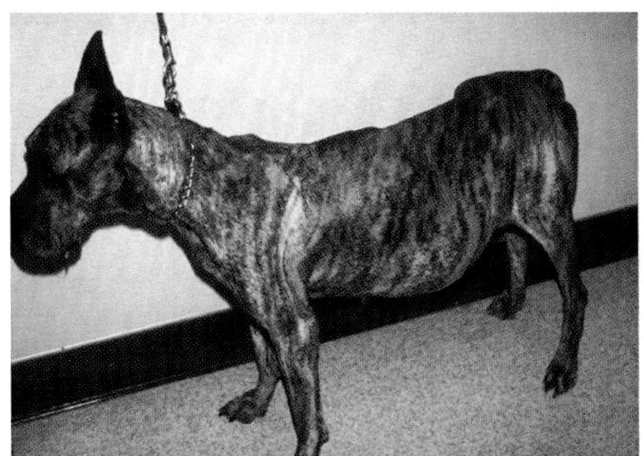

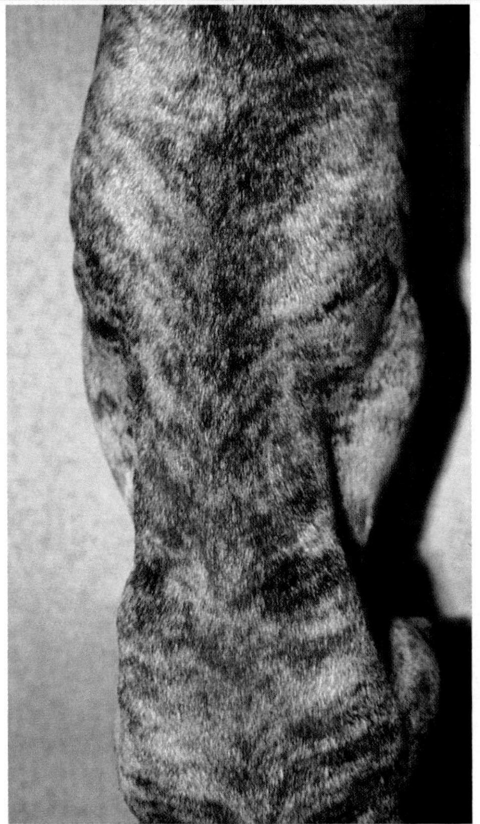

Figure 1-2. Great Dane with cardiac cachexia secondary to dilated cardiomyopathy.

Box 1-6 Problems Contributing to Cardiac Cachexia in the Dog

Ascites
Cardiac medications causing anorexia and vomiting
Electrolyte imbalance causing anorexia
Increased energy use by the body
Increased tumor necrosis factor
Malabsorption
Maldigestion
Protein losing enteropathy

- Malabsorption caused by the congestion of the intestines secondary to the ascites.
- Congestion of the pancreas, which may decrease its function of secreting enzymes for digestion, resulting in maldigestion.
- Systemic venous and lymphatic hypertension from right-heart failure causing a secondary intestinal lymphangiectasia that results in a protein-losing enteropathy.
- Increased effort to breath and increased myocardial oxygen consumption that result from the decreased cardiac output. These two problems result in an increased use of energy and therefore calories by the heart and lungs. The activation of the sympathetic nervous system, which also results from the decreased cardiac output, causes increased energy use by the rest of the body.
- Use of cardiac medications such as digoxin, mexiletine, quinidine, procainamide, diltiazem, and occasionally other drugs that can cause anorexia and/or vomiting. Digoxin also has a direct effect on the small bowel, where it inhibits sugar and amino acid transport.
- Electrolytes, especially sodium and potassium, are adversely affected by diuretics, angiotensin converting enzyme inhibitors, and digoxin. When

KEY POINT

Weight loss and cardiac cachexia are due to multiple factors. It is very important to make sure that an animal with ascites is being treated appropriately for heart failure and that the animal's digoxin levels, electrolytes, and renal function are being monitored. It is also important to calculate the animal's caloric requirement and make sure it is eating enough to meet its requirements. Special high caloric diets and multiple small meals may be needed to insure adequate caloric intake. Appetite stimulants have been tried with varying success.

potassium levels are abnormal, they contribute to anorexia.

- Dogs with chronic congestive heart failure have increased tumor necrosis factor that inhibits the activity of lipoprotein lipase (hydrolyzes chylomicrons) and therefore interferes with the conversion of triglycerides to free fatty acids.

Paresis

- Cats with acute, posterior paresis (Figure 1-3) or paresis of one front leg (Figure 1-4) often have thromboembolism secondary to cardiomyopathy. The thrombi tend to form in the dilated left atrium or left ventricle, and pieces break off and lodge in the distal aorta or other artery. When the thrombus lodges in the aortic bifurcation, the cat will exhibit severe pain in the first few hours after the embolism and the distal limbs will be cold and may be slightly swollen. The pads on the rear feet will be cyanotic (Figure 1-5). The cat's pulses cannot be detected, and the nails on the affected legs do not bleed when cut short.
- Acute, posterior paresis is rare in dogs but it has been associated with emboli from severe, vegetative endocarditis of the aortic or mitral valve.
- Shifting leg lameness in dogs has also been associated with bacterial endocarditis.

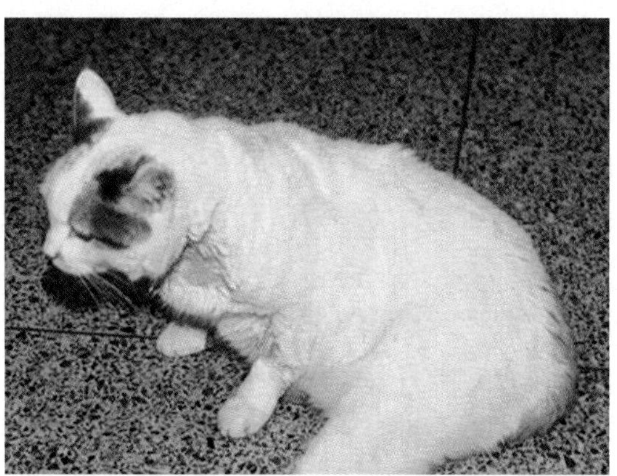

Figure 1-3. Cat with a saddle thrombus secondary to a left atrial thrombus due to hypertrophic cardiomyopathy.

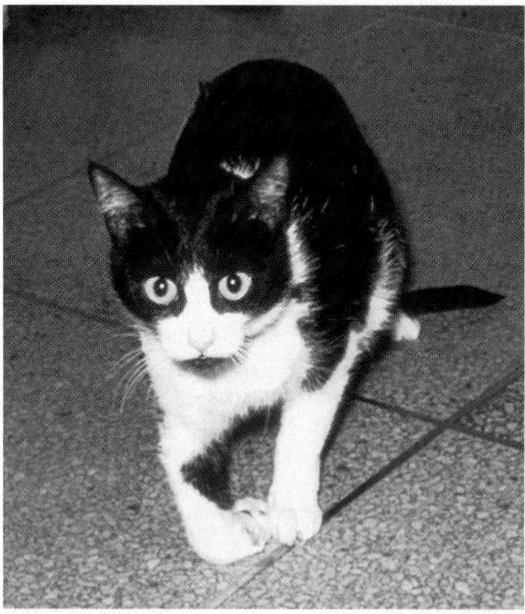

Figure 1-4. Cat with a front leg thrombus secondary to a left atrial thrombus due to hypertrophic cardiomyopathy.

KEY POINT

Paresis in the rear limbs of the cat is usually due to emboli that form in the left atrium secondary to left atrial enlargement secondary to cardiomyopathies. Shifting leg lameness or posterior paresis in the dog can be due to emboli from vegetations on either the mitral or aortic valve.

PHYSICAL EXAMINATION

Observation

- The animal's attitude and behavior can give clues as to the severity and kind of problems that the animal is having. It is important to note whether the animal is depressed or alert, and listless or active.

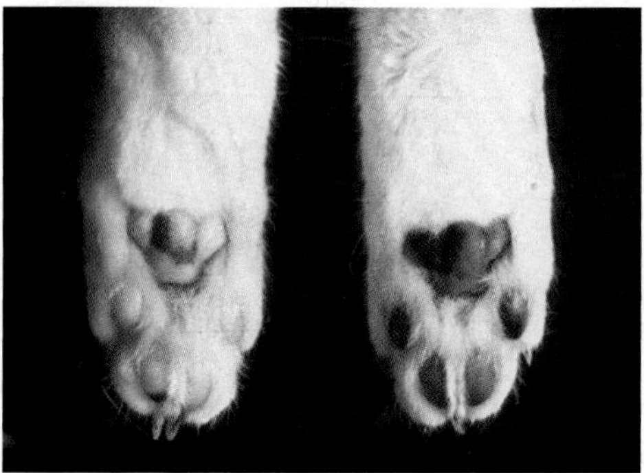

Figure 1-5. Comparison of the front and rear leg footpads in a cat with a saddle thrombus. Note the purple color of the rear leg due to the complete occlusion of blood flow to the rear limbs secondary to the saddle thrombus and constriction of the collateral circulation.

- An animal that refuses to lie down may have severe pulmonary edema, pleural effusion, pericardial effusion, pneumothorax, diaphragmatic hernia, or respiratory disease (Box 1-7).
- An animal that stands with elbows abducted and head extended as well as open-mouth breathing with flared nostrils has severe respiratory distress and needs immediate therapy.
- The rate and rhythm of respirations can help determine the underlying problem. Tachypnea and panting are usually due to excitement; however, expiratory dyspnea usually indicates lower airway disease, and inspiratory dyspnea usually indicates upper airway disease.
- The nature and type of coughing is helpful if it occurs during the course of the physical exam.
- The presence of dependent ventral edema can give the clinician an idea as to the source of the animal's problem. If edema is present in the neck, head, and forelimbs only, then it usually indicates an obstruction of the cranial vena cava or a mediastinal mass. If edema is present in the entire body, then pleural effusion with or without ascites is usually present. Other causes of edema (e.g., hypoproteinemia) should also be considered.
- Elevated temperature may be seen with an infectious disease or subacute bacterial endocarditis.

KEY POINT

By observing an animal, the presence and severity of a respiratory problem can be determined quickly. Animals with severe dyspnea should be handled gently to avoid stress and should be treated immediately.

Head

- Check for any asymmetry and swellings.
- The eyes should be examined for changes that could indicate systemic diseases.

Box 1-7 Reasons an Animal Will Not Lie Down

Diaphragmatic hernia
Pneumothorax
Severe pericardial effusion
Severe pleural effusion
Severe pulmonary edema
Severe respiratory disease

- Hypertension in cats will cause decreased pupillary responses due to retinal detachment or hemorrhage. Also, a fundic exam may reveal papilledema (swelling of the optic disc) along with hemorrhage or retinal detachment.
- Retinal hemorrhages also can occur with polycythemia and bacterial endocarditis.
- Central retinal degeneration occurs in about one third of cats with dilated cardiomyopathy caused by taurine deficiency. The areas of degeneration are horizontal, linear, and hyperreflective.
- The ears have no significant changes associated with the cardiovascular system.
- Cyanosis can sometimes be recognized by evaluating the color of the pinna.
- Examine the nose for signs of disease and for patency.
- In the mouth, mucous membrane color and perfusion should be noted. A perfusion time of greater than 2 seconds suggests decreased cardiac output; however, most animals with congestive heart failure have normal mucous membrane color until their heart failure is severe. So, mucous membrane color and perfusion are very insensitive ways to evaluate adequate circulation.
- Cyanosis is due to hypoventilation or poor diffusion across the alveoli produced by multiple different factors (see history section discussed previously).
- Hyperemic mucous membranes (dark red to muddy) may indicate an increased packed cell volume (polycythemia), which can be secondary to a chronic right-to-left vascular shunt (Figure 1-6).
- Pale mucous membranes indicate anemia or poor perfusion.
- The mucous membranes of the mouth should be compared with the posterior membranes

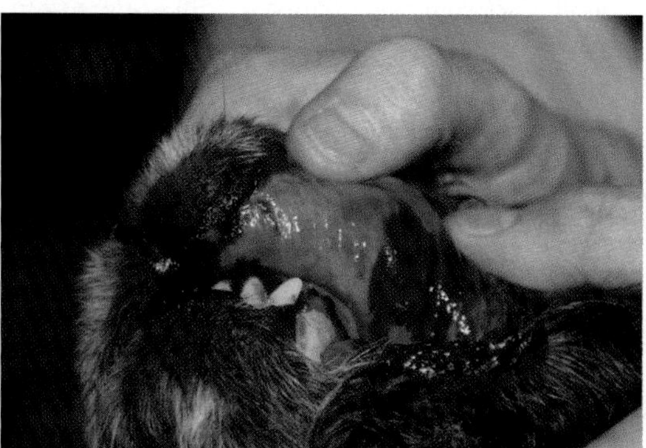

Figure 1-6. Hyperemic mucous membranes in a dog with polycythemia due to Tetralogy of Fallot.

(e.g., vagina, prepuce), because differential cyanosis can occur in a right-to-left shunting PDA.

- Check the oral cavity for severe dental tartar, gingivitis, or pyorrhea, which can serve as sources of sepsis leading to bacteremia and possibly endocarditis.

KEY POINT

Mucous membrane color and perfusion are insensitive signs of cardiac function, so when they are abnormal, the animal's cardiac or respiratory problem is severe.

Neck

- The jugular pulse should be evaluated while the animal is standing with its head in a normal position. Any pulse going over one third of the way up the neck is abnormal and can be due to any of several factors. See Box 1-8 for causes of abnormal jugular pulses.
- Abnormal jugular pulses occur in right-heart failure due to tricuspid regurgitation or dilated cardiomyopathy, when the right ventricle contracts and the blood flows back into the right atrium and up the jugular veins due to the insufficient tricuspid valve.
- Abnormal jugular pulses occur with pulmonic stenosis and pulmonary hypertension, when the right atrium contracts against a hypertrophied, noncompliant right ventricle so that only some of the blood enters the right ventricle and the rest goes back up the jugular veins.
- With heartworm disease, abnormal jugular pulses occur because there is both a stiff, hypertrophied right ventricle and tricuspid regurgitation which both contribute to the jugular pulses.
- Arrhythmias such as second or third degree heart block or premature beats cause abnormal jugular pulses because the sequence of atrial and ventricular activation is disrupted so that the atrium contracts against a closed tricuspid valve sending blood back up the jugular veins.

Box 1-8 Causes of Abnormal Jugular Pulses

Arrhythmias
Heartworm disease
Pulmonary hypertension
Pulmonic stenosis
Right-heart failure (e.g., tricuspid regurgitation, dilated cardiomyopathy)

- The entire jugular vein can be distended indicating increased systemic venous pressure caused by right-heart failure, pericardial disease, or obstruction of the cranial vena cava (e.g., heart base tumor). Only about 70% of dogs with right-heart failure have distended jugular veins, and cats rarely have distended jugular veins with right-heart failure. See Box 1-9 for causes of jugular distension.
- Mediastinal masses such as lymphosarcoma can compress the cranial vena cava causing a distended jugular vein; however, they also usually cause pleural effusion and head and neck edema.
- Arterial pulses can mimic a jugular pulse; however, when light pressure is applied to the area of the jugular pulse, the arterial pulse will continue, whereas the jugular pulse will stop.
- The hepatojugular reflex is a distension of the jugular veins that occurs when the abdomen is compressed for 10 to 30 seconds. It is caused by an increased return of blood to the right heart from the abdomen. However, the right heart is not normal and cannot handle the increased venous return, so the blood from the cranial vena cava cannot enter the heart and the jugular veins become distended. This reflex is present with both right- and left-heart failure and indicates increased blood volume in the peripheral venous system due to an inability of the heart to circulate the blood properly.
- Cats with left-heart failure may have distended jugular veins only when lying down and the jugular veins return to normal when they sit or stand.

Box 1-9 Causes of Distended Jugular Veins

Right-heart failure (e.g., tricuspid regurgitation, dilated cardiomyopathy)
Pericardial diseases
Heart base tumor
Mediastinal mass

KEY POINT

Jugular vein distention can be present with both right- and left-heart failure, but may be present in only 70% of these cases. Abdominal ultrasound is a sensitive, noninvasive method of determining increased venous pressure by detecting distended hepatic veins; however, the ultrasound only confirms the presence of increased venous pressure and not the cause of it.

- A central venous pressure can be obtained on animals with distended jugular veins. It is most useful in the diagnosis of restrictive pericardial disease where less invasive tests have not confirmed the diagnosis.
- A young dog with regurgitation due to a megaesophagus may have a congenital vascular ring anomaly.

Tracheal Palpation

- The trachea should be palpated for abnormalities such as collapsing, masses, or increased sensitivity.
- This step is best postponed until after auscultation of the thorax, because a cough may be elicited that makes auscultation difficult.
- Lymph nodes should be palpated to see if they are enlarged.
- The thyroids may be enlarged in cats with hyperthyroidism (thyroid slip).
- An old dog having a mass near the larynx with an associated thrill usually has thyroid carcinoma with an arteriovenous fistula causing the thrill (murmur that can be felt as well as heard).

KEY POINT

Palpation of the neck can reveal primary or secondary problems that affect the heart and can mimic heart disease (collapsing trachea).

Thoracic Palpation

- The apex beat (sometimes called the point of maximum intensity [PMI]) is where the cardiac impulse is felt strongest on the chest wall. It should be on the left side of the thorax between the fourth and sixth intercostal spaces. Shifting of the PMI is due to cardiac enlargement, masses displacing the heart, collapsed lung lobes allowing the heart to shift, diaphragmatic hernias, pleural effusions associated with collapsed lung lobes or fibrin, or lying down in right lateral recumbency such that the heart falls to the right. Pectus excavatum, a deformity of the sternum, can also shift the heart to the right (Box 1-10).
- A decreased intensity of heartbeat or heart sounds may be due to obesity, pleural effusion, pericardial effusion, thoracic masses, pneumothorax, emphysema, diaphragmatic hernias, or decreased left ventricular contractility with decreased cardiac output (Box 1-11).
- There can be an increased intensity of the PMI or heart sounds in young, thin animals or in animals with increased heart rates or with hyperdynamic states such as anemia, hyperthyroidism, or fever.
- The heart sometimes appears to be beating on the chest wall. The heart is not actually hitting the chest wall; the appearance is due to the increased wall tension of the thoracic wall for an indeterminate reason. It does not mean that the heart is contracting normally or better than normal.
- Loud cardiac murmurs can be palpated as thrills, which are due to vibrations caused by blood flow. A thrill is always located where a murmur is loudest.

Box 1-10 Causes of Shifting of the Palpable Apex Beat or Point of Maximum Intensity

Cardiac enlargement
Collapsed lung lobes on the right
Diaphragmatic hernias
Pectus excavatum
Lying down
Masses displacing the heart
Pleural effusions

Box 1-11 Causes of Changes in Heart Sounds

Decreased intensity due to:
- Decreased left ventricular contractility
- Diaphragmatic hernias
- Emphysema
- Obesity
- Pleural or pericardial effusions
- Pneumothorax
- Thoracic masses

Increased intensity due to:
- Hyperdynamic states (e.g., anemia, hyperthyroidism, fever)
- Increased heart rates
- Young, thin animals

KEY POINT

It is important to locate both the PMI of the heartbeat and the presence of thrills due to heart murmurs on the thoracic wall.

Abdominal Palpation

- Abdominal palpation is done to check for ascites, the presence of fluid in the abdomen. Ascites can be due to right-heart failure but also can be due to multiple other causes.

- The presence of ascites can be difficult to ascertain in obese animals. The clinician should put one hand on one side of the abdomen and the other hand on the other side, and then tap the abdomen. If a fluid wave is felt by the hand on the opposite side of the abdomen, then ascites is present.
- Check for signs of hepatomegaly and splenomegaly. The presence of ascites, splenomegaly and hepatomegaly, usually indicates right-heart failure due to dilated cardiomyopathy, tricuspid regurgitation, heartworm disease, pericardial disease, or congenital heart disease. Another possibility is an obstruction of the posterior vena cava.
- Palpate for any masses.
- Palpate the kidneys as chronic renal failure can lead to systemic hypertension that can affect the heart.
- Most ascites due to right-heart failure is a modified transudate on cytology and accumulates slowly.

KEY POINT

Ascites can be due to right-heart failure or other heart problems such as pericardial effusion; however, it can also be due to other noncardiac problems. Further tests are indicted to determine the cause of ascites.

Skin

- Palpate for evidence of edema due to right-heart failure or venous obstruction.

Femoral Pulses

- Both pulses should be felt with the dog or cat standing, and they should be compared to each other because one could be obstructed.
- It is difficult to palpate the femoral pulse in a normal cat; therefore, the absence of palpable femoral pulses in a cat should not be interpreted as definite arterial obstruction.
- Partial or complete occlusion of the pulses so that they cannot be felt is usually due to thromboembolism. In dogs this can occur with bacterial endocarditis of the mitral or aortic valves, hyperadrenocorticism, and protein-losing glomerulonephritis (especially amyloidosis). Cavalier King Charles Spaniels with mitral regurgitation sometimes lack a pulse for unknown reasons. In cats, absent pulses are associated with cardiomyopathy but can also occasionally be due to bacterial endocarditis or extra cardiac disease.
- The femoral pulse rate should be taken. Normal rates in dogs are 70 to 180 beats per minute (bpm). Puppies can have a normal rate of 220 bpm. Normal rates in cats are 160 to 240 bpm.
- The rhythm of the pulses should be noted. There should be a pulse for every heartbeat. Pulse deficits usually indicate incomplete ventricular filling, as seen in arrhythmias.
- Arterial pulse pressure (femoral pulse quality) is the difference between the arterial systolic pressure and the diastolic pressure. Pulse quality can normally vary depending on the animal's conformation, age, hydration, heart rate, cardiac function, and level of excitement or activity.
- The intensity of the pulse should be palpated. Normal pulses are strong and have a rapid rate of rise and fall.
- Table 1-3 lists the pulse quality and the cause for each type of pulse.
- Hypokinetic (weak) pulses are due to decreased cardiac output (e.g., congestive heart failure, hypovolemia), decreased peripheral vascular resistance, increased arterial compliance, or slower rate of rise due to delayed emptying of the left ventricle (e.g., subaortic stenosis). Dogs will have normal pulses until the stroke volume is markedly decreased with severe congestive heart

Table 1-3 Types of Pulses and Their Associated Causes

Pulse	Cause
Absent pulses	Thromboembolism
Abrupt pulses	Mitral regurgitation Ventricular septal defects
Erratic pulses	Atrial fibrillation
Hypokinetic pulses	Heart failure Hypotension Hypovolemia Subaortic stenosis
Hyperkinetic pulses	Aortic regurgitation Fear Fever Patent ductus arteriosus Severe anemia Severe bradycardia Thyrotoxicosis
Pulse deficits	Arrhythmias
Pulsus alternans	Severe dilated cardiomyopathy
Pulsus bigeminus	Arrhythmias
Pulsus paradoxus	Cardiac tamponade

failure so pulses are an insensitive indicator of cardiac output.

- Hyperkinetic (strong) pulses rise and fall quickly and are due to large left ventricular stroke volumes with rapid diastolic runoffs (e.g., PDA, aortic regurgitation). They are called "B-B shot" or "water-hammer" pulses. Fear, fever, severe bradycardia, thyrotoxicosis, and anemia can also produce this type of pulse.
- The pulses can be abrupt or jerky with mitral regurgitation and ventricular septal defects as a greater volume of blood is ejected in early systole.
- Pulsus alternans occurs when the pulse is alternately weak and then strong in patients with normal sinus rhythm. It is frequently associated with severe myocardial failure (e.g., dilated cardiomyopathy).
- Pulsus bigeminus occurs when weak pulses alternate with strong pulses. This is associated with arrhythmias such as ventricular bigeminy where a normal heart beat alternates with a ventricular premature beat. The weak pulses occur because the premature beat causes the ventricles to contract before they are adequately filled so a smaller than normal volume of blood is ejected by the left ventricle, causing weak pulses. The difference between the normal and abnormal pulses may be accentuated due to the fact the ventricles have more time to fill on the normal beats so that the normal pulses feel even stronger.
- Pulsus paradoxus is an alteration of the pulse strength during respiration due to changes in ventricular filling. There is an increase in pulse strength on expiration and a decrease in strength on inspiration in normal animals; however, this change is exaggerated and easier to feel when cardiac tamponade is present.
- Pulses feel erratic when an animal has atrial fibrillation.

KEY POINT

The quality of an animal's pulse is not a good indication of the severity of its cardiac problem because only very advanced heart disease will cause weak pulses; however, pulse deficits are very good indicators of the presence of an arrhythmia.

Percussion

- Percussion can be used to determine the presence of masses or fluid lines, especially in the thorax. It will elicit a hollow sound (hyperresonance) over the lungs and a dull sound over solid structures (hyporesonant).
- If an area, especially dorsally, in the thorax sounds hyperresonant, then pneumothorax may be present.
- If an area, especially ventrally, sounds hyporesonant, then pleural effusion may be present.

KEY POINT

Percussion can be a rapid way of determining the presence or absence of pleural effusion.

Stethoscope

- The main components of the stethoscope are the bell, diaphragm, tubing, and ear pieces. The bell transmits both low-frequency (20 to 300 cycles per second [cps]) sounds when light pressure is used and high-frequency (300 to 1000 cps) sounds when firm pressure is used to apply it to the thorax. It is best for hearing third and fourth heart sounds. The diaphragm attenuates low frequencies and selectively transmits the high frequencies. It is best for hearing the first and second heart sounds.
- Most stethoscopes combine the bell and diaphragm into a dual-sided, combination-style chest piece. Some stethoscopes have the bell and diaphragm as one piece. With these stethoscopes, simple fingertip pressure allows one to switch from low- to high-frequency sounds. There is no interruption in sound as there is in a traditional two-sided stethoscope, resulting in added convenience and efficiency in auscultation.
- A practical tubing length on a stethoscope is approximately 14 to 18 inches. If the tubing is too long, then it will attenuate all the heart and lung sounds.
- Ear tubes should angle forward to conform to the anatomy of the ear canals. A stethoscope with variable sizes of ear pieces is ideal because each person can find the correct size earpiece that fits comfortably in the ear canal and shuts out extraneous sounds.
- For dogs and cats less than 15 pounds, a pediatric stethoscope that has a smaller headpiece should be used.
- Electronic stethoscopes have improved dramatically in the past 10 years. In addition to electronic amplification of heart sounds and murmurs, most electronic stethoscopes currently allow the user to record and play back sounds at either normal or half speed. This feature is useful for judging and timing the shape or quality of murmurs in tachycardic patients and for judging the timing of transient heart sounds such as clicks or gallops. Some models also provide the ability to record graphic representations of sounds in a digital file format

(i.e., a phonocardiogram) that can be stored on a computer, possibly even becoming part of the patient's medical record. A new electronic stethoscope (Figure 1-7), the 3M Littman Model 3000, features useful ambient noise reduction circuitry that appears to overcome most if not all of the problems of background noise amplification that plagued previous models.

KEY POINT

Not every stethoscope is ideal for everyone. Ideally, a clinician should try various stethoscopes to find the one that works best for him or her.

Auscultation

- This is the most helpful part of the cardiac examination; it should be done carefully and systematically. The animal should be standing so that the heart is in its normal position. This avoids the problem of positional murmurs caused by the heart rubbing against the chest wall when an animal is lying down.
- Common artifacts heard include respiratory clicks and murmurs, rumbles due to shivering and twitching, and movement sounds such as crackling due to the rubbing of hair. Extraneous sounds will occur if auscultation is not performed in a quiet area.
- Auscult the heart and lungs separately.
- Auscult the entire thorax on both sides.
- The areas of auscultation of the heart are shown in Figure 1-8. Table 1-4 lists the areas of auscultation.
- The pulmonic valve area is on the left side. In the dog, it is between the second and the fourth intercostal spaces just above the sternum. In the

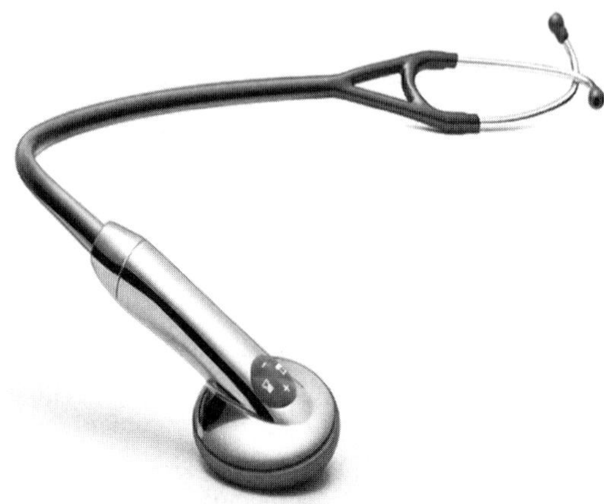

Figure 1-7. 3M Littman electronic stethoscope. (Courtesy 3M Health Care, St. Paul, Minn.)

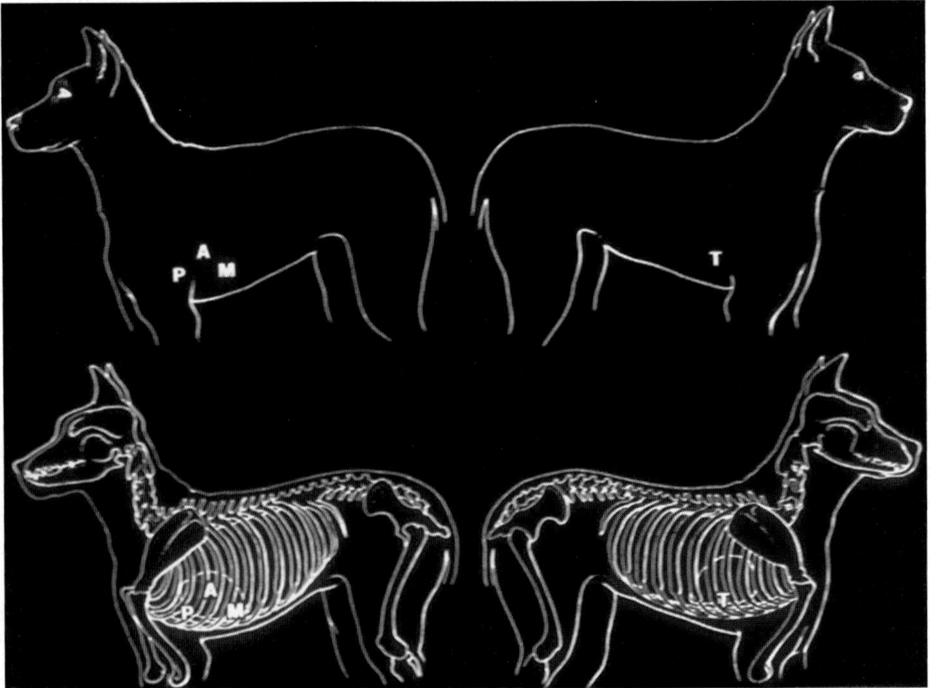

Figure 1-8. Areas of auscultation in the dog. M is the mitral valve area, A is the aortic valve area, P is the pulmonic valve area, and T is the tricuspid valve area. (From Gompf RE: The clinical approach to heart disease: history and physical examination. In Fox PR, ed: Canine and feline cardiology. New York, 1988, Churchill Livingstone.)

Table 1-4 Areas of Auscultation in the Dog and Cat

Structure	Location
Mitral valve	Dog—left side, fifth intercostal space at the costochondral junction Cat—left side, fifth to sixth intercostal space near sternum
Aortic valve	Dog—left side, fourth intercostal space just above costochondral junction Cat—left side, second to third intercostal space just dorsal to pulmonic area
Pulmonic valve	Dog—left side, between second and fourth intercostal space just above the sternum Cat—left side, second to third intercostal space one-third way up from sternum
Tricuspid valve	Dog—right side, third to fifth intercostal space near costochondral junction Cat—right side, fourth to fifth intercostal space near sternum

cat, it is located at the second to the third intercostal space one third to one half of the way up the thorax from the sternum.

- The aortic valve area is on the left side. In the dog, it is at the fourth intercostal space just above the costochondral junction. In the cat, it is at the second to the third intercostal space just dorsal to the pulmonic area.
- In cats and small dogs, it may be impossible to distinguish the pulmonic and aortic areas, so these two areas are referred to as the left heart base.
- The mitral valve area is on the left side. In the dog, it is at the fifth intercostal space at the costochondral junction. In the cat, it is at the fifth to the sixth intercostal space one fourth of the way up the thorax from the sternum. In cats and small dogs, this area may also be referred to as the left heart apex.
- The tricuspid valve area is on the right side. In the dog, it is at the third to the fifth intercostal space near the costochondral junction. In the cat, it is at the fourth or fifth intercostal space, at a level opposite the mitral area.
- The areas in which murmurs are loudest (PMI) and to which they radiate should be noted. This can help identify the heart problem.
- Alternate areas of auscultation include the thoracic inlets for radiation of the murmur of subaortic stenosis and the left axillary area for the murmurs of PDA.
- Heart rate and rhythm should be identified. The effects of inspiration and expiration on heart rate, rhythm, and heart sounds should be noted.
- The presence or absence of heart sounds should be noted.

KEY POINT

The lungs and heart should be ausculted separately to avoid missing or confusing any abnormal sounds. All valve areas should be ausculted in all animals. Congenital heart defects have been missed when clinicians only listen to the mitral valve area in a young animal.

Normal Heart Sounds

- Heart sounds are due to the abrupt acceleration or deceleration of blood and the vibrations of the heart and vessels.
- The first heart sound (S_1) (Figure 1-9) is due to passive closure of the mitral (left AV) and tricuspid (right AV) valves resulting in the sudden acceleration and deceleration of blood. It has four parts that can be seen on a phonocardiogram.
- S_1 is longer, louder, duller, and lower-pitched than the second heart sound. It is loudest over the mitral and tricuspid areas. It is loudest in young, thin animals and those with high sympathetic tone (e.g., fear), tachycardia, systemic hypertension, anemia, or mitral regurgitation.
- The intensity of S_1 decreases owing to obesity, pleural or pericardial effusion, thoracic masses, diaphragmatic hernias, bradycardia, emphysema, shock and insufficient filling of the ventricles.
- S_1 varies in intensity with arrhythmias.
- Splitting of S_1 (see Figure 1-9) is due to asynchronous closure of the mitral and tricuspid valves. It can be split normally in large breeds of dogs or abnormally with right bundle branch block, atrial or ventricular premature beats, cardiac pacing, or stenosis of the mitral or tricuspid valve.
- Box 1-12 lists the causes of changes in the first heart sound.
- The second heart sound (S_2) (see Figure 1-9) is produced by passive closure of the aortic and pulmonic valves. It is short, high pitched, and sharp. It is loudest over the aortic and pulmonic areas.
- A split S_2 (see Figure 1-9) is due to closure of the pulmonic valve after the aortic valve. This occurs in pulmonary hypertension (e.g., severe

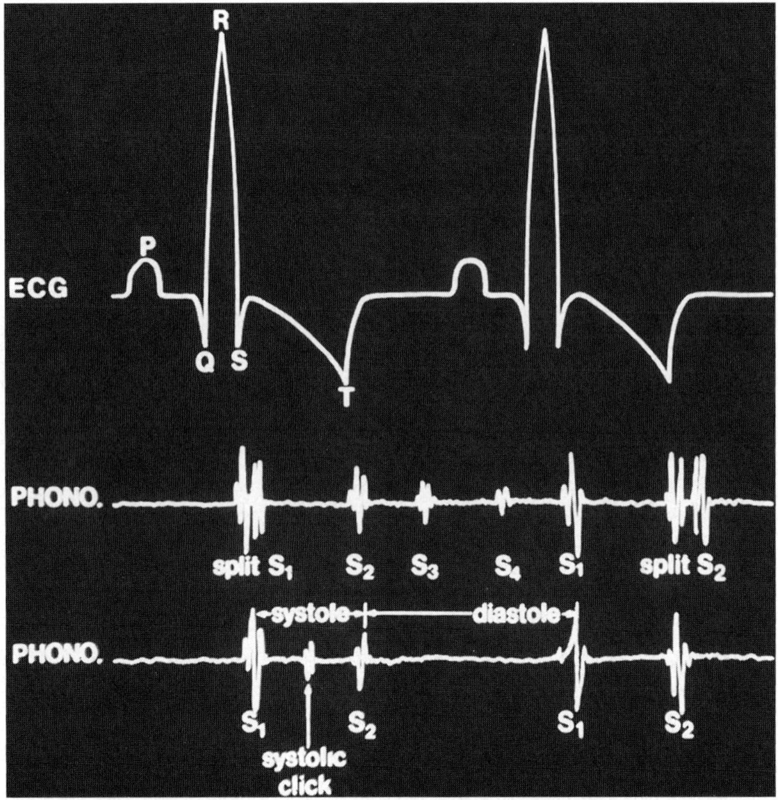

Figure 1-9. Heart sounds and their relationship to the ECG. The first heart sound is S_1. The second heart sound is S_2. The third heart sound is S_3 and the fourth heart sound is S_4. (From Gompf RE: The clinical approach to heart disease: history and physical examination. In Fox PR, ed: Canine and feline cardiology. New York, 1988, Churchill Livingstone.)

heartworm disease or right-to-left PDA), right bundle branch block, ventricular premature beats originating in the left ventricle, atrial septal defect, pulmonic stenosis, and mitral stenosis.

- Paradoxical splitting of S_2 is due to delayed closure of the aortic valve. This results from left bundle branch block, premature beats originating from the right ventricle, subaortic stenosis, severe systemic hypertension, and left ventricular failure.
- S_2 may be absent in arrhythmias where there is incomplete filling of the ventricles and insufficient pressure to open the semilunar valves.
- Box 1-13 lists the causes of changes in the second heart sound.

KEY POINT

It is critical to identify the first and second heart sounds in all patients in order to use auscultation as an effective tool in the diagnosis of heart disease. If extraneous sounds are present, then the clinician may need to move to another area of the thorax in order to identify these sounds properly.

Abnormal Heart Sounds

- The third heart sound (S_3) (Figure 1-9) is due to rapid ventricular filling and is not heard in normal dogs or cats. It is lower pitched than the second heart sound. It is heard best in the mitral valve area and occurs during diastole after the second heart sound (S_2).
- An S_3 in dogs indicates dilated ventricles, which most commonly occur with dilated cardiomyopathy, decompensated mitral or tricuspid regurgitation, large ventricular or atrial septal defects, and large PDA. In cats it is associated with dilated cardiomyopathy, severe anemia, and severe hyperthyroidism.
- Table 1-5 lists the causes of abnormal heart sounds.
- The fourth heart sound (S_4) (see Figure 1-9) is due to atrial contraction into an already over-distended ventricle or into a stiff ventricle in dogs and cats. It is heard best over the aortic or pulmonic areas but sometimes can be heard over the mitral valve area as well. It occurs in diastole just prior to the first heart sound.
- An S_4 is present in dogs or cats when the atria dilate in response to ventricular diastolic dysfunction,

Box 1-12 Causes of Changes in the First (S_1) Heart Sound

Loud S_1
- Anemia
- Excitement
- Exercise
- Fear
- Fever
- Hyperthyroidism
- Mitral regurgitation
- Positive inotropic agents
- Pregnancy
- Systemic hypertension
- Tachycardia
- Thin animals

Soft S_1
- Bradycardias
- Decreased cardiac output
- Diaphragmatic hernias
- Emphysema
- Hypothyroidism
- Left bundle branch block
- Negative inotropic agents
- Obesity
- Pericardial effusion
- Pleural effusion
- Severe aortic or mitral regurgitation
- Severe heart failure
- Shock
- Thoracic masses

Variable S_1
- Arrhythmias

Split S_1
- Atrial or ventricular premature beats
- Cardiac pacing
- Right bundle branch block
- Stenosis of mitral or tricuspid valve

Box 1-13 Causes of Changes in the Second (S_2) Heart Sound

Loud S_2
- Atrial septal defect
- Mild valvular pulmonic stenosis
- Patent ductus arteriosus
- Pulmonary embolism
- Pulmonary hypertension
- Systemic hypertension
- Valvular aortic stenosis
- Ventricular septal defect

Soft S_2
- Dilated cardiomyopathy
- Hypothyroidism
- Marked aortic regurgitation
- Shock
- Significant pulmonic stenosis
- Valvular aortic stenosis

Split S_2
- Atrial septal defect
- Heartworms
- Mitral stenosis
- Pulmonary hypertension—moderate to severe
- Pulmonic stenosis
- Right bundle branch block
- Right to left patent ductus arteriosus
- Ventricular premature beat from left ventricle

Paradoxical split S_2
- Left bundle branch block
- Left ventricular failure
- Severe systemic hypertension
- Significant aortic regurgitation
- Subaortic stenosis
- Ventricular premature beats from the right ventricle

Absent S_2
- Arrhythmias

such as hypertrophic cardiomyopathy or third degree heart block. It may also be heard in dogs with ruptured chordae tendineae.

- A gallop rhythm is an S_3, S_4, or combination (summation) of the two. Gallops are of a low frequency and can be difficult to hear. A gallop can be a very early sign of heart failure, preceding clinical signs.
- Systolic clicks are short, mid- to high-frequency clicking noises that occur in systole between S_1 and S_2 (see Figure 1-9). They are usually loudest over the mitral and tricuspid areas. A systolic click may come and go and may change its position in systole (gets closer to or further away from S_2) and may change its intensity.
- A systolic click can be hard to differentiate from a gallop, especially if the animal's heart rate is fast.
- The precise cause of the click is unknown, but it may be due to the mitral valve buckling into the left atrium (mitral valve prolapse) in dogs with early mitral regurgitation because many of these animals develop a mitral regurgitation murmur later in life. This is a benign finding and is not usually associated with heart failure.
- Ejection sounds are high frequency sounds generated in early systole due to hypertension, dilation of the great vessels, or opening of abnormal semilunar valves such as in valvular pulmonic stenosis.

KEY POINT

The presence of a gallop is an indication of cardiac disease in small animals.

Table 1-5 Causes of Abnormal Heart Sounds

Sound	Cause
Gallop sounds	
S_3	Decompensated mitral or tricuspid regurgitation
	Dilated cardiomyopathy
	Large atrial septal defect
	Large patent ductus arteriosus
	Large ventricular septal defect
	Severe anemia in cats
	Severe hyperthyroidism in cats
	Significant aortic regurgitation
S_4	Anemia
	Hypertrophic cardiomyopathy
	Dogs with ruptured chordae tendineae
	Pulmonary hypertension
	Systemic hypertension
	Third degree heart block
	Thyrotoxicosis
Systolic click	Mitral valve prolapse
Ejection sounds	Anemia
	Atrial septal defect
	Dilation of great vessels
	Exercise
	Heartworms
	Hyperthyroidism
	Pulmonary embolism
	Pulmonary hypertension
	Systemic hypertension
	Valvular aortic stenosis
	Valvular pulmonic stenosis

Arrhythmias Heard on Auscultation

- Arrhythmias that increase the heart rate (tachycardias) include both atrial and ventricular arrhythmias.
- Animals with atrial fibrillation have a rapid, irregular rhythm with heart sounds that vary in intensity. Pulse deficits are present. It has been described as being irregularly irregular and rarely is mistaken for other tachycardias.
- Ventricular tachycardias are usually intermittent and tend to be more regular than atrial fibrillation. Pulse deficits are frequently present.
- Sinus and atrial tachycardias are rapid and regular. All the heart sounds are of a uniform intensity, but an atrial tachycardia tends to be intermittent.
- An electrocardiogram is necessary to distinguish among sinus, atrial, and ventricular tachycardia.
- Atrial and ventricular premature beats generate extra sounds that mimic S_3 and S_4. It is difficult to differentiate between the two types of premature beats as well as S_3 and S_4 on physical examination. An electrocardiogram and phonocardiogram may be necessary.
- Both atrial and ventricular premature beats interrupt the normal rhythm and are usually followed by a pause. Usually only an S_1 is heard with a premature beat and S_2 is absent. However, sometimes S_1 and S_2 can be heard very close together. Premature beats can also cause a split S_1 or S_2.
- Sinus arrhythmia has a cyclical pattern. The heart rate will increase during inspiration and decrease during expiration owing to changes in vagal tone. The intensity of the pulse and heart sounds may vary. It is normal in dogs, but in cats it is usually associated with heart disease. Sinus arrhythmia occurs at normal heart rates in dogs and cats and tends to disappear as the heart rate increases.
- Arrhythmias that decrease the heart rate are called bradycardias and examples include both sinus bradycardia and heart blocks.
- Sinus bradycardia has a very slow rhythm. The heart sounds may vary. The heart rate in dogs is between 50 to 70 bpm, depending on the size of the dog. The heart rate in cats is less than 120 bpm.
- Second and third degree heart blocks result in slow heart rates. The heart sounds will vary in intensity. A fourth heart sound may be present in third degree block. The pulses will be slow and hyperkinetic, but there are no pulse deficits. A jugular pulse is usually present. Extra sounds may be generated by escape beats.
- An electrocardiogram is necessary to diagnose the type of bradycardia present.
- Unexpected pauses can occur with sinoatrial (SA or sinus) arrest. Sinus arrest occurs when an impulse does not leave the SA node. The pause continues until the next normal beat or an escape beat occurs. The heart sound following a pause may be louder than usual as the ventricles have had longer to fill and eject a larger amount of blood. An electrocardiogram is necessary to diagnose sinus arrest.

Murmurs

- Murmurs are caused by turbulent blood flow through the heart and vessels. The turbulence can be caused by disruptions of blood flow through holes in the heart (e.g., ventricular septal or atrial septal defect), a stenotic valve (e.g., aortic, pulmonic, mitral or tricuspid stenosis), an insufficient valve (e.g., mitral, tricuspid, aortic, or pulmonic regurgitation), an abnormal arterial venous connection near the heart (e.g., PDA), or can be due to altered blood viscosity or changes in blood vessel diameter.

- Functional murmurs are divided into physiologic and innocent murmurs.
- Physiologic murmurs have a known cause such as increased cardiac output or decreased blood viscosity and occur with anemia, hypoproteinemia, fever, increased blood pressure, pregnancy, hyperthyroidism, and an athletic heart. These are high frequency murmurs occurring in the early to mid-systolic phase, are loudest over the aortic and pulmonic areas and rarely radiate to other areas. Table 1-6 lists the types of murmurs and their causes.
- Innocent murmurs have no known cause and are not associated with any cardiac problem. These murmurs are soft systolic murmurs (no louder than grade 3) and usually just occur in young animals. They can be located over any valve area but are most frequent over the mitral and aortic areas. Also, these murmurs should disappear by the time of the animal's last vaccinations (5 months of age).
- Pathologic murmurs are caused by underlying heart or vessel disease such as stenosis of valves or outflow tract or great vessels, valvular regurgitation, or abnormal intracardiac or extracardiac shunts. Refer to individual defects in the following chapters for a description of the murmurs associated with each defect.

Table 1-6 Types of Heart Murmurs and Their Causes

Murmur	Cause
Physiologic	Anemia Athletic heart Fever Hypoproteinemia Hypertension Hyperthyroidism Pregnancy
Innocent	No known cause
Pathologic	Aortic regurgitation Aorticopulmonary septal defect Arteriovenous fistula Atrial septal defect Mitral dysplasia Mitral regurgitation Mitral stenosis Patent ductus arteriosus Pulmonic regurgitation Pulmonic stenosis Subaortic stenosis Tetralogy of Fallot Tricuspid Dysplasia Tricuspid regurgitation Tricuspid stenosis Ventricular septal defect

- The loudness of a murmur does not indicate the severity of the underlying problem.
- A murmur should be described by using the following classification. First, the murmur should be identified as to its timing in the cardiac cycle (e.g., systolic, diastolic, continuous). Also, the duration of the murmur (e.g., early systolic, holosystolic, pansystolic) should be noted (Figures 1-10 and 1-11).
- Next the site at which the murmur is loudest (PMI) (e.g., valve area) and where it radiates due to blood flow through the defect (e.g., other valve areas where it can be heard) should be noted.
- The intensity or loudness of the murmur can be evaluated based on the following scale: grade I/VI can only be heard after listening for several minutes and sounds like a prolonged first heart sound; grade II/VI is very soft, but can be heard immediately; grade III/VI is low to moderate in intensity; grade IV/VI is very loud, but a thrill cannot be palpated on the thorax; grade V/VI is very loud, and a thrill can be palpated on the thorax; grade VI/VI can be heard without the use of a stethoscope or with the stethoscope slightly off the thoracic wall.
- The quality or shape of the murmur is subjective, but can be evaluated according to graphic appearance on phonocardiogram (see Figures 1-10 and 1-11). Regurgitant murmurs are plateau shaped (e.g., equal loudness throughout). Ejection murmurs are usually decrescendo, crescendo, or diamond shaped. Machinery or continuous murmurs are diamond-shaped and peak at S_2, continuing through all of systole and most of diastole. Blowing murmurs are decrescendo murmurs (e.g., decrease in intensity).
- The pitch or frequency of the murmur can also be described. Some murmurs are high, medium or low pitched, or a mix. Also, they can be harsh, blowing, or musical.

Other Sounds Auscultated in the Thorax

- Normal respiratory sounds include referred sounds from the trachea that are commonly heard over the lungs. Vesicular sounds are due to air moving through the small bronchi and are louder on inspiration. Bronchial sounds are due to air moving through the large bronchi and trachea and are heard best on expiration. Bronchovesicular sounds are the combination of the above two and are heard best over the hilar area.
- Abnormal respiratory sounds include attenuated sounds as well as increased, abnormal sounds.

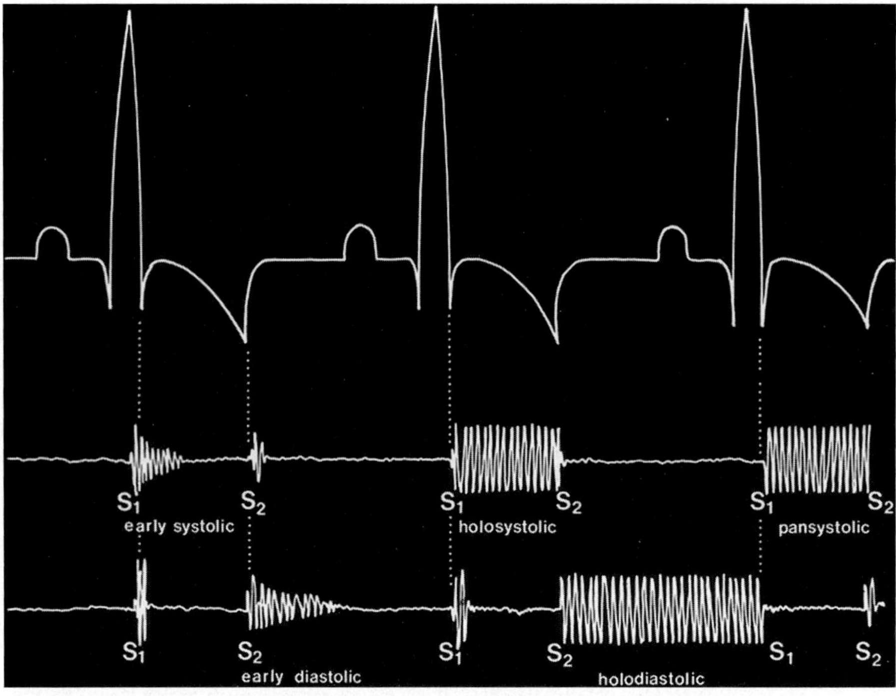

Figure 1-10. Timing and duration of murmurs. (From Gompf RE: The clinical approach to heart disease: history and physical examination. In Fox PR, ed: Canine and feline cardiology. New York, 1988, Churchill Livingstone.)

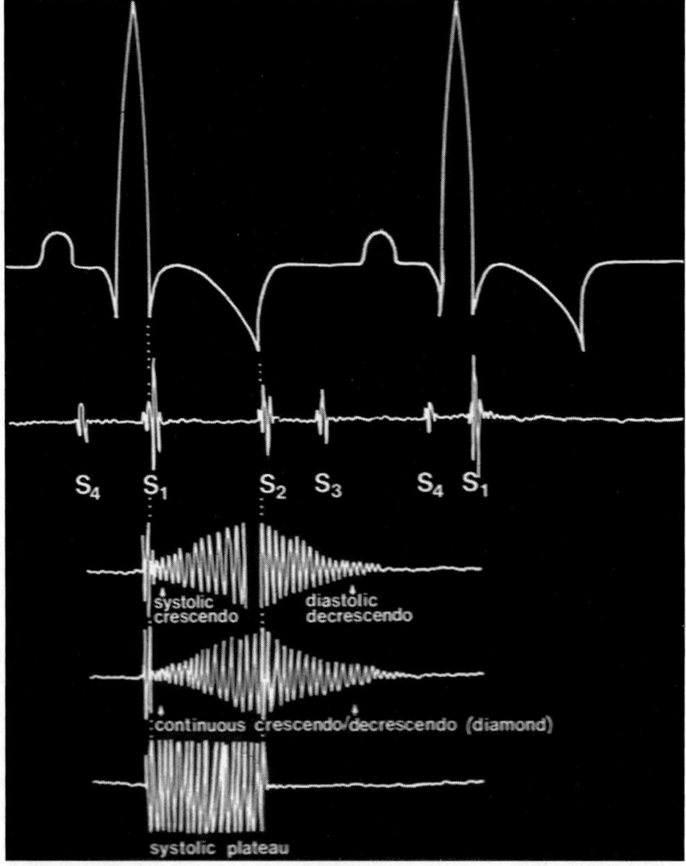

Figure 1-11. Timing and quality of murmurs. (From Gompf RE: The clinical approach to heart disease: history and physical examination. In Fox PR, ed: Canine and feline cardiology. New York, 1988, Churchill Livingstone.)

- Attenuated bronchovesicular lung sounds are due to thoracic masses, pleural effusion, pneumothorax, obesity, pneumonia, shallow breathing, or early consolidation of the pulmonary parenchyma.
- Rhonchi are due to air passing through partially obstructed airways in the bronchial tubes or smallest airways. Rhonchi from the large bronchi are low pitched, sonorous, and almost continuous. They are heard best on inspiration. Rhonchi from the small bronchi are high pitched, sibilant, or squeaky, and are heard best on expiration.
- Crackles are interrupted, crepitant, inspiratory sounds heard in many disease conditions and are not pathognomonic for pulmonary edema. They are due to opening of alveoli or airways that are collapsed or partially filled with fluid or bubbles bursting in the airways. They are further defined as fine or coarse in quality.
- Other sounds which can be ausculted include pleural friction rubs. Pleural friction rubs are grating, rubbing sounds heard during inspiration and expiration owing to the moving of two relatively dry, roughened pleural surfaces against each other. Pericardial friction rubs are short, scratchy noises produced by pericarditis and heart movement. Pericardial knocks are diastolic sounds that occur in animals with constrictive pericarditis. Wheezes are relatively high pitched, musical sounds and are often a sign of pulmonary pathology.

SUGGESTED READINGS

Buchanan J: Prevalence of cardiovascular disorders. In Fox PR, Sisson DD, Moise NS, eds: Textbook of canine and feline cardiology, ed 2, Philadelphia, 1992, WB Saunders.

Gompf RE: The clinical approach to heart disease: history and physical examination. In Fox PR, ed: Canine and feline cardiology. New York, 1988, Churchill Livingstone.

Kittleson MD: Signalment, history, and physical examination. In Kittleson MD, Kienle RD, eds: Small animal cardiovascular medicine. St Louis, 1998, Mosby.

Sisson DD, Ettinger SJ: The physical examination. In Fox PR, Sisson DD, Moise NS, eds: Textbook of canine and feline cardiology, ed 2, Philadelphia, 1999, WB Saunders.

Smith FWK, Keene B, Tilley LP: Heart sounds. In Smith FWK, Keene B, Tilley LP, eds: Interpretation of heart sounds, murmurs, arrhythmias, and lung sounds: a guide to cardiac auscultation in dogs and cats—CD ROM and manual. Philadelphia, 2006, WB Saunders.

CHAPTER 2

Radiology of the Heart

Brian A. Poteet

INTRODUCTION

Thoracic radiography is a key component of the cardiovascular evaluation. Careful attention to proper positioning is of primary importance to the use of radiographic guidelines for interpretation. Radiographic interpretation relies heavily on possible disease considerations (i.e., differential diagnosis) derived from signalment, physical examination, and clinical pathology. Radiographic findings are not consistently specific enough to lead to the derivation of a definitive diagnosis without supportive clinical evidence. The radiographic study isolated from clinical information will not provide a diagnosis. The clinician must be aware of certain parameters and guidelines for interpretation in order to derive information from the radiographic image.

RADIOGRAPHIC TECHNIQUE

Exposure Technique and Film Quality

- Exposure technique will vary depending on equipment and film-screen combinations. The current standard for veterinary radiographic equipment is a 300 mA/125 to 75 kVp machine.
- The current standard for economic film-screen combination imaging systems is the rare earth systems. Because of the motion created by respiration, relatively high-speed (400) film-screen combinations that allow shorter exposure times are best suited for thoracic radiography.
- Use of a grid is imperative for adequate image quality when chest thickness exceeds 10 cm. Table 2-1 is a representative thoracic technique chart using a 400-speed imaging system and 300 mA/125 kVp radiographic equipment.

Radiographic Projections

Lateral Projection

- There are subtle differences in cardiac conformation and position when comparing the right versus the left lateral radiographic projection. These differences are not significant enough to warrant further discussion except to note that the same projection should be used on all serial radiographic examinations when repeated evaluation is required.
- Patient positioning and adequate radiographic exposure are critical to an accurate radiographic interpretation in the lateral projection.

KEY POINT

A normal heart can appear diseased and vice versa when positioning is not adequate.

Guidelines for proper exposure and positioning of a lateral thoracic radiograph (Figure 2-1) include:

- Radiographic exposure should be adequate to define the dorsal spinous process of the cranial thoracic vertebrae superimposed on the scapula.
- To ensure a lateral projection, the dorsal heads of the ribs should be superimposed.

TABLE 2-1 Small Animal Thoracic Radiographic Technique Chart Using a 400-Speed Film-Screen System and Standard Radiographic Equipment*

	mA	Time	mAs	Thickness (cm) / kVp												
Table Top																
Thorax	100	1/60	1.7	3	4	5	6	7	8	9	10 cm					
				48	50	52	54	56	58	60	62					
In the Table (using Grid)																
Thorax	200	1/60	3.3	4	5	6	7	8	9	10	11	12	13	14	15	16 cm
				52	54	56	58	60	62	64	66	68	70	72	74	76
	300	1/60	5	17	18	19	20	21	22	23	24	25	26	27		28 cm
				76	78	80	82	84	86	88	90	92	95	90		101

Technique rules of thumb: Change exposure—(1) 10% KVp; (2) two thirds of mAs.
*Single-phase fully rectified 300mA 125 KVp generator focal-film distance = 38".

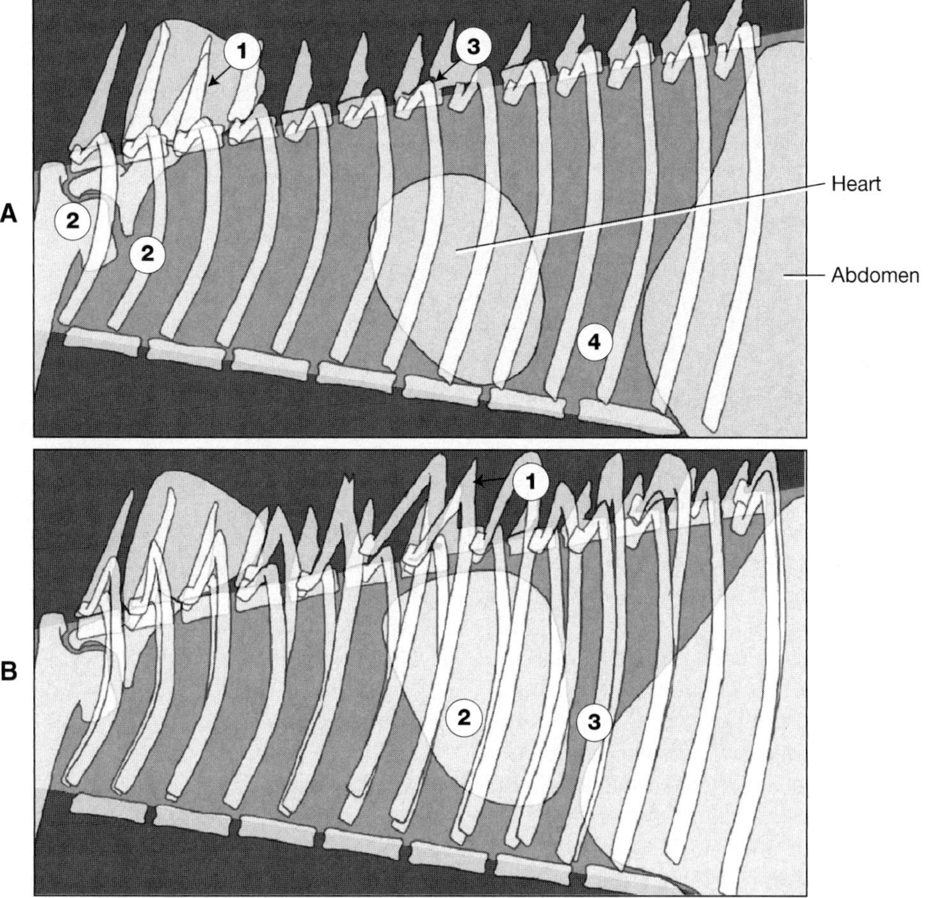

Figure 2-1. **A,** Guidelines for proper exposure and positioning of a lateral thoracic radiographic projection. (1) Exposure should allow delineation of the thoracic vertebral dorsal spinous process superimposed over the scapula. (2) The forelimbs should be pulled forward to provide an unsuperimposed view of the cranial thorax. (3) The dorsal rib heads should be superimposed (compare with **B**). (4) The exposure should be performed during inspiration, which provides maximum separation between caudal cardiac margin and diaphragmatic cupula. **B,** Improperly positioned lateral thoracic radiographic projection (compare with **A**). (1) Nonsuperimposed left and right rib heads. (2) The oblique projection markedly distorts cardiac silhouette conformation and intrathoracic position. (3) Expiratory phase radiographic exposure with poor lung volume between caudal cardiac margin and cupula of the diaphragm.

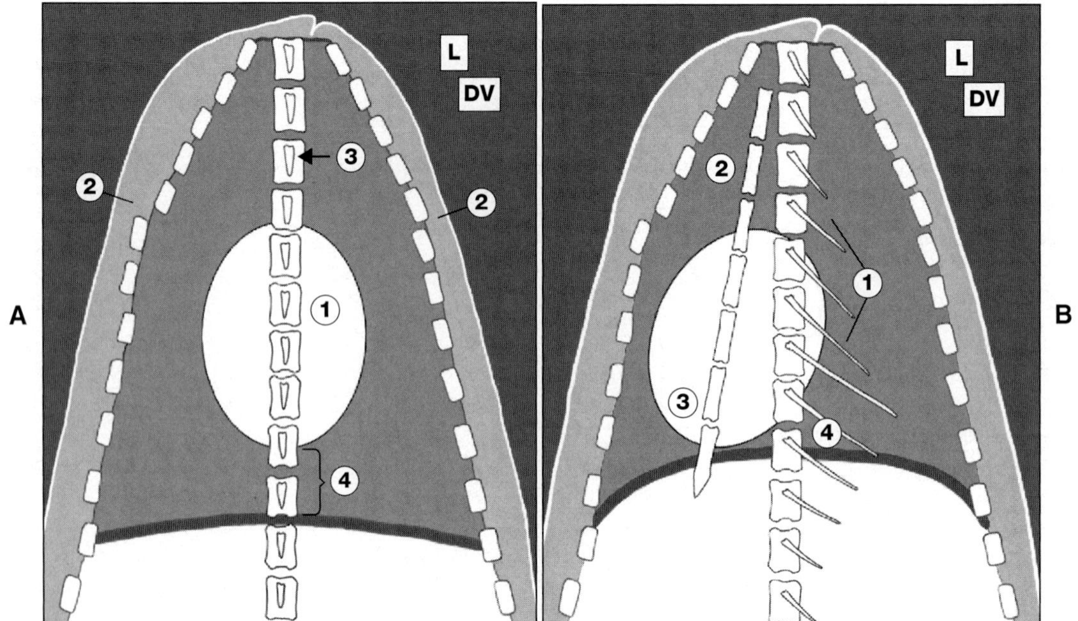

Figure 2-2. A, Guidelines for proper exposure and positioning of a dorsoventral/ventrodorsal thoracic radiographic projection. *L*, Lateral; *DV*, dorsoventral. (1) The radiographic exposure should provide outline definition of thoracic vertebra superimposed over the cardiac silhouette. (2) Exposure should be increased (usually a 10% kVp increase with obesity as suggested by an increase in thoracic body wall thickness). (3) The thoracic vertebral dorsal spinous processes should be superimposed over the body portions for the entire length of the thoracic spine. (4) Adequate lung volume between caudal cardiac margin and cupula indicates an inspiratory phase radiographic exposure. **B,** Improperly positioned dorsoventral radiographic projection. Thoracic vertebral dorsal spinous processes projected over the left hemithorax (1) and the sternal vertebra projected over the right hemithorax (2), indicating an oblique thoracic dorsoventral radiographic projection. A lack of lung volume between caudal cardiac margin (3) and cupula (4) indicates an expiratory phase radiographic exposure.

- The forelimbs should be pulled forward so that they are not superimposed over the cranial thorax or cranial margin of the heart.
- The radiographic exposure is taken during full inspiration, identified as an adequate lung field spacing between the caudal margin of the heart and the cupula of the diagram. Two primary disease considerations for consistent expiratory phase radiographs are:
  - Obesity and Pickwickian syndrome, where the overabundance of abdominal fat prevents adequate inspiratory distraction of the diaphragm
  - Upper airway disease, which most commonly causes obstruction during the inspiratory phase of respiration

Dorsoventral/Ventrodorsal Projection

- The dorsoventral (DV) radiographic projection is preferred over the ventrodorsal (VD) for cardiac evaluation for two reasons:
- The anatomic positioning of the heart in the DV projection is less dependent on thoracic cavity conformation (deep-chested vs. barrel-chested breeds).
- The dorsal lung fields are hyperinflated, and the vessels to the caudal lung fields are magnified owing to increased object-film distance. This produces an improved radiographic definition of the large pulmonary arteries and veins of the caudal lung fields. The DV projection also allows increased detection of early pulmonary infiltrates (most commonly with cardiac disease in the hilar and caudodorsal lung fields). However, an improperly positioned DV/VD projection is worthless for cardiac radiographic interpretation.

KEY POINT

Although the DV projection is preferred, a straight (symmetric) projection is the ultimate goal, with patient compliance determining which projection (DV vs. VD) is attainable.

Guidelines for proper exposure and positioning for the DV/VD projections (Figure 2-2) include:

- Radiographic exposure should be sufficient to define the outline of the thoracic vertebrae superimposed over the cardiac silhouette.
- The kVp should be increased 10% from technique-chart values for obese patients. Examination of the thoracic body wall thickness on the VD view should assist in evaluation of obesity.
- The dorsal spinous processes of the thoracic vertebrae should be centered over the vertebral bodies along the full length of the thoracic spine. The thoracic sternal vertebrae also should be superimposed over the thoracic spine and be essentially indistinguishable radiographically.
- The radiograph is taken during full inspiration, identified as an adequate lung field spacing between caudal cardiac margin and cupula of the diaphragm.

PROJECTION SELECTION IN CARDIAC-RELATED PATHOLOGY

Pulmonary Edema

- The DV is preferred over the VD projection for radiographic detection of pulmonary edema. The DV view accentuates pathology in the dorsal lung field, which is the most common location for the formation of early cardiogenic pulmonary edema. Adequate exposure is critical to ensure definition of caudal pulmonary vasculature superimposed over the cupula of the diaphragm.
- The radiographic detection of caudodorsal pulmonary vasculature is the best objective parameter for the detection of pulmonary edema. Vessels in the normal lung are detected by their soft tissue opacity contrasting with the normal radiolucent gas-filled lung parenchyma surrounding them. As pulmonary parenchyma (interstitial spaces as well as alveoli) become filled with edema fluid, the normal radiographic soft tissue–gas contrast is lost, and delineation of the vessels diminishes. In other words, the vessels start to "disappear" from radiographic detection with the increased opacity of the surrounding edematous lung parenchyma (Figure 2-3).
- The phase of inspiration is critical when using this method for interpretation both in the DV/VD and in the lateral projections. Pulmonary pathology can be mimicked when underinflation decreases the parenchymal gas content per unit volume, thus decreasing the radiographic contrast between lung parenchyma and associated vasculature. This is especially true in older patients, which already have slightly increased pulmonary

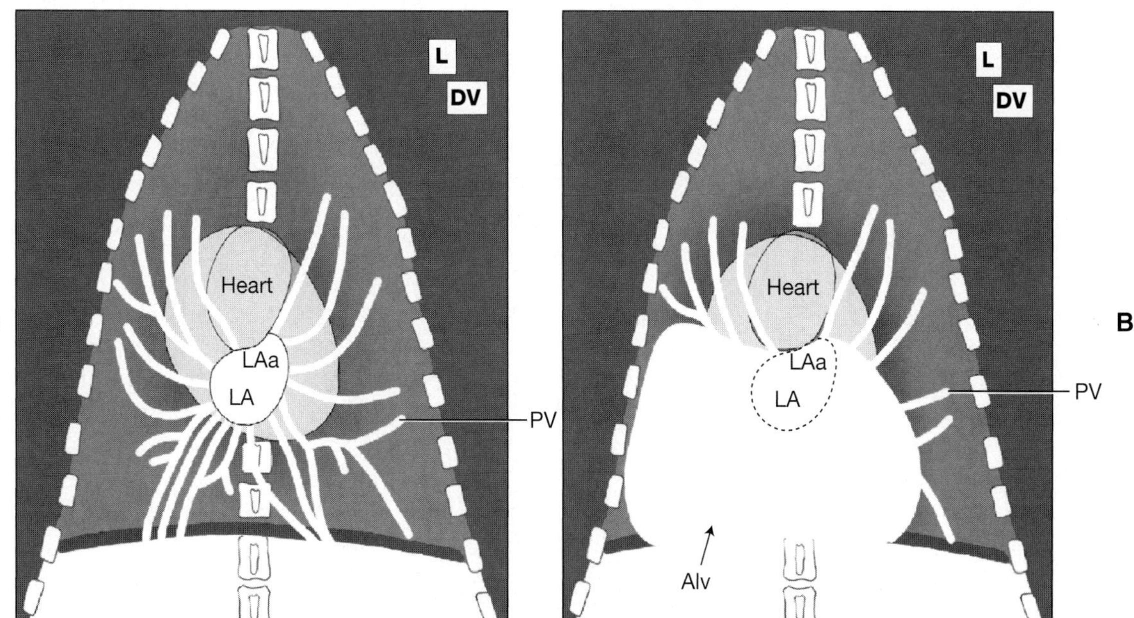

Figure 2-3. **A,** Normal radiographic definition and contrast of pulmonary venous vasculature (PV) with surrounding normal radiolucent lung parenchyma. *L,* Lateral; *DV,* dorsoventral; *LA,* left atrium; *LAa,* left atrial auricular appendage. **B,** Radiographic obliteration of pulmonary venous vasculature *(PV)* by alveolar consolidation *(Alv)* of hilar and caudal lung lobes, a characteristic distribution for cardiogenic pulmonary edema.

parenchymal radiographic opacity owing to age-related pulmonary degenerative changes (interstitial fibrosis, bronchial mineralization, heterotopic pulmonary bone formation).

Pleural Effusion

- Pleural effusion is radiographically evident as focal areas of increased soft tissue opacity located within the thoracic cavity. It causes separation of lung lobes from both the thoracic wall and the adjacent lobes. This is seen on the lateral projection as an increase in the soft tissue thickness of the caudodorsal thoracophrenic angle and diaphragm as well as linear soft tissue opacities (pleural fissures) at anatomic locations comparable with interlobar fissures (Figure 2-4). Pleural effusion also contributes to loss of definition of the cranial and caudal margins of the heart, producing a radiographic positive-silhouette sign.
- In cases of pleural effusion, the VD projection is much preferred over the DV view for detection and delineation of cardiac size and shape. If intrathoracic fluid volumes are severe enough, the heart can effectively disappear on the DV view because of the relative distribution of the fluid and heart in the thoracic cavity. The positive-silhouette phenomenon is accentuated in the DV compared with the VD view (Figure 2-5). However, patient positioning for the DV projection puts less physiologic demand on the patient compromised by pleural effusion and thus is favored over the VD projection. The patient's physiologic stability and degree of respiratory compromise should always be assessed prior to thoracic imaging.
- If significant amounts of pleural effusion are suspected, increasing radiographic exposure to abdominal technique-chart levels results in better intrathoracic radiographic contrast. When possible, thoracocentesis and fluid drainage prior to radiography is always preferred.

RADIOGRAPHIC ANATOMY

Lateral Thoracic Radiographic Projection

Cardiac Parameters

Even though the lateral radiographic projection defines the cranial-caudal and dorsal-ventral dimensions of the thorax, the anatomy of the heart of the dog and the cat as it resides in the thorax also allows this projection to detail the left and right aspects of the heart. This is because in the dog and the cat the heart is slightly rotated along its base-apex axis, such that the right cardiac chambers are positioned more cranially and the left chambers positioned more caudally. Thus, the cardiac silhouette as it appears on the lateral projection defines the right side of the heart along the cranial margin and the left side is defined by its caudal margin (Figures 2-6 to 2-8).

The canine and feline heart shape or radiographic silhouette is ovoid, with the apex more pointed in conformation than the broader base. This base-apex difference in conformation is accentuated in the cat. The heart axis is defined by drawing a

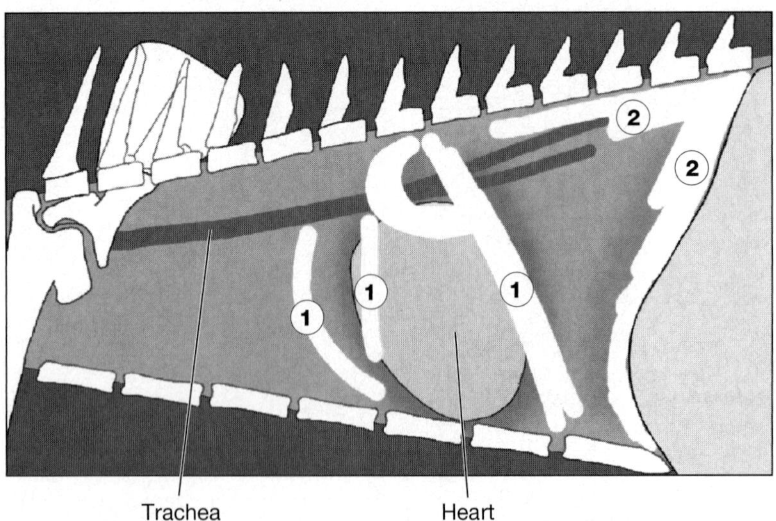

Figure 2-4. Lateral thoracic radiographic projection of pleural effusion. Intrathoracic fluid accumulation causes separation of adjacent lung lobes by (1) linear interlobar opacities, radiographically defined as pleural fissures, and (2) separation of lung lobes from the thoracic wall.

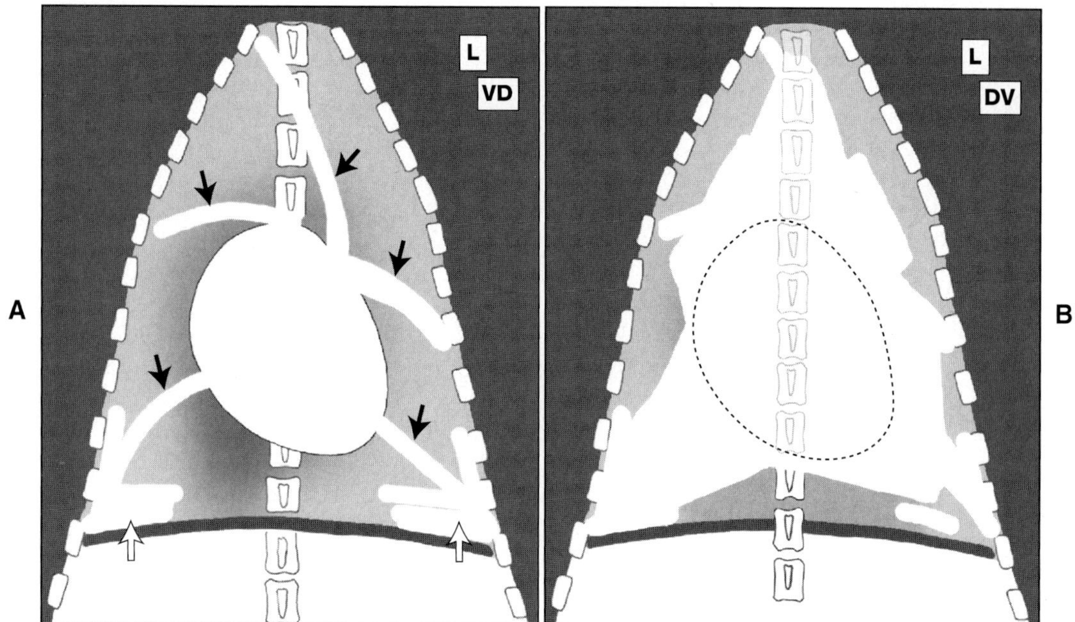

Figure 2-5. **A,** Ventrodorsal *(VD)* thoracic radiographic projection of pleural effusion consisting of pleural fissure lines *(closed arrows)* with blunting of the thoracophrenic angles *(open arrows)*. Note that the cardiac silhouette is still well outlined. **B,** Dorsoventral *(DV)* thoracic radiographic projection of pleural effusion. The intrathoracic fluid distribution creates a "positive silhouette sign" where a complete loss of the cardiac silhouette has occurred. Thus, the VD projection (**A**) is preferred for cardiac silhouette definition in the presence of pleural effusion. *L,* Lateral.

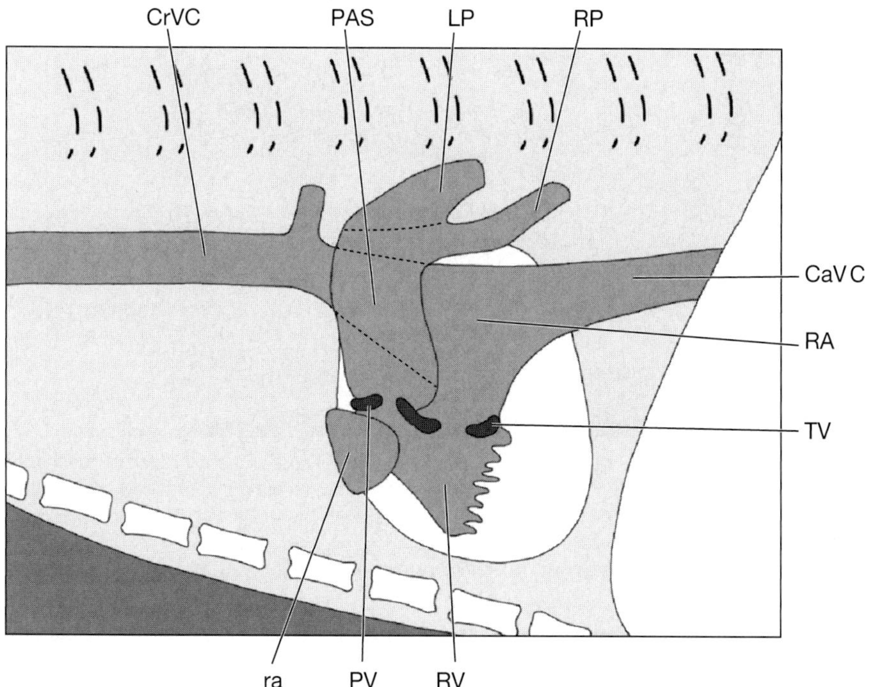

Figure 2-6. Schematic lateral thoracic radiographic projection of the relative position and size of the right-side structures of the heart. Note the more cranial position of the right chambers of the heart. *CrVC,* Cranial vena cava; *PAS,* main pulmonary artery; *PV,* pulmonic valve; *ra,* right atrial auricular appendage; *RV,* right ventricle; *RA,* right atrium; *LP,* left pulmonary artery; *RP,* right pulmonary artery; *TV,* tricuspid valve; *CaVC,* caudal vena cava.

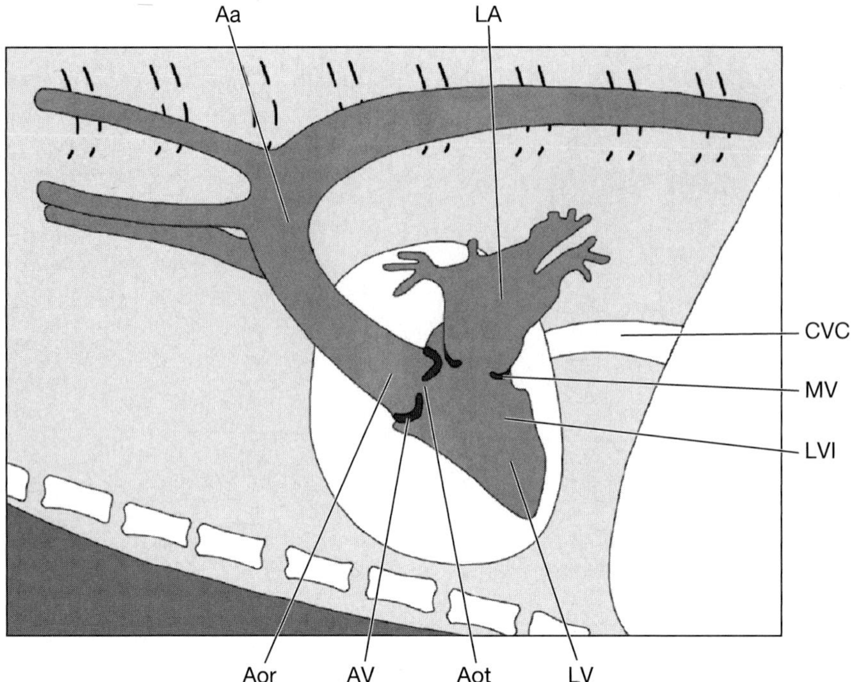

Figure 2-7. Schematic lateral thoracic radiographic projection of the relative position and size of the left-side structures of the heart. Note the more caudal position of the left chambers of the heart. *Aa*, Aortic arch; *AOr*, aorta; *AV*, aortic valve; *Aot*, aortic outflow tract; *LV*, left ventricle; *LVi*, left ventricular inflow tract; *LA*, left atrium; *MV*, mitral valve; *CVC*, caudal vena cava.

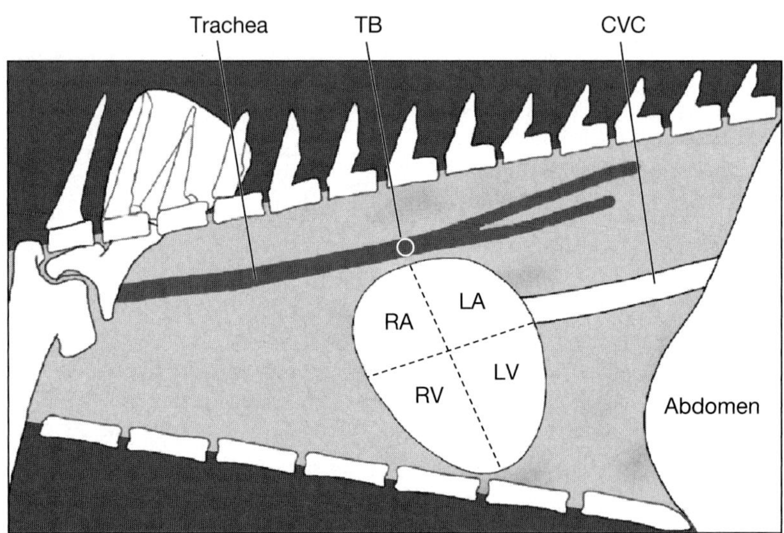

Figure 2-8. Schematic lateral thoracic radiographic projection outlining the approximate location of the four heart chambers. *TB*, Tracheal bifurcation; *CVC*, caudal vena cava; *RA*, right atrium; *LA*, left atrium; *RV*, right ventricle; *LV*, left ventricle.

line from the tracheal bifurcation (carina) to the apex at an angle approximately 45 degrees to the sternal vertebrae. This angle can decrease in the cat with age and is often called a "lazy" heart. It has been postulated that this may be related to a loss of aortic connective tissue elasticity. This is most often seen in cats older than 7 years. Shallow, barrel-chested dog breeds (Dachshund, Lhasa Apso, Bulldog) tend to have more globular-shaped hearts, with increased sternal contact of the cranial margin of the heart. The heart chambers can be roughly defined by a line connecting the apex to the tracheal bifurcation and a second line perpendicular to the base-apex axis and positioned at the level of the ventral aspect of the caudal vena cava (see Figure 2-8).

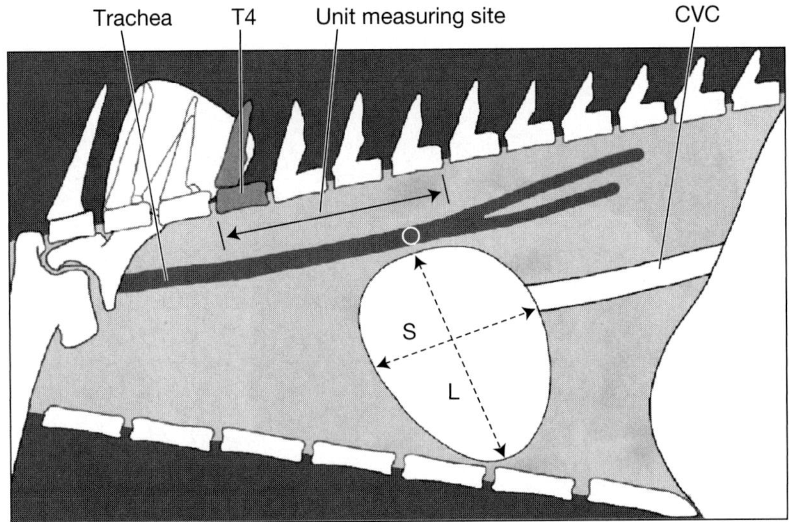

Figure 2-9. Schematic representation parameters for the vertebral scale system of cardiac size. The vertebral heart sum *(VHS)* is the sum of the long axis cardiac dimension *(L)* and the maximal perpendicular short axis dimension *(S)*. S and L are measured in vertebral units beginning at T4. *CVC,* Caudal vena cava.

The dorsal cardiac margin includes both atria, pulmonary arteries and veins, the cranial and caudal vena cavae, and the aortic arch (see Figures 2-6 to 2-8). The cranial border is formed by both the right ventricle and the right atrial appendage, resulting in the radiographically defined "cranial waist" (see Figures 2-6 and 2-8). The caudal margin is formed by the left atrium and left ventricle, with the atrioventricular junction defined as the radiographic "caudal waist."

The base-to-apex cardiac dimension or length occupies approximately 70% of the DV distance of the thoracic cavity at its position within the thorax. For objective measurements it is important to measure thoracic cavity distance between the thoracic spine and the sternum *at an axis perpendicular to the thoracic spine*.

The cranial-caudal dimension or width as it appears on the lateral projection is measured at its maximum width (which is usually at the level of the ventral aspect of the insertion of the caudal vena cava) and perpendicular to the base-apex axis. This classically has been defined as between 2.5 (deep-chested conformation breeds [Setters, Afghans, Collies]) and 3.5 (barrel-chested conformation breeds [Dachshunds, Bulldogs]) intercostal spaces (ICS) in the dog and 2.5 to 3.0 ICS in the cat. The ICS measurement is made at an axis *perpendicular to the long axis of the ribs*. Thus, the cardiac width distance determination may have to be shifted in axis angle before comparison to ICS length.

A more objective determination of cardiac size has been formulated for the dog and uses a vertebral scale system in which cardiac dimensions are scaled against the length of specific thoracic vertebrae (Figure 2-9). In lateral radiographs the long axis of the heart (L) is measured with a caliper extending from the ventral aspect of the left main stem bronchus (tracheal bifurcation hilus, carina) to the left ventricular apex. The caliper is repositioned along the vertebral column beginning at the cranial edge of the fourth thoracic vertebra. The length of the heart is recorded as the number of vertebrae caudal to that point and estimated to the nearest tenth of a vertebra. The maximum perpendicular short axis (S) is measured in the same manner beginning at the fourth thoracic vertebra. If obvious left atrial enlargement is present, the short axis measurement is made at the ventral juncture of left atrial and caudal vena caval silhouettes.

The lengths in vertebrae (v) of the long and short axes are then added to obtain a vertebral heart sum (VHS), which provides a single number representing heart size proportionate to the size of the dog. The average VHS in the dog is 9.7 v (range 8.5 to 10.5 v). Caution must be exercised in some breeds that have excessively disproportionate skeletal–body weight conformations. An example is the English Bulldog, which has relatively small thoracic vertebrae and commonly has hemivertebrae as well; thus, a normal heart may be interpreted

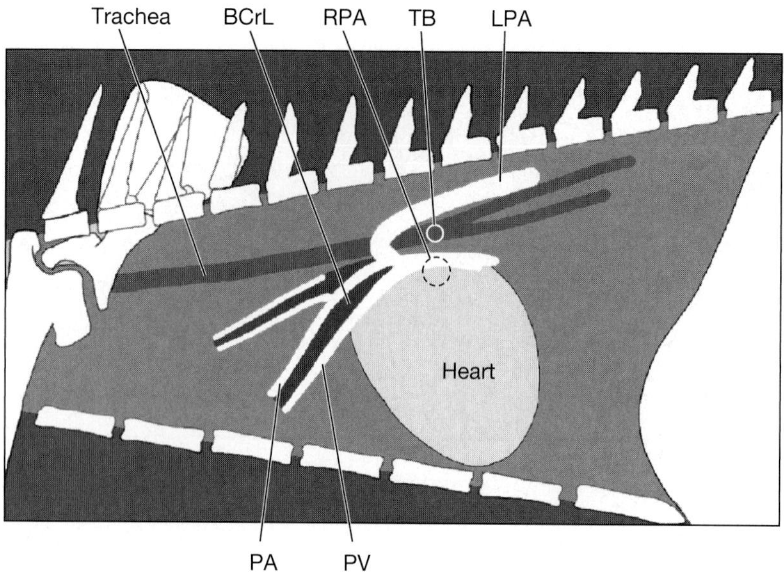

Figure 2-10. Pulmonary vascular anatomy in the lateral thoracic projection. Cranial lung lobe branch of the pulmonary artery *(PA)*, cranial lung lobe branch of the pulmonary vein *(PV)*, end-on view of the right main pulmonary artery *(RPA)* as it traverses the thorax from left to right, and left main pulmonary artery *(LPA)*. TB, tracheal bifurcation (carina); *BCrL*, Bronchus to a cranial lung lobe.

as large with the VHS method. Although the VHS concept is more precise, clinical judgment is still necessary to avoid over diagnosing or under diagnosing heart disease.

Vessel Parameters

The main pulmonary artery (pulmonary trunk) cannot be seen on the lateral projection owing to a positive-silhouette sign with the craniodorsal base of the heart. The left pulmonary artery can sometimes be seen extending dorsal and caudal to the tracheal bifurcation (carina). The right pulmonary artery is frequently seen end-on as it leaves the main pulmonary artery immediately ventral to the carina (Figure 2-10). This end-on appearance may be confused with a mass lesion on normal radiographs and is accentuated in cases of pulmonary hypertension such as heartworm disease. The pulmonary veins are best identified as they enter the left atrium caudal to the heart base.

Using the larger, more proximal segments of the mainstem bronchi as a reference, the pulmonary arteries are dorsal to the bronchus, and the pulmonary veins are ventral to the bronchus (see Figure 2-10).

The vessels to the cranial lung lobes are usually seen as two pairs of vessels, each with their respective bronchi. The more cranial pair of vessels generally corresponds to the side on which the lateral projection was made. Thus, in the right lateral projection, the right cranial lobar vessels are more cranial than vessels of the left cranial lung lobe. The pulmonary arteries and veins should be equal in size. The width of the vessels where they cross the fourth rib should not exceed the width of the narrowest portion of that rib at its juncture with the rib head (the dorsal aspect of the rib near the thoracic spine). The dorsal section of the rib is used as a reference to adjust for radiographic magnification owing to thoracic conformation.

Dorsoventral and Ventrodorsal Projections

Cardiac Parameters

The heart is rotated on its long axis such that the right chambers are oriented both right and cranially, and the left chambers reside both left and caudal. The degree of rotation is less in the cat. The cranial-caudal rotation is most significant when defining the location of the left and right atria, respectively.

The canine heart appears radiographically as an elliptical opacity with its base-apex axis orientation approximately 30 degrees to the left of the midline. The width of the heart across its widest point is usually 60% to 65% of the thoracic width at its location within the thorax. In the cat the cardiac axis is most commonly on or close to midline, and its width does not usually exceed 50% of the width of the thoracic cavity during full inspiration. The cardiac silhouette may be artificially increased in the obese patient owing to an excessive amount of pericardial fat. In these cases, the cardiac silhouette margin appears to be less well defined or blurred because the margin of contrast between soft tissue

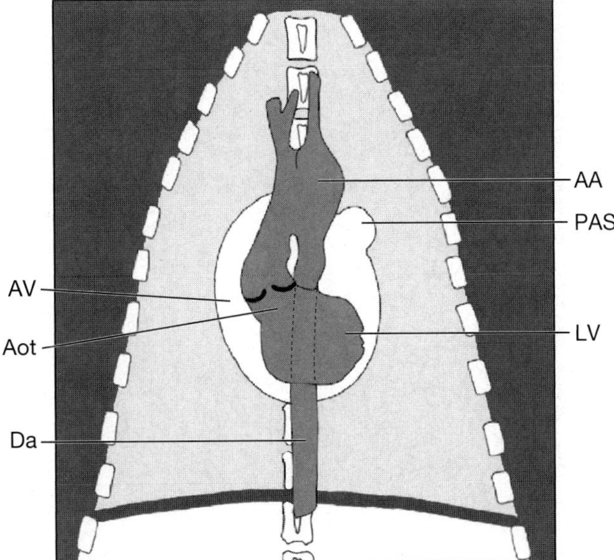

Figure 2-11. Schematic anatomy of the chambers and vasculature of the left ventricular outflow tract of the heart in the dorsoventral radiographic projection. *LV*, Left ventricle; *Aot*, aortic outflow tract; *AV*, aortic valve; *AA*, aortic arch; *PAS*, pulmonary artery segment; *Da*, descending aorta.

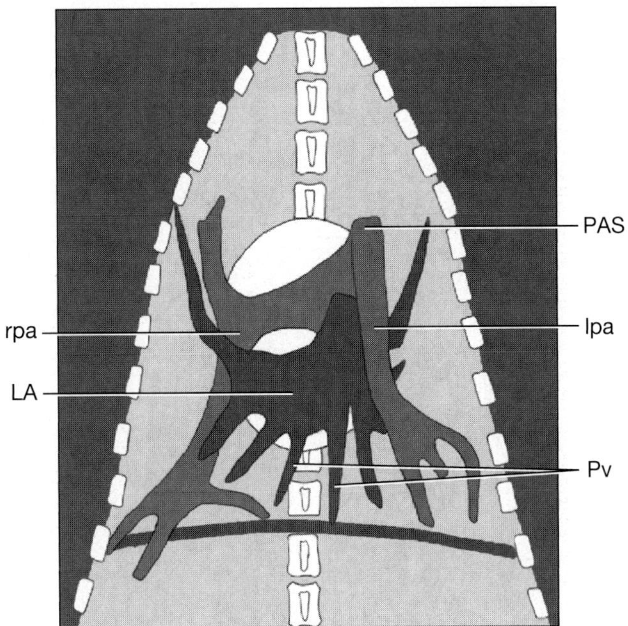

Figure 2-12. Schematic anatomy of the pulmonary vasculature in the dorsoventral projection. *PAS*, Main pulmonary artery (radiographic description—pulmonary artery segment); *lpa*, left pulmonary artery; *rpa*, right pulmonary artery; *LA*, left atrium; *Pv*, pulmonary veins.

(heart), fat (pericardial), and air is not as distinct as that between soft tissue and air.

Evaluating the obesity of the patient by evaluating the thickness of the abaxial thoracic wall and width of the mediastinum (as well as examining the patient) will assist in the determination of pericardial fat contribution to cardiac size. In deep, narrow-chested breeds, the heart stands more vertical in the thorax and thus produces a smaller and more circular cardiac silhouette conformation. The broad, barrel-chested breeds produce a radiographic silhouette that appears wider than that of standard breeds.

The margins of the heart that create the cardiac silhouette contain a number of structures that often overlap. A clock face analogy can be used to

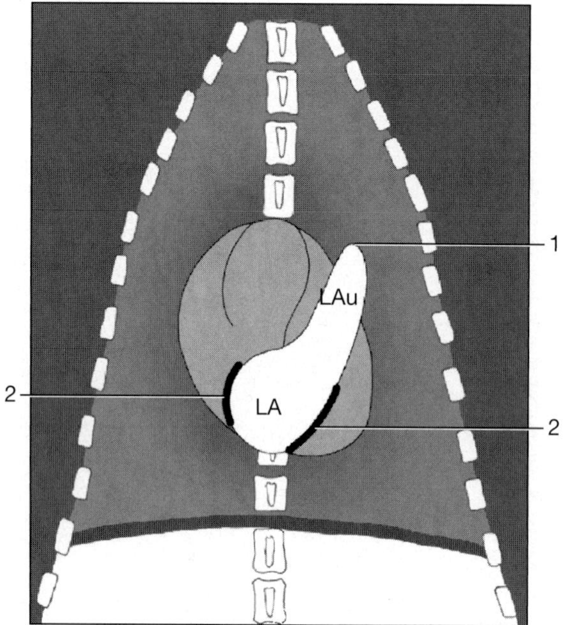

Figure 2-13. Dorsoventral thoracic radiographic projection of a dog with severe left atrial *(LA)* enlargement. The left atrial auricular appendage *(LAu)* contributes to the cardiac silhouette at the 2 to 3 o'clock position (1). The body of the left atrium superimposed over the caudal cardiac silhouette produces a radiolucent "mach" line, a radiographic edge effect caused by an acute change in soft tissue thickness (2).

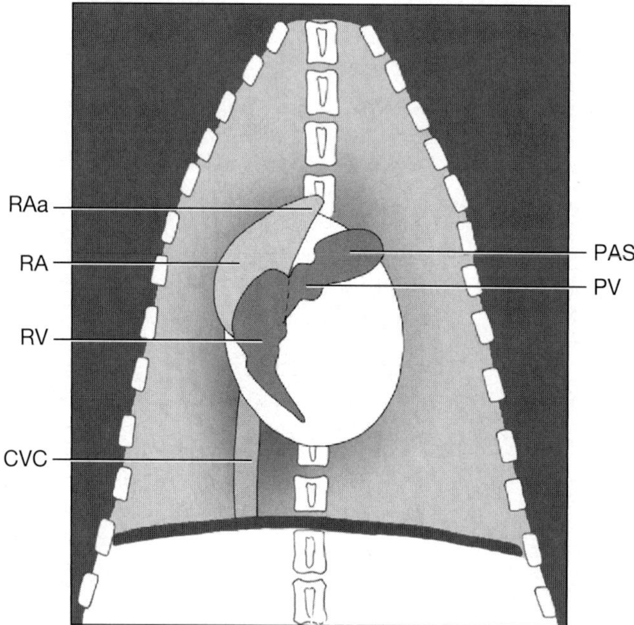

Figure 2-14. Schematic anatomy of the chambers and outflow tract of the right side of the heart in the dorsoventral radiographic projection. *RV,* Right ventricle; *RA,* right atrium; *RAa,* right atrial auricular appendage; *PV,* pulmonic valve; *PAS,* mainstem pulmonary artery segment; *CVC,* caudal vena cava.

simplify the location of these structures. The aortic arch extends from the 11 o'clock to 1 o'clock position (Figure 2-11). The main pulmonary artery is located from the 1 to 2 o'clock position, with its radiographic designation as the pulmonary artery segment (PAS) (Figures 2-12 and 2-13). In the cat, the body of the left atrium proper forms the 2 to 3 o'clock position of the cardiac silhouette. In the dog, the left atrium is superimposed over the caudal portion of the cardiac silhouette in the DV projection (see Figure 2-12). With severe cases of left atrial enlargement in the dog, the left auricular appendage contributes to the definition and enlargement of the cardiac silhouette at the 2 to 3 o'clock position (Figure 2-13). The left ventricle forms the left heart margin from the 2 to 6 o'clock position (see Figure 2-11). The right ventricle is located from the 7 to 11 o'clock position (the right ventricle does not extend to the apex of the heart) (Figure 2-14). The right atrium is located at the 9 to 11 o'clock position (see Figure 2-14). Pericardial fat in the dog can asymmetrically contribute to cardiac silhouette enlargement at the 4 to 5 o'clock and 8 to 11 o'clock positions.

Vessel Parameters

The pulmonary arteries originate from the main pulmonary artery or the PAS with the right branch coursing transversely, superimposed over the cranial portion of the heart silhouette, extending beyond the right heart margin at approximately the 8 o'clock position (see Figure 2-12). The left pulmonary artery branch courses caudally, superimposed over the caudal left ventricular portion of the heart, and extends beyond the left heart margin at approximately the 4 o'clock position. The pulmonary veins are best seen as they enter the left atrium along the caudal margin of the cardiac silhouette (see Figure 2-12). Compared with the pulmonary arteries, they are clustered in a more axial position. Thus, the pulmonary arteries extend to both the cranial and caudal lung fields in a more abaxial position relative to the pulmonary veins.

The aortic arch is within the cranial mediastinum at the cranial heart margin and is normally not visible. The descending aorta is superimposed over the heart and extends caudally, dorsally, and medially. The left lateral margin of the aorta can be seen to the left of the vertebral column on both DV and VD views (see Figure 2-11). The caudal vena cava courses cranially from the diaphragm to the right of midline and into the right caudal margin of the heart (see Figure 2-14). This is one of the most useful landmarks for determination of proper orientation of the DV radiograph on a viewbox.

RADIOGRAPHIC INTERPRETATION

A systematic evaluation of the entire thoracic cavity involves adherence to and inclusion of the following steps with each radiographic interpretation. Abnormalities supportive of disease should be substantiated on multiple radiographic views where applicable.

- Evaluate the radiographs for technical quality, positioning, and proper exposure. *If the study is substandard, then stop right here and repeat the radiographic study.*
- Determine the phase of respiration.
- Review the entire thoracic cavity: spine, sternum, diaphragm, thoracic wall, ribs, cranial and caudal mediastinum, conformation and position of the diaphragm.
- Review the portion of the cranial abdomen included in the projection. Thoracic radiographic exposure is usually *half* of that required for abdominal imaging but a cursory evaluation of abdominal contrast, detail, and hepatic size (using gastric axis) can be performed.
- Evaluate the position, course, and diameter of the trachea and mainstem bifurcations.
- Evaluate the position of the cardiac apex and caudal mediastinum.
- Evaluate the size, shape, and course of the main pulmonary artery and peripheral pulmonary arteries and veins.
- Evaluate the lung fields for hyperinflation or underinflation and for distribution and pattern of increased or decreased opacity.
- Evaluate the cardiac margin (cranial, caudal, right, left, "clock position" segmentation) for enlargement, abnormal position, or conformation.

NONCARDIAC–RELATED VARIABLES THAT CAN MIMIC RADIOGRAPHIC SIGNS OF CARDIAC DISEASE

Cardiac Position

- Pulmonary pathology (such as lung consolidation, atelectasis, or pleural disease) can cause a mediastinal shift and alter the position and axis of the heart in the thoracic cavity.
- Mediastinal mass lesions can affect the cardiac position and axis, as well as obscure the cranial and cardiac margins when in contact with the heart, by producing a radiographic positive-silhouette sign.
- Pneumothorax can produce disproportionate hemithoracic volume changes, altering cardiac position and axis. Pneumothorax commonly produces elevation of the cardiac apex from the sternum. This is supported by other radiographic signs of pneumothorax:
    - Premature termination of lung vasculature into the periphery of the thoracic cavity

- Lung lobe margin detection as it contrasts with nonparenchymal free intrathoracic gas
- Sternal conformational abnormalities due to congenital defects or previous trauma can alter cardiac position and axis.

Cardiac Size and Lateral Projection

- Younger animals appear to have larger hearts relative to their thoracic size than do mature patients.
- The heart appears smaller on inspiration than on expiration. During expiration increased sternal contact of the right heart margin and dorsal elevation of the trachea occurs, falsely suggesting right-heart enlargement.
- Anemic or emaciated patients often have small hearts owing to hypovolemia and are hyperinflated to compensate for hypoxemia. In deep-chested conformation breeds, the cardiac apex can be elevated far enough from the sternum to mimic pneumothorax.

Cardiac Position, Dorsoventral/ Ventrodorsal Projection

Malposition of the Cardiac Apex to the Right or Left

- Malposition of the heart to the right is normal variant in the cat.
- Uneven lung inflation secondary to disease or previous lobectomy can produce a mediastinal shift and resultant apex shift.
- If radiographs are taken on diseased, recumbent patients or patients during or immediately following general anesthesia, then hypostatic congestion and atelectasis of the dependent lung fields can produce a mediastinal shift, altering cardiac position.
- Pectus excavatum or "funnel chest" sternal conformation due to congenital deformities

EVALUATION OF HEART CHAMBER ENLARGEMENT

Right Atrial Enlargement

Radiographic Signs

- Lateral projection (Figure 2-15):
  - Elevation of the trachea as it courses dorsally over the right atrium
  - Accentuation of the cranial waist. Preferential enlargement of the more dorsal margin of the cranial margin of the cardiac silhouette defines selective enlargement of the right atrial auricular appendage.
  - Increased soft tissue opacity of the cranial aspect of the cardiac silhouette owing to increased soft tissue thickness of the right atrium superimposed over the right ventricle

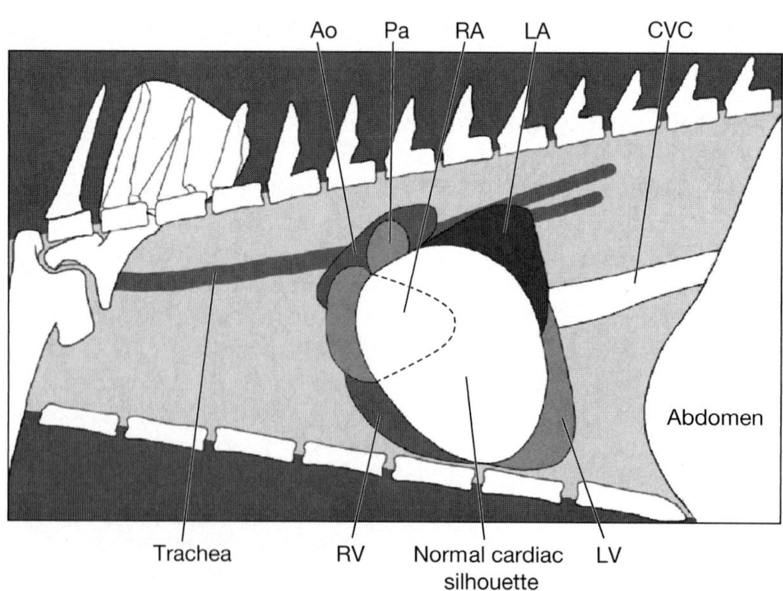

Figure 2-15. Cardiac silhouette changes associated with vessel and chamber enlargement in the lateral thoracic radiographic projection. *Ao,* Aortic arch; *Pa,* main pulmonary artery; *RA,* right atrium; *LA,* left atrium; *RV,* right ventricle; *LV,* left ventricle; *CVC,* caudal vena cava. *Dotted line,* area of right atrial superimposition over the right ventricle.

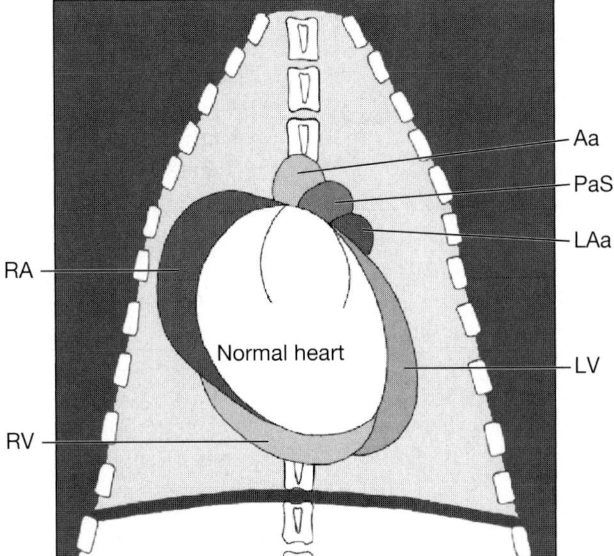

Figure 2-16. Cardiac silhouette changes associated with vessel and chamber enlargement in the dorsoventral radiographic projection. *Aa,* Aortic arch; *PaS,* main pulmonary artery; *LAa,* left atrial auricular appendage; *LV,* left ventricle; *RV,* right ventricle; *RA,* right atrium.

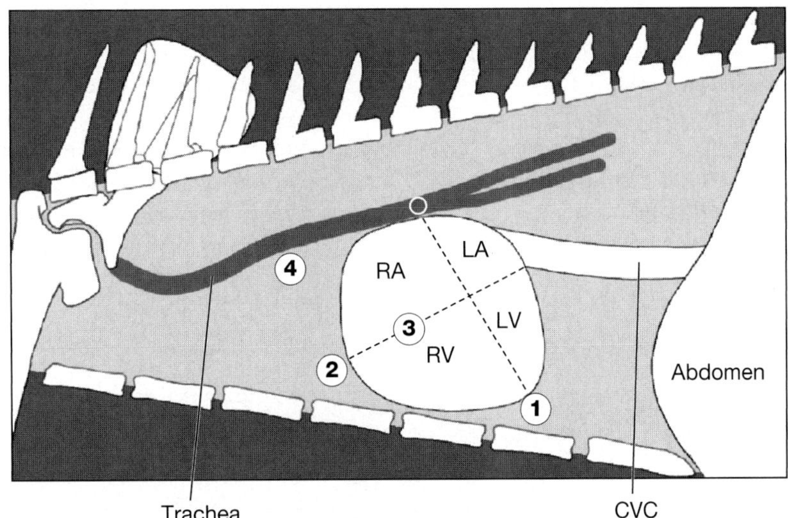

Figure 2-17. Schematic representation of radiographic signs associated with right- heart enlargement in the lateral projection. (1) Dorsal lifting of apex from sternum. (2) Increased sternal contact of cranial cardiac margin. (3) Disproportionate enlargement of the cranial portion of the cardiac silhouette when empirically divided into its right and left chambers. (4) Elevation of the trachea as it courses dorsally over the right atrium. *RA,* Right atrium; *RV,* right ventricle; *LA,* left atrium; *LV,* left ventricle; *CVC,* caudal vena cava.

- DV projection (Figure 2-16):
  - Enlargement of the cardiac margin at 9 to 11 o'clock
  - Enlargement can be dramatic in severe cases (especially in the cat) and can be easily mistaken for pulmonary hilar mass lesion.

Causes of Right Atrial Enlargement

- Right-heart failure
- Tricuspid insufficiency
- Cardiomyopathy
- Right atrial neoplasia (e.g., hemangiosarcoma)

Differential Diagnosis

- Cranial mediastinal mass
- Heart base neoplasia (most common in brachycephalic breeds)
- Tracheobronchial lymphadenopathy
- Superimposition of the aortic arch or main pulmonary artery

- Right cranial or middle lobar pulmonary alveolar consolidation or mass lesion

Right Ventricular Enlargement

Radiographic Signs

- Lateral projections (see Figure 2-15)
  - Increased sternal contact of cranial cardiac margin
  - Elevation of the cardiac apex from the sternum
  - Rounding of the conformation of the entire cardiac silhouette; increased cardiac width
  - Disproportionate enlargement of the cranial portion of the cardiac silhouette when empirically divided into its right and left chambers (Figure 2-17)
  - Dorsal elevation of the caudal vena cava
- DV projection (see Figure 2-16)
  - Cardiac silhouette enlargement at the 6 to 11 o'clock position
  - Given the enlargement and rounded conformation of the right margin, the left margin in comparison assumes a more straightened conformation; an overall "reverse-D" conformational appearance of the cardiac silhouette results
  - Shift of cardiac apex to the left

Causes of Right Ventricular Enlargement

- Secondary to left-heart failure
- Tricuspid insufficiency
- Cardiomyopathy
- Cor pulmonale
- Dirofilariasis
- Congenital heart disease: pulmonic stenosis, patent ductus arteriosus (PDA), ventricular septal defects, tetralogy of Fallot, tricuspid valve dysplasia

Left Atrial Enlargement

Radiographic Signs

- Lateral projection (see Figure 2-15)
  - Dorsal elevation of the caudal portion of trachea and carina
  - Disproportionate dorsal elevation of the mainstem bronchi (the two will no longer be superimposed; the left bronchus will appear more dorsal than the right bronchus)
  - Enlargement and straightening of the caudodorsal portion of the cardiac silhouette with almost a right-angle margin conformation (Figure 2-18); straightening of the caudal margin of the heart and loss of the caudal waist (determined by the atrioventricular junction)
- DV projection (see Figure 2-16)
  - The dog
    - Enlargement of the atrial auricular appendage, which now produces a noticeable focal "bulge" enlargement at the 2 to 3 o'clock position (see Figures 2-13 and 2-16)

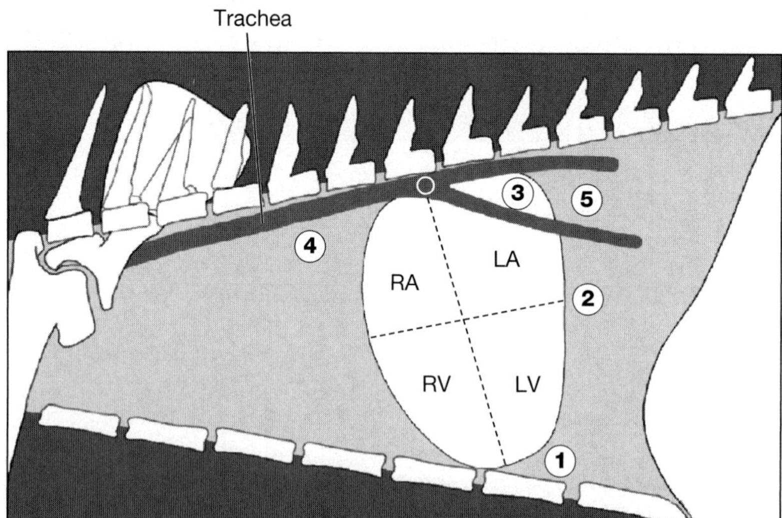

Figure 2-18. Schematic representation of radiographic signs associated with left- heart enlargement in the lateral projection. (1) Rounding and widening of the cardiac apex conformation. (2) Straightening and increased vertical axis of the caudal cardiac margin. (3) Left atrial enlargement with characteristic right-angular caudodorsal margin conformation. (4) Dorsal elevation of the intrathoracic portion of the trachea, carina, and mainstem bronchi. The angle between the thoracic spine axis and the trachea is diminished to the point of becoming parallel. (5) Separation of normally superimposed caudal mainstem bronchi. Left more dorsal in position than the right. *RA*, Right atrium; *RV*, right ventricle; *LA*, left atrium; *LV*, left ventricle.

- A double opacity of the atrial body over the caudal aspect of the cardiac silhouette; the body of the left atrium superimposed over the caudal cardiac silhouette produces a radiolucent "mach" line, a radiographic edge effect caused by an acute change in soft tissue thickness (see Figure 2-13)
- The cat
  - Enlargement if the cardiac margin at the 2 to 3 o'clock position of the silhouette

Causes of Left Atrial Enlargement
- Mitral insufficiency
- Cardiomyopathy
- Congenital heart disease; mitral valve dysplasia, PDA, ventricular septal defects, atrial septal defects
- Left ventricular failure

Differential Diagnosis
- Hilar lymphadenopathy
- Pulmonary mass adjacent to hilus

Left Ventricular Enlargement

Radiographic Signs
- Lateral projection (see Figure 2-15)
  - Loss of the caudal waist
  - Caudal cardiac margin straighter and more vertical than normal
  - Dorsal elevation of the intrathoracic portion of the trachea, carina, and mainstem bronchi; the angle between the thoracic spine axis and trachea is diminished to the point of becoming parallel
  - Disproportionate enlargement of the caudal portion of the cardiac silhouette when empirically divided into its right and left cardiac chambers (see Figure 2-18)
- DV projection (see Figure 2-16)
  - Rounding and enlargement of left ventricular margin
  - Rounding and broadening of the cardiac apex conformation
  - Shift of the cardiac apex to the right

Causes of Left Ventricular Enlargement
- Mitral insufficiency
- Cardiomyopathy
- Congenital heart disease: PDA, aortic stenosis, ventricular septal defects
- High-output cardiac disease: fluid overload, chronic anemia, peripheral arteriovenous fistula, obesity, chronic renal disease, hyperthyroidism

Enlargement of the Aortic Arch and Aorta

Radiographic Signs
- Lateral projection (see Figure 2-15)
  - Widening of the dorsal aspect of the cardiac silhouette
  - Enlargement of the craniodorsal cardiac margin
- DV projection (see Figure 2-16)
  - Widening and increased cranial extensions of the cardiac margin between the 11 and 1 o'clock positions.

Causes of Aortic Arch Enlargement
- PDA; enlargement more abaxial (1 o'clock)
- Aortic stenosis with poststenotic enlargement of the aortic arch; enlargement more axial and cranial (11 o'clock)
- Aortic aneurysm (very rare)

Differential Diagnosis
- Normal variation in some dogs
- Very common variant in older cats with "lazy" heart conformation; very prominent on the DV projection
- Cranial mediastinal mass
- Thymus, or the "sail-sign" in young dogs
- Cranial mediastinal fat in obese brachycephalic dogs

Enlargement of the Pulmonary Artery

Radiographic Signs
- Lateral projection (see Figure 2-15)
  - Protrusion of the craniodorsal heart border
- DV projection (see Figure 2-16)
  - Lateral bulge of the cardiac margin at 1 to 2 o'clock position
  - Radiographically defined as the pulmonary artery segment (PAS)

Causes of Pulmonary Artery Segment Enlargement
- Dirofilariasis
- Pulmonary thrombosis and thromboembolism
- Cor pulmonale
- Congenital disease: pulmonic stenosis, PDA, septal defects both ventricular and atrial with left-to-right shunting

Differential Diagnosis
- Previous dirofilariasis infection and treatment
- Rotational (oblique) positional artifact (usually on VD projection) most commonly experienced with deep-chested conformation dogs

EVALUATION OF THE PULMONARY CIRCULATION

Undercirculation

Radiographic Signs

- Lung field more radiolucent than normal owing to lack of pulmonary vascular volume
- Hyperinflation due to hypoxemia or ventilation/perfusion mismatch
- Pulmonary arteries smaller than normal; may be smaller in size when compared with corresponding pulmonary veins

Causes of Pulmonary Undercirculation

- Congenital disease: pulmonic stenosis, tetralogy of Fallot, reverse PDA (right-to-left shunting)

Differential Diagnosis

- Emphysema, chronic obstructive pulmonary disease
- Hyperinflation
- Pneumothorax
- Overexposure
- Pulmonary thromboembolism
- Hypovolemia, shock (the heart will also be smaller than normal)
- Hypoadrenocorticism (Addison's disease); the heart may also be smaller than normal

Overcirculation

Radiographic Signs

- Both the pulmonary arteries and the veins are enlarged
- Arteries are frequently larger than the veins
- Pulmonary thoracic opacity is increased because of larger vascular volume

Causes of Pulmonary Overcirculation

- Dirofilariasis (arteries are larger than corresponding veins)
- PDA: both arteries and veins enlarged
- Left-to-right shunts (ventricular and atrial septal defects): both arteries and veins enlarged
- Congestive heart failure: veins may be larger than arteries if mainly left sided; both arteries and veins enlarged with concurrent left- and right-sided failure
- Fluid overload

Differential Diagnosis

- Underexposure
- Expiratory phase of respiration

RADIOGRAPHIC DIAGNOSIS OF HEART FAILURE

The radiographic diagnosis of heart failure is dependent upon recognition of imbalances in the blood and fluid distribution within the body. This circulatory imbalance is the result of diminished cardiac output into the pulmonary or systemic vascular systems or reduced acceptance of blood by the failing ventricle (hypertrophy), or both. Depending on which side of the heart is most severely affected, blood is shifted from the systemic to the pulmonary circulation (left-heart failure) or from the pulmonary to the systemic circulation (right-heart failure).

Right-Heart Failure

Physiologic Phenomenon

- In right-heart failure, an inadequate right ventricular output into the pulmonary arteries exists concurrently with a reduced acceptance of blood from the systemic veins. The blood volume and pressure in the splanchnic and systemic veins are elevated. The venous congestion causes hepatomegaly.
- With further progression of right-heart failure, a progression of systemic hypertension leads to increased amounts of fluid, solutes, and protein escaping from the capillary beds of the major organs. The lymphatic circulation is overtaxed, and fluid exudes into the serosal cavities, producing ascites, pleural, and even pericardial effusions.
- The extracardiac radiographic signs of progressively worsening right-heart failure are hepatomegaly, ascites, and then pleural effusion.

Radiographic Signs

- Right-sided cardiomegaly (see Figures 2-15 through 2-17). Patients with concentric cardiac hypertrophy (e.g., pulmonic stenosis), thin-walled cardiomyopathy, or acute arrhythmias often may not have dramatic radiographic cardiomegaly. Thus, subtle cardiac silhouette changes in both the DV and the lateral projections must be considered significant with supportive clinical evidence of cardiac disease.
- Hepatomegaly: rounded liver margin, which extends caudal to last rib; displacement of stomach caudally and to the left
- Ascites: abdominal distention; diffuse loss of intra-abdominal detail
- Pleural effusion
  - Generalized increase in thoracic opacity

- Visualization of interlobar pleural fissures (see Figures 2-4 and 2-5, *A*)
- Obliteration of cardiac silhouette definition (best demonstrated on the DV projection) (see Figure 2-5, *B*)
- Separation of pulmonary visceral pleural margin away from thoracic wall (see Figures 2-4 and 2-5)

Causes of Pleural Effusion Secondary to Right-Heart Failure

- Decompensated mitral and tricuspid insufficiency
- Decompensated pulmonic stenosis, tetralogy of Fallot
- Dirofilariasis (caval syndrome)
- Pericardial effusion with tamponade
- Restrictive pericarditis

Differential Diagnosis

- Pleuritis
- Chylothorax
- Hemothorax
- Pyothorax
- Hypoproteinemia
- Neoplasia (pleural, mediastinal, cardiac, pulmonary, primary, or metastatic)

Left-Heart Failure

Physiologic Phenomenon

- In left-heart failure, inadequate left ventricular output into the aorta occurs, and a diminished acceptance of blood from the pulmonary veins entering the left atrium results. This causes pulmonary venous congestion and leakage of fluid into the pulmonary interstitium, with progression to flooding of the alveoli.
- Clinically, this evolves as a progression of physiologic events: pulmonary venous congestion, interstitial pulmonary edema, alveolar edema, and lung consolidation.

Radiographic Signs

- Left-sided cardiomegaly (see Figure 2-18). Patients with concentric cardiac hypertrophy (e.g., aortic stenosis), thin-walled cardiomyopathy (large- and giant-breed dogs), or acute arrhythmias often may not have dramatic radiographic cardiomegaly. Thus, subtle cardiac silhouette changes in both the DV and lateral projections as well as noncardiac changes (pulmonary vascular changes, pulmonary edema, etc.) must be evaluated.
- Pulmonary venous congestion
  - Engorgement and distention of the pulmonary veins, especially in the hilar area as they enter the left atrium. On the DV view these are identified as the more axial of the caudal vasculature (see Figure 2-12).
  - The diameter of the pulmonary veins is greater than that of their corresponding pulmonary arteries (best seen on the lateral projection with cranial lobar vessels) (see Figure 2-10).
  - The radiopacity of the lung parenchyma distal and peripheral to the hilus is unchanged.
- Interstitial edema
  - Diffuse increased radiopacity of the lung fields owing to a hazy interstitial opacity is apparent.
  - The margins of the pulmonary veins and arteries are indistinct owing to perivascular edema. As the lung parenchyma surrounding the pulmonary vasculature fills with fluid, the normal pulmonary radiographic contrast between gas (air-filled lung) and soft tissue (blood-filled vessels) is lost. Thus, the pulmonary vasculature becomes indistinct and begins to disappear in the surrounding, fluid-filled lung parenchyma.
  - In some patients, fluid accumulates around major bronchi, producing prominent peribronchial markings.
- Alveolar edema
  - Radiographic signs
    - Fluid enters the alveolar air spaces and peripheral bronchioles, causing a coalescent fluffy alveolar infiltrate. Air bronchograms (black tubes in a white radiopaque background) and air alveolograms (lung parenchyma with the radiopacity of *liver* containing no vascular markings) are present. In the cat, cardiogenic alveolar consolidations can appear as a very well margined, "cloudlike" conformation area of increased pulmonary radiopacity.
    - The margins of the pulmonary vessels are usually completely obscured (see Figure 2-3, *B*). The alveolar infiltrate is of greatest opacity in the perihilar area, fading peripherally. In the dog, alveolar edema can be asymmetrical, with the right lung fields more severely affected than the left (best seen on the DV projection).
  - Differential diagnosis for pulmonary edema
    - Neurogenic: electrocution, head trauma, post seizure, encephalitis, brain neoplasm
    - Hyperdynamic (excessive negative intrathoracic pressures): choking, strangulation, upper airway obstructions

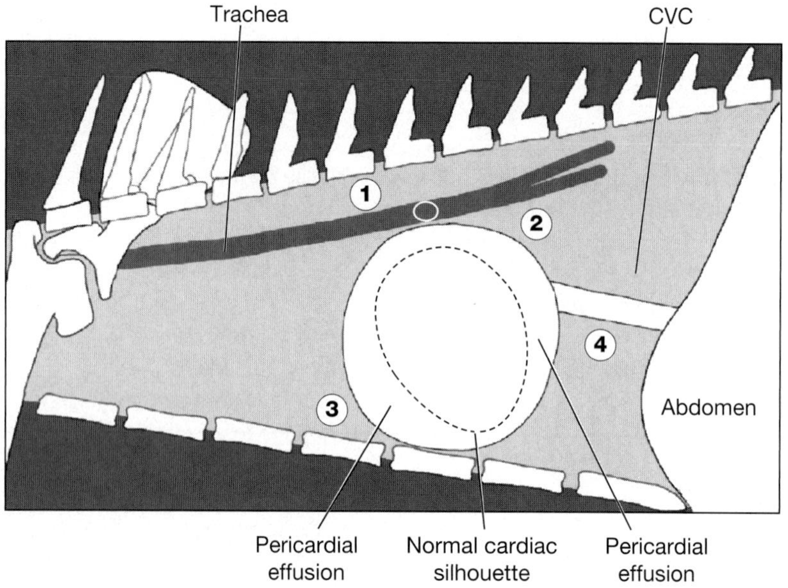

Figure 2-19. Schematic representation of radiographic signs associated with pericardial effusion. (1) Dorsal elevation of the intrathoracic portion of the trachea, carina, and mainstem bronchi. The angle between the thoracic spine axis and the trachea is diminished to the point of becoming parallel. (2) Convex enlargement of the caudodorsal cardiac margin without a "right-angle" conformation characteristic for left atrial enlargement. (3) Increased sternal contact of cranial margin. (4) Dorsal elevation and enlargement of the caudal vena cava *(CVC)*. The cardiac silhouette takes on a smoothly contoured circular conformation with obliteration of normal cardiac contour.

    - Fluid overload: overhydration
    - Toxicity
    - Systemic shock
    - Hypersensitization
    - Drowning
- Increased bronchial markings in some cases
- Pleural effusion
  - In the dog, this can occur only in very progressive or severe forms of left-heart failure; this usually indicates early concurrent left- and right-heart failure.
  - In the cat, pleural effusion is very common with only left-heart failure; this can be separated from right-heart failure by the absence of accompanying hepatomegaly and ascites.

RADIOGRAPHIC DIAGNOSIS OF PERICARDIAL EFFUSION

- Generalized enlargement of cardiac silhouette in a "basketball" conformation, with elimination of all normal cardiac margin contours on all views
- Increased sternal contact of the cranial margin and convex bulging of the caudal margin, without the angular conformation and straightening characteristic for left atrial and ventricular enlargements (Figure 2-19)
- Elevation and enlargement of the caudal vena cava
- Dorsal elevation of the trachea (similar to left-side enlargement)
- Hepatomegaly, ascites, and pleural effusion secondary to cardiac tamponade (see Figures 2-4 and 2-5)

SUMMARY OF RADIOGRAPHIC SIGNS

The clinician must be armed with both potential radiographic parameters and a clinically derived differential diagnostic list for cardiac disease before the radiographic image can begin to provide useful information. Table 2-2 summarizes the radiographic signs associated with congenital and acquired heart diseases. Awareness of noncardiac and artifactual conditions that can present with the same radiographic signs is also paramount to a correct diagnosis.

INTRODUCTION TO DIGITAL RADIOGRAPHY

Digital radiography is a relatively new technology that is becoming common place in veterinary medicine. It is been used in human medicine for over 20 years and has been thoroughly tested and proven. There are many advantages to digital radiography beyond the excellent image quality (Figure 2-20) which include:

TABLE 2-2 Summary of Radiographic Signs of Congenital and Acquired Cardiac Disease

Lesion	RA	RV	LA	LV	Aorta	MPAs	PAb	PV	VC	Failure/Side	Failure/Type
Congenital defects											
Patent ductus arteriosus	N	In	In	In	In	In	In	In	N/In	Left	Volume
Pulmonic stenosis	In	In	N/De	N/De	N	In	N/De	N/De	In	Right	Pressure
Aortic stenosis	N	N/In	N/In	In	In	N	N	N/In	N	Left	Pressure
Ventricular septal defect	N	In	In	In	N	N/In	In	In	N/In	Left	Volume
Tetralogy of Fallot	N/In	In	N/De	N/De	N	De/N/In	De	De	N	Right	Pressure
Atrial septal defect	In	In	N/In	N	N	N/In	N/In	N/In	N/In	Left	Volume
Acquired heart disease											
Mital insufficiency	N	N/In	In	In	N	N	N	In	N	Left	Fluid
Tricuspid insufficiency	In	In	N	N	N	N	N	N	In	Right	Fluid
Aortic insufficiency	N	N	In	In	N/In	N	N	In	N	Left	Fluid
Hypertrophic cardiomyopathy	In	In	In	In	N	N	N/In	N/In	N/In	Left > Right	Myocardial
Dilated cardiomyopathy	In	In	In	In	N	N	N/In	N/In	N/In	Right > Left	Myocardial
Pericardial effusion	In	In	In	In	N	N	N/De	N/De	In	Right	Tamponade

RA, Right atrium; *RV,* right ventricle; *LA,* left atrium; *LV,* left ventricle; *MPAs,* main pulmonary artery segement; *PAb,* pulmonary artery branches; *PV,* Pulmonary vein; *VC,* caudal vena cava; *In,* enlarged or increased; *De,* smaller or decreased; *N,* normal.

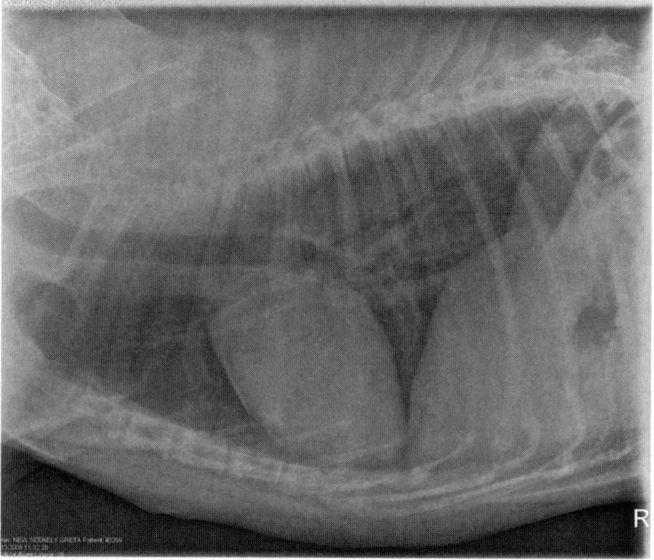

Figure 2-20. Right lateral view of the thorax taken with a flat panel detector system (DR). Note that all structures (bone, lung, pulmonary vessels, spine, etc) are visible in the same image. There are no areas of overexposure or underexposure.

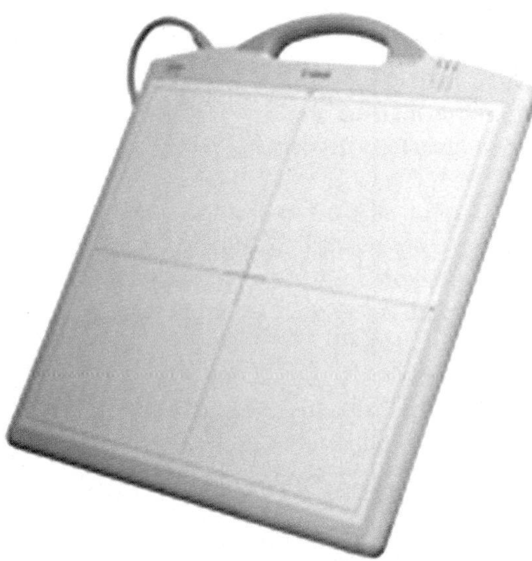

Figure 2-21. Flat panel detector (DR plate) made by Canon® (CXDI-50G). This plate is mounted out of sight under the x-ray table top in the location of the Bucky tray. The plate converts x-ray photon energy to an electrical pulse which is then interfaced with an acquisition station computer.

- No lost films
- No film degradation over time
- The ability to view images on any networked computer at your clinic or home
- The ability to easily send images to specialists for consultation

- There are several types of digital acquisition systems, including flat panel radiology, computed radiography, and charge-coupled device systems.
- Other devices such as film scanners and digital cameras can be used to digitize conventional x-ray film that allows the image to be stored on a computer. Once the image is acquired and stored it can be manipulated by the user to taste.
- There are financial savings over time including:
  - No cost for radiology disposable (film, chemicals)
  - No expense for processor maintenance, film jackets and storage space
  - Perhaps the most significant means of recouping revenue pertains to the fact there will be a significant reduction in the number of retakes because there should be little to no need to retake images due to under or overexposure.
- Flat panel technology (also known as digital radiography [DR] or direct digital radiography [DDR] [Figure 2-21]) is the most expensive form of digital radiography; however, this technology results in the highest quality image. These systems consist of a DR plate that is physically mounted in the area of the Bucky tray under the x-ray table top. The plate is then electronically interfaced to both the x-ray machine and a dedicated computer (acquisition station). Of the three forms of digital radiography, DR systems are extremely forgiving as far as technique (kVp and mAs settings) (Figure 2-22). This in turn simplifies a typical technique chart to essentially three or four settings (small, medium, large and extra large) no matter if you are imaging bone, thorax, or abdomen. Another advantage of DR systems include extremely quick image time (3 to 8

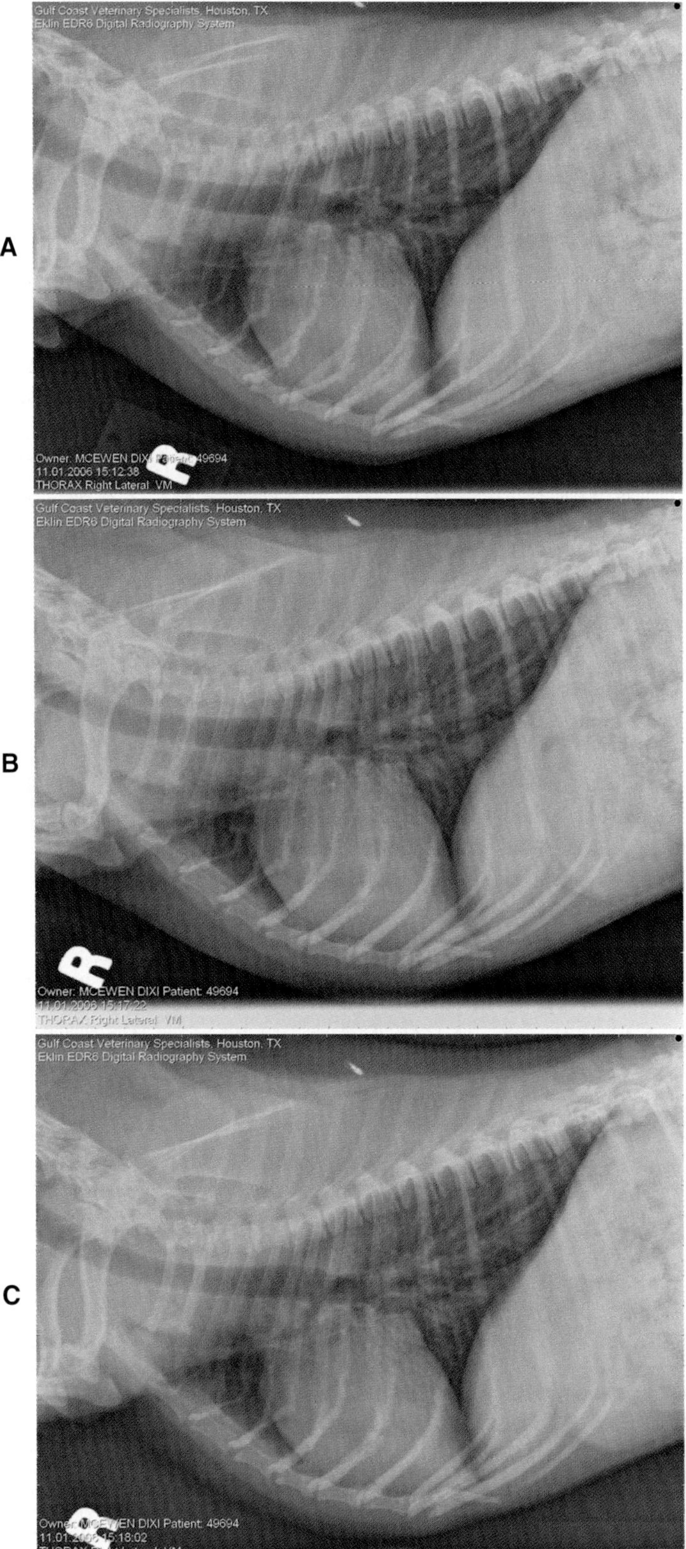

Figure 2-22. Technique independence. These three exposures were made with different mAs settings and identical kVp (90). **A,** 1.8 mAs. **B,** 2.5 mAs. **C,** 5.0 mAs. Note that all three exposures appear similar and are diagnostic. The computer software corrects for under or overexposure automatically. This decreased the number of retakes and increases productivity. On the other hand, if image **A** is magnified, it will appear much grainier than the other images.

seconds before the image is seen on a computer monitor) which allows the user to either save or delete the image immediately if it is not satisfactory (rotated, crooked, etc).

- Computed radiography (CR) systems use imaging plates that resemble traditional x-ray cassettes. The major difference is that the intensifying screen and film within the cassette is replaced by a flexible phosphor plate that has the ability to store a latent image. These storage phosphor plates operate similarly to the screen inside a conventional cassette in that they emit light (scintillate) in response to incident x-ray energy. However, unlike an x-ray screen, a storage phosphor plate retains a portion of the energy as a latent image, which is extracted ("read out") by a CR reader. In general, the image quality from a CR system is very high (similar to that of DR); however, CR is typically less forgiving as far as technique (compared to DR) which necessitates a more complicated technique chart. The image time for most CR systems range from about 55 to 90 seconds. CR systems are less expensive than DR systems, however.
- Charge-coupled device systems consist of a phosphor storage plate mounted under the x-ray table top that is in turn interfaced with a small light sensitive chip (CCD chip) similar to that found in digital cameras and video cameras. These CCD chips are commonly about 2 cm in size and may have thousands of individual light sensitive elements on them. Because of the small size of the chips, the aerial image (14 × 17, etc.) must be minified down to the size of the CCD chip. This is usually accomplished using a series of mirrors and lenses, which unfortunately results in a significant loss (90%) of the photon data. This loss of data can often make the resultant image appear "grainy" or pixilated on the computer monitor which is accentuated if the image is electronically magnified. On the other hand, CCD systems have fast image time (similar to DR systems) and are less expensive than DR systems. Because of the nature of these systems, they are usually sold as a complete system that includes the x-ray machine.
- Dedicated x-ray film scanners (Figure 2-23) and digital cameras are not forms of digital radiography. Both of these methods only reproduce the traditional hard copy radiograph, and in general do a poor job of image reproduction. Even expensive multi-megapixel digital cameras now available do a poor job of converting an analog x-ray image into a digital format without the loss of significant grey scale data. Because of this fact, the use of film scanners and digital cameras are not recommended as a means of sending images for consultation (teleradiology).

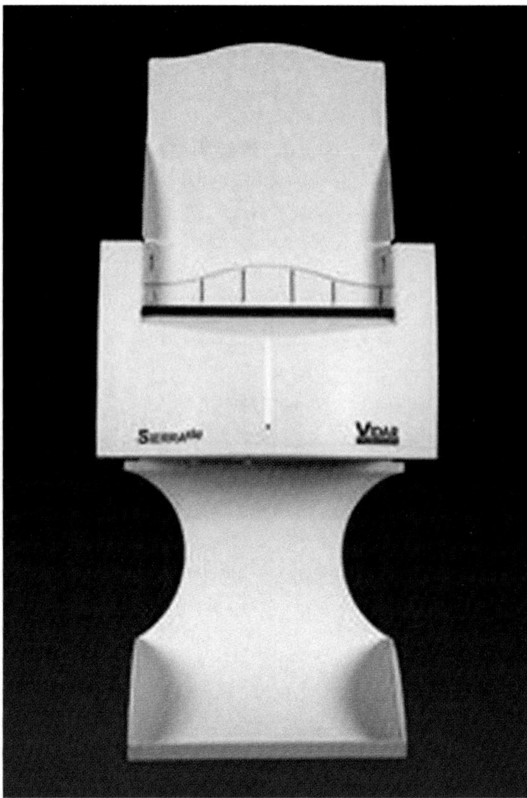

Figure 2-23. Dedicated x-ray film scanner (Vidar Sierra). An x-ray film is fed into the machine, and it is converted to a digital image that can be stored on a computer.

KEY POINTS

- Digital Radiography (DR) is extremely fast, is technique independent, has the highest image quality but is the most expensive method.
- Computed Radiography (CR) is slower, is somewhere between conventional film-screen technology and DR as far as reliance on x-ray technique, has high image quality, and is moderately expensive.
- Charged Coupled Devices (CCD) systems are fast, are similar to CR systems as far as technical factors, have the poorest image quality, and are the least expensive.
- Film scanners and digital cameras are not forms of digital radiography and have a limited role.

INTRODUCTION TO TELERADIOLOGY

- Teleradiology (telemedicine) offers the practitioner quick access to board certified specialists for case consultation. Once the radiographic images are in a digital format, they can be sent to any specialist for review via the World Wide Web. There are several methods of accomplishing this including using dedicated teleradiology companies, emailing images directly to specialists, or by using DICOM.
- At this time, there are four or five companies in the United States that cater to veterinary telemedicine. In general, these companies provide the necessary software that allows the veterinarian to upload digital images to the company's server and they in turn send those images to affiliated radiologists, internists, etc. The referring practice pays a fee to the teleradiology company which in turn pays the specialists to read their images. The disadvantage of this type of service is that the referring veterinarian often pays a premium fee (more than they would pay if they could send the images directly to the specialist), they may not have any or little input on exactly which specialist their images are sent to and they may have little ability to directly communicate with that specialist.
- Submission of images via standard email can be simple, but it is not recommended. Because of the very large image size of digital radiographs (a 14 × 17 radiograph of the thorax can be 14 megabytes of information) these images must be compressed or saved in a "lossy" format (such as jpg) before emailing, thus making the transmitted image of poor quality. Also, in the author's experience, these images are often submitted with a lack of necessary patient information and history.
- DICOM (Digital Image Communication in Medicine) is a proven and world wide recognized method of transmitting high-quality, lossless, digital radiographs (and other medical images such as ultrasound) from one place to another. DICOM images are embedded with very specific information regarding patient data as well as the type of system that the images were acquired on and this information cannot be altered. Also, DICOM allows transmission of images without the need for proprietary software that is vendor specific. For example, if you have a GE brand ultrasound machine, the images can be read by any radiologist with a DICOM viewer (which can be found for free) and they do not need to have specific GE software to view the images. DICOM allows the practicing veterinarian to send non-lossy, high-quality images that incorporate patient data directly to any radiologist of their choosing. Although DICOM "compliance" initially met with resistance (mostly from vendors), it has become common place in veterinary medicine and will continue to flourish.

Frequently Asked Questions

A Weimaraner dog is being anesthetized. Because of a murmur and mild coughing episodes, the heart and especially lung fields are of interest. The DV radiograph is not too light, and not too dark. This judgment is determined by the:

1. Inability to see the bony column details (very white), but a light (white) appearance of the lung fields to increase detail visualization there.
2. Ability to see the outline of the heart clearly against the lungs.
3. Ability to see the thoracic vertebrae in the area where they overlap the cardiac silhouette.
4. The appearance of the lungs as a dark air density, and full visualization of the bony structures.

The most correct answer is #3. This indicates the appropriate technique. The first option indicates that this is too light a technique. This is common where the technique has not been adjusted in obese patients. In #2, seeing the outline of the heart clearly against the lungs is not necessarily associated with technique, but may be due to pathology in the area. The #4 answer is burning through the soft tissues and is not appropriate for heart and lung studies.

A new digital radiography system has just been installed. The practice has opted for the flat panel technology. It does not appear that the image is different even when thin, obese or barrel shaped dogs are imaged using the same settings. This means:

1. Further staff training is needed.
2. This is normal—only four basic settings will be needed with digital radiography, and that is why we chose the system!
3. The chart needs to be evolved further, because something must be wrong if the same setting works for a large range of animals.
4. The equipment is working better than promised.

Answer #2 is most correct. Answer #1 is not probably an issue because this is the most forgiving of the imaging systems, digital or traditional.

Answer #3 is not relevant because only three or four settings will capture all dog breeds and body condition scores. Answer #4 is normal for this system. Though most expensive, this digital radiography system is known to be the most forgiving and is known to produce the highest quality images.

The thoracic radiographs for this patient are not easily interpreted so the plan is to:

1. Take another view and use foam supports to help stabilize the body in a fully vertical position, to ensure sternum and spine are superimposed which gives a better image. This still does not provide a clear answer, so "no significant findings" is placed on the medical record, assuming that the standard of care has been met due to acquisition of the best possible radiographs.
2. Follow the steps in answer #1 and send a jpg to the telemedicine group for a radiologist opinion.
3. Follow the steps in answer #1 and send a DICOM image to the telemedicine group for a radiologist's opinion.

Answer #3 is the best option as a lossless format, and an expert opinion will provide best practices here. Answer #2 is going to degrade the image—if an important detail is lost during image compression, it could compromise patient care. #1 is a good first step, but if the attending clinician does not have a confident interpretation, then use of a specialist will provide the gold standard for care. Generalist practitioners cannot be the master of all trades, and with the ability to transmit high-quality images of reasonable size, questionable interpretations for radiographs should always be referred for a specialist evaluation via telemedicine.

SUGGESTED READINGS

Animal Insides. *http://www.animalinsides.com* (accessed October, 2006).

Buchanan JW, Bucheler J: Vertebral scale system to measure canine heart size in radiographs. J Am Vet Med Assoc 206:194-199, 1995.

Bushberg JT, Seibert JA, Leidholdt EM, et al: The essential physics of medical imaging, Philadelphia, 2002, Lippincott, Williams & Wilkins.

Ettinger SJ, Suter PF: Canine cardiology. Philadelphia, 1970, WB Saunders.

Kittleson MD, Kienle RD: Small animal cardiovascular medicine. St Louis, 1998, Mosby.

Lord PF, Suter PF: Radiology. In Fox PR, Sisson D, Moiuse NS, eds: Textbook of canine and feline cardiology. ed 2, Philadelphia, 1999, WB Saunders.

Matton JS: Digital radiography, Vet Comp Orthop Traumatol, 19:123-132, 2006.

Owens JM: Radiographic interpretation for the small animal clinician, St Louis, 1982, Ralston Purina Co.

CHAPTER 3

Electrocardiography

Larry P. Tilley and Francis W. K. Smith, Jr.

INTRODUCTION

Electrocardiography in clinical practice is the recording at the body surface of electrical fields generated by the heart. Specific waveforms represent stages of myocardial depolarization and repolarization. The electrocardiogram is a basic and valuable diagnostic test in veterinary medicine and is relatively easy to acquire. The electrocardiogram is the initial test of choice in the diagnosis of cardiac arrhythmias and may also yield information regarding chamber dilation and hypertrophy.

INDICATIONS AND ROLE OF THE ELECTROCARDIOGRAM IN CLINICAL PRACTICE

Documentation of Cardiac Arrhythmias

- An electrocardiogram should be recorded when an arrhythmia is detected during physical examination. This may include bradycardia, tachycardia, or irregularity in rhythm that is not secondary to respiratory sinus arrhythmia.
- Animals presenting with a history of syncope or episodic weakness may have cardiac arrhythmias, and an electrocardiogram is indicated in these cases. Arrhythmias in such cases may be transient—a normal electrocardiogram does not rule out transient arrhythmias. In some cases, long-term electrocardiographic monitoring (Holter monitor or cardiac event recorder) is warranted.
- Arrhythmias often accompany significant heart disease and may significantly affect the clinical status of the patient. An electrocardiogram should be recorded in animals with significant heart disease.
- The electrocardiogram is also used to monitor efficacy of antiarrhythmic therapy and to determine whether arrhythmias may have developed secondary to cardiac medications (e.g., digoxin).
- Significant arrhythmias may also occur in animals with systemic disease, including those diseases associated with electrolyte abnormalities (hyperkalemia, hyponatremia, hypercalcemia, and hypocalcemia), neoplasia (particularly splenic neoplasia), gastric dilatation-volvulus, and sepsis.

Assessment of Chamber Enlargement Patterns

- Changes in waveforms may provide indirect evidence of cardiac chamber enlargement. The electrocardiogram may be normal, however, in cases with chamber enlargement. Right ventricular hypertrophy most consistently results in waveform changes.
- As heart disease progresses, waveform changes may indicate progressive chamber enlargement.
- Thoracic radiography and, ideally, echocardiography, should be performed for definitive assessment of chamber enlargement.

Miscellaneous Indications for Electrocardiography

- The electrocardiogram may provide evidence of pericardial effusion (electrical alternans, low-amplitude complexes).

- Electrocardiographic abnormalities are often present with hypothyroidism and hyperthyroidism.
- A pronounced sinus arrhythmia may be present in animals with elevated vagal tone (often seen with diseases affecting the respiratory tract, central nervous system, and gastrointestinal tract).

PRINCIPLES OF ELECTROCARDIOGRAPHY

Surface Electrodes are Placed in a Designated Fashion to Obtain Standard Electrocardiographic Leads

- A lead consists of the electrical activity measured between a positive electrode and a negative electrode.
- Electrical impulses with a net direction toward the positive electrode will generate a positive waveform or deflection. Electrical impulses with a net direction away from the positive electrode will generate a negative waveform or deflection. Electrical impulses with a net direction perpendicular to the positive electrode will not generate a waveform or deflection (isoelectric).
- Standard electrocardiographic lead systems are used to create several angles of assessment. A single lead would provide information on only one dimension of the current (e.g., left vs. right). Two leads would allow two-dimensional information (e.g., left vs. right and cranial vs. caudal). As many as 12 leads may be acquired simultaneously.

Standard Lead Systems

- The standard leads are I, II, III, aVR, aVL, and aVF (Figure 3-1, Box 3-1). Placement of electrodes to generate each lead is illustrated in Figure 3-2.
- Leads I, II, and III are bipolar limb leads. These are termed bipolar because the electrocardiogram is recorded from two specific electrodes.
- Leads aVR, aVL, and aVF are augmented unipolar leads. To generate these, two electrodes are electrically connected (as a negative electrode) and compared with the single electrode (positive).
- Precordial chest leads are obtained using an exploring unipolar positive electrode at specific locations on the chest. These leads may provide additional information or supportive evidence of cardiac chamber enlargement. They are also useful in evaluating for the P wave when limb leads are equivocal.
- The base-apex lead is often used in equine electrocardiography and may also be used in small-animal practice for rhythm assessment. A positive electrode is placed on the left side of the chest, over the heart, and the negative electrode is placed in the area of the right shoulder or neck.
- Esophageal ECG electrode lead for surgical monitoring (Figure 3-3.) This technique is very useful as complexes recorded are increased in size, providing an increased accuracy for diagnosing an arrhythmia during surgery.
- Hand-held, wireless ECG and ECG real time computer display represents new technology for recording electrocardiograms (Figures 3-4 and 3-5.)

RECORDING THE ELECTROCARDIOGRAM

- The electrocardiogram should be recorded in an area as quiet and as free of distraction as possible. Noises from clinical activity and other animals may significantly affect rate and rhythm. Any use of electrically operated equipment, such as clippers, may cause interference and should be minimized during the electrocardiogram. In some cases, fluorescent lighting may result in electrical interference.
- The patient should ideally be placed in right lateral recumbency.
  - Electrocardiographic reference values were obtained from animals in right lateral recumbency.
  - Limbs should be held perpendicular to the body. Each pair of limbs should be held parallel, and limbs should not be allowed to contact one another.
  - The animal should be held as still as possible during the electrocardiogram. When possible, panting should be prevented.
  - When dyspnea or other factors prevent standard positioning, the electrocardiogram may be recorded while the animal is standing, or, less ideally, sitting.
- Electrode placement
  - Alligator clips or adhesive electrodes may be used. To reduce discomfort, teeth of alligator clips should be blunted and the spring should be relaxed.
  - Limb electrodes are placed either distal or proximal to the elbow (caudal surface) and over the stifle. Electrodes placed proximal to the elbow may increase respiratory artifact.
  - Each electrode should be wetted with 70 % isopropyl alcohol to ensure electrical contact.
- Recording the electrocardiogram
  - Approximately three to four complete complexes should be recorded from each lead at 50 mm/s.

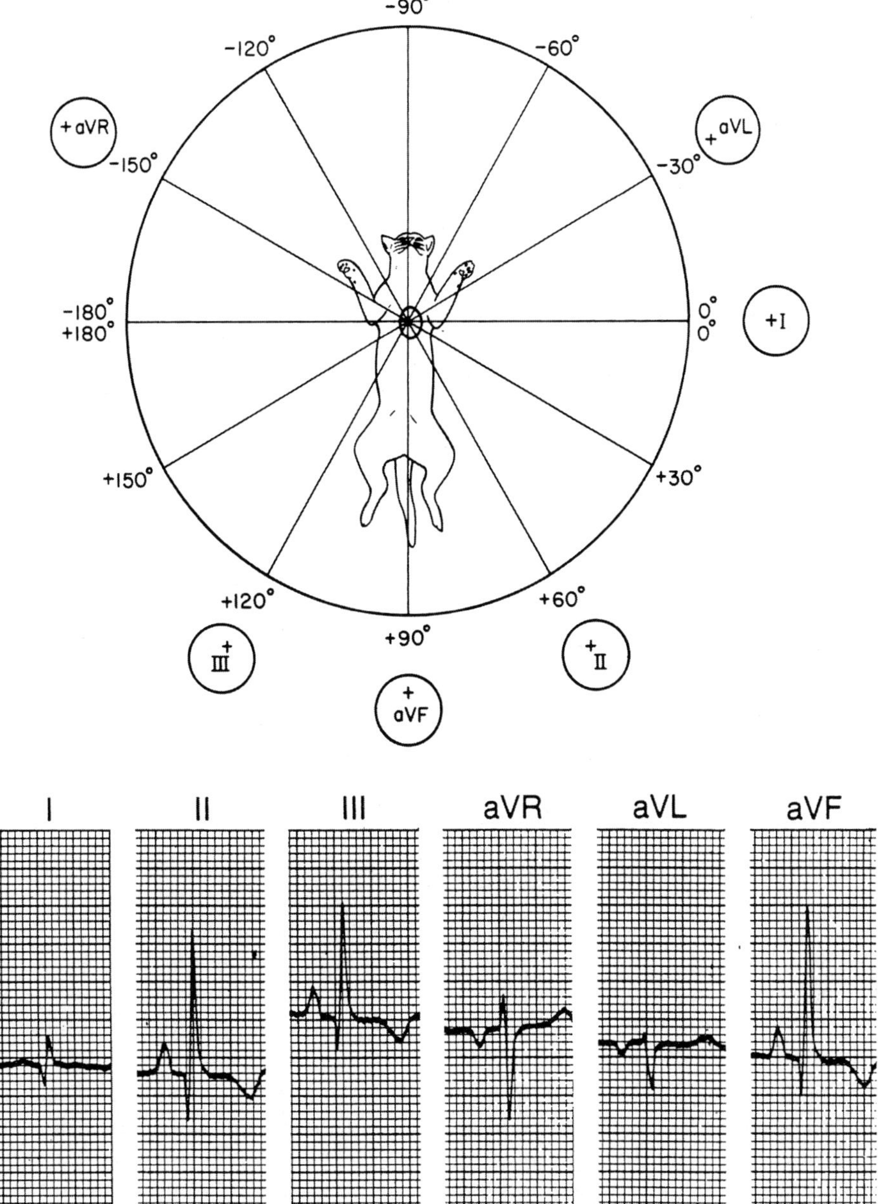

Figure 3-1. The limb leads (I, II, III, aVR, aVL, aVF) surround the heart in the frontal plane as shown in the top part of the figure (feline). The circled limb lead names indicate the direction of electrical activity if the QRS is positive in that lead. The mean electrical axis in this canine ECG (bottom part of the figure) is +90. Lead I is isoelectric. The lead perpendicular to lead I is aVF (see axis chart on top). Lead aVF is positive, making the axis +90. If lead aVF had been negative, the axis would have been −90. (From Tilley LP: Essentials of canine and feline electrocardiography. ed 3, Malvern, Penn: 1992, Lea & Febiger.)

- A lead II rhythm strip should then be recorded at 25 mm/s or 50 mm/s.

KEY POINT

The 1 mV standardization marker should be recorded at the onset of the electrocardiogram and any time the sensitivity is changed.

CARDIAC CONDUCTION AND GENESIS OF WAVEFORMS

- The function of the cardiac conduction system is to coordinate the contraction and relaxation of the four cardiac chambers (Figures 3-6 and 3-7).
- For each cardiac cycle, the initial impulse originates in the sinoatrial (SA) node located in the wall of the right atrium near the entrance of the cranial vena

Box 3-1 Lead Systems Used in Canine and Feline Electrocardiography

Bipolar limb leads
- I: Right thoracic limb (–) compared with left thoracic limb (+)
- II: Right thoracic limb (–) compared with left pelvic limb (+)
- III: Left thoracic limb (–) compared with left pelvic limb (+)

Augmented unipolar limb leads
- aVR: Right thoracic limb (+) compared with average voltage of left thoracic limb and left pelvic limb (–)
- aVL: Left thoracic limb (+) compared with average voltage of right thoracic limb and left pelvic limb (–)
- aVF: Left pelvic limb (+) compared with average voltage of right thoracic limb and left thoracic limb (–)

Unipolar precordial chest leads plus exploring electrode
- CV_5RL (rV_2): Right fifth intercostal space near the sternum
- CV_6LL (V_2): Left sixth intercostal space near the sternum
- CV_6LU (V_4): Left sixth intercostal space near the costochondral junction
- V_{10}: Over the dorsal process of the seventh thoracic vertebra

Base-apex bipolar lead
Record in lead I position on ECG machine with leads placed as follows
- LA electrode over left sixth intercostal space at costosternal junction
- RA electrode over spine of right scapula near the vertebra

cava. This impulse is rapidly propagated through the atrial myocardium, resulting in depolarization of the atria. Depolarization of the atria results in the P wave and atrial contraction. The initial SA nodal impulse is small and does not produce an electrocardiographic change on the body's surface.
- Immediately after atrial depolarization, the impulse travels through the atrioventricular (AV) node, located near the base of the right atrium. Conduction is slow here, which allows atrial contraction to be completed before ventricular depolarization occurs. As the impulse travels through the AV node, there is no electrocardiographic activity on the body's surface—rather the PR interval is generated.
- Upon leaving the AV node, conduction velocity increases significantly, and the impulse is rapidly spread through the bundle of His, bundle branches, and Purkinje system. This results in rapid and nearly simultaneous depolarization of the ventricles. Depolarization of the ventricles results in the prominent QRS complex and causes ventricular contraction.
  - The Q wave represents initial depolarization of the interventricular septum and is defined as the first *negative* deflection following the P wave and occurring before the R wave. A Q wave may not be identified in all animals.
  - The R wave represents depolarization of the ventricular myocardium from the endocardial surface to the epicardial surface. The R wave is the first *positive* deflection following the P wave and is usually the most prominent waveform.
  - The S wave represents depolarization of the basal sections of the ventricular posterior wall and interventricular septum. The S wave is defined as the first negative deflection following the R wave in the QRS complex.
- Ventricular repolarization quickly follows ventricular depolarization and results in the T wave. The delay in repolarization results in the ST segment on the surface electrocardiogram.

EVALUATION OF THE ELECTROCARDIOGRAM

- The electrocardiogram should be evaluated from left to right.
- Areas of artifact should be identified and avoided in the evaluation.
- Calculate the heart rate.
  - Determine the number of R waves (or R-R intervals) within 3 seconds and multiply by 20 to obtain beats per minute (bpm) (for an electrocardiogram recorded at 50 mm/s, vertical timing marks above the gridlines occur every 1.5 seconds).
  - If the rhythm is regular, the heart rate may be derived by determining the number of small boxes in one R-R interval and dividing 3000 by that number (for paper speed of 25 mm/s, use 1500). The method is also useful for determining the rate of paroxysmal ventricular tachycardia and other arrhythmias lasting less than 3 seconds.
- Obtain measurements for the waveforms and intervals (Figure 3-8).
  - P wave height and width
  - Duration of PR interval
  - Duration of QRS complex and height of R wave
  - Duration of QT segment
- Determine the approximate mean electrical axis (MEA)
  - The *MEA* refers to the direction of the net ventricular depolarization and refers solely to the QRS complex. If there is significant right ventricular hypertrophy, then the MEA

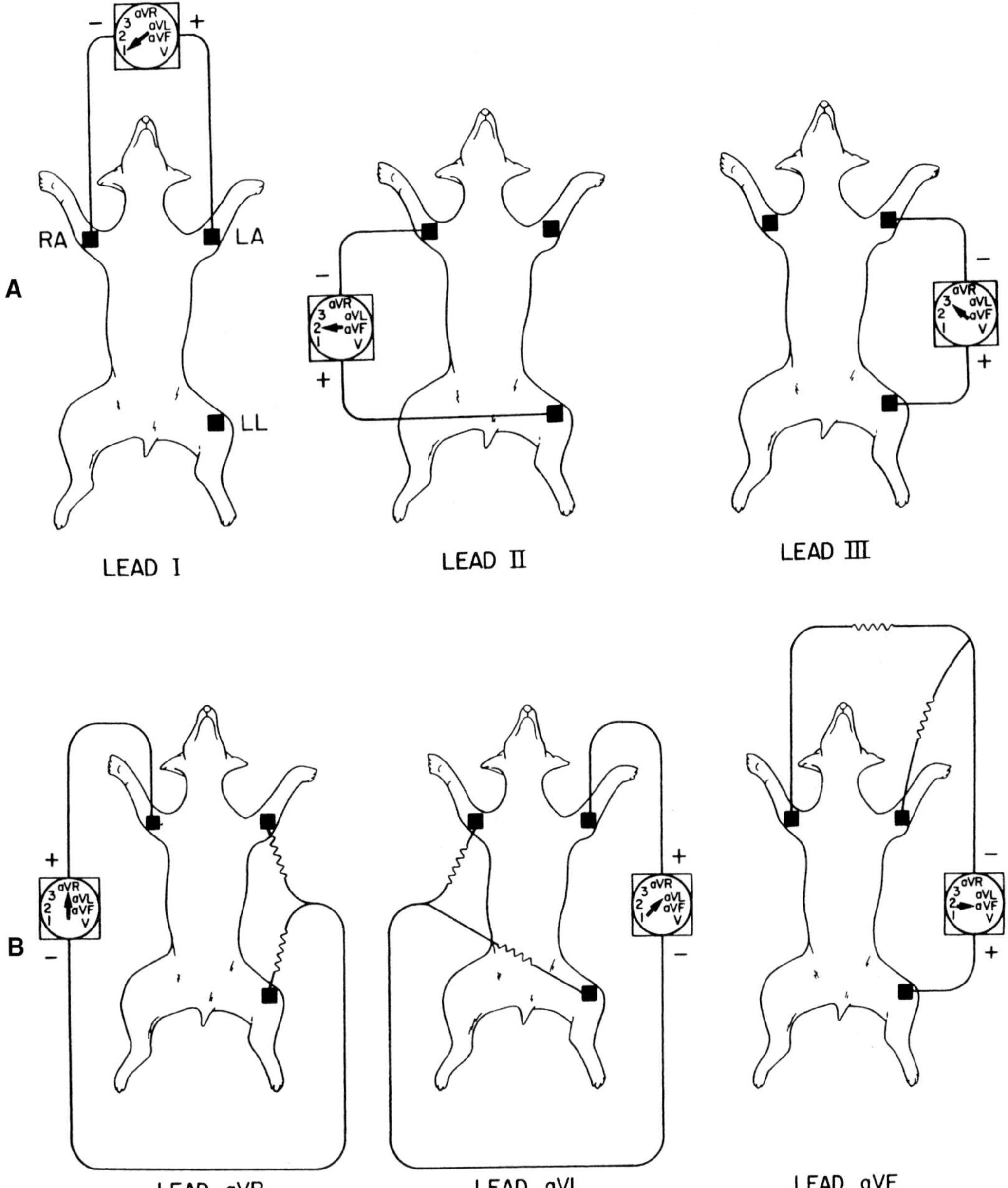

Figure 3-2. **A,** Three bipolar standard leads. By means of a switch incorporated in the instrument, the galvanometer can be connected across any pair of several electrodes. Each pair of electrodes is called a lead. The leads illustrated here are identified as I, II, and III. **B,** Augmented unipolar limb leads aVR, aVL, and aVF. (From Tilley LP: Essentials of canine and feline electrocardiography: interpretation and treatment, ed 3, Malvern, Penn, 1992, Lea & Febiger.)

will shift to the right. Because the left ventricle is normally the dominant ventricle, the normal MEA is to the left. A degree system is used—if the MEA is directly to the left, then it is said to be 0 degrees; if the MEA is directly downward, then it is 90 degrees, and if it is directly to the right, then it is 180 degrees. The MEA of the normal dog is 40 to 100 degrees. For the cat, the MEA is more variable, ranging from 0 to 160 degrees.

- The MEA may be determined using the six standard leads and the Bailey axis system (see Figure 3-1). If there is a lead with isoelectric QRS complexes, then the MEA equates to the lead on the Bailey axis perpendicular to the isoelectric lead.
- The MEA may also be determined by plotting the net amplitude of a lead I QRS complex (horizontal axis) and the net amplitude of a lead aVF QRS (vertical axis). The intersection will provide the vector equal to the MEA (see Figure 3-1).

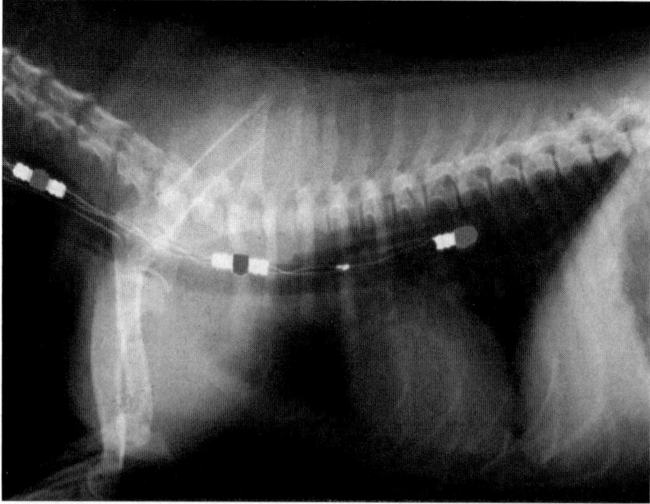

Figure 3-3. Esophageal ECG electrode and temperature probe positioned for surgical monitoring. This technique is very useful as complexes recorded are increased in size, providing an increased accuracy for diagnosing an arrhythmia during surgery.

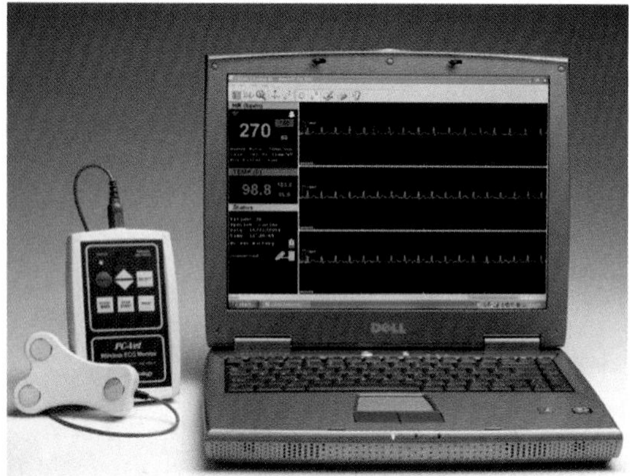

Figure 3-4. Hand-held, wireless ECG and ECG real time computer display. (Courtesy Vmed Technology, Redmond, Wash. www.vmedtech.com.)

- The MEA may be approximated by inspecting leads I and aVF.
  - If the net direction of the lead I QRS is positive, then the MEA is to the left. If the net deflection of the lead I QRS is negative, then the MEA is to the right.
  - If the net direction of the lead aVF QRS is positive, then the MEA is downward or caudal. If the net deflection of the lead aVF QRS is negative, then the MEA is upward or cranial.
  - The approximate angle can be estimated by examining the relative amplitudes of leads I and aVF.
- Determine the rhythm.
- Compare patient values with reference values (Table 3-1).

EVALUATION OF WAVEFORMS

P Wave

- Atrial enlargement patterns (Figure 3-9)
  - The P wave is generated by atrial depolarization. Atrial enlargement may result in an increase in width or height of the P waves recorded in lead II.
  - Enlargement of the right atrium may result in an increased P wave height. This is referred to as P-pulmonale. The height of the P wave should not exceed 0.4 mV (dog) or 0.2 mV (cat). Chronic pulmonary disease may result in P-pulmonale in the absence of heart disease.
  - Enlargement of the left atrium may result in an increased P wave width or duration. This is referred to as P-mitrale. The duration of the P wave should not exceed 0.04 second (dog or cat). Left atrial enlargement may also result in notching of the P wave.
- Presence or absence of P waves
  - There is no minimum height or duration for the P wave. In some cases, P waves may be indistinct. In this situation, carefully evaluate all leads for P wave activity. If P waves cannot be discerned in any of the limb leads, evaluation of chest leads is recommended.
  - P waves may be absent in several arrhythmias, including atrial fibrillation and atrial standstill. P waves may be superimposed on other waveforms in ventricular tachycardia and supraventricular tachycardia (SVT).
  - Variation of P wave height is a normal finding in the dog and a manifestation of alterations in vagal tone.

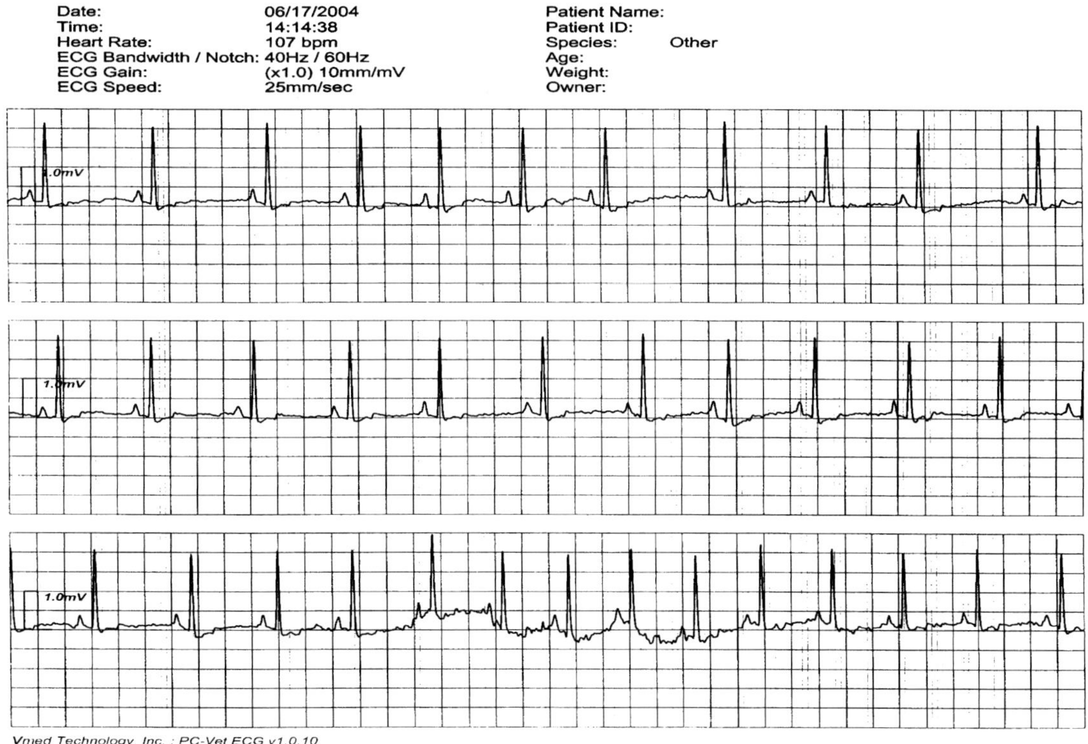

Figure 3-5. Wireless ECG printout report from laptop computer software system in Figure 3-4. (Courtesy Vmed Technology, Redmond, Wash. www.vmedtech.com.)

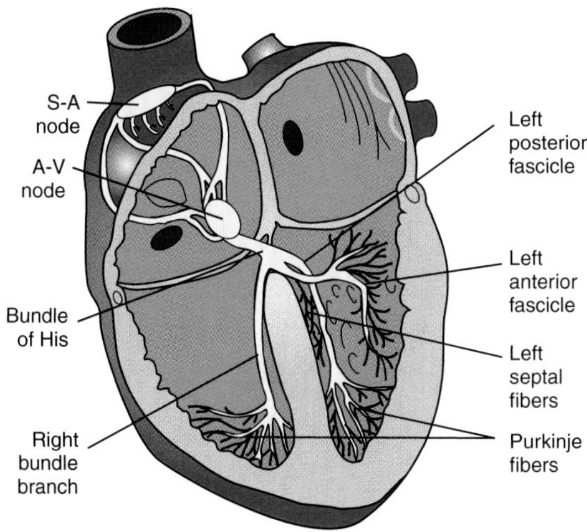

Figure 3-6. Anatomy of the cardiac conduction system. *S-A,* Sinoatrial; *A-V,* atrioventricular. (Modified from Tilley LP: Essentials of canine and feline electrocardiography: interpretation and treatment, ed 2, Philadelphia, 1985, Lea & Febiger.)

PR Interval

- The PR interval reflects the slowed conduction through the AV node. The normal PR interval is 0.06 to 0.13 second for dogs and 0.05 to 0.09 second for cats.
- A significantly shortened PR interval may occur when an accessory pathway allows conduction to bypass the AV node.
- Prolongation of the PR interval represents first degree AV block.
- Variation of the PR interval may occur with alterations in vagal tone or secondary to the presence of ectopic beats causing dissociation of atrial and ventricular activity.

QRS Complex

- The QRS complex is generated by ventricular depolarization (left ventricle, interventricular septum, and right ventricle). Ventricular enlargement may result in changes in the QRS complex.
- Left ventricular enlargement pattern
  - Increased amplitude of the R wave
    - Dog
      - Amplitude of R wave greater than 3.0 mV (2.5 mV in small-breed dogs) in leads II, aVF, and the precordial chest leads CV_6LU, CV_6LL and CV_5RL
      - Amplitude of R wave greater than 1.5 mV in lead I

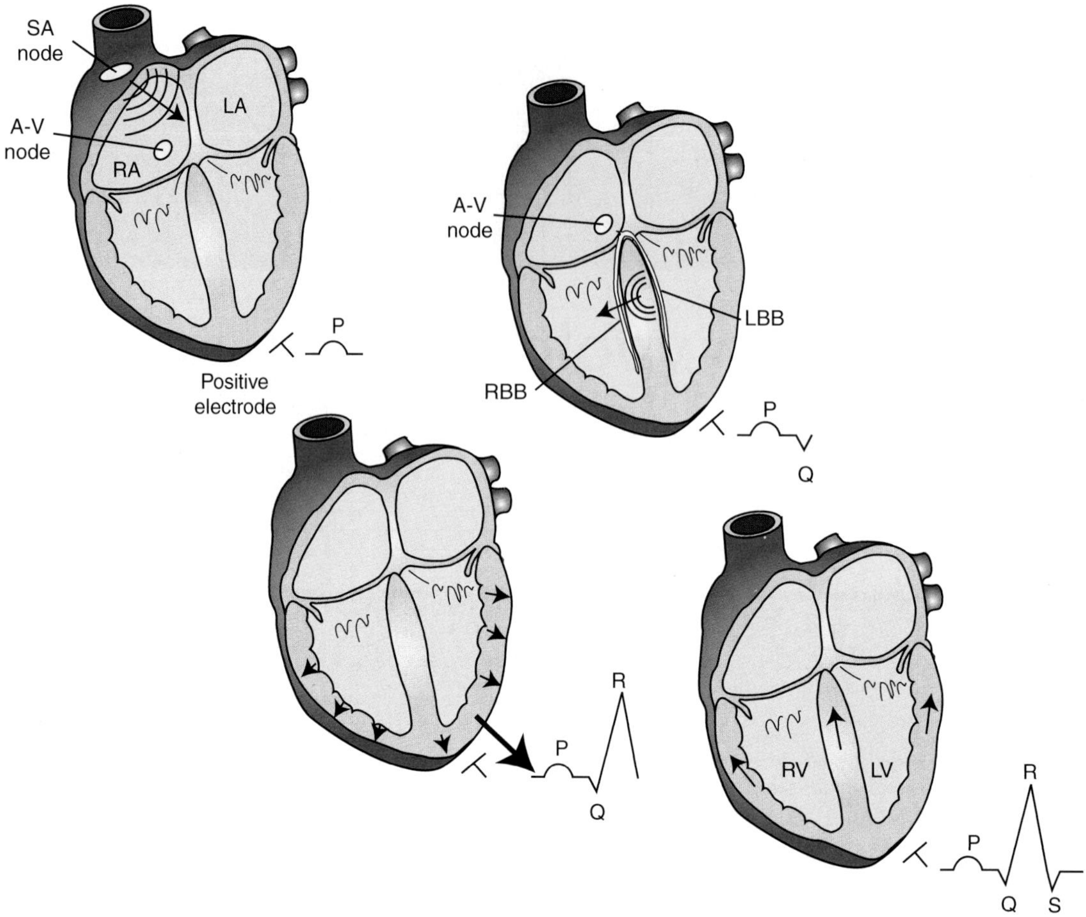

Figure 3-7. Sequence of electrical impulse conduction and cardiac chamber activation as it relates to the electrocardiogram. (Modified from Tilley LP: Essentials of canine and feline electrocardiography: interpretation and treatment, ed 3, Philadelphia, 1992, Lea & Febiger.)

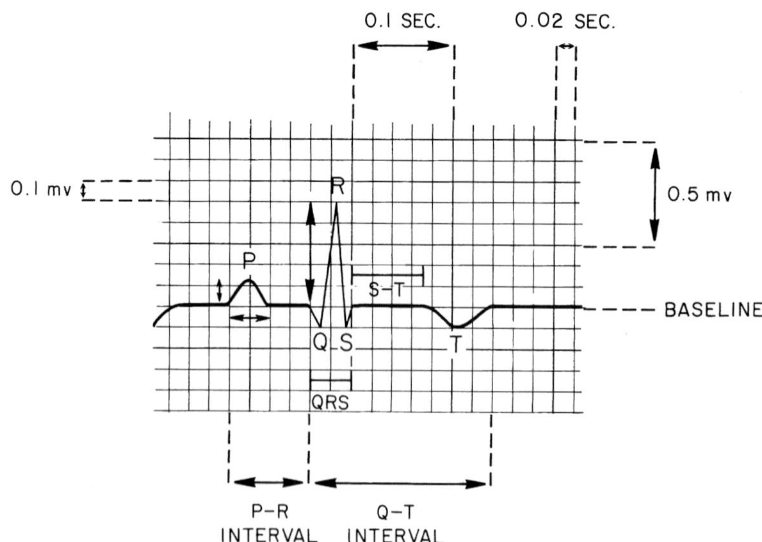

Figure 3-8. Close-up of a normal feline lead II P-QRS-T complex with labels and intervals. Measurements for amplitude (millivolts) are indicated by positive (+) and negative (–) movement; time intervals (hundredths of a second) are indicated from left to right. Paper speed, 50 mm/s; sensitivity 1 cm = 1 mV. (From Tilley LP: Essentials of canine and feline electrocardiography: interpretation and treatment, ed 2, Philadelphia, 1985, Lea & Febiger.)

Table 3-1 Normal Canine and Feline ECG Values*

	Canine	Feline
Heart rate (HR)	Puppy: 70-220 bpm	120-240 bpm
	Toy breeds: 70-180 bpm	
	Standard: 70-160 bpm	
	Giant breeds: 60-140 bpm	
Rhythm	Sinus rhythm	Sinus rhythm
	Sinus arrhythmia	
	Wandering pacemaker	
P wave		
Height	Maximum: 0.4 mV	Maximum: 0.2 mV
Width	Maximum: 0.04 s (Giant breeds 0.05 s)	Maximum: 0.04 s
PR interval	0.06-0.13 s	0.05-0.09 s
QRS		
Height	Large breeds: 3.0 mV maximum†	Maximum: 0.9 mV
	Small breeds: 2.5 mV maximum	
Width	Large breeds: 0.06 s maximum	Maximum: 0.04 s
	Small breeds: 0.05 s maximum	
ST segment		
Depression	No more than 0.2 mV	None
Elevation	No more than 0.15 mV	None
QT interval	0.15-0.25 s at normal HR	0.12-0.18 s at normal HR
T waves	May be positive, negative, or biphasic	usually positive and < 0.3 mV
	Amplitude range ± 0.05-1.0 mV in any lead	
	Not more than ¼ of R wave amplitude	
Electrical axis	+40 to + 100	0 ± 160
Chest leads		
CV_5RL (rV_2)	T positive; R < 3.0 mV	
CV_6LL (v_2)	S < 0.8 mV; R < 3.0 mV	R < 1.0 mV
CV_6LU (V_4)	S < 0.7 mV; R < 3.0 mV	R < 1.0 mV
V_{10}	QRS negative; T negative except in Chihuahua	T negative. R wave/Q wave < 1

S, Second.
*Measurements are made in lead II unless otherwise stated.
†Not valid for thin, deep-chested dogs under 2 years old.

- Sum of R wave amplitudes in leads I and aVF greater than 4.0 mV
- Cat
- Amplitude of R wave greater than 0.9 mV in lead II
- Amplitude of R wave greater than 1.0 mV in CV_6LU and CV_6LL
    - R wave/Q wave > 1.0 in lead V_{10}
- QRS duration greater than 0.06 second (large dogs), 0.05 second (small dogs), or 0.04 second (cats)
- ST slurring or coving
- Shift in the MEA to the left (less than 40 degrees for dog, less than 0 degrees for cat)

- Right ventricular enlargement pattern (Figure 3-10)
  - Increased amplitude of S waves
    - Dog
      - Presence of S waves in leads I, II, III, and aVF
      - S wave in lead I > 0.05 mV
      - S wave in lead II > 0.35 mV
      - S wave in lead CV_6LL > 0.8 mV
      - S wave in lead CV_6LU > 0.7 mV
    - Cat
      - Presence of S waves in leads I, II, III, and aVF
      - Prominent S waves in CV_6LU and CV_6LL
      - T wave positive in lead V_{10} (except Chihuahua)
      - W-shaped QRS complex in V_{10} (dog)
    - R:S ratio < 0.87 in CV_6LU
    - Shift in the MEA to the right (more than 100 degrees for the dog or more than 160 degrees for the cat)
- Widening of the QRS complexes may occur with left ventricular enlargement, right or left bundle branch block (LBBB), and complexes of ventricular origin (ventricular premature complexes [VPCs] or ventricular escape complexes).
- Electrical alternans (Figure 3-11, *A*)
  - In electrical alternans, there is a pattern of regular variation in the amplitude of normal electrocardiographic complexes (excluding ventricular ectopy). This is usually manifested by an alteration in R wave height, although variation in other waveforms may be seen. The amplitude may change significantly with every complex and alternate short-tall.
  - Electrical alternans is most often associated with pericardial effusion. A severe pleural effusion may cause electrical alternans.
  - SVT may result in an electrical alternans pattern.
- Low-amplitude QRS complexes
  - The minimum height for the normal R wave in the dog is 0.05 mV to 1.0 mV.

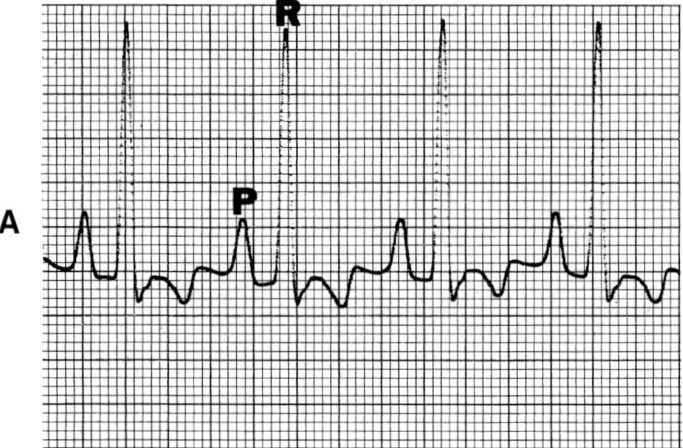

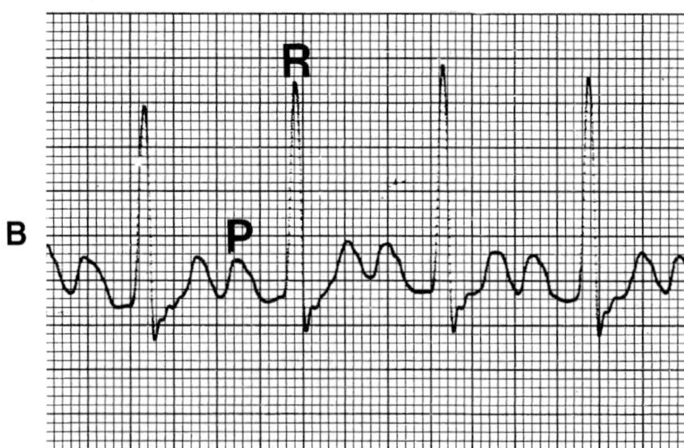

Figure 3-9. **A,** Biatrial enlargement in a small-breed dog with a collapsed trachea and compensated mitral regurgitation. The P wave is 0.5 mV tall (P pulmonale) and 0.05 sec wide (P mitrale). **B,** Left atrial enlargement in a geriatric, small-breed dog with chronic acquired valvular disease (mitral insufficiency). P waves are wide (0.075 second), notched, and equivocally tall. (From Fox PR, Sisson D, Moise NS, eds: Textbook of Canine and Feline Cardiology. Philadelphia, 1999, WB Soundes.)

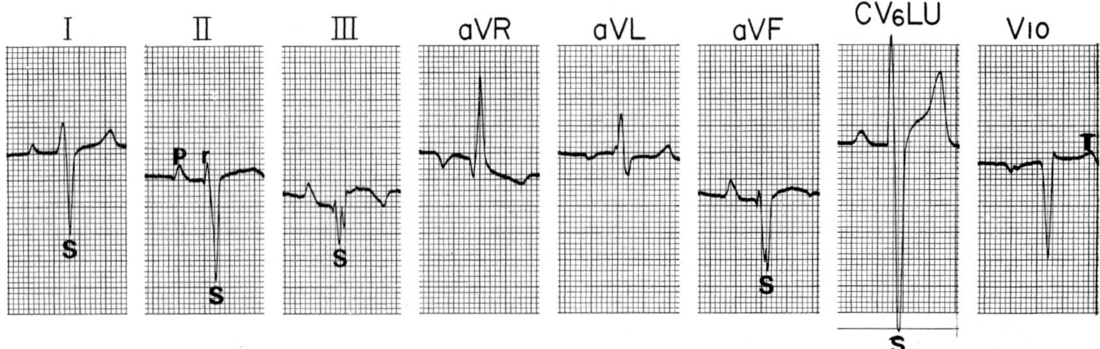

Figure 3-10. Severe right ventricular enlargement in a dog with pulmonic stenosis. There is a right axis deviation of approximately −110 degrees. Note the deep S waves in leads I, II, III, aVF, and CvsLU. The T wave is positive in V10. (From Tilley LP: Essentials of canine and feline electrocardiography: interpretation and treatment, ed 3, Philadelphia, 1992, Lea & Febiger.)

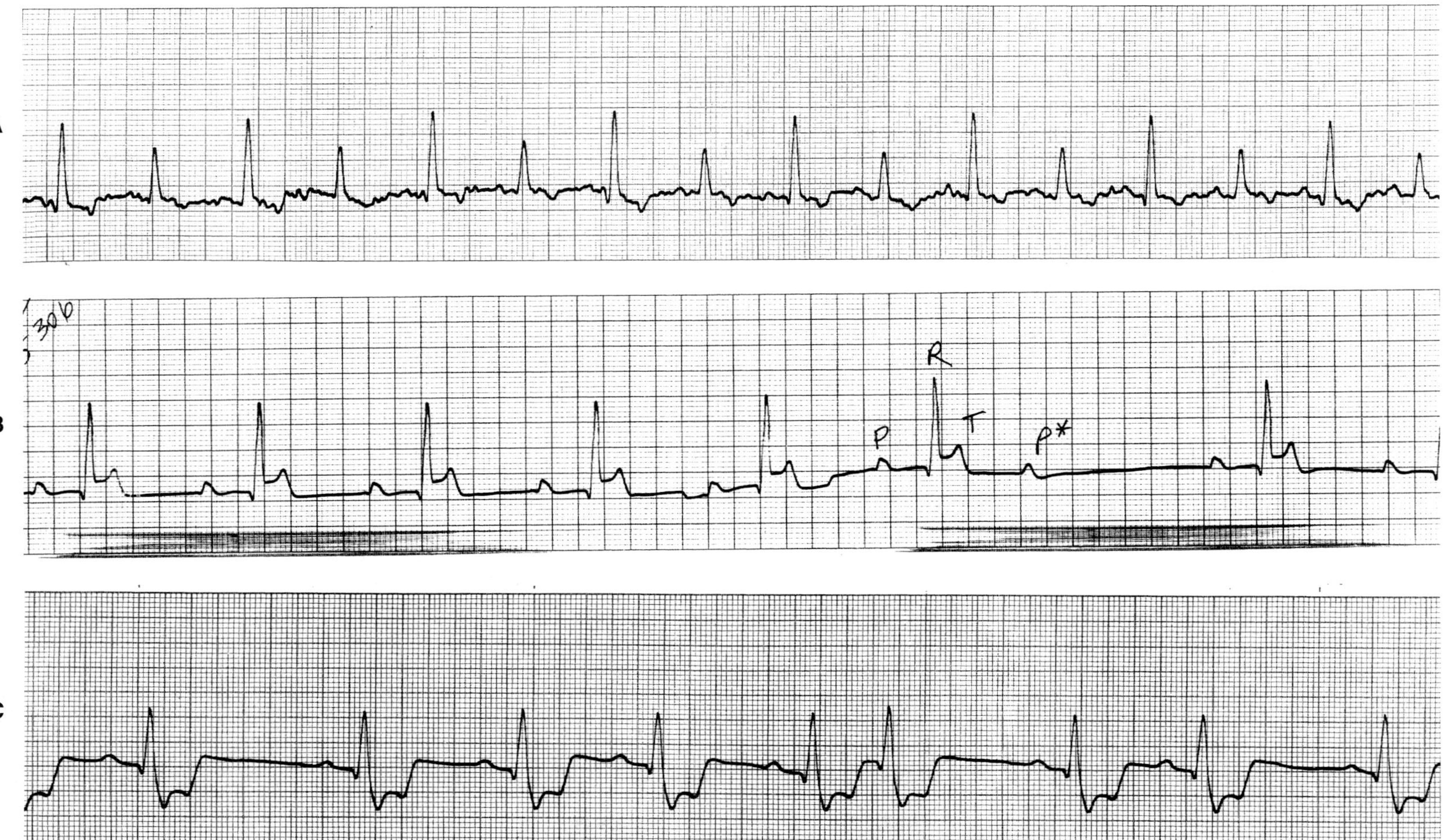

Figure 3-11. **A,** Electrocardiogram—electrical alternans. **B,** Electrocardiogram—ST segment elevation. **C,** Electrocardiogram—ST segment depression.

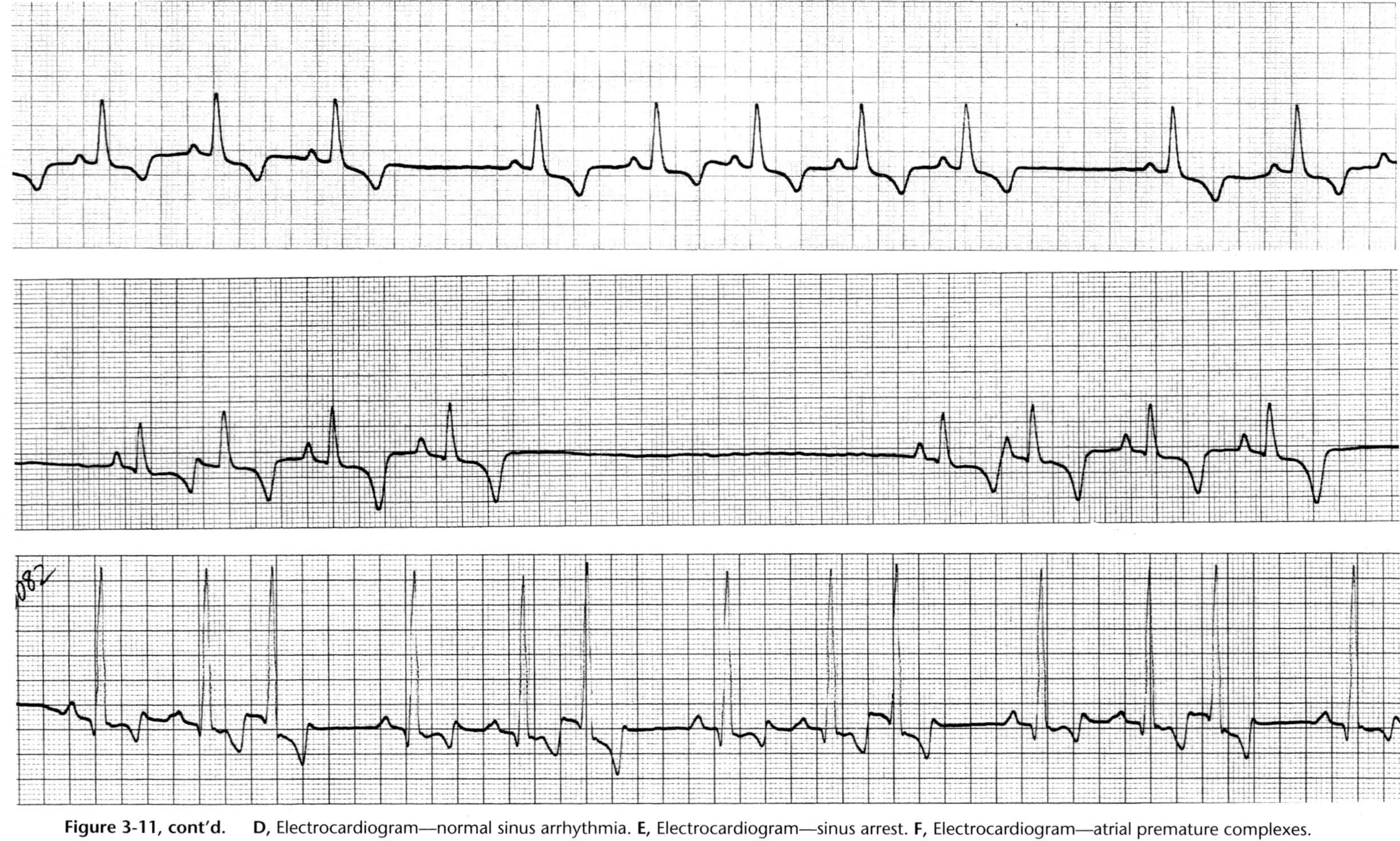

D

E

F

Figure 3-11, cont'd. **D,** Electrocardiogram—normal sinus arrhythmia. **E,** Electrocardiogram—sinus arrest. **F,** Electrocardiogram—atrial premature complexes.

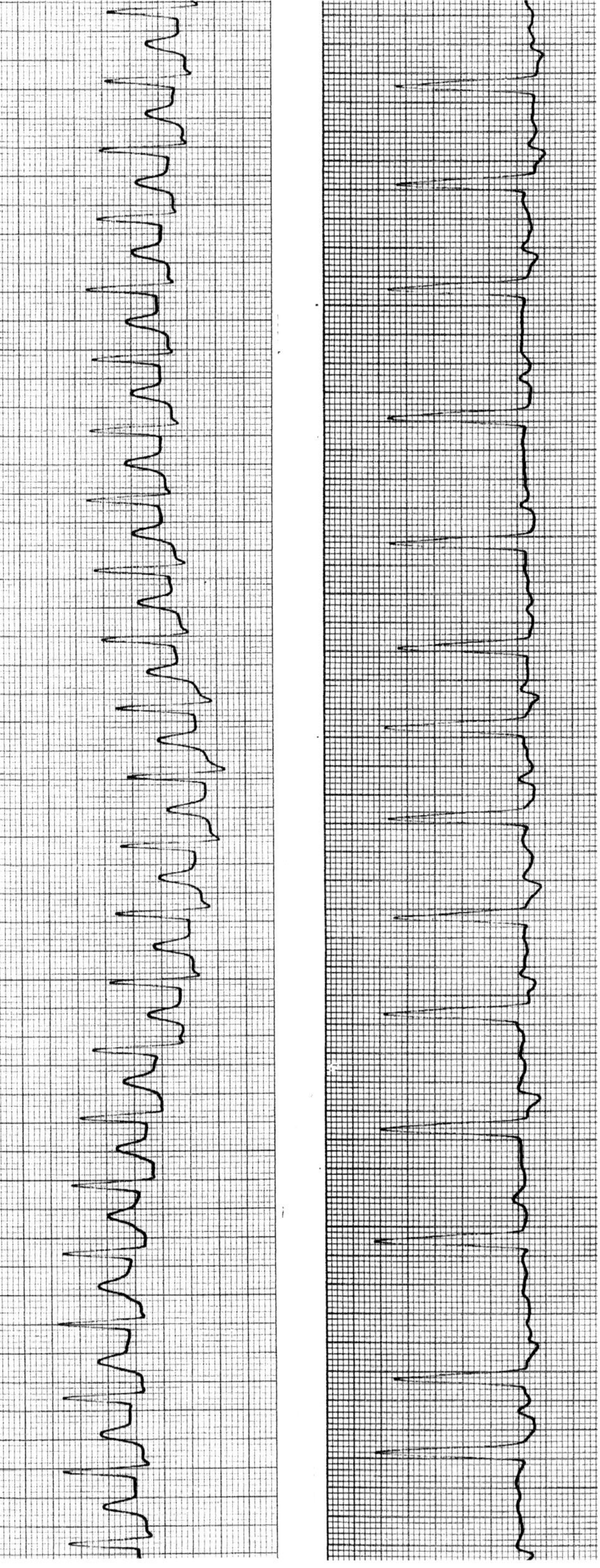

Figure 3-11, cont'd. **G,** Electrocardiogram—atrial tachycardia. **H,** Electrocardiogram—atrial fibrillation.

- Low-amplitude R waves may occur when transmission of the cardiac electrical impulse to the skin is hindered. This may occur with pericardial effusion, pleural effusion, obesity, or subcutaneous edema. Pneumothorax and pulmonary edema may also decrease R wave height.
- Hypothyroidism may result in low-amplitude R waves (usually with accompanying slow rate).

ST Segment

- ST segment elevation (Figure 3-11, *B*)
  - Elevation of the ST segment greater than 0.15 mV in leads II, III, or aVF is abnormal in the dog. Any ST segment elevation in the cat is abnormal.
  - ST segment elevation may be caused by myocardial hypoxia, transmural myocardial infarction, pericardial effusion, see pericarditis. In cats, digoxin toxicity may cause ST segment elevation.
- ST segment depression (Figure 3-11, *C*)
  - Depression of the ST segment greater than 0.2 mV in leads II, III or aVF is abnormal in the dog. Any ST segment depression in the cat is abnormal.
  - ST segment depression may be caused by myocardial hypoxia, hyperkalemia, hypokalemia, subendocardial myocardial infarction, or digoxin toxicity.
  - Pseudodepression due to prominent T_a waves (atrial repolarization) caused by atrial disease or tachycardia also causes ST segment depression.
- Miscellaneous ST segment changes
  - ST segment changes may occur secondary to bundle branch blocks, myocardial hypertrophy, or VPCs. The changes in the ST segment are in the opposite direction from the main QRS deflection.

KEY POINT

Baseline artifact may mimic changes with the ST segment.

QT Interval

- The normal QT interval is 0.15 to 0.25 second (dog) and 0.12 to 0.18 second (cat). The QT interval tends to increase with slow heart rates and decrease with rapid rates. In general, the QT interval should be less than half of the preceding R-R interval.
- The length of the QT interval is chiefly determined by an interplay of autonomic influences. Heart rate and QT interval are governed separately by different sympathetic neurons that may or may not be activated together. Corrections of the QT interval (QT_c) for heart rate appear to be applicable under circumstances, such as exercise.
- Within the past two decades, the overall ventricular repolarization and its relationship to the QT_c interval has led to studies for using the QT_c interval as a prognostic marker of ventricular tachyarrhythmias and death. Class IA or class III antiarrhythmic drugs, such as quinidine and sotalol, are known to prolong myocardial repolarization. This may either provide a protective effect against arrhythmias or lead to an increased occurrence of QT_c interval-related arrhythmias, including torsade de pointes ventricular tachycardia.

Box 3-2 Classification of Cardiac Arrhythmias

Normal sinus impulse formation
- Normal sinus rhythm
- Sinus arrhythmia
- Wandering sinus pacemaker

Disturbances of sinus impulse formation
- Sinus arrest
- Sinus bradycardia
- Sinus tachycardia

Disturbances of supraventricular impulse formation
- Atrial premature complexes
- Atrial tachycardia
- Atrial flutter
- Atrial fibrillation
- Atrioventricular junctional rhythm

Disturbances of ventricular impulse formation
- Ventricular premature complexes
- Ventricular tachycardia
- Ventricular asystole
- Ventricular fibrillation

Disturbances of impulse conduction
- Sinoatrial block
- Persistent atrial standstill (“silent” atrium)
- Atrial standstill (hyperkalemia)
- Ventricular pre-excitation
- First-degree AV block
- Second-degree AV block
- Complete AV block (third degree)
- Bundle branch blocks

Disturbances of both impulse formation and impulse conduction
- Sick sinus syndrome
- Ventricular pre-excitation and the Wolff-Parkinson-White (WPW) syndrome
- Atrial premature complexes with aberrant ventricular conduction

Escape rhythms
- Junctional escape rhythms
- Ventricular escape rhythms (idioventricular rhythm)

- Torsades de pointes (turning about a point) is a rare arrhythmia in the dog. It is a form of polymorphic ventricular tachycardia or flutter in which the amplitude of the complexes increases and decreases in size so that they appear to twist around the baseline. Human patients with torsades de pointes are at risk for sudden death.

Possible Formulas for Corrected QT intervals.

- Many formulas and methods for correcting the QT interval for the effects of heart rate, including logarithmic, hyperbolic, and exponential functions, but they also have limitations. These limitations result from both physiological and computational problems. The Bazett's formula, for example, predicts an ever-increasing increment in the QT interval as the heart rate slows and an ever-decreasing increment as the rate rises, both of which are physiologically improbable. In addition, all these formulas do not account for the effects of autonomic tone on the QT interval independent of the effects on rate. They also do not account for the relatively slow adaptation of repolarization to changes in rate. Fridericia's formula (QT divided by the cube root of the R-R interval) is a modification of Bazett's formula. This modification is important, because Bazett's formula will overcorrect for rates higher than 60 bpm. Van de Water formula (study was done in dogs) involves regression analysis yielding the following equation: QT_c = Van de Water formula = QT − 87(60/HR − 1). Recent publications have recommended the use of the log-log formula for correcting the QT interval for heart rate (Linear regression with $\log_c$HR as the covariate: QT = a + b ($\log_c$HR); a & b are constants).
- Prolongation of the QT interval may occur with interventricular conduction disturbances that are associated with prolongation of the QRS complexes, bradycardia, ethylene glycol toxicity, strenuous activity, or CNS disturbances. QT prolongation has been reported with many drugs and electrolyte imbalances. These include hypokalemia, hypocalcemia, quinidine, procainamide, bretylium, tricyclic antidepressants and many anesthetics.
- Shortening of the QT interval may occur with hypercalcemia, hyperkalemia, or digoxin therapy.

T Wave

- The T wave is quite variable in the dog and cat. In most leads, the T wave may be positive, negative or biphasic. The height of the T wave should not exceed one-fourth the height of the R wave, one-fourth the height of the Q wave (if Q wave is greater than R wave), or 0.5 mV to 1.0 mV in any lead.
- The T wave should be positive in CV_5RL in dogs 2 months of age and should be negative in V_{10}, except in the Chihuahua.
- Prominent T waves may occur with myocardial hypoxia, interventricular conduction disturbances, ventricular enlargement, and in some animals with heart disease and bradycardia.
- Prominent and peaked T waves are associated with hyperkalemia.
- Small, biphasic T waves may occur with hypokalemia.
- Nonspecific T wave changes may occur with metabolic disturbances (hypoglycemia, anemia, shock, fever), drug toxicity (digoxin, quinidine, procainamide), and neurologic disease.
- T wave alternans has been reported secondary to hypocalcemia, increased circulating catecholamines, and sudden increases in sympathetic tone.

ARRHYTHMIAS AND CONDUCTION DISTURBANCES

- An arrhythmia (or dysrhythmia) refers to an irregularity in the cardiac rhythm. In general, an arrhythmia denotes an abnormality of the cardiac rhythm, although in the dog the term normal sinus arrhythmia is used to describe the normal variation in heart rate associated with respiration (see Box 3-2).
  - Arrhythmias may be classified according to their **origin**.
    - Supraventricular arrhythmias arise from the atria or AV node.
    - Ventricular arrhythmias arise from the ventricles.
  - Arrhythmias may be classified according to their **rates**.
    - Arrhythmias with slow rates are referred to as bradyarrhythmias.
    - Arrhythmias with rapid rates are referred to as tachyarrhythmias.
  - Arrhythmias may be classified according to their **regularity**.
    - Fibrillation is an irregular, chaotic rhythm.
    - Tachycardia is a regular (non irregular) rhythm.
  - Examples: Atrial fibrillation is an irregular, chaotic arrhythmia originating from the atria; ventricular tachycardia is a regular arrhythmia originating from the ventricles.

- There are several pathophysiologic causes of arrhythmias.
  - Abnormal automaticity of normal pacemaker cells
  - Shift of the pacemaker from the SA node to other areas of the heart
  - Conduction blocks that terminate or slow normal conduction through the heart
  - Abnormal pathways of impulse conduction through the heart
  - Spontaneous impulse formation in any area of the heart
- Systemic approach to arrhythmia recognition and evaluation
  - Any lead may be used for arrhythmia evaluation—lead II is generally used as waveforms are usually best defined in this lead. A significant duration of artifact-free lead II should be carefully evaluated.
  - Determine if P waves are present. Examine all leads—P waves may be small or isoelectric in several leads. You must distinguish baseline motion (artifact) from P waves. P waves are generally consistent in size and distance from associated QRS complex. The presence of P waves indicates a sinus (originating from SA node) rhythm.
  - Determine if an atrial (P wave) and ventricular (QRS complex) association exists. There should be a P wave for every QRS complex. If there are a greater number of P waves or QRS complexes, then an arrhythmia exists.
    - P waves should slightly precede QRS complexes.
    - If P waves follow the QRS complex, then AV dissociation exists, and the rhythm is ventricular or junctional rather than sinus.
    - There should be a QRS complex following each P wave. If not, then a conduction disturbance is present.
  - Determine the regularity of the rhythm.
    - Normal sinus rhythm—insignificant (less than 10%) variation in the P-P or R-R intervals
    - Normal sinus arrhythmia—significant (more than 10%) variation in the P-P or R-R intervals
      - A pattern of irregularity is usually noted—the heart rate increases during inspiration and decreases during expiration in a cyclical pattern.
      - This may be referred to as a respiratory sinus arrhythmia.
  - Check for pauses in the rhythm—periods of inactivity greater than two R-R intervals.
  - Check for P waves occurring prematurely (occurring earlier than expected)—distinguish from normal sinus arrhythmia, where P wave rate increases during inspiration. Premature P waves will noticeably break the rhythm. Premature P waves indicate the presence of atrial premature complexes (APCs).
  - Check for QRS complexes occurring prematurely. These may occur without preceding P wave, may be superimposed on P wave, or may follow P wave with shortened PR interval. Premature QRS complexes indicate presence of VPCs.

KEY POINT

Remember, a ventricular *premature* complex is *premature*. A ventricular complex occurring after a pause is *not* premature—it is a ventricular escape complex.

- Evaluation of PR interval
  - PR interval may vary slightly with changes in vagal tone—this would also result in a sinus arrhythmia.
  - Progressive prolongation of the PR interval signals first degree AV block.
  - P waves without associated QRS complexes are usually indicative of second degree AV block
  - Shortened PR interval may be seen with increased sympathetic tone and pre-excitation syndromes (presence of accessory pathway bypassing AV node).
- Evaluation of QRS complexes
  - Height of R wave and duration of QRS complex
  - Presence of prominent S waves
  - Morphology of QRS complexes should not vary significantly. Variation may be caused by:
    - VPCs or ventricular escape complexes
    - Fusion beats—simultaneous occurrence of VPC and normal QRS
    - Electrical alternans
    - Intermittent bundle branch block
    - Artifact
  - Premature QRS complexes suggest VPCs; QRS complexes without P waves and occurring after a pause suggest ventricular escape complexes.

- Note morphology of any premature complexes—APCs have a QRS of normal morphology; VPCs have a QRS that is significantly different from the normal QRS.

KEY POINT

QRS complexes should not vary in their morphology in a normal animal.

NORMAL RHYTHMS

Normal Sinus Rhythm

- Normal rhythm in the dog and cat
- P wave for every QRS complex, regular rhythm
- Rate between 60 bpm and 180 bpm for the dog, depending on size of dog and degree of anxiousness
- Rate between 140 bpm and 240 bpm for the cat, depending on degree of anxiousness
- Rate and rhythm dependent on SA nodal discharge. This is highly influenced by changes in autonomic tone. An elevated sympathetic tone will increase rate of SA nodal discharge; an elevated parasympathetic (vagal) tone will decrease rate of SA nodal discharge.

Normal Sinus Arrhythmia

- Normal in the dog, generally abnormal in the cat
- A pattern of irregularity is present—the heart rate increases during inspiration and decreases during expiration in a cyclical pattern (Figure 3-11, *D*).
- Irregularity is secondary to fluctuations in vagal tone associated with the respiratory cycle.
- When respiratory effort is increased (brachycephalic breeds, animals with respiratory disease), fluctuations in vagal tone may be dramatic, producing a pronounced sinus arrhythmia.
- Normal sinus arrhythmia is a rhythm of high vagal tone and low sympathetic tone—this situation is rare in dogs with congestive heart failure. The presence of a sinus arrhythmia in a dog with severe cough is more supportive of primary respiratory disease rather than congestive heart failure.

Wandering Sinus Pacemaker

- The origin of SA nodal discharge may change as a consequence of alterations in vagal tone. This is noted on the electrocardiogram as a cyclical change in the height of the P wave. At times, the P wave may become isoelectric and not detectable.
- Often associated with normal sinus arrhythmia or pronounced sinus arrhythmia.

KEY POINT

Sinus arrhythmia is NOT expected in the cat, but is normal, and the result of variations in vagal tone in dogs.

DISTURBANCES OF SINUS IMPULSE FORMATION

Sinus Arrest

- When the SA node fails to discharge as expected, a pause in the rhythm will occur. The duration of the pause is at least twice the preceding R-R interval. When severe, pause duration may be 5 to 12 seconds (Figure 3-11, *E*).
- For survival, the pause is ended by a ventricular escape complex, junctional escape complex, or normal complex.
- Causes include fibrosis of the SA nodal tissue, greatly increased vagal stimulation, drug influences (digoxin, beta blockers), and rarely neoplasia.
- If severe and frequent, intermittent weakness or syncope may occur.

Sinus Bradycardia

- A sinus rhythm with an abnormally slow rate
- May be physiologic—during sleep, the heart rate of many dogs drops to 30 to 40 bpm. Calm animals or athletic animals at rest may have a physiologic sinus bradycardia.
- Elevated vagal tone may result in a sinus bradycardia.
- Drug-induced—anesthetics and sedatives, digoxin, calcium channel blockers, beta blockers
- Pathologic—hypothermia, hypothyroidism, sick sinus syndrome (SSS)
- Specific therapy for sinus bradycardia is not warranted unless clinical signs (weakness, reduced cardiac output) have developed as a result of the arrhythmia.

Sinus Tachycardia

- A sinus rhythm with an abnormally rapid rate
- May be physiologic—associated with exercise, stress, anxiousness, pain
- Drug-induced—atropine or glycopyrrolate, methylxanthines (theophylline), excessive thyroid supplementation, catecholamines (epinephrine, dobutamine)
- Pathologic—fever, shock, hyperthyroidism, anemia, hypoxia, and congestive heart failure
- Specific therapy for sinus tachycardia is usually indicated for rate control in congestive heart failure patients.

KEY POINT

The underlying cause of the sinus tachycardia should be identified and addressed if necessary.

DISTURBANCES OF SUPRAVENTRICULAR IMPULSE FORMATION

Atrial Premature Complexes

- An APC is an abnormal beat occurring prematurely and originating in atrial tissue
- Electrocardiographic features Figure 3-11, *F*
  - Presence or absence of ectopic P wave—P wave is usually of normal morphology
  - Ectopic P wave may be superimposed on preceding T wave.
  - Premature QRS with identical or nearly identical appearance to normal QRS
  - A compensatory pause may follow the APC.
  - If the APC occurs when the ventricles are refractory, then an isolated ectopic P wave will be noted—it is nonconducted owing to the refractoriness of the ventricles.
- Causes generally include any disease associated with atrial enlargement, such as degenerative valve disease, congenital heart disease, or cardiomyopathy. Other causes include hypoxia, atrial neoplasia, and chronic obstructive pulmonary disease.
- Therapy is not generally warranted for infrequent APCs. Antiarrhythmic therapy may be needed if APCs are frequent and thought to be compromising cardiac output, or if there is a concern of impending atrial tachycardia or atrial fibrillation.

Atrial Tachycardia

- A paroxysmal tachycardia originating from atrial tissue (other than SA node)
- Electrocardiographic features (Figure 3-11, *G*)
  - Rapid rate—from 200 to 350 bpm
  - Usually a regular rhythm. If originating from multiple atrial sites, then an irregular rhythm may occur.
  - P waves may be difficult to discern. QRS complexes are generally normal but may widen, or electrical alternans may develop.
  - Sudden onset and sudden termination of arrhythmia
  - May occur as a reentrant arrhythmia within the AV node
- Causes are the same as for APCs.
- May be clinically significant depending on rate, frequency of runs, and length of runs

Atrial Flutter

- An uncommon arrhythmia characterized by a rapid atrial rate (greater than 250 bpm) and altered atrial depolarization resulting in bidirectional saw-toothed atrial complexes (F waves). Ventricular rate varies depending on refractoriness of AV node.
- Usually a result of severe structural heart disease
- Clinical significance depends on ventricular rate. If excessive, then cardiac output is reduced.

Atrial Fibrillation

- A common arrhythmia in the dog characterized by lack of P waves, rapid ventricular rate, and irregularity of ventricular depolarizations. In atrial fibrillation, there are numerous sites of ectopic atrial depolarization and varying AV nodal refractoriness (Figure 3-11, *H*). Atrial fibrillation is uncommon in the cat.
- Baseline may be flat or may exhibit fine fibrillation potentials.
- Causes include
  - Structural heart disease (advanced degenerative valve disease, dilated cardiomyopathy, atrial neoplasia, congenital heart disease)
  - Lone atrial fibrillation—occurs in large- to giant-breed dogs without structural heart disease
  - May occur as a complication of noncardiac disease, such as gastric dilatation-volvulus or other disorders altering vagal tone
  - May be drug-induced, for example, digoxin
- Clinical significance depends on ventricular rate in most cases. With atrial fibrillation there is also loss of atrial contraction (atrial kick), which may reduce ventricular performance. If the rate is not controlled, then lone atrial fibrillation may cause myocardial deterioration and secondary dilated cardiomyopathy.

Junctional Premature Complexes

- A junctional premature complex is an abnormal beat occurring prematurely and originating in the AV nodal area.
- Electrocardiographic characteristics include abnormal-appearing P wave (often inverted), which may precede QRS, be superimposed on QRS, or follow QRS complexes. The QRS complex is usually unaffected.
- Causes are the same as for APCs.
- Clinical significance is the same as APCs.

Atrioventricular Junctional Tachycardia

- A paroxysmal or sustained rhythm originating from AV nodal tissue
- Electrocardiographic features
  - Rate is greater than 60 bpm (inherent rate of AV nodal tissue is approximately 40 bpm to 60 bpm)
  - A regular rhythm
  - Abnormal appearing P wave (often inverted in lead II), which may precede QRS, be superimposed on QRS, or follow QRS complexes
  - QRS complexes may be normal or may be widened secondary to aberrant conduction.
- Causes include digoxin toxicity and structural heart disease
- May be clinically significant depending on ventricular rate

Supraventricular Tachycardia

- *SVT* refers to a rapid arrhythmia originating from supraventricular tissue, but in which the exact site of origin cannot be determined. Atrial tachycardia and AV junctional tachycardia are often indistinguishable, so the term SVT may be more precise in these cases.

> **KEY POINT**
>
> AV junctional tachycardia may be difficult to distinguish from atrial tachycardia

DISTURBANCES OF IMPULSE CONDUCTION

Sinus Block

- The SA node discharges normally, but the impulse is blocked by neighboring tissue.
- Produces a pause equal to twice the preceding R-R interval, with immediate restoration of rhythm
- Causes are the same as for sinus arrest
- Usually not clinically significant

Atrial Standstill

- Atrial standstill is characterized by an absence of P waves and can be temporary in nature or persistent. The most common cause of temporary atrial standstill is hyperkalemia. Persistent atrial standstill is due to an atrial muscular dystrophy, most commonly occurring in English Springer Spaniels.
- In atrial standstill due to hyperkalemia, SA nodal discharge occurs, but atrial depolarization is blocked by the effects of hyperkalemia. As there is no atrial depolarization, P waves are absent. The impulse originating from the SA node reaches the AV node by way of internodal fibers. Hyperkalemia also slows the rate of SA nodal discharge and affects ventricular depolarization and repolarization.
- Electrocardiographic characteristics of persistent atrial standstill
  - Absence of P waves
  - Heart rate usually slow (< 60 bpm)
  - Rhythm regular with supraventricular-appearing QRS complexes
  - Heart rate does not increase with atropine administration
- Electrocardiographic characteristics of atrial standstill due to hyperkalemia (Figure 3-12, *A*)
  - As serum potassium increases, P wave amplitude diminishes. Absence of P waves occurs when the potassium approaches 8.0 mEq/L.
  - Slow ventricular rate—the rhythm is termed sinoventricular, and the rate is approximately 20 to 40 bpm.
  - As serum potassium increases, T wave amplitude increases and becomes peaked.
  - QRS duration progressively increases and R wave height decreases as serum potassium levels increase.
  - Heart rate may increase slightly with atropine administration
- Causes of hyperkalemia include hypoadrenocorticism, anuric or oliguric renal failure, uncontrolled diabetic ketoacidosis, metabolic acidosis, urethral obstruction, rupture of the urinary bladder.

> **KEY POINT**
>
> Atrial standstill due to hyperkalemia is usually life threatening.

Ventricular Pre-Excitation Syndrome

- In these syndromes, an abnormal accessory pathway exists, which bypasses the AV node. This results in a shortening or loss of the PR interval due to premature activation of the ventricles. With an accessory pathway, there are two electrical connections between the atria and the ventricles, and both may simultaneously be relaying impulses. There also exists the potential for reentry as the impulse may leave the atria through one pathway and immediately reenter through the other. The accessory pathway may connect the atria to the distal AV node, bundle of His, or directly to ventricular tissue.
- Electrocardiographic features (Table 3-2 and Figure 3-13)

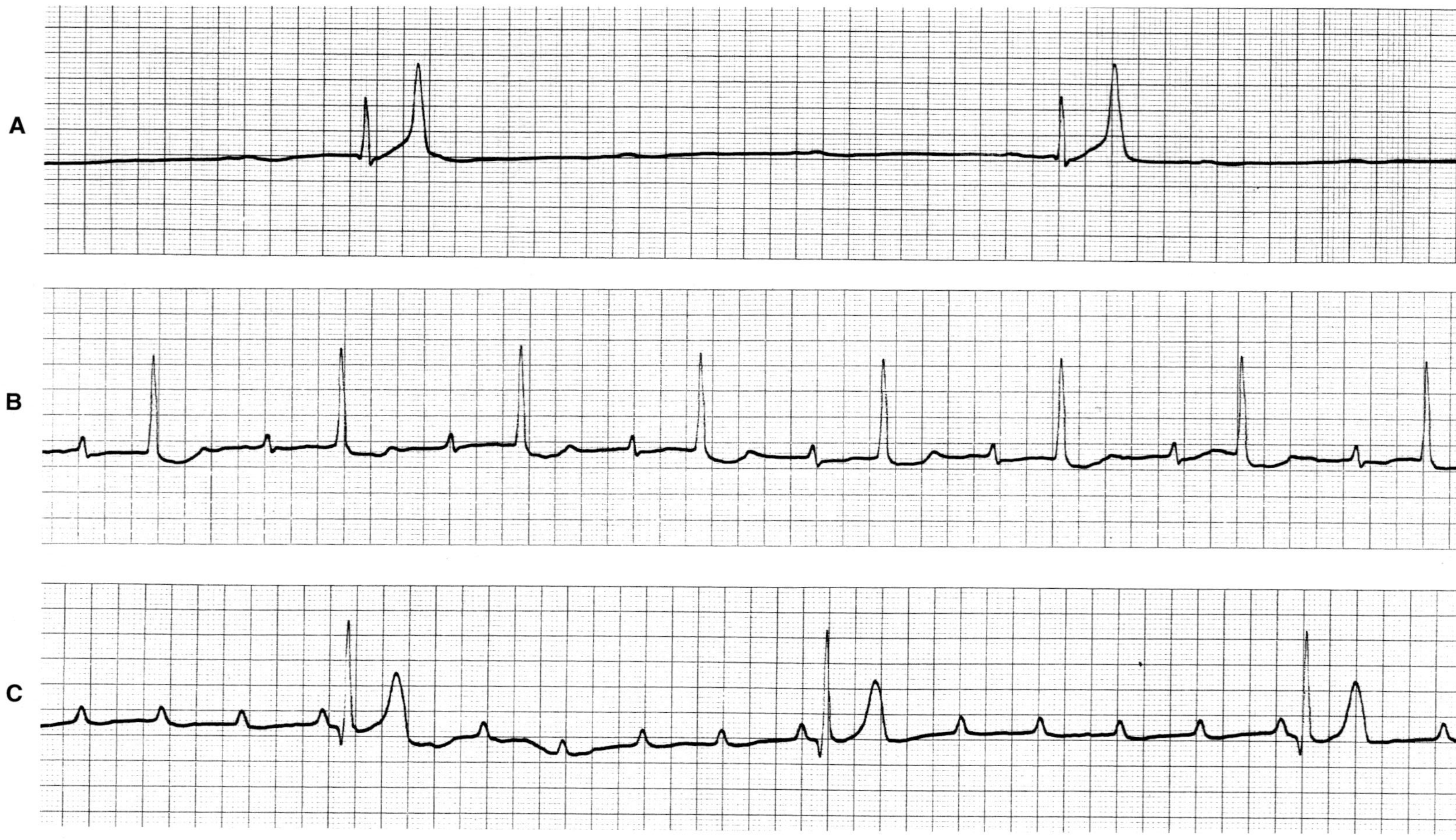

Figure 3-12. A, Electrocardiogram—atrial standstill. **B,** Electrocardiogram—first-degree AV block. **C,** Electrocardiogram—second-degree AV block.

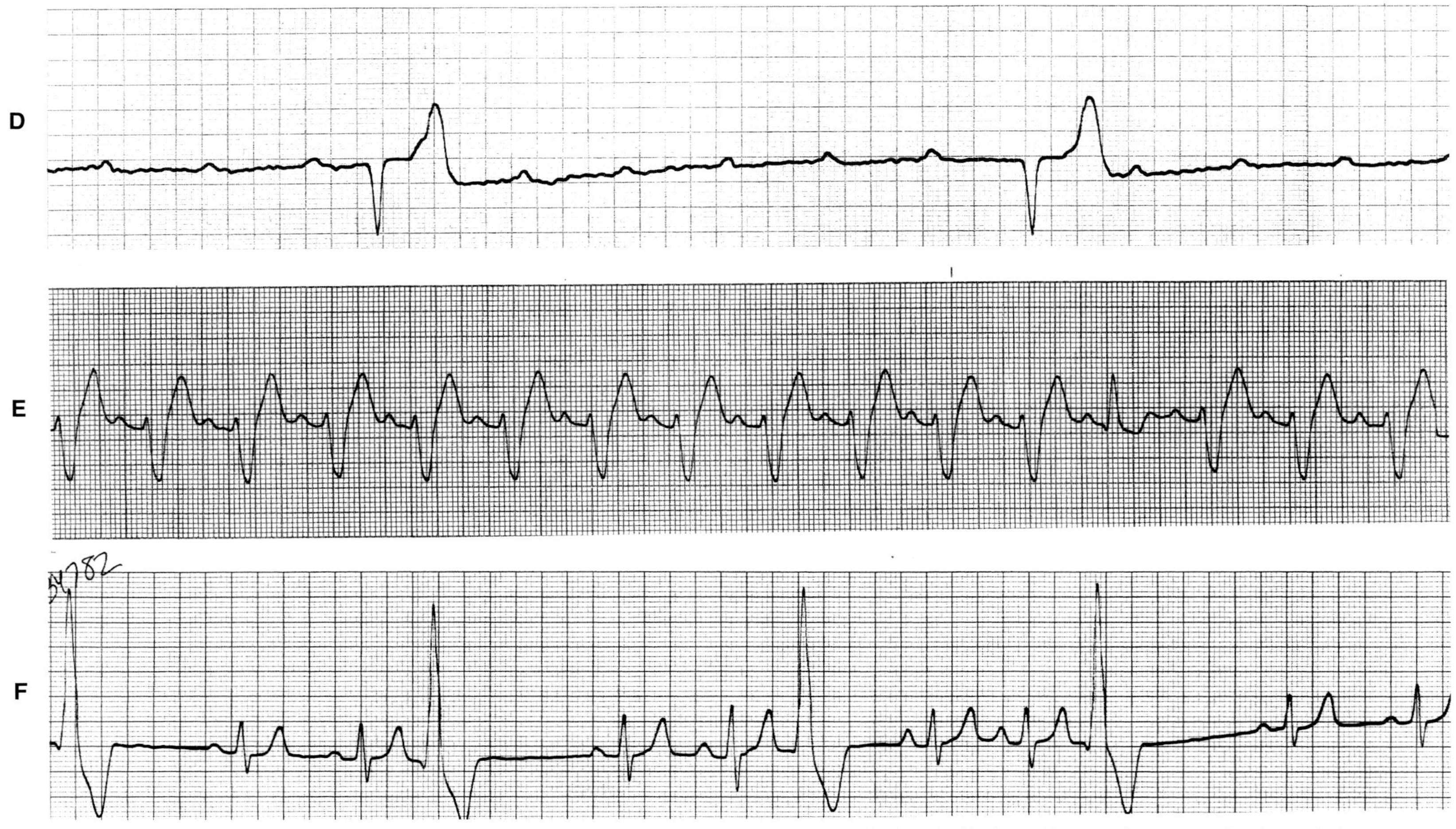

Figure 3-12, cont'd. D, Electrocardiogram—third-degree AV block. **E,** Electrocardiogram—right bundle branch block. **F,** Electrocardiogram—unifocal ventricular premature complexes.

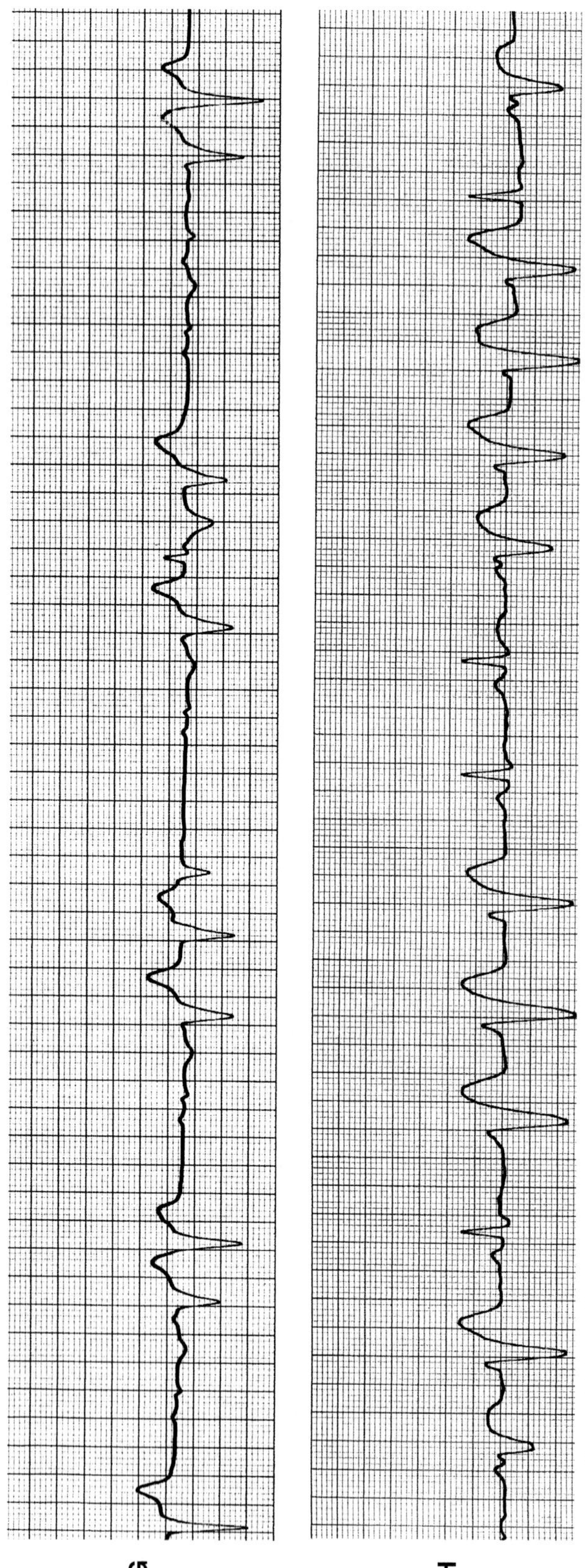

Figure 3-12, cont'd. **G,** Electrocardiogram—multiform ventricular premature complexes. **H,** Electrocardiogram—run of ventricular premature complexes.

Table 3-2 Summary of Pre-Excitation Syndrome

Cardiac Sequence	Mechanism	ECG
Sinus impulse	Normal	—
Atrial depolarization	Normal	Normal P wave
AV node accessory pathways	Relatively rapid conduction, skirting the A-V nodal system	Short PR interval
Early ventricular depolarization	One ventricle activated early	Initial QRS slurred (delta wave) (∴ widened QRS)
Retrograde conduction from ventricles to atria	Atrial re-entry impulse	Tendency to supraventricular paroxysmal arrhythmias
Late ventricular depolarization	Fusion between normal and anomalous ventricular activation	Delay, often with altered direction, of terminal QRS

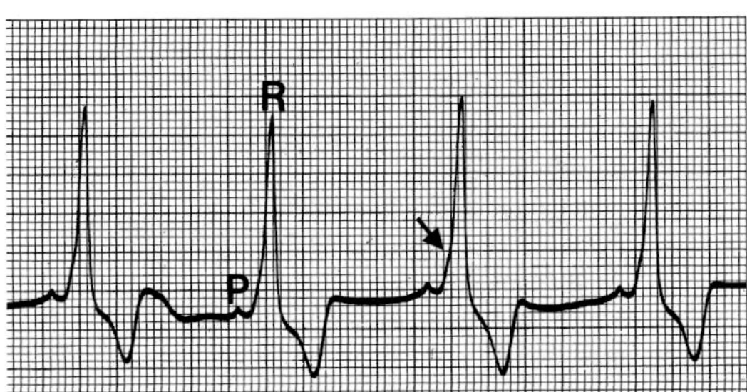

Figure 3-13. Ventricular pre-excitation in a dog. A short P-R interval and a widened QRS complex with slurring or notching *(arrow)* of the upstroke ("delta" wave) are present. (From Fox PR, Sisson D, Moise NS, eds: Textbook of canine and feline cardiology, St Louis, 1999, Elsevier.)

    - A shortened PR interval
    - If the accessory pathway terminates in ventricular tissue, then initial slurring of the QRS complex (delta wave) occurs.
    - Paroxysmal reentrant tachycardia in some cases
- Causes include congenital anomalies, feline hypertrophic cardiomyopathy, and other structural heart diseases.
- Clinical significance depends on the frequency and severity of secondary tachycardia resulting from the accessory pathway.

First-Degree Atrioventricular Block

- Conduction through the AV node is delayed.
- Produces prolongation of the PR interval (more than 0.13 second for the dog, more than 0.09 second for the cat) (see Figure 3-12, *B*).
- Causes include fibrosis of the AV node, vagal stimulation, and drug-induced (digoxin) and electrolyte imbalance.
- Isolated first degree AV block is not clinically significant but may be an early indicator of progressive AV nodal dysfunction.

Second-Degree Atrioventricular Block

- There is intermittent blockage of conduction through the AV node.
- Following discharge of the SA node and atrial depolarization, there is no associated ventricular depolarization.
- Electrocardiographic features include absence of QRS-T complexes following P wave (see Figure 3-12, *C*).
    - In Mobitz type I (Wenckebach) block, there is progressive prolongation of the PR interval, followed by occurrence of second degree AV block.
    - In Mobitz type II block, there is second degree AV block without preceding prolongation of the PR interval.
    - A pattern of block may exist—a 2:1 AV block would refer to the presence of two P waves for every QRS complex.
    - Advanced or high-grade AV block consists of more than two consecutive blocked atrial depolarizations.
- Causes are identical to those of first-degree AV block.
- High-grade AV block may reduce cardiac output and result in clinical signs.

KEY POINT

Second-degree block may progress to complete AV block. This is more common with Mobitz type II AV block.

Third-Degree Atrioventricular Block (Complete Heart Block)

- All conduction through the AV node is blocked. Atrial and ventricular depolarizations are no longer coordinated and occur independently of one another. Ventricular depolarization is initiated by discharge of a ventricular escape focus.
- Electrocardiographic features (see Figure 3-12, *D*)
  - There is no association between P waves and QRS-T complexes.
  - P waves are of normal morphology and usually occur at a normal rate.
  - QRS complexes are of ventricular origin morphology.
  - Ventricular rate is typically 30 to 50 bpm.
- Causes include fibrosis of the AV node, drug-induced (digoxin), infiltrative disease, Rickettsial myocarditis, hyperkalemia.
- Usually associated with clinical signs of weakness or collapse. Complete AV block warrants implantation of a permanent pacemaker in most cases.

Left Bundle Branch Block

- A conduction delay or block in both the left posterior and the left anterior fascicles of the left bundle. A supraventricular impulse activates the right ventricle first through the right bundle branch. Left ventricular depolarization is delayed.
- Electrocardiographic features (Figure 3-14)
  - Prolongation of QRS duration (> 0.08 second for the dog; > 0.06 second for the cat)
  - QRS wide and positive in leads I, II, III, and aVF
  - Unlike VPCs, the QRS complex is associated with a preceding P wave.
  - May be difficult to distinguish from left ventricular enlargement pattern
- Causes include structural heart disease (cardiomyopathy, congenital anomalies, neoplasia, trauma, fibrosis)
- The presence of an LBBB does not impair cardiac performance directly, but is a marker of significant heart disease.

KEY POINT

Complete heart block will occur if right bundle branch block (RBBB) develops in an animal with LBBB.

Left Anterior Fascicular Block

- There is a block in the left anterior fascicle of the left bundle branch slowing depolarization of the left ventricle.
- Electrocardiographic features
  - QRS duration is within normal limits
  - Left axis deviation (dog less than 40 degrees, cat less than 0 degrees)
  - Small Q wave and tall R wave in leads I and aVL (small Q wave not consistent)
  - Deep S waves in leads II, III, and aVF (exceeding R wave)
  - Associated with feline hypertrophic cardiomyopathy, other diseases associated with left ventricular hypertrophy, hyperkalemia, ischemia, and post-cardiac surgery

KEY POINT

Left anterior fascicular block does not directly impair cardiac function, but if present, then one should look for underlying etiologies.

Right Bundle Branch Block

- There is block of the right bundle branch, delaying depolarization of the right ventricle.
- Electrocardiographic features (Figure 3-12, *E*)
  - QRS duration increased
  - Prominent S waves in leads I, II, III, and aVF

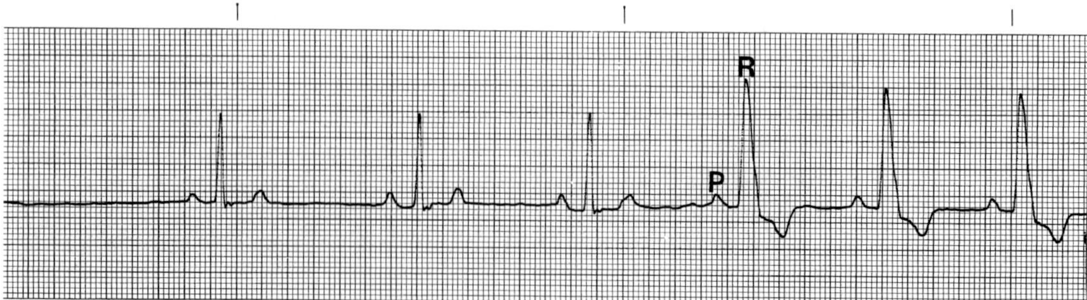

Figure 3-14. Intermittent left bundle branch block in a dog. The QRS complexes are wider and taller than normal in the fourth, fifth, and sixth complexes. (From Fox PR, Sisson D, Moise NS, eds: Textbook of canine and feline cardiology, St Louis, 1999, Elsevier.)

- Right axis shift
- Associated with structural heart disease, Chagas disease, heartworm disease, acute pulmonary thromboembolism, hypokalemia.

KEY POINT

As in the case of LAFB, RBBB does not significantly impair cardiac function, but one should look for underlying etiologies.

DISTURBANCES OF VENTRICULAR IMPULSE FORMATION

Ventricular Premature Complexes

- An abnormal beat originating in the ventricles and occurring earlier than expected in relation to the existing rhythm. A compensatory pause often follows a VPC.
  - Unifocal VPCs occur from one ventricular site and have identical morphologies (see Figure 3-12, *F*).
  - Multifocal VPCs usually occur from more than one ventricular site and have differing morphologies. Electrophysiologic studies have demonstrated that a single ventricular site may produce VPCs of differing morphology—this is due to altered conduction of the VPCs rather than multiple ectopic sites. It is more precise, therefore, to use the term multiform rather than multifocal (see Figure 3-12, *G*).
  - When the VPC does not alter the underlying normal rhythm, it is said to be interpolated.
  - When normal ventricular depolarization is interrupted by a VPC, a fusion beat occurs—this is essentially the electrocardiographic merging of a normal QRS and VPC.
- Electrocardiographic features (Figures 3-12, *F* to *H*)
  - As the site of depolarization is ventricular, there is no AV association. P waves are not associated with the QRS complexes of the VPCs.
  - QRS complexes wide and bizarre, consistent with ventricular origin
  - T wave polarity often reversed
  - Compensatory pause following VPC is typical.
  - Patterns of VPCs
    - Two consecutive VPCs are referred to as a couplet
    - Three or more consecutive VPCs is a salvo or run (see Figure 3-12, *H*).
    - When every other complex is a VPC, ventricular bigeminy exists.
    - When every third complex is a VPC, ventricular trigeminy exists.
    - R-on-T phenomenon occurs when the VPC occurs immediately following a normal beat within the T wave. This may predispose to the development of ventricular tachycardia.
- Causes are numerous and include structural heart disease, familial in young German Shepherds, arrhythmogenic right ventricular cardiomyopathy (boxer cardiomyopathy), hypoxia, anemia, uremia, gastric dilatation-volvulus, splenic torsion and splenic neoplasia, pancreatitis, myocarditis, and drug induced (digoxin, anesthesia).
- Clinical significance depends on the frequency of VPCs, pattern of ectopy, and cause of the arrhythmia.
  - Isolated VPCs usually pose no significant problems but may signal the presence of progressive disease and potential for more serious arrhythmia.
  - Runs of VPCs do suggest the potential for ventricular tachycardia and possibly ventricular fibrillation.

KEY POINT

The finding of isolated VPCs in a young to middle-aged Doberman Pinscher or Boxer is highly suggestive of occult dilated cardiomyopathy or arrhythmogenic right ventricular cardiomyopathy respectively.

Ventricular Tachycardia

- Runs of VPCs occurring in succession at a rate of usually greater than 100 bpm. The inherent discharge rate of the ventricle is approximately 40 to 50 bpm (seen with complete heart block). In normal animals, this is overdriven by the sinus rhythm. An accelerated idioventricular rhythm refers to a ventricular rhythm at a rate of 60 to 100 bpm. Ventricular tachycardia may be sustained or paroxysmal.
- Electrocardiographic features (Figure 3-15, *A*)
  - P waves not associated with QRS complexes
  - QRS complexes wide and bizarre, consistent with ventricular origin
  - Regular rhythm, as contrasted with atrial fibrillation and RBBB
- Causes are the same as for VPCs.
- Ventricular tachycardia indicates significant heart disease or systemic disease. Cardiac

output may be significantly impaired, and the arrhythmia predisposes to ventricular fibrillation.

Ventricular Fibrillation

- Completely irregular, chaotic variable fibrillation potentials, indicating lack of organized ventricular depolarization and impending death
- Electrocardiographic features (Figure 3-15, *B*)
  - There is no evidence of organized cardiac depolarization (absence of P-QRS-T waves)
  - Wavy, undulating baseline
  - Coarse ventricular fibrillation is characterized by large wavelets.
  - Fine ventricular fibrillation is characterized by small wavelets.

KEY POINT

Ventricular fibrillation indicates cardiopulmonary arrest, and immediate restoration of rhythm is required to preserve life.

Ventricular Asystole

- Lack of any significant ventricular electrical activity
- Electrocardiogram demonstrates flat baseline—occasional ventricular escape complexes may occur
- A terminal rhythm requiring immediate restoration of rhythm to preserve life

DISTURBANCES OF BOTH IMPULSE FORMATION AND IMPULSE CONDUCTION

Sick Sinus Syndrome

- SSS is a progressive heart disease characterized by a variety of arrhythmias, including sinus bradycardia, sinus arrest, paroxysmal atrial tachycardia (bradycardia-tachycardia syndrome), intermittent AV nodal block, and lack of ventricular escape complexes (Figure 3-15, *C*).
- Breeds predisposed include Miniature Schnauzers, Cocker Spaniels, Dachshunds, Pugs, West Highland White Terriers. SSS is most common in older female dogs.
- The cause is unknown but likely involves idiopathic degeneration of the conduction system.
- Most cases are presented with a history of intermittent weakness and collapse.
- Medical therapy may be successful in some cases; many require pacemaker implantation.

Atrial Premature Complexes with Aberrant Conduction

- When the impulse of an APC encounters an area of refractoriness (AV node, bundle of His, or ventricular myocardium), it may terminate or continue with aberrant conduction. The latter may result in a wide and bizarre QRS configuration resembling a beat of ventricular origin.
- Most often occurs at slow heart rates
- QRS may take the form of RBBB.

ESCAPE RHYTHMS

Junctional Escape Beat

- When not activated by atrial depolarization, the junctional AV nodal area may spontaneously discharge. This impulse results in ventricular depolarization in a normal fashion. Junctional escape beats may occur when there is a significant pause in the sinus rhythm.
- Electrocardiographic features
  - Inverted P wave, occurring before, during, or just after QRS complex
  - Normal or relatively normal QRS complex
  - Occurs after significant pause in sinus rhythm
- Clinical significance—this complex is adaptive and helps to maintain cardiac output in the face of a slow rate or sinus arrest.

KEY POINT

Junctional escape beats should not be suppressed.

Junctional Rhythm

- Succession of junctional escape beats in absence of adequate sinus node function
- Rate of junctional escape rhythm is typically 40 to 60 bpm.
- This rhythm is adaptive and should not be suppressed. Correction of the cause of sinus node dysfunction is warranted.

Ventricular Escape Beat

- When not activated by atrial depolarization, a ventricular focus may spontaneously discharge. This impulse results in an abnormal ventricular depolarization, but contraction is not affected. Ventricular escape beats may occur when there is a significant pause in the sinus rhythm and lack of junctional escape complexes.
- Electrocardiographic features
  - Ventricular escape beat occurs following a pause in the rhythm

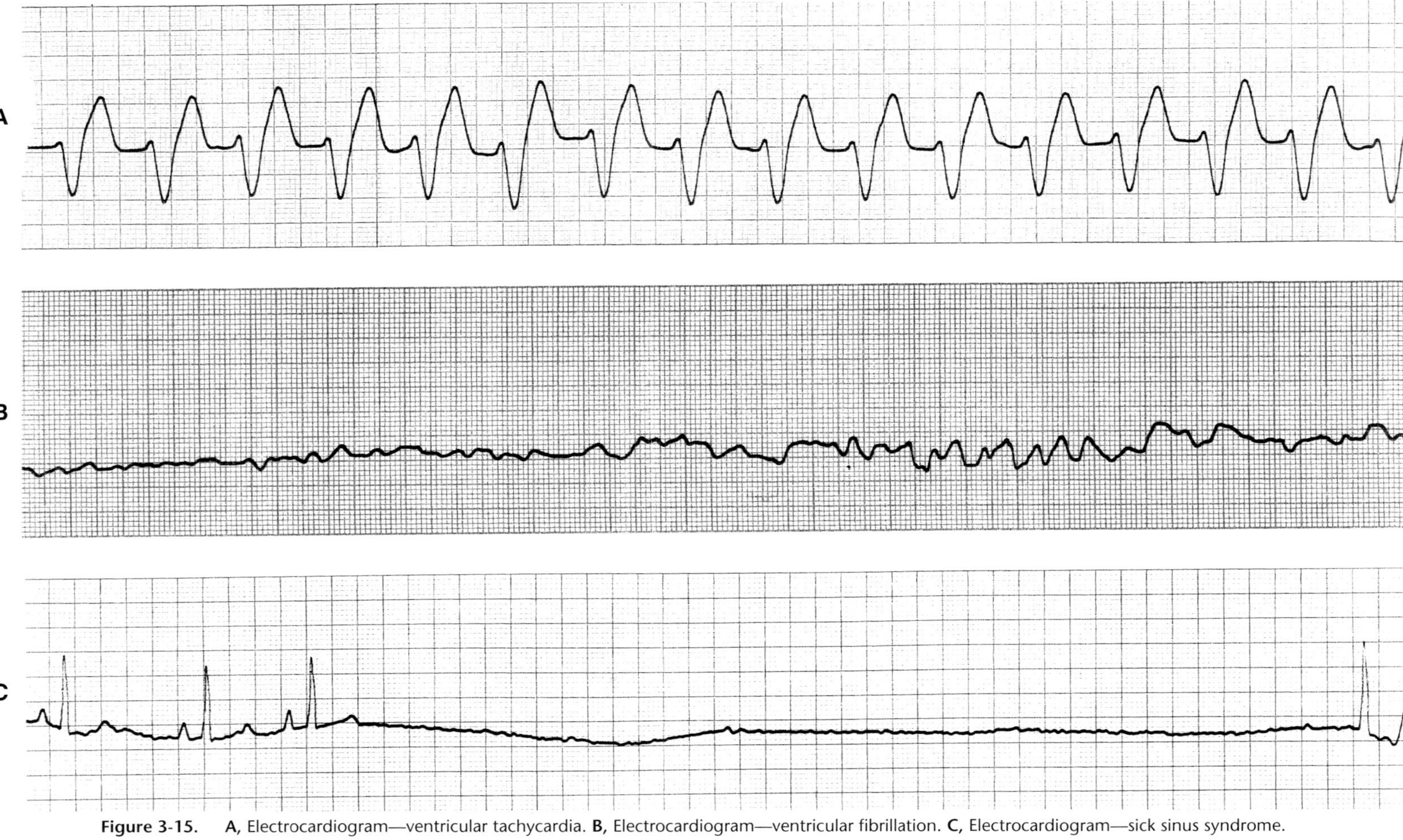

Figure 3-15. **A,** Electrocardiogram—ventricular tachycardia. **B,** Electrocardiogram—ventricular fibrillation. **C,** Electrocardiogram—sick sinus syndrome.

- QRS wide and bizarre, consistent with ventricular origin
- Clinical significance—this complex is adaptive and helps to maintain cardiac output in the face of a slow rate or sinus arrest.

Ventricular Escape Rhythm

- Succession of ventricular escape beats in absence of adequate sinus node function
- Rate of ventricular escape rhythm is typically 30 to 40 bpm.
- This rhythm is adaptive and should not be suppressed. Correction of the cause of sinus node dysfunction is warranted.

KEY POINT

These ventricular escape beats should not be suppressed.

MISCELLANEOUS

Artificial Pacemaker

- A permanent pacemaker is used to control bradyarrhythmias that caused clinical signs and were unresponsive to medical therapy.
- Transvenous implantation with an endocardial lead is the preferred means and is much less invasive than abdominal surgery and epicardial lead implantation.
- Most pacemakers used in dogs are set at 100 bpm.
- Electrocardiographic features
  - If the sinus node is functioning and the heart rate is greater than 100 bpm (or discharge rate of pacemaker), then there will be no electrocardiographic changes.
  - Once the heart rate decreases below the pacemaker's minimum rate, a pacing spike will appear followed by a wide and bizarre QRS (ventricular origin of impulse).

KEY POINT

Ashman's aberrance may mimic a VPC.

Parasystole

- In parasystole, there is an independent focus discharging spontaneously. There is an entrance block, so the focus is not overdriven by the normal cardiac impulse. The parasystolic focus will discharge at a regular rate and may cause complete depolarization of the atria or ventricles.
- Atrial parasystole focus is located within atrial myocardium and produces small P waves, usually unassociated with QRS complexes.
- Ventricular parasystole focus is located within ventricular myocardium and produces regularly spaced QRS complexes. When the focus discharges during the ventricle's refractory period, a QRS will not be created.

Ashman's Phenomenon

- Tendency of premature supraventricular beats to have aberrant ventricular conduction when a short cycle follows a long one.

KEY POINT

The beats generated by the pacemaker are not of normal morphology—this is expected.

Frequently Asked Questions

If a veterinarian auscults an abnormality that comes and goes, and the ECG does not show an arrhythmia, then what should be done?

Repeat ECGs may be required to pick up changes in heart activity occurring only in a paroxysmal pattern. In some cases, a Holter monitor must be used for a 24-hour recording so that the pattern and frequency of abnormality can be properly tracked.

Interference is occurring on an ECG tracing; it appears to be 60 cycle (small waveforms) and is not improved when the fluorescent bulbs and all electrical equipment in the room are turned off. What could cause this ongoing interference?

Sometimes, interference may travel through the walls from the adjacent room and close proximity to power supply in the wall could also send off interference. Electrical supply to the facility must be properly grounded and so if the problem persists when all of those factors have been controlled, then an electrician should examine the electrical system of the building.

We must do a surgery that requires an unusual position for the dog. Will abnormal relative and absolute position of the clips interfere with our routine intra-operative monitoring?

Position is not critical for routine intra-operative electrocardiography, as opposed to position required for a primary ECG with multiple leads for diagnostic purposes, and so a useful capture can be done in spite of unorthodox limb or animal position. Any position for the recording will still always give an analysis of an arrhythmia and/or conduction abnormality. It is important to watch that the extreme positioning required will not lead to the lead wires or clips touching a metal surgical table since that can cause interference.

SUGGESTED READINGS

Davis AS, Middleton, BJ: Relationship between QT interval and heart rate in Alderley Park beagles, Record, 145:248-250, 1999.

Detweiler DK: The dog electrocardiogram: a critical review. In MacFarlane, PW, Lawrie, TDV, eds: Comprehensive electrocardiography: theory and practice in health and disease, New York, 1998, Pergamon Press.

Ettinger SJ Le Bobinnec G, Cote E: Electrocardiography. In Ettinger SJ, Feldman EC, eds: Textbook of Veterinary internal medicine, ed 5, St Louis, 2000, WB Saunders.

Finley MR, Lillich JD, Gilmour RF, Freeman LC: Structural and functional basis for the long QT syndrome: relevance to veterinary patients. J Vet Med 17:473-488, 2003.

Kittleson MD: Electrocardiography. In Kittleson MD, Kienle RD, eds: Small animal cardiovascular medicine, St Louis, 1998, Mosby.

Miller MS, Tilley LP, Smith FWK Jr, Fox PR, Electrocardiography. In Fox PR, Sisson D, Moise NS, eds: Textbook of canine and feline cardiology, St Louis, 1999, Elsevier.

Miller MS, Tilley LP, Detweiler DK: Cardiac electrophysiology. In Duke's physiology of domestic animals, ed 11, Ithaca, NY, 1993, Cornell.

Redfern WS, Carlsson L, Davis AS, Lynch WG, MacKenzie I, et al: Relationships between preclinical cardiac electrophysiology, clinical QT interval prolongation and torsade de pointes for a broad range of drugs: evidence for a provisional safety margin in drug development. Cardiovasc Res, 58, 32-45, 2003.

Smith, FWK, Tilley, LP, Miller, MS: Disorders of cardiac rhythm. In Brichard, SJ, Sherding, RG, eds: Manual of small animal practice, ed 3, St Louis, 2007, WB Saunders.

Smith FWK, Tilley, LP, Miller, MS. Electrocardiography. In Brichard, SJ, Sherding, RG, eds: Manual of small animal practice, ed 3, St Louis, 2007, WB Saunders.

Tilley LP: Essentials of canine and feline electrocardiography, ed 3, Ames, Iowa, 1992, Blackwell.

Tilley LP, Miller MS, Smith FW, Jr: canine and feline cardiac arrhythmias: self-assessment. Ames, Iowa, 1993, Blackwell.

CHAPTER 4

Echocardiography and Doppler Ultrasound

Virginia Luis Fuentes

INTRODUCTION

Echocardiography has become the most important diagnostic technique for the diagnosis of canine and feline heart disease. The interaction between ultra-high-frequency sound waves and the heart allows the depiction of cardiac morphology, information on the movement of myocardium and valves, and blood flow within the heart. Echocardiography is complementary to physical examination, radiography and electrocardiography (ECG) and has replaced invasive techniques such as cardiac catheterization for all but a few specific indications.

TYPES OF IMAGING

Two-Dimensional Echocardiography

- A sector-shaped beam of ultrasound waves is reflected by the interfaces of cardiac tissue to provide a two-dimensional (2D) cross-sectional (tomographic) image (Figure 4-1).

Applications
- Demonstrating cardiac morphology
- Increasingly important in quantification of chamber dimensions (as machines become capable of faster frame rates)

M-Mode Echocardiography

- M-mode uses a single narrow beam of ultrasound, but displays the resulting echoes as a distance-time graph (Figure 4-2). The time resolution is superior to that obtained with 2D, so that the frame is updated thousands of time per second rather than the 40 to 200 times per second obtained with 2D.

Applications
- Time-dependent measurements (chamber dimensions, wall motion)

Doppler Echocardiography

- Doppler echocardiography uses the *Doppler principle*: the frequency of a reflected sound wave depends on the direction and velocity of the reflector and the transmitted frequency (producing a *Doppler shift*).
- If the transmitted ultrasound frequency and the velocity of sound in soft tissue and blood are known, then the velocity of red blood cells can be calculated.

KEY POINT

The angle of the incident ultrasound beam is critical: *the ultrasound beam must be parallel with flow* (or less than 20° from the direction of flow) or the velocity will be underestimated.

There are several modes of Doppler echocardiography:
- *Spectral Doppler*, where the velocity of blood flow is calculated in a region of interest selected by moving a cursor (Figure 4-3)
- *Color Doppler*, where the blood flow is coded in red (toward the transducer) or blue (away from the transducer) and superimposed on the black-and-white 2D image (Figure 4-4)

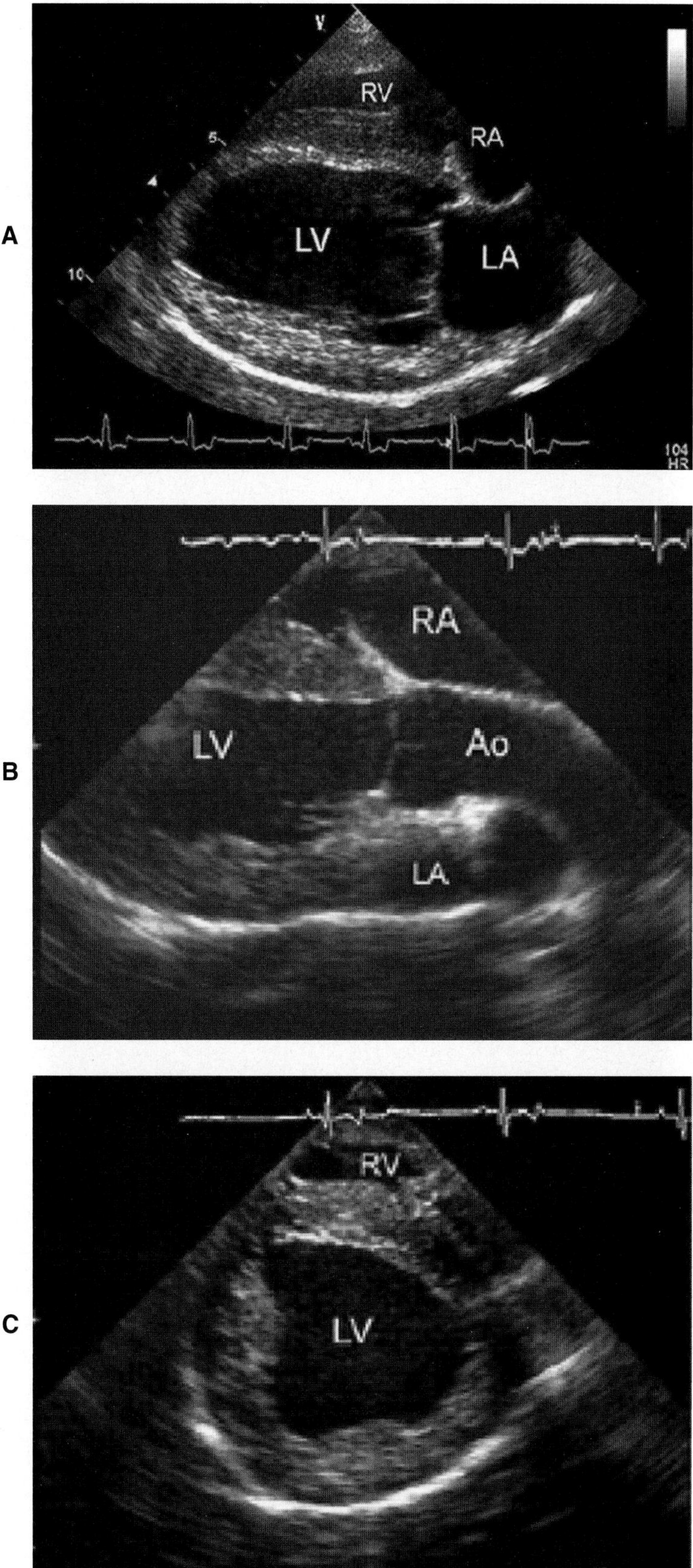

Figure 4-1. Right parasternal echocardiographic views. **A,** Long-axis four-chamber view optimized for left ventricular inlet. **B,** Long-axis view optimized for left ventricular outflow tract. **C,** Short-axis view at the papillary muscle level.

Continued

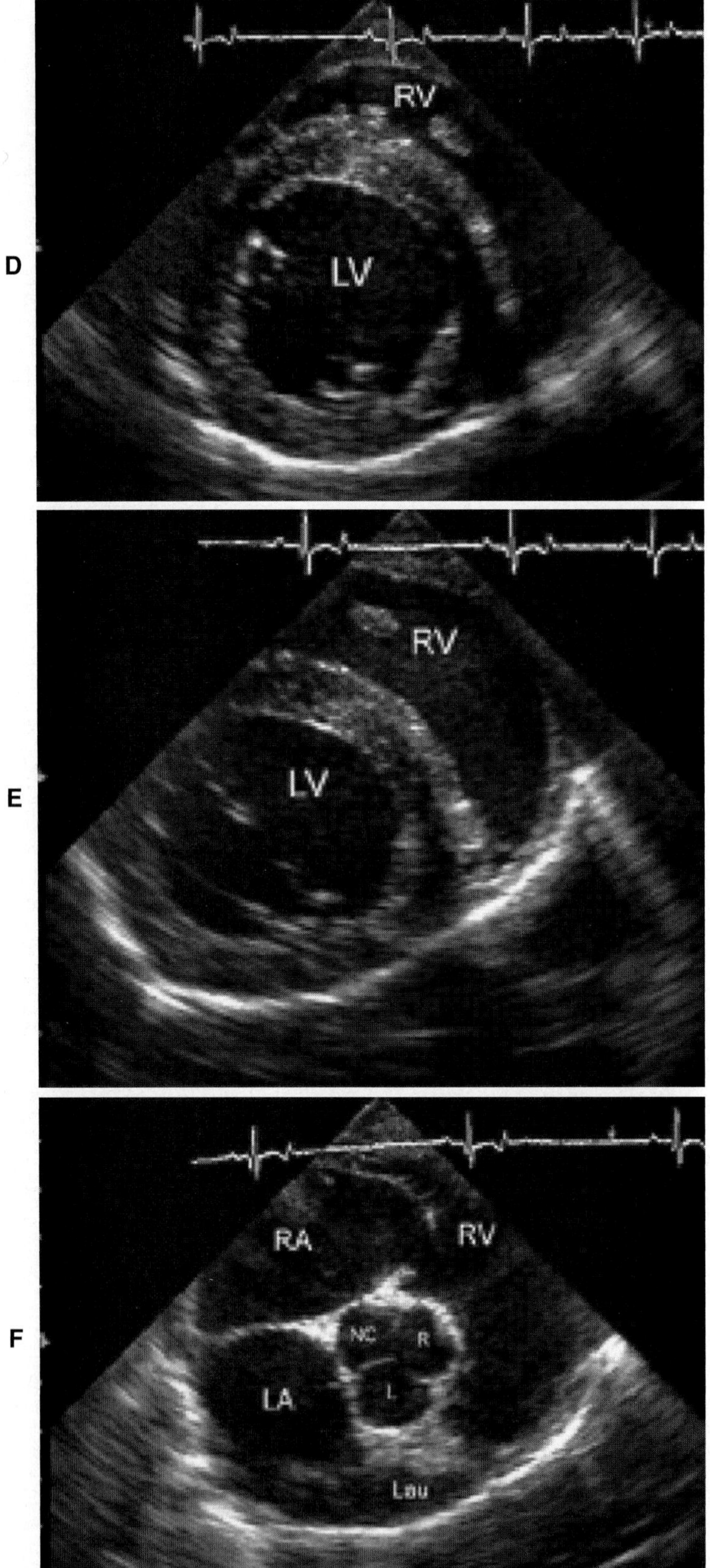

Figure 4-1. cont'd. **D,** Short-axis view at chordal level. **E,** Short-axis view at mitral valve level. **F,** Short-axis view at the heart base, optimized for left atrium and aortic valve.

Continued

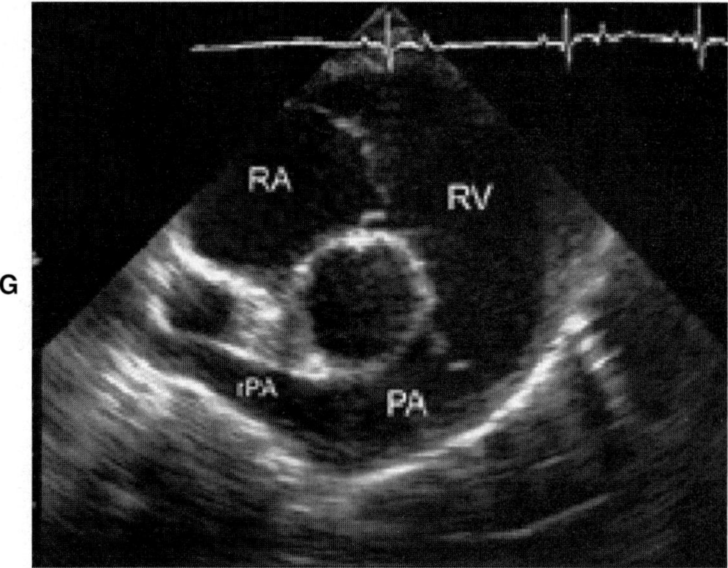

Figure 4-1. cont'd. **G,** Short-axis view at the heart base, optimized for pulmonary artery. *LA,* Left atrium; *LV,* left ventricle; *RA,* right atrium; *RV,* right ventricle; *Ao,* aorta; *R,* right coronary sinus of Valsalva; *L,* left coronary sinus of Valsalva; *NC,* noncoronary sinus of Valsalva; *PA,* pulmonary artery; *rPA,* right pulmonary artery.

- *Tissue Doppler imaging (TDI)*, where the velocity of myocardial motion is displayed (Figure 4-5, *E*)

Spectral Doppler Echocardiography

- A graph of blood flow velocity against time is shown, usually with a simultaneous ECG display.
- Blood flow velocities toward the transducer are displayed as positive (above the baseline), and blood flow velocities away from the transducer are displayed as negative (below the baseline).
- The Doppler shift can also be represented by an audible sound, because the shift in frequency is usually quite small and within the audible range (around 10 kHz), so that most machines will show a visual spectral display with a simultaneous audible signal.
- Spectral Doppler is usually recorded with guidance from two-dimensional echocardiographic images (2D-Doppler, or Duplex Doppler). This allows a cursor to be superimposed over a 2D image, showing the angle of interrogation of the Doppler beam in two dimensions.
- Spectral Doppler can be further subdivided into pulsed wave, continuous wave, and high-pulse repetition frequency.

Pulsed Wave Doppler

- The ultrasound waves are transmitted as pulses of waves, with the transducer acting at different times as a receiver or transmitter of ultrasound waves, allowing the interrogation of blood flow velocities within a specific region of interest.
- This region of interest is represented as a *sample volume* on the cursor.
- Pulsed wave Doppler has limitations in the maximum velocities that it can display without ambiguity: high velocities result in "aliasing," where blood flow will be displayed as both positive and negative velocities (i.e., signal wraps around the baseline).
- The velocity at which aliasing will occur depends on the *Nyquist limit* (half the pulse repetition frequency), with higher velocities without aliasing achieved at lower transducer frequencies, and reduced depth from the transducer.

Continuous Wave Doppler

- In contrast, with continuous wave (CW) Doppler, ultrasound waves can be transmitted and received simultaneously. This allows much higher velocities to be displayed, but it is not possible to draw any conclusions about the depth along the cursor from where these velocities are originating (i.e., there is *range ambiguity*).

High-Pulse Repetition Frequency Doppler

- High-Pulse repetition frequency Doppler is a form of pulsed Doppler that shares some similarities with CW Doppler. Frequent pulses of ultrasound waves are produced so that a number of sample volumes will be superimposed on the 2D image.

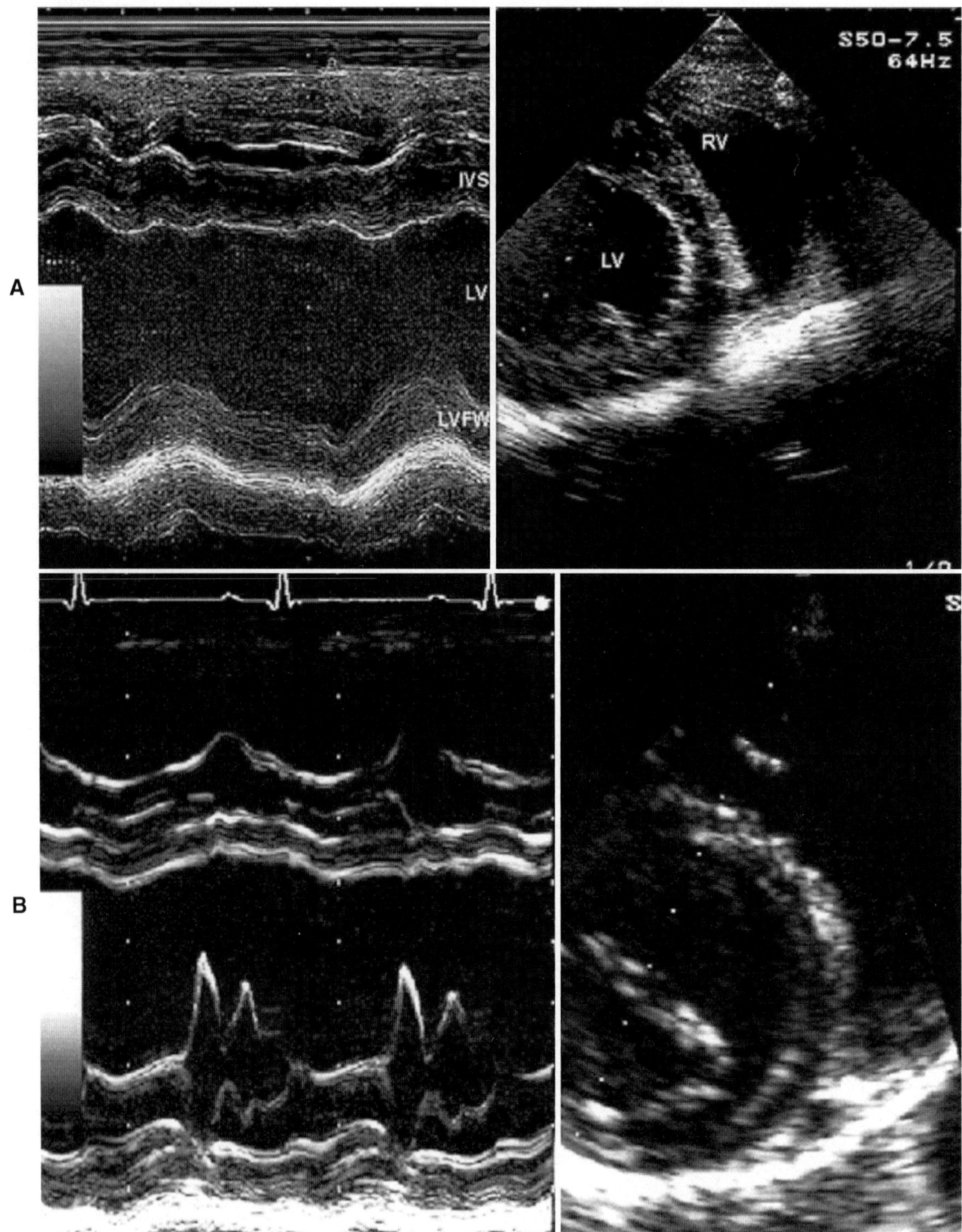

Figure 4-2. M-mode echocardiograms of the left heart at the mitral valve chordal level (note that the 2D image is moved to the left of the screen to allow correct placement of the cursor) **(A)**; mitral valve leaflet level **(B)**; aortic valve level.

Continued

C

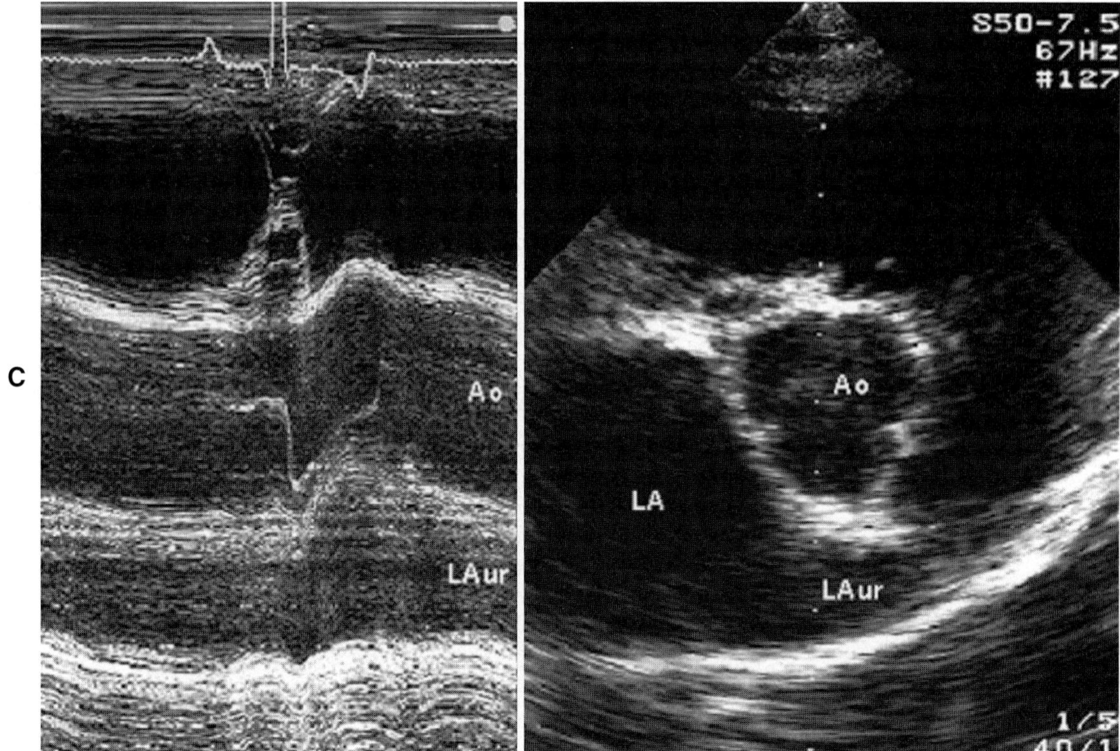

Figure 4-2. cont'd. (C). *IVS,* Interventricular septum; *LV,* left ventricle; *LVFW,* left ventricular free wall; *RV,* right ventricle; *Ao,* aorta; *LA,* left atrium; *LAur,* left auricle.

This not only allows the display of higher velocities without aliasing, but also increases the number of possible sites from which the velocities are being recorded.

Color Flow Doppler

- Color flow Doppler represents the velocity and direction of blood flow in color, superimposed on a black-and-white 2D image. In effect, the color is displayed within a very large sample volume superimposed on the 2D image. Blood flow away from the transducer is shown in blue, and blood flow toward the transducer is displayed in red ("BART:" blue away, red toward). Disturbed or turbulent flow may be displayed in green or yellow. Aliasing may also occur in color flow Doppler.

Tissue Doppler Imaging

- More sophisticated machines may include facilities for recording the velocity of myocardial motion. The signals reflected by the moving myocardium are high amplitude, but low velocity. These myocardial velocities can be displayed in spectral format, as a color display, or as color M-mode. It is believed that TDI indices may have advantages over conventional echocardiographic indices, because they may be less influenced by loading conditions.

Applications

- Doppler echocardiography is most often used to characterize abnormal direction or velocity of blood flow, or to indicate the origin of turbulent blood flow. This is invaluable in valve disease or congenital heart disease, but Doppler echocardiography may also be used to estimate flow volumes, to assess systolic and diastolic function, and to obtain information about intracardiac pressures.
- *Abnormal blood flow direction* may be noted with conditions such as valvular insufficiency.
- *Abnormal blood flow velocity* may be a clinically useful finding, as the velocity of blood flow across an orifice is chiefly determined by the difference in pressure. If there is a large difference in the pressures in the chambers on each side of a valve, then the velocity of flow across the valve will be high. For example, during systole the pressure in the left ventricle is very high, and the pressure in the left atrium is very low. If the mitral valve is incompetent and regurgitation occurs, then the velocity of the regurgitant jet traveling from the left ventricle to the left atrium will be very high, reflecting the large difference in pressures.

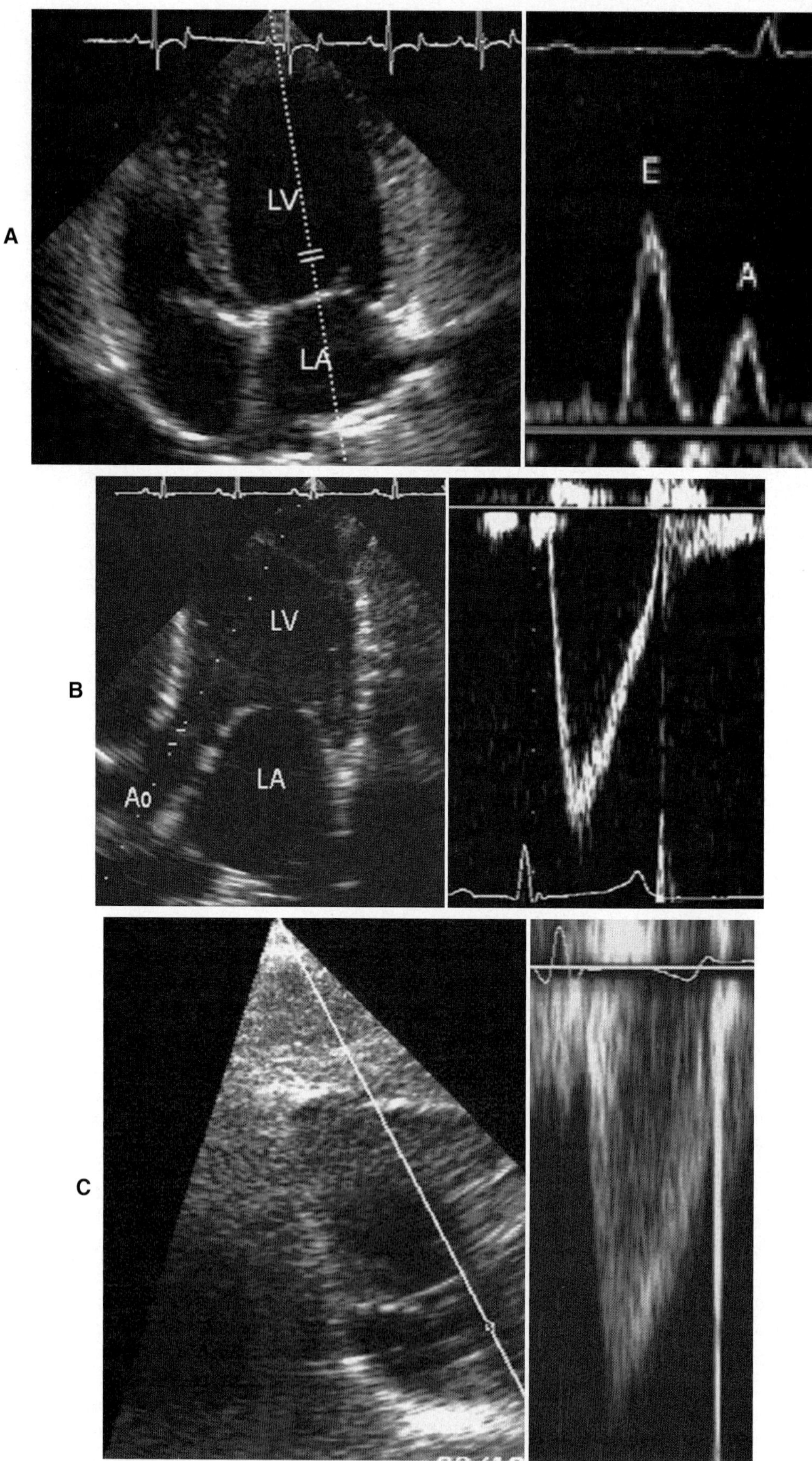
A
LV
LA
E
A
B
LV
LA
Ao
C

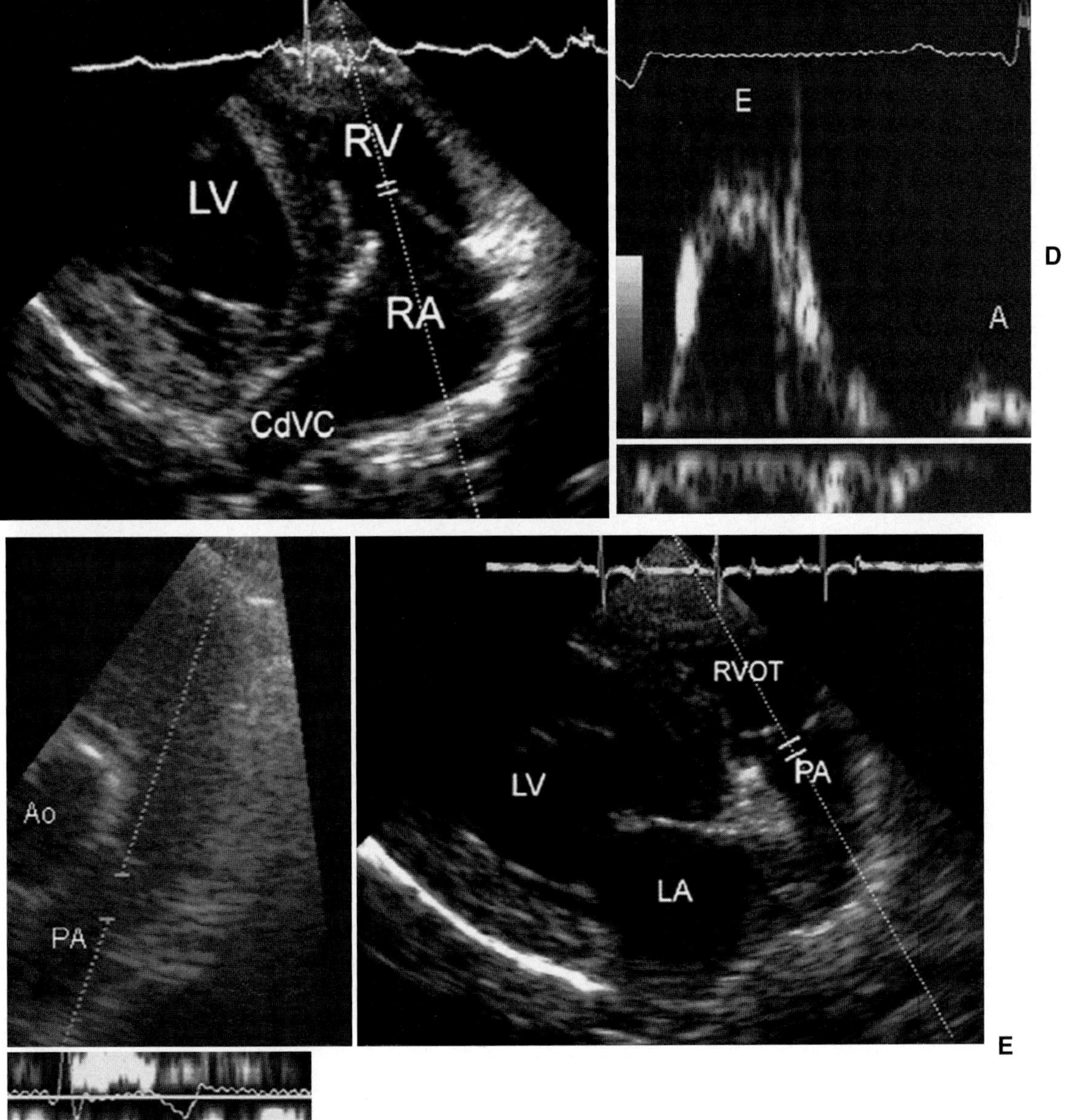

Figure 4-3. Doppler echocardiographic studies. **A,** Mitral inflow obtained from the left caudal parasternal (apical) four-chamber view, with the cursor placed parallel with mitral inflow, and a small sample volume placed at the tips of the mitral valve leaflets when the mitral valve is open. The typical spectral Doppler waveform of mitral inflow displays an early diastolic *(E)* wave and an atrial contraction *(A)* wave of filling. **B,** Aortic flow obtained from the left caudal parasternal (apical) "five-chamber" view, showing left ventricular outflow tract and placement of pulsed wave sample volume in ascending aorta. The typical spectral Doppler waveform of aortic flow is displayed. **C,** Aortic flow obtained from the subcostal view, showing continuous wave cursor positioned in ascending aorta. The typical spectral Doppler waveform of aortic flow is displayed. **D,** Tricuspid valve flow obtained the left cranial parasternal view optimized for right ventricular inflow. The pulsed wave sample volume is placed at the tricuspid leaflet tips, with the probe in a cranial position. The spectral waveform is similar to that of mitral inflow, although sometimes an additional systolic forward flow wave is recorded. **E,** Pulmonary artery flow from the right parasternal short-axis view optimized for right ventricular outflow (left panel) with the pulsed wave sample volume positioned in the main pulmonary artery, and from the left cranial parasternal view optimized for the pulmonary artery (middle panel). The typical spectral Doppler waveform of pulmonary artery flow is displayed. *LA,* Left atrium; *LV,* left ventricle; *RA,* right atrium; *RV,* right ventricle; *CdCV,* caudal vena cava; *Ao,* aorta; *RVOT,* right ventricular outflow tract; *PA,* pulmonary artery.

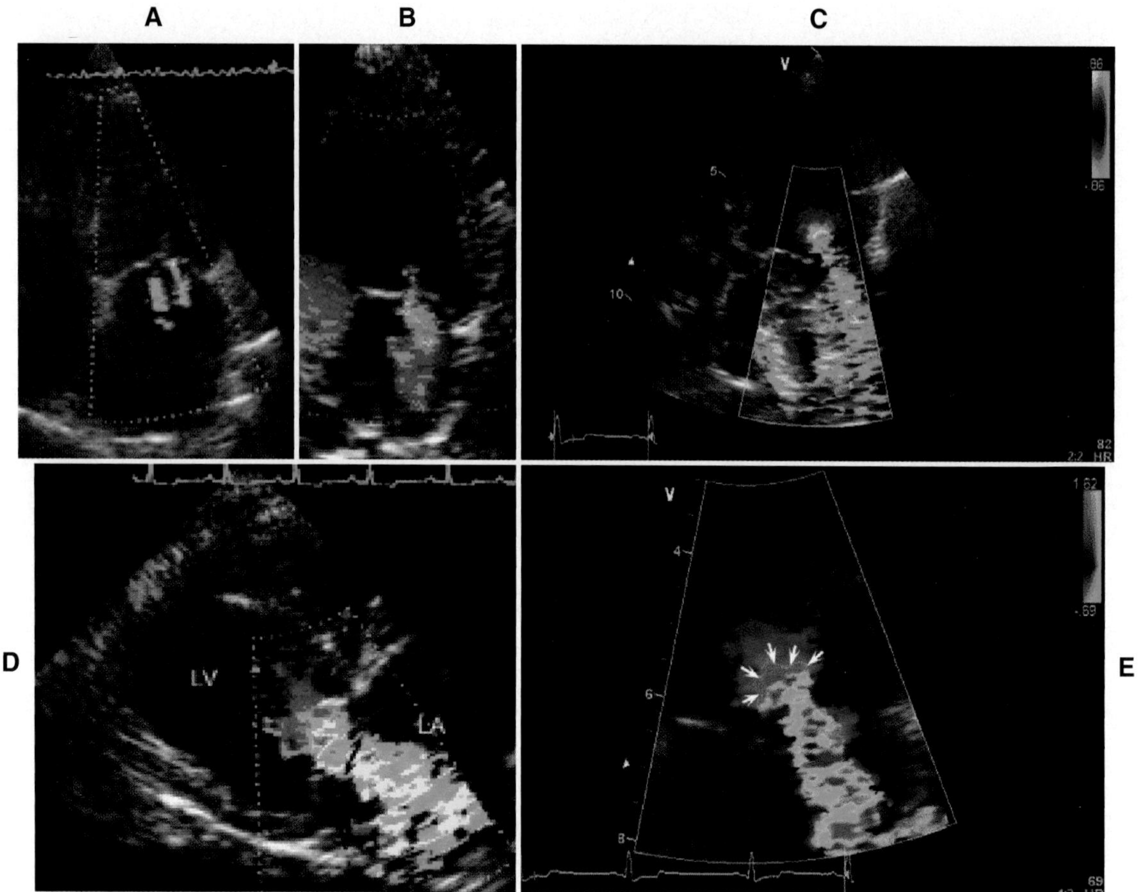

Figure 4-4. Color flow echocardiographic studies of mitral regurgitation. **A,** Mild mitral regurgitation. The color jet occupies < 20% of the left atrial area. **B,** Moderate mitral regurgitation. The color mitral regurgitation jet occupies 20% to 40% of the left atrial area. **C,** Severe mitral regurgitation. The color jet occupies > 40% of the left atrial area (the jet is rebounding from the dorsal LA wall in red), the vena contracta is wide, and a proximal flow convergence region can be seen. **D,** Right parasternal long-axis view of a dog with severe mitral regurgitation, showing a large vena contracta width *(black arrow)*. **E,** Left apical view of a dog with severe mitral regurgitation, showing a large proximal flow convergence region. The white arrows indicate the borders of the hemisphere where aliasing is occurring. The larger the hemisphere's diameter for a particular aliasing velocity (in this case 69 cm/s), the more severe the mitral insufficiency.

Conversely, for much of diastole, the pressure in the left atrium is only slightly higher than the pressure in the left ventricle, so the velocity of the early filling (E) wave is fairly low. This velocity information can therefore be used to derive information about intracardiac pressures.

- *Turbulent blood flow* is relatively uncommon in the normal heart, but when present, is most likely to occur where velocity is highest (i.e., within the aorta). Even in a normal heart, vigorous ejection into the aorta can sometimes result in signal aliasing on color Doppler. Blood flow will be turbulent whenever velocity is high, and valvular insufficiency or stenosis almost inevitably results in turbulent blood flow. Turbulent blood flow may be displayed in a different color (green/yellow) or color distribution (mosaic pattern); this is termed *variance*. In most cases, turbulent flow will be present when a murmur is audible, making Doppler echocardiography particularly useful in conditions where a murmur is present.
- *Estimation of flow volumes* is possible using Doppler echocardiography combined with 2D measurements. Flow is the product of cross-sectional area multiplied by the area under the spectral Doppler curve (velocity time integral).
- *Assessment of pressure gradients* is possible using the modified Bernoulli equation, where $[4 \times (\text{blood flow velocity})^2]$ gives the difference in pressure across a valve or between chambers.
- *Diastolic dysfunction* can also be assessed with Doppler echocardiography, although many measurements are influenced by loading conditions. Evaluation of transmitral and pulmonary venous flow in conjunction with TDI indices can suggest abnormal left ventricular (LV) relaxation and filling pressures.

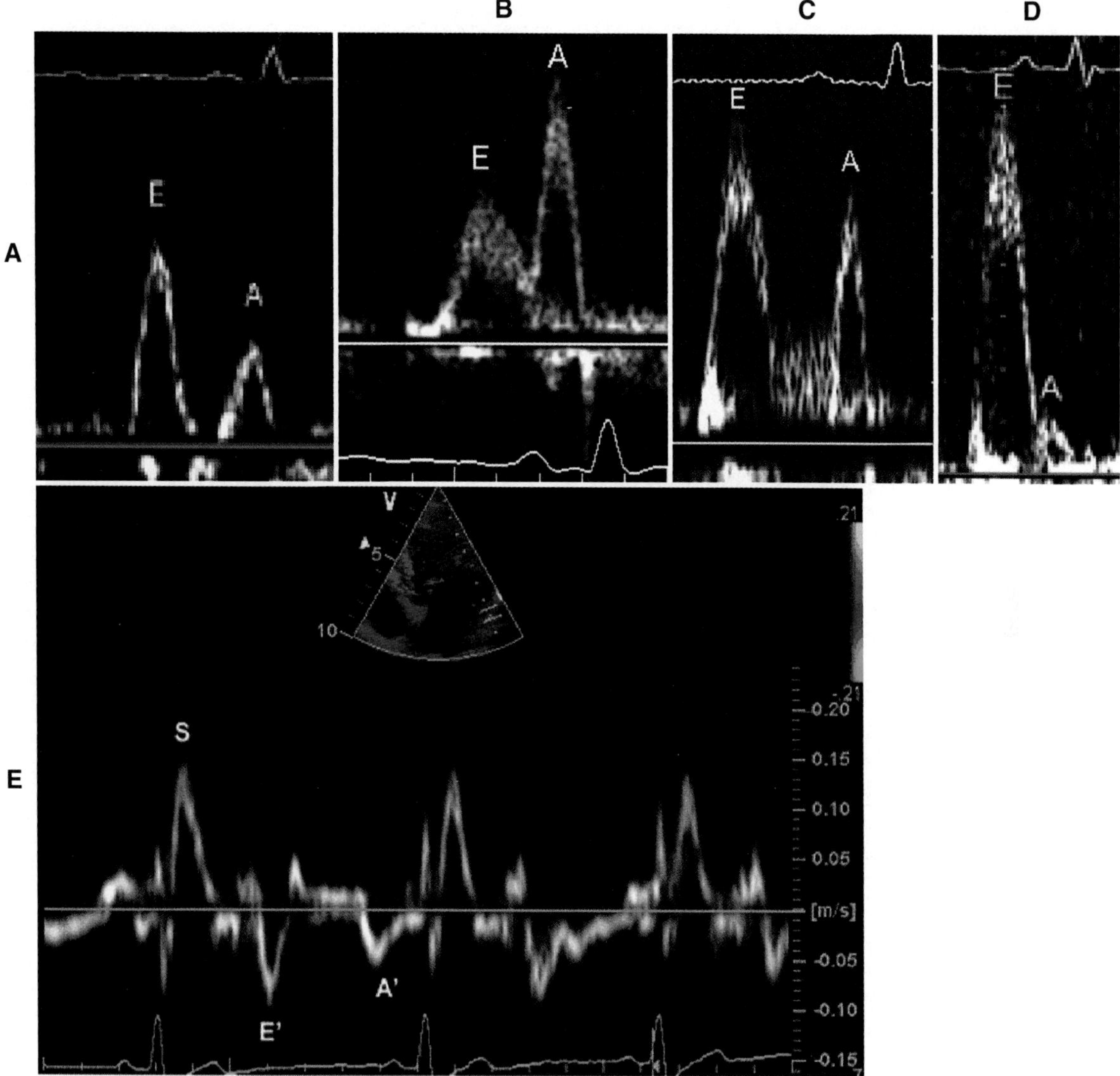

Figure 4-5. Echocardiographic evaluation of ventricular diastolic function. **A,** Normal transmitral flow pattern demonstrating an early filling wave *(E)* with higher velocity than the atrial contraction wave *(A)*. **B,** Delayed relaxation transmitral flow pattern demonstrating reduced amplitude and prolonged duration of the E wave. **C,** Pseudonormal transmitral flow pattern demonstrating a normal E:A velocity ratio, but this is the result of the combined effects of delayed relaxation, increased LA pressures and increased LV stiffness. **D,** Restrictive transmitral flow pattern. High LA pressures result in increased E wave amplitude despite delayed relaxation. Decreased LV compliance (sometimes with atrial systolic dysfunction) results in a diminished A wave. **E,** Pulsed wave tissue Doppler (TDI) image of mitral annulus velocity, displaying a systolic wave *(S)*, early diastolic wave *(E')* and atrial wave *(A')*.

ECHOCARDIOGRAPHIC TECHNIQUE

Equipment

Echocardiographic Machines

- Echo machines are becoming increasingly affordable for many practices. Almost all machines have appropriate software for cardiac measurements and will be capable of 2D and M-mode imaging. Many machines will also have Doppler capabilities, with spectral and CW as well as color Doppler. Image quality remains the most important feature, although this will also be affected by the choice of transducer. High-end machines may have additional options such as TDI or even 3D echocardiography.

Transducers

- Linear scanners are unsuitable for echocardiography because of the limited acoustic window available between ribs.
- Sector probes produce a fan-shaped arc of ultrasound waves, and so they will provide a wide image of the far field from a small acoustic window. These are ideal for cardiac applications.

- Types of sector probes include:
  - *Mechanical* transducers, where the crystal is oscillated back and forth to produce the arc-shaped ultrasound beam. These are more common with basic machines.
  - *Curvilinear* probes are similar to linear probes, but have a rounded surface. They tend to produce good images when the footprint is placed between ribs, but rib shadows are a problem when they are rotated through 90°.
  - *Phased array* transducers are also available and have an array of crystals that are electronically fired in sequence to produce the fan-shaped wavefront. They are more expensive, but they have better beam focusing.
- Some commercially available transducers have a wide frequency bandwidth that allows a single probe to operate at more than one frequency, for example, 2.5 and 3.5 MHz, or 5 and 7.5 MHz.
- Higher-end machines may have *harmonic imaging*, which results in a better signal to noise ratio.

KEY POINT

Low-frequency transducers have high penetrating power but poor resolution. They produce better Doppler signals.

High-frequency transducers have low penetrating power but high resolution. The higher the frequency, the better the imaging (providing the tissue can be penetrated and signal strength is adequate).

The Echo Table

- The majority of echocardiographers position animals in lateral recumbency and approach from underneath, with the probe on the dependent chest wall. This minimizes air artifact in the lung tissue between the probe and the heart. The ideal table will have a wedge-shaped cut-out rather than a circular hole, and should be covered with a comfortable but hygienic surface.

Patient Preparation

Clipping

- Most dogs will need to be clipped for echocardiography. In some short-coated breeds and cats, good acoustic contact may be obtained with liberal use of alcohol and acoustic gel (but check first that the transducer used is not damaged by alcohol).

Sedation

- The ideal is to echo patients without sedation, but a sedated patient may be better than a restless one, because it can be impossible to obtain the necessary images without adequate patient cooperation. A reasonable compromise for most canine and feline patients is a combination of low-dose acepromazine and an opiate. This may have a mild effect on some blood flow velocities, but is less likely to affect cardiac dimensions and will not affect lesions. General anesthesia and alpha-2 agonists will affect systolic function and may affect ventricular dimensions.

Electrocardiography

- An ECG should be obtained simultaneously. ECGs allow a much longer time period of screening for arrhythmias than would be normally practicable with an ECG machine and a paper trace. An ECG also allows accurate timing of measurements. Adhesive ECG electrodes are more comfortable than traditional alligator clips and can be attached with tape or bandage, and electrical contact can be maintained by using additional alcohol, if necessary.

ECHOCARDIOGRAPHIC VIEWS

Two-Dimensional Imaging

- It is worthwhile to adopt a consistent technique so that the same views are obtained in the same sequence with each study. Some views may be more difficult to obtain in some patients. The most commonly used imaging planes are obtained with the transducer on the right side of the chest (right parasternal views; see Figure 4-1). Views obtained from the left apical windows (caudal and cranial left parasternal views; see Figure 4-3) are mainly used for Doppler echocardiography applications, but as with radiography, it is helpful to confirm lesions in more than one view.

Doppler Imaging

- Most Doppler recordings can be made from the left parasternal views, with the subcostal view preferred for aortic velocities. Color Doppler used in the right parasternal views can be used for screening for mitral and aortic insufficiency. The features of blood flow across each valve are listed in the following sections. Normal values for blood flow velocity are derived from several studies (See reference list) and are summarized below.

Pulmonary Artery Flow

- Recorded from the right parasternal short-axis view or the left cranial parasternal position (see Figure 4-3, *E*). Both should be recorded, in an attempt to record the highest velocity. A large sample volume should be used to minimize aliasing.
- There is usually one single systolic envelope, away from the transducer, with peak velocities < 1.5 m/s.
- There may be some positive flow (toward the transducer) during diastole associated with pulmonic insufficiency. A small amount of pulmonic insufficiency is common in healthy dogs and *is usually considered a normal finding*.

Aortic Flow

- Recorded from the left caudal parasternal (apical) 5 chamber (see Figure 4-3, *B*) or from the subcostal position (see Figure 4-3, *C*). The subcostal view usually allows the best alignment with flow. A large sample volume should be used to minimize aliasing.
- There should be one single systolic envelope, away from the transducer, with peak velocities < 1.7 m/s (left caudal parasternal view) or < 2.0 m/s (subcostal).

Mitral Inflow

- Recorded from the apical four- or two-chamber view (see Figure 4-3, *A*). As small a sample volume as possible should be used, with the sample volume placed at the leaflet tips during diastole.
- Two peaks of flow are generally recorded, corresponding to early passive filling at the start of diastole (the E wave: 0.5 to 1.0 m/s) and filling across the mitral valve during atrial contraction (the A wave: 0.3 to 0.6 m/s).

Tricuspid Inflow

- Tricuspid flow is recorded one or two intercostal spaces cranial to the position for mitral inflow (see Figure 4-3, *D*). As small a sample volume as possible should be used.
- Two peaks of flow are recorded, corresponding to early passive filling at the start of diastole (the E wave: 0.3 to 0.9 m/s) and filling across the tricuspid valve during atrial contraction (the A wave: 0.3 to 0.6 m/s). In addition, a systolic forward wave is sometimes recorded corresponding to vena caval inflow.

ECHOCARDIOGRAPHIC MEASUREMENTS

- Echocardiography is ideally suited to identification of structural lesions, but quantitative assessment of cardiac dimensions and function is also important. Echocardiography allows quantification of chamber dimensions, systolic and diastolic performance, valve function and hemodynamic estimates (e.g., intracardiac pressures).

Chamber Dimensions

- LV diameter
- LV wall thickness
- Left atrial (LA) and aortic dimensions

Left Ventricular Diameter

- LV diameter is typically measured from M-mode images (see Figures 4-2, *A*, and 4-6, *A*).

M Mode Measurement Technique

- Measure from “leading edge” to “leading edge”
- Diastolic measurements made at onset of QRS (LVDd)
- Systolic measurements made at peak excursion (LVDs)
- Average several beats, particularly if the rhythm is irregular

Problems with Left Ventricular Dimension Measurements

- Poor alignment may result in diameter inaccuracies
- Difficulties in establishing normal values for a widely varying canine population
- One suggestion is to divide every measurement by the aortic diameter in the same animal—this should “normalize” for body size, although normal reference ranges derived for specific breeds are the ideal.

Index of Sphericity

- One solution to the problem of identifying LV dilation (eccentric hypertrophy) in a wide range of breeds is to measure the long axis from a 2D image and divide by the M-mode LV diameter, as LV dilation usually results in a more spherical chamber (due to a bigger increase in diameter than length). The LV length: diameter ratio should be > 1.65.

Left Ventricular Wall Thickness

- This is more important in cats than in dogs, as detection of LV hypertrophy is an important clinical goal in feline myocardial disease. In cats, M-mode imaging planes may miss localized areas of hypertrophy, or erroneously include papillary muscles, so that wall thickness may be best measured from 2D images. 2D echocardiography has the advantage of allowing measurements irrespective of the location of hypertrophy.

KEY POINT

Measurements *must* be made at end-diastole, when the walls are at their thinnest. There is a risk of overestimating wall thickness from 2D images with machines with slow frame rates.

Left Atrial Diameter

- LA size can be estimated from M-mode, 2D short axis, or 2D long axis.

M-Mode Measurements

- The aortic diameter is measured in diastole (Ao), and the LA diameter is measured in systole. The LA:Ao ratio should be approximately 1.0, but in many dogs alignment is difficult, so that the left auricle is measured rather than the left atrium. In cats, the cursor is more likely to cross the main body of the LA rather than the auricle, so that M-mode measurements may more accurately reflect LA size than in dogs (see Figures 4-2, *C*, and 4-6, *C*).

Two-Dimensional Measurements

- ***Short axis:*** the LA:Ao ratio should be < 1.6. Measurements are usually made in diastole. There can be problems avoiding pulmonary veins, and the LA size may vary throughout diastole (Figure 4-7, *A*).
- ***Long axis:*** the LA:Ao ratio should be < 2.5, where the aortic diameter is measured from a right parasternal long-axis view at the valve level during systole (Figure 4-1, *B,* and 4-7, *B*).
- In cats, there is no need to normalize the LA diameter to the aortic diameter; absolute diameter should be < 1.6 cm (note, however, that this is a technically difficult view to achieve in cats).

Systolic Function

- Many different echocardiographic measurements can be made to assess systolic performance, but virtually all are affected by loading conditions.

Left Ventricular Fractional Shortening

- LV fractional shortening (FS%) is the most commonly used echo index of systolic function (Figure 4-8, *A*).
- Calculated using the following formula: $FS\% = [(LVDd - LVDs) / LVDd] \times 100$
- FS% will increase with improved contractility, increased preload, or decreased afterload, and only assesses shortening in the minor axis dimension.
- Normal reported *mean* values range from 25% to 39% or 40%. Note that individual normal dogs may have values less than 25%.

E Point to Septal Separation

- E point to septal separation (EPSS) may be increased with reduced systolic function. It is unreliable in the presence of mitral stenosis or aortic regurgitation.
- Measured from an M-mode recording at the mitral valve level as the distance between the septum and peak opening of the anterior mitral valve leaflet (see Figure 4-6, *B*).
- Normal reported mean values range from 5 mm to 8 mm in giant breeds.

End-Systolic Volume Index

- End-systolic volume index (ESVI) should be measured from 2D images, *not* from indices derived from M-mode such as with the Teichholz formula
- Endocardial borders of left ventricle are traced in a right parasternal long-axis or left caudal parasternal view, and an area-length formula or modified Simpson's rule are generally used to calculate LV volumes (see Figure 4-8, *B*).
- ESVI is end-systolic volume divided by body surface area
- Normal ESVI is often quoted as 30 ml/m^2, although this value has been extrapolated from human reference ranges and relationship with bodyweight may not be linear.

Ejection Fraction

- Calculation of LV volumes allows calculation of ejection fraction (EF%).

  $EF\% = [(\text{end-diastolic volume} - \text{end-systolic volume}) / \text{end-diastolic volume}] \times 100$

- Normal EF% in dogs is 50% to 65%

Systolic Time Intervals

- The ratio of pre-ejection period (PEP) and LV ejection time (LVET) is another global index of systolic function, and can be measured from the spectral Doppler aortic velocity waveform (see Figure 4-8, *C*). Normal PEP/LVET should be < 0.40.

Diastolic Function

- Diastolic function is complex: clinically relevant aspects of diastolic function include LV relaxation, LV compliance, LA pressures, LA systolic function and heart rate and rhythm. Clearly, no single echocardiographic measurement will provide a complete overview of diastolic function. However, a range of Doppler measurements can be used to give a composite assessment of diastolic function or highlight specific aspects, and Doppler echocardiography has become the technique of choice for evaluation of diastolic function in human patients.

Transmitral Flow

- Transmitral flow reflects the instantaneous pressure gradient across the mitral valve. There is a progressive change in the ventricular filling pattern with advancing disease across a range of underlying cardiac diseases (see Figure 4-5, *A* through *D*). The principal difficulty with use of transmitral flow patterns is the confounding effect of a "pseudonormal" phase, where the transmitral flow pattern is similar to that seen in the normal animal. Transmitral flow patterns should therefore be interpreted in the context of other clinical and echocardiographic findings. Pulmonary venous flow patterns and Doppler tissue imaging of mitral annular velocities (see Figure 4-5, *E*) have been used to distinguish pseudonormal filling from normal.

Valve Function

- Color Doppler can be used as a quick screen for valve function, but caution should be used in determining severity of valvular regurgitation on regurgitant jet size alone, or in relying on the presence of turbulent signals to identify valvular stenosis.

Mitral Insufficiency

- 2D echocardiography should be used to determine whether the underlying cause of mitral insufficiency is structural valve disease or whether the mitral regurgitation is functional (i.e., secondary to diseases such as dilated cardiomyopathy [DCM]). Functional mitral regurgitation often results in a central jet, whereas the jet is often eccentric or multiple with myxomatous valve disease.

Mitral insufficiency can be graded as mild, moderate, or severe (see Figure 4-4, *A* through *C*). The grade of mitral regurgitation can be assumed to be severe when the following criteria are present:

- Large regurgitant jet area compared with LA area
- Increased width of the vena contracta (see Figure 4-4, *D*)
- Presence of large proximal flow convergence region (see Figure 4-4, *E*)
- High-intensity CW spectral Doppler signal
- Increased mitral E wave velocity
- Chamber remodeling (dilated left atrium or left ventricle)
- Similar principles apply to tricuspid regurgitation.

Aortic Insufficiency

Less common than mitral insufficiency, aortic insufficiency is considered severe when the following criteria are present:

- Large insufficiency jet size compared with LV area
- Increased width of vena contracta
- Rapid deceleration of aortic insufficiency spectral Doppler signal

Aortic and Pulmonic Stenosis

- The severity of aortic or pulmonic stenosis is generally assessed in terms of the magnitude of the pressure gradient across the stenosis.

Assessment of Pressure Gradients

- Pressure gradients (PGs) across a valve or between chambers can be estimated by using the modified *Bernoulli equation* (Figure 4-9).

$$PG(\text{in mm Hg}) = 4 \times (V^2)$$

where V = velocity of blood flow distal to the orifice (m/s). For example, if the velocity in the aorta is 5 m/s, then the pressure gradient can be estimated as $4 \times (5^2)$, or $4 \times 25 = 100$ mm Hg.

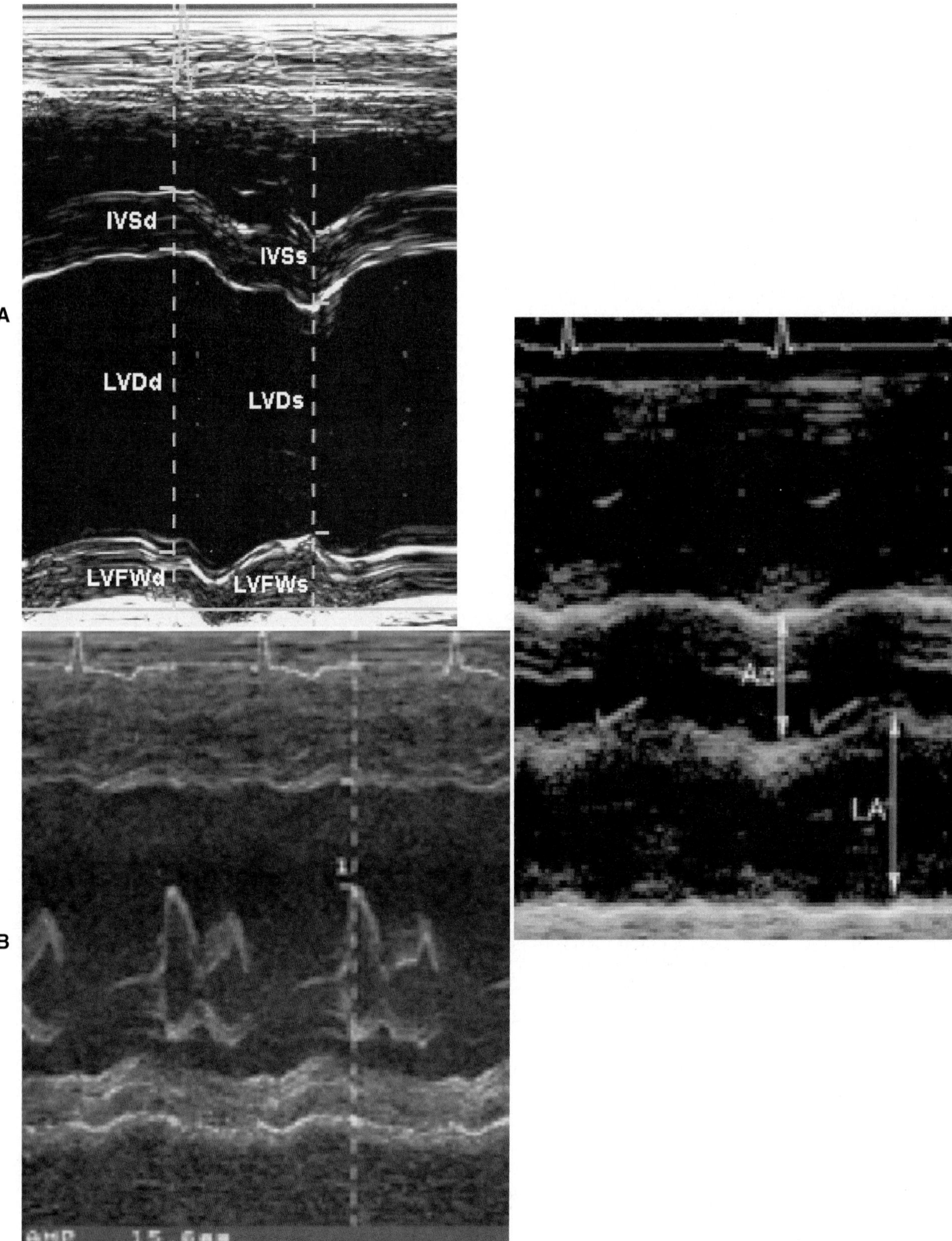

Figure 4-6. M-mode measurements of the left heart and aorta. **A,** M-mode at chordal level, showing measurements at end-diastole (onset of QRS) and end-systole (peak septal motion). Septal thickness in diastole *(IVSd)*, left ventricular diameter in diastole *(LVDd)*, left ventricular free wall in diastole *(LVFWd)*, septal thickness in systole *(IVSs)*, left ventricular diameter in systole *(LVDs)*, left ventricular free wall in systole *(LVFWs)*. **B,** M-mode measurements at mitral valve level, showing an increased E-point to septal separation *(EPSS)* of 15.6 mm. **C,** M-mode measurements at the atrial and aorta level showing measurement of left atrial *(LA)* and aortic *(Ao)* diameter.

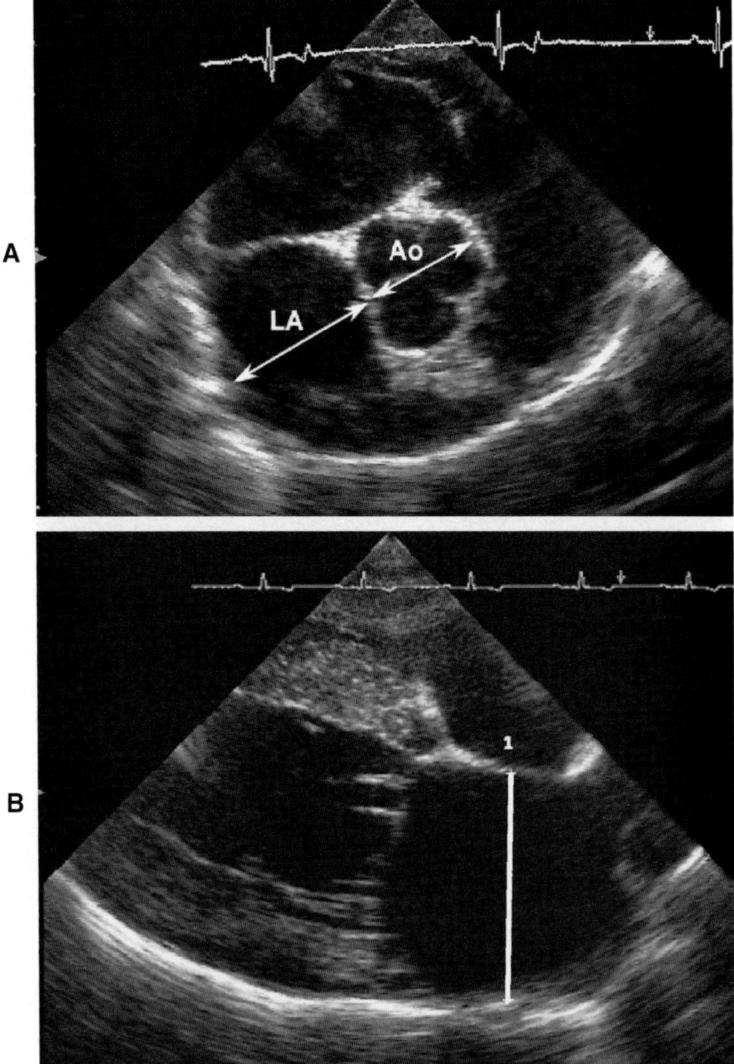

Figure 4-7. Measurement of the left atrial *(LA)* and aortic *(Ao)* diameters from the right parasternal short-axis view **(A)** and LA diameter from the right long-axis view optimized for the left ventricular inlet **(B)**.

COMMON ACQUIRED CARDIAC CONDITIONS

Degenerative (Myxomatous) Mitral Valve Disease

- Degenerative mitral valve disease (endocardiosis) must be distinguished from mitral infectious endocarditis, although this generally occurs in dogs with a different signalment and presenting signs, as well as differing subtly in lesion morphology.

Two-Dimensional Changes

- Thickened, distorted mitral leaflets (Figure 4-10)
- The mitral valve motion is usually abnormal—often with prolapse or flail with chordal rupture
- Dilation of LA and LV
- The LV systolic function usually appears hyperdynamic (see Figure 4-8, *A*)
- Tricuspid valve may also be affected, with prolapse or flail leaflets sometimes seen

KEY POINT

Infectious endocarditis usually does not result in mitral valve prolapse and is more likely to result in oscillating focal vegetations than degenerative mitral valve disease.

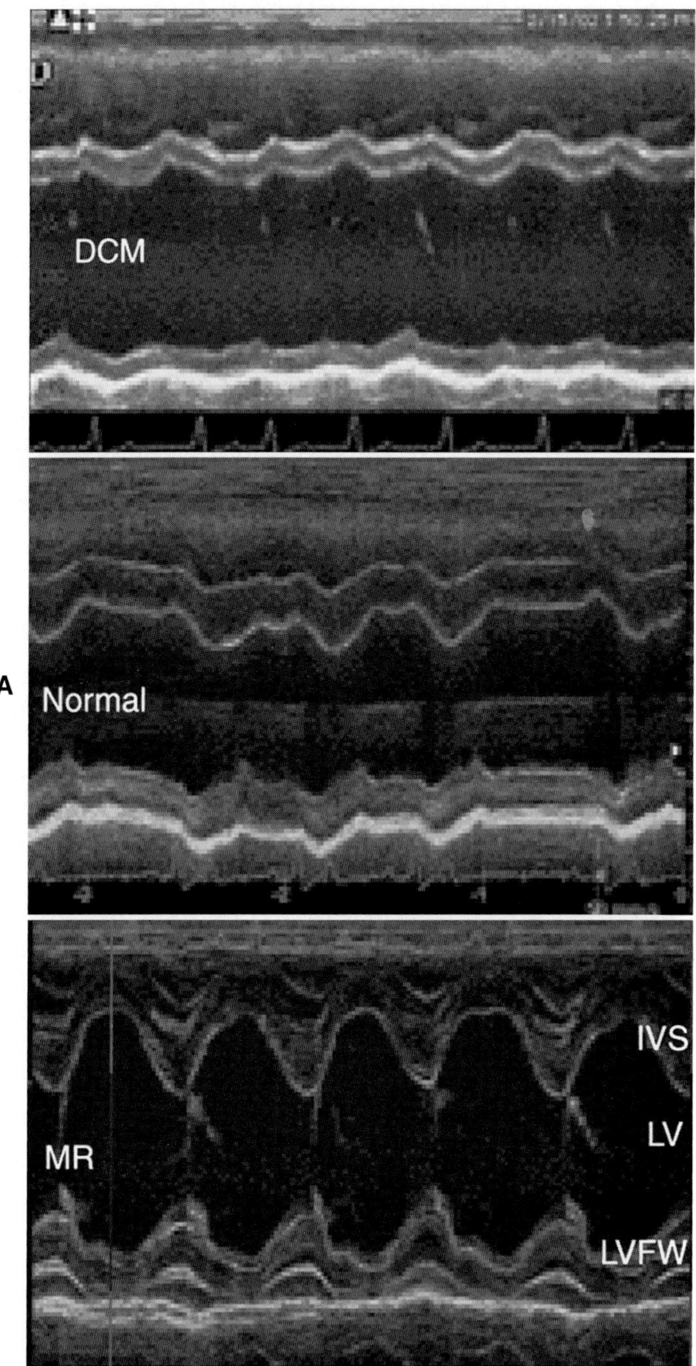

Figure 4-8. Echocardiographic evaluation of ventricular systolic function. **A,** M-mode of ventricular hypokinesis from a dog with dilated cardiomyopathy *(DCM) (left panel),* normal ventricular motion from a healthy dog *(middle panel),* and ventricular hyperkinesis from a dog with mitral regurgitation *(MR) (right panel).*

Continued

Dilated Cardiomyopathy

- Overt DCM is a relatively easy diagnosis to make, with global hypokinesis of a dilated heart in the absence of any other lesions (Figure 4-11). Occult DCM may be more difficult, and caution is required in diagnosing DCM in asymptomatic dogs on the basis of a low fractional shortening value alone (especially in dogs of nonpredisposed breeds).
- Dilation of LA and LV
- ± Dilation of RA and RV
- LV hypokinesis (↓ FS%, EF%)
- ↑ EPSS

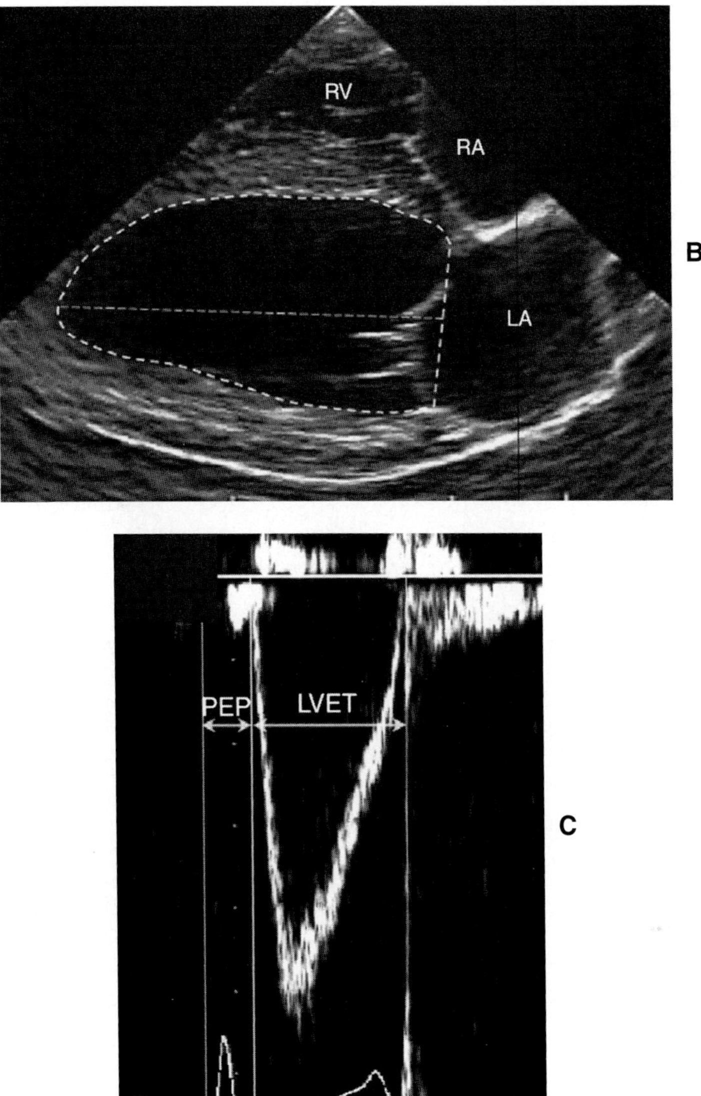

Figure 4-8. Cont'd. B, Measurement of left ventricular volume from a right parasternal long-axis view. The endocardial borders are traced, with the left ventricular length measured from a line drawn across the mitral annulus to the apex. *LA,* Left atrium; *RA,* right atrium; *RV,* right ventricle. **C,** Spectral Doppler aortic blood flow velocity, showing preejection period *(PEP)* and LV ejection time *(LVET)*.

Hypertrophic Cardiomyopathy

- Feline hypertrophic cardiomyopathy (HCM) is very common, and a spectrum of disease exists. Severe HCM is easy to diagnose (Figure 4-12), but mild HCM may be very difficult (focal hypertrophy may be the only recognizable feature that distinguishes mild HCM from a normal heart with a functional murmur).
- Septal or free wall thickness in diastole > 6.0 mm on 2D and/or M-mode
- LA may or may not be dilated (depending on degree of hemodynamic compromise)
- Systolic anterior motion of the mitral valve often present (hypertrophic obstructive cardiomyopathy)
- Thrombus or spontaneous echocontrast ("smoke") may be present in left auricle

Pericardial Disease

- *Pericardial effusions* can be identified as an echo-free space around the heart, although they may be confused with pleural effusions. Tamponade may be suggested by collapse of the right atrial wall. The heart may be affected by a number of different neoplasms which can result in pericardial effusions, and these may be best imaged while some pericardial fluid is present.

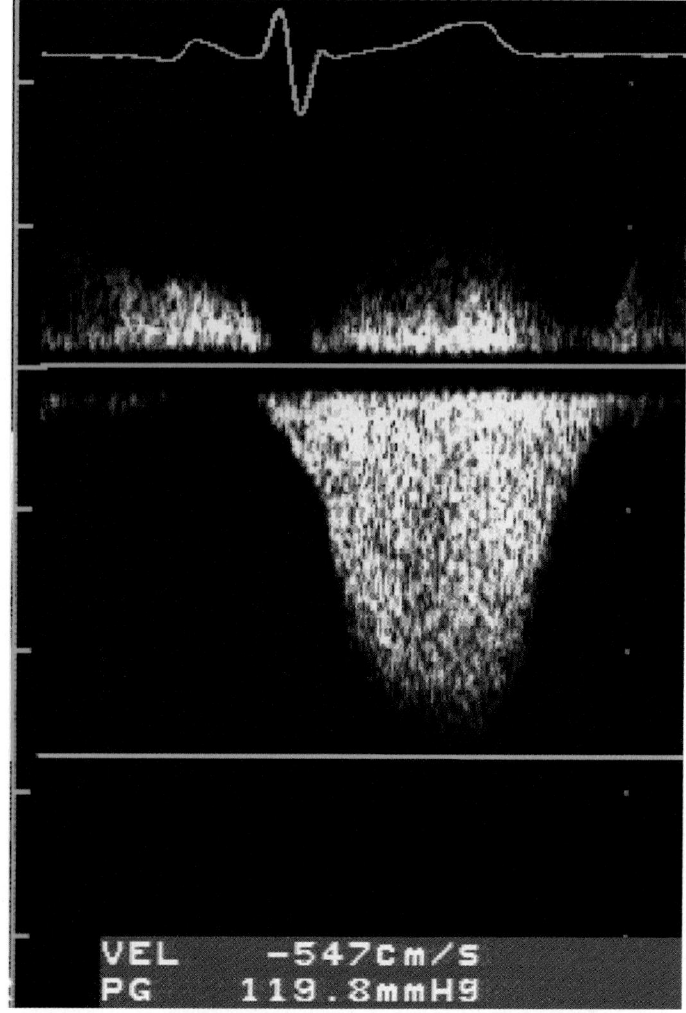

Figure 4-9. CW spectral Doppler recording of high-velocity flow in pulmonary artery in a dog with severe pulmonic stenosis. The measured peak velocity of 5.47 m/s corresponds with a pressure gradient of 119.8 mm Hg across the pulmonic valve.

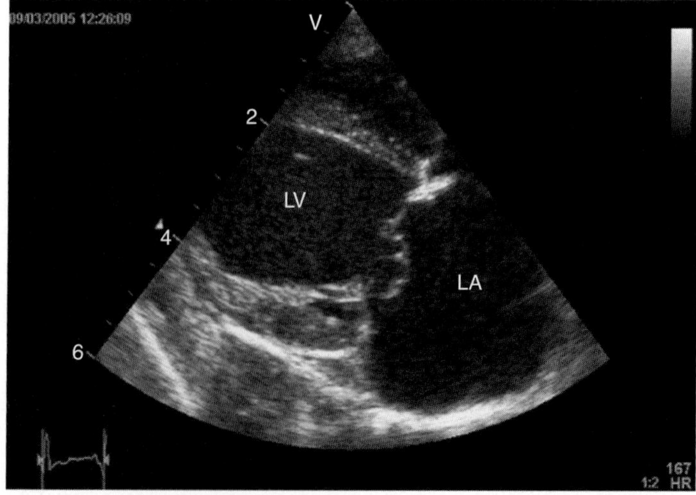

Figure 4-10. Right parasternal long-axis view of dog with myxomatous mitral valve disease, showing thickened, distorted mitral leaflets with prolapse of the anterior leaflet.

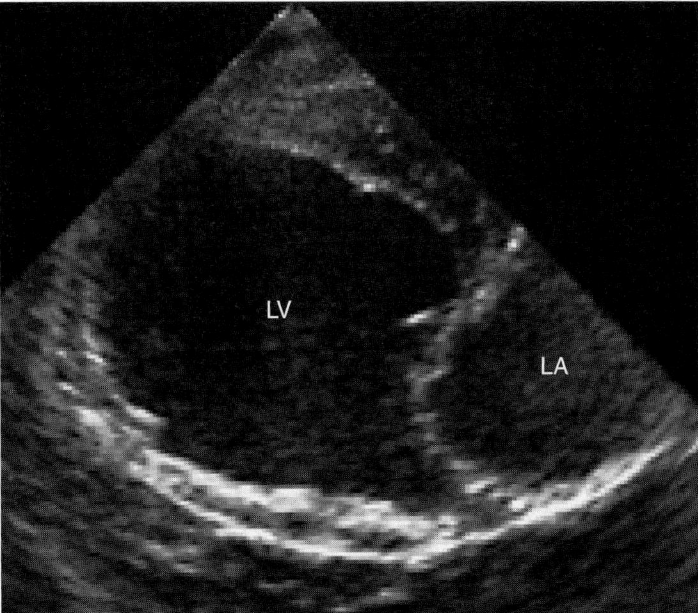

Figure 4-11. Right parasternal long-axis view of a dog with dilated cardiomyopathy, showing a rounded LV with normal mitral valve morphology (and no mitral valve prolapse).

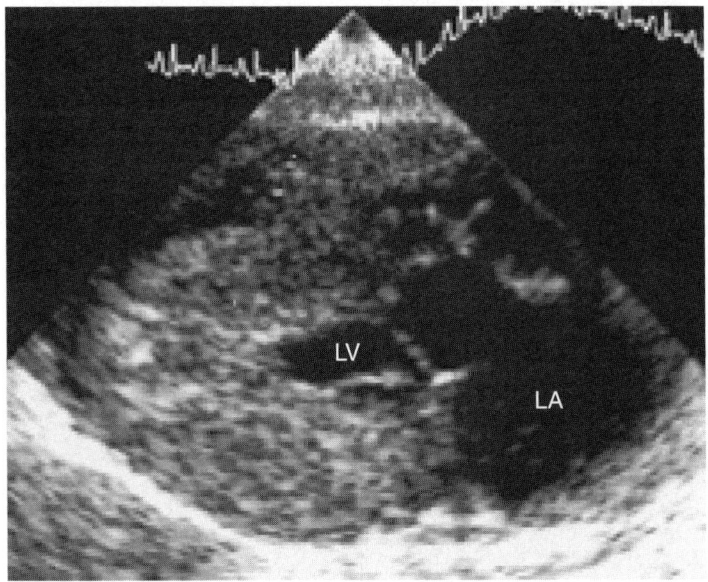

Figure 4-12. Right parasternal long-axis view of a cat with hypertrophic cardiomyopathy, showing marked LV hypertrophy.

- *Chemodectomas* generally involve the heart base and may be imaged as homogeneous soft tissue densities encircling the aortic and pulmonary artery roots. They may be associated with pericardial effusion.
- *Hemangiosarcomas* frequently affect the right atrium, although they can be very difficult to image at this site. They may also infiltrate other areas of the heart (such as the septum and ventricular walls) where they may have an irregular echotexture compared with surrounding myocardium. Right atrial hemangiosarcomas are often associated with pericardial effusions.

Frequently Asked Questions

1. *How can you tell when the left ventricle is dilated when there are no breed-specific normal reference values?*

   A. A number of approaches can be used when there are no breed-specific reference intervals. Reference intervals based simply on bodyweight are not reliable, because the relationship between LV dimensions and bodyweight is not linear. One solution has been to reference the LV diameter to another dimension, such as aortic diameter. An alternative solution is to look for signs of chamber remodeling. A decrease in the index of sphericity to < 1.65 would support a suspicion of LV dilation (eccentric hypertrophy).

2. *How does one interpret a low value for fractional shortening in an otherwise healthy dog?*

   A. Caution should be used when making a diagnosis of DCM in an asymptomatic dog based on a fractional shortening value < 25%. Multiple other variables should be assessed, including evidence of chamber dilation, any increase in end-systolic volume index, whether the EF% is also subnormal, and systolic time intervals (PEP/LVET). Guidelines have been proposed for a scoring scheme for diagnosis of DCM in asymptomatic dogs (see Dukes-McEwan J, et al. in Suggested Readings).

3. *Does an increased aortic blood flow velocity always indicate aortic stenosis?*

   A. A fixed LV outflow tract obstruction such as subaortic stenosis will result in increased blood flow velocity, with the velocity correlating with the severity of obstruction. The velocity recorded also depends on *flow*, so with increased blood flow, the velocity will be increased even without any decrease in LV outflow tract diameter. An extreme example is the increased aortic blood flow velocity often recorded with patent ductus arteriosus, where the left-to-right shunting across the ductus leads to an increased volume of blood flowing through the aortic valve, sometimes resulting in dramatically elevated aortic velocities (which return to normal after ductal ligation). Other conditions with increased stroke volume (e.g., anemia, bradycardias) may also result in increased aortic blood flow velocity. A diagnosis of subaortic stenosis is supported by the presence of anatomic lesions imaged with 2D echocardiography.

SUGGESTED READINGS

Bonagura JD, et al: Doppler echocardiography I: pulsed and continuous wave studies, Vet Clin N Am Small Anim Pract 28:1325, 1998.

Boon JA: Manual of veterinary echocardiography, Baltimore, 1998, Williams & Wilkins.

Brown DJ, Rush JE, MacGregor J, et al: M-mode echocardiographic ratio indices in normal dogs, cats, and horses: a novel quantitative method, J Vet Intern Med 17:653, 2003.

Brown DJ, et al: M-mode echocardiographic ratio indices in normal dogs, cats, and horses: a novel quantitative method, J Vet Intern Med 17:653, 2003.

Bussadori C, et al: Guidelines for the echocardiographic studies of suspected subaortic and pulmonic stenosis, J Vet Cardiol 2:17, 2000.

Dukes-McEwan J, Borgarelli M, Tidholm A, et al: Proposed guidelines for the diagnosis of canine idiopathic dilated cardiomyopathy, J Vet Cardiol 5:7, 2003.

Hansson K, Haggstrom J, Kvart C, et al: Left atrial to aortic root indices using two-dimensional and M-mode echocardiography in cavalier King Charles spaniels with and without left atrial enlargement, Vet Radiol Ultrasound 43:568, 2002.

O'Grady MR, Bonagura JD, Powers JD, et al: Quantitative cross-sectional echocardiography in the normal dog, Vet Radiol 27:34, 1986.

Thomas WP, Gaber CE, Jacobs G, et al: Recommendations for standards in transthoracic two-dimensional echocardiography in the dog and cat, J Vet Intern Med 7:247, 1993.

Yuill CDM, O'Grady MR: Doppler-derived velocity of blood flow across the cardiac valves in the normal dog, Can J Vet Res 55:185, 1991.

CHAPTER 5

Special Diagnostic Techniques for Evaluation of Cardiac Disease*

Meg M. Sleeper

INTRODUCTION

Many special diagnostic techniques are available for evaluation of animals with cardiovascular disease. Ambulatory electrocardiographic equipment is available through various services, continuous in-hospital electrocardiographic monitoring equipment is widely available, and several large diagnostic laboratories provide specialized clinical pathology services. Additionally, veterinary cardiology referral centers are increasingly available for special diagnostic techniques such as cardiac catheterization.

CONTINUOUS IN-HOSPITAL ELECTROCARDIOGRAPHIC MONITORING

Continuous electrocardiographic monitoring is recommended for hospitalized patients at risk of heart rate or rhythm disturbances. These patients include:

- Patients with congestive heart failure
- Patients hospitalized with clinical signs (e.g., syncope) secondary to arrhythmia
- Patients with systemic disease that puts them at risk for arrhythmias (e.g., shock, sepsis, gastric dilation-volvulus, etc.)

Technique

- Continuous electrocardiographic monitoring requires an ECG unit with an oscilloscope or light-emitting diode (LED) display.
- Use of a chest lead configuration with adhesive electrode patches will minimize artifacts on the tracing while allowing the patient the most freedom for mobility.
- Clip two 2- to 3-cm square areas at the left apex and the heart base (where the apex beat is palpable on the left chest and at the heart base caudal to the right or left scapula).
- Clean and de-fat the area with 70% isopropyl alcohol. Allow to dry.
- Place the positive electrode patch at the left apical site and the negative electrode at the heart base site. A ground electrode may be placed at either site (Figure 5-1).
- Apply a light chest wrap to secure the electrodes and wires.
- If a multiple-lead electrocardiographic (ECG) unit is being used, then use the left arm electrode for the positive electrode, the right arm electrode for the negative electrode lead, and lead I for display/recording.
- If the patient is recumbent and unlikely to move, leads attached directly to the patient limbs can be used.
- Depending on the unit available, the signal is transmitted to the machine by cables or by radiotelemetry.

*John Karl Goodwin contributed to previous versions of this chapter.

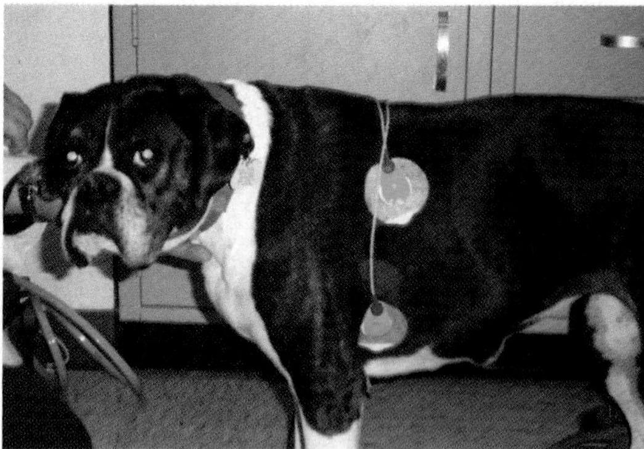

Figure 5-1. Chest lead preparation in a Boxer. The negative lead should be placed in the upper patch behind the scapula and the positive lead should be placed at the left apex (behind the elbow). This configuration can be used for in hospital continuous ECG monitoring or ambulatory monitoring.

- Many ECG units will print out an ECG strip, which can be added to the permanent patient record.

Limitations

- Excessive patient motion may result in displacement of electrodes or motion artifact in the ECG.
- Adhesive patches may occasionally result in contact dermatitis.

PROVOCATIVE ELECTROCARDIOGRAPHIC TECHNIQUES

In some patients, the history or baseline ECG is suggestive of pathologic arrhythmias, but a definitive diagnosis is elusive. In these cases, vagal stimulation or abolition may be informative. A provocative vagal maneuver will transiently elevate parasympathetic tone. In normal animals, the technique typically slows the heart rate or has no effect. However, when there is sinoatrial or atrioventricular (AV) nodal dysfunction, or an abnormal sensitivity to parasympathetic tone, transient sinus arrest or significant AV block may occur. Similarly, a vagal maneuver may be diagnostic and/or therapeutic for an ectopic supraventricular tachycardia. A sinus tachycardia typically slows over several seconds while an ectopic supraventricular tachycardia may terminate abruptly (see Frequently Asked Questions).

An ECG recorded immediately post exercise may demonstrate cardiac arrhythmias associated with increased sympathetic tone. Likewise, an atropine response test can be used to determine if a slow heart rate is associated with elevated vagal tone, as can occur with respiratory disease, gastrointestinal disease or neurologic disease, or is associated with primary cardiac conduction system disease. If the bradycardia is due to elevated vagal influence, then atropine administration or exercise will result in its abolition.

Vagal Maneuver

- The techniques listed below can be used for elevating vagal tone. The patient should be restrained and calm so that a good quality lead II ECG is obtained prior to and during the technique.

Ocular Pressure

- Moderately firm digital pressure is applied over the closed eyelid to one or both eyes for a period of 5 to 10 seconds or until significant slowing of the heart rate occurs.

Carotid Body Massage

- The carotid bodies are located in the area behind the larynx. Apply moderate digital pressure around the larynx while monitoring the ECG. Initiation of a gag response or a cough yields similar results and suggests adequate pressure has been applied.

Inhibition of Vagal Tone

- Two techniques are possible for abolishing vagal tone and are useful if the patient is suspected to have a vagally mediated bradycardia. With either technique, it is important to first obtain a baseline ECG.

Postexercise Electrocardiography

- Typically, strenuous leash running is used; however, the duration of exercise is not standardized. Evidence of exertion, such as panting, is sufficient to stop exercise and an immediate post-exercise ECG is obtained. A delay of as little as 30 seconds may alter results, and heavy panting can result in artifacts making the ECG difficult to interpret.

Atropine Response Test

- Atropine (0.04 mg/kg IV or IM) will result in abolition of vagal influence. An ECG should be obtained 10 to 15 minutes after administration of the drug for comparison with the baseline ECG.

Clinical Utility

Vagal Maneuver

Clinically useful in two scenarios:

- In the evaluation of dogs with a history of syncope, a vagal maneuver may demonstrate sinus arrest or AV block, suggestive of parasympathetic hypersensitivity or primary nodal disease.

- In dogs with tachycardia, abrupt termination of the arrhythmia with a vagal maneuver suggests an ectopic supraventricular origin because ventricular tachycardias are not usually sensitive to vagal tone; however, lack of response is not helpful in differentiating the origin of the tachycardia. The maneuver can also be useful to differentiate sinus tachycardia (no response or gradual slowing of heart rate) from pathologic ectopic supraventricular tachycardia (no responce or abrupt termination of tachycardia).

Postexercise Electrocardiography

- This test can be performed in the evaluation of dogs with subaortic stenosis or occult cardiomyopathy. In affected dogs, the combination of exercise, myocardial disease and left ventricular hypertrophy may result in electrocardiographic indicators of myocardial ischemia (i.e., ST segment depression or ventricular ectopy). Lack of response does not necessarily rule out heart disease. In dogs with bradycardia, abolition of the arrhythmia after exercise suggests a vagally mediated etiology. The increased availability of ambulatory ECG recordings has markedly reduced the use of post exercise ECGs in clinical practice.

Atropine Response Test

- Sinus tachycardia with a heart rate greater than 135 beats per minute suggests normal sinus node function in the dog. Additionally, this response suggests that medical management with vagolytic therapy may be effective if the bradycardia is associated with clinical signs such as syncope or collapse and implantation of a pacemaker is not possible.

KEY POINT

Provocative ECG techniques are easily performed, relatively inexpensive, and can be very helpful for diagnostic and therapeutic purposes in animals with bradycardias and/or tachycardias.

AMBULATORY ELECTROCARDIOGRAPHY (HOLTER MONITORING AND CARDIAC EVENT RECORDING)

Indications

Routine in-hospital electrocardiography only provides a glimpse of the daily electrocardiographic activity. Moreover, arrhythmia detection may be confounded by iatrogenic changes in the autonomic nervous system activity. A 24-hour ambulatory (Holter) recording of the ECG increases the sensitivity of arrhythmia detection. Major indications include:

- Detection of transient arrhythmias associated with syncope or periodic weakness.
- Screening of high-risk breeds for cardiomyopathy (e.g., Boxers, Doberman Pinschers).
- Evaluation of frequency, severity, and significance of arrhythmias detected on in-hospital ECG.
- Monitoring efficacy of antiarrhythmic therapy (e.g., control of heart rate in patients with chronic atrial fibrillation).
- Determining the true incidence and type of arrhythmia in heart disease patients.

Technique

Modern Holter monitors use a high-fidelity digital recorder to capture and store the cardiac electrical activity for 24 hours. Some digital recorders are now capable of monitoring the patient for up to 7 days. Two to three simultaneous ECG chest leads are typically recorded.

- Electrode sites are prepared by clipping, shaving, cleaning and drying the chest.
- Adhesive patches are firmly adhered to the skin (see Figure 5-1).
- A chest wrap is essential for securing electrodes, wires and the recorder. A vest or harness can also be used (Figure 5-2).
- Once the monitor has been applied, the animal returns home to resume normal activity. Very small dogs and cats that find it cumbersome to ambulate with the monitor in place may respond better to hospitalization with cage restraint during the 24-hour recording session.

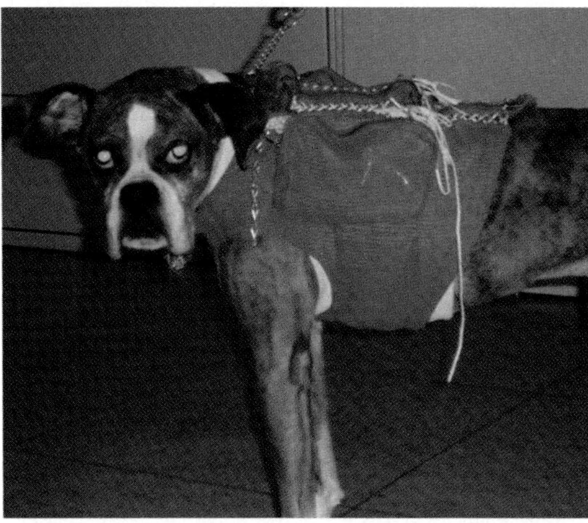

Figure 5-2. A vest can be placed over the light wrap, which secures Holter or CER monitor electrodes in place. The vest has pockets to hold the monitor and helps keep the device in place.

- Owners or caretakers should maintain a diary of significant changes in activity, such as sleeping, exercising, and so on. Any clinical signs such as syncopal events must be noted.
- At least 24 hours should be evaluated in order to assess a full circadian cycle.
- At the conclusion of the recording period, the components are removed and the monitor is analyzed with the aid of automated computer-based software. Operator interaction and editing is essential for diagnostically accurate results.
- Consultation with a veterinary cardiologist is recommended regarding the significance of arrhythmias found and the need for therapy. Many normal dogs will have infrequent ventricular premature complexes and/or sinus pauses noted during a 24 hour period. Assessment of arrhythmia significance and risk/benefit ratio of anti-arrhythmic medications is essential.

Cardiac Event Recorders

The cardiac event recorder (CER) is an ambulatory microprocessor with a solid-state memory loop capable of storing portions of ECG tracings when activated. The CER is lightweight, activated by a person witnessing an event (e.g., weakness or syncope) and can be worn by small dogs and cats without restricting activity. Unlike most 24 hour Holter monitors, which are worn for only 1 day, the CER can be worn for up to a week, increasing the diagnostic yield in animals with infrequent clinical signs.

- CERs can be programmed to store up to five separate, one minute duration, single channel ECGs, or fewer ECGs of longer duration.
- Recording is activated by pressing the event button on the device. The CER utilizes a memory loop to store the ECG (most commonly 30 seconds before activation to 30 seconds after activation); however, these times may be changed as indicated for the individual patient.
- After one or more events, the CER is detached and the stored ECG is transmitted and downloaded to a receiving station for computer-based analysis and interpretation.

Application

- The CER uses two adhesive electrodes in a base-apex configuration and is relatively easy to apply.
- A light chest wrap is used to secure the unit over the dorsum. As with Holter monitoring, the patient may be discharged to resume routine activity.

Use of Cardiac Event Recorders

- The CER will not store an ECG unless the activation button is pressed; therefore, the event must be witnessed by the owner. If an event does not occur during the time the unit is worn, then a definitive diagnosis is not possible.
- CERs may be rented from a commercial service or the patient may be referred to a specialty practice offering this service.

Implantable Cardiac Event Recorders

- Implantable loop recorders are available for those unusual cases in which syncope is very rare and difficult to capture with a 7 day CER. These devices are small enough to implant subcutaneously in most dog or cat patients. They are capable of monitoring the ECG for longer than 18 months, and can be activated to store the ECG by a person observing an episode, or can be programmed to store the ECG if the heart rate is slower or faster than the programmed limits (set at the time of implantation). The device is interrogated by a radiotelemetry device (similar to those used for pacemakers) to determine if unobserved episodes occurred. The devices are expensive; however, they can be very helpful in cases with rare clinical signs.

> **KEY POINT**
>
> If syncope is very infrequent, then a CER is much more likely to result in definitive diagnosis than a 24-hour Holter recording.

NONSELECTIVE ANGIOGRAPHY

Indications

- Nonselective angiography is occasionally helpful to identify congenital and/or acquired abnormalities of intracardiac or intravascular blood flow. Abnormalities of the right side of the heart (e.g., right atrium, right ventricle, pulmonary arteries) are most readily identified by this technique; however, echocardiography and ultrasound have superseded the need for this technique at most facilities.

Technique

- Sedation or a light plane of anesthesia is usually necessary.
- A large bore catheter (18 gauge or larger) is placed intravenously (preferably in the jugular vein).
- The animal is placed in the most appropriate position for opacification of the structures of interest (i.e., lateral recumbency for most cardiac

defects, sternal recumbency to visualize pulmonary arteries).

- A large bolus of contrast is rapidly injected intravenously. Typically, 1 ml of radiopaque contrast per kg of body weight is used for the injection. Alternatively, the dose of iodine to be injected can be calculated using 400 mg iodine/kg body weight as the desirable dose.
- A fluoroscopy unit allows continuous assessment. If fluoroscopy is not available, radiographic exposures are obtained 2 to 8 seconds after the injection is initiated (depending on the structures of interest and cardiovascular performance). Shorter times should be used for evaluation of the right heart and pulmonary arteries, longer times for evaluation of structures on the left side of the heart or animals with heart failure and slow circulation.

Clinical Utility

- Nonselective angiography is an alternative technique primarily used to evaluate lesions that involve the right side of the heart, particularly when echocardiography or cardiac catheterization is either not an option or is inconclusive.

Limitations, Risks, and Costs

- Dilution of contrast material occurs as it moves through the circulation. Thus, nonselective angiography results in poor opacification of structures that are very distal to the site of injection (e.g., left heart and systemic arteries).
- Timing of radiographs is difficult to predict and several attempts are often required unless fluoroscopy is available.
- Intravenous contrast agents may result in transient hypotension, cardiac arrhythmias, nephrotoxicity (especially in patients with pre-existing renal dysfunction), and allergic reactions.

> **KEY POINT**
>
> Nonselective angiography is significantly limited, particularly in the assessment of left heart structures. Echocardiography and/or ultrasound are preferred diagnostics.

CARDIAC CATHETERIZATION

Indications

- Generally, cardiac catheterization is defined as a combined angiographic and hemodynamic study undertaken for therapeutic or diagnostic purposes. The standard cardiac catheterization procedure for evaluation of congenital or acquired cardiac diseases typically includes measurement of intracardiac pressures, blood oximetry, and selective angiocardiography. The most common indication for cardiac catheterization is to ameliorate congenital heart disease (e.g., pulmonic stenosis or patent ductus arteriosus). For the purposes of diagnosis, advances in echocardiography have markedly reduced the need for routine cardiac catheterization.

Technique

- Anesthesia is usually required.
- Surgical preparation of the neck (carotid artery or jugular vein) or inguinal area (femoral vein or artery) is required.
- Vascular access can be obtained by dissecting down to the vessel or with a percutaneous catheter introducer system using a modified Seldinger technique.
- Catheter advancement to the chamber of interest is performed under fluoroscopic or pressure wave form guidance (Figure 5-3).
- Intravascular pressures are recorded from chambers of interest. Pressures are typically recorded before and after therapeutic interventions (e.g., balloon valvuloplasty) to assess procedure efficacy.

Oximetry

- Blood samples are obtained from various cardiac or great vessel locations to measure oxygen saturation and to calculate shunt fraction in animals with congenital shunting defects.

Angiocardiography

- Radiopaque contrast material is injected through the catheter(s) located at the appropriate areas of interest, and the image is recorded on videotape, radiographic film, by cineangiography or is digitally stored (Figure 5-4). Post processing can be performed on digital images using digital subtraction techniques. The primary advantage over nonselective angiography involves superior opacification of structures of interest.
- Cardiac output may be determined using thermodilution or indicator dye techniques.
- Additional procedures such as balloon valvuloplasty, patent ductus arteriosus coil occlusion, endomyocardial biopsy, heartworm retrieval, and cardiac pacing can be performed.

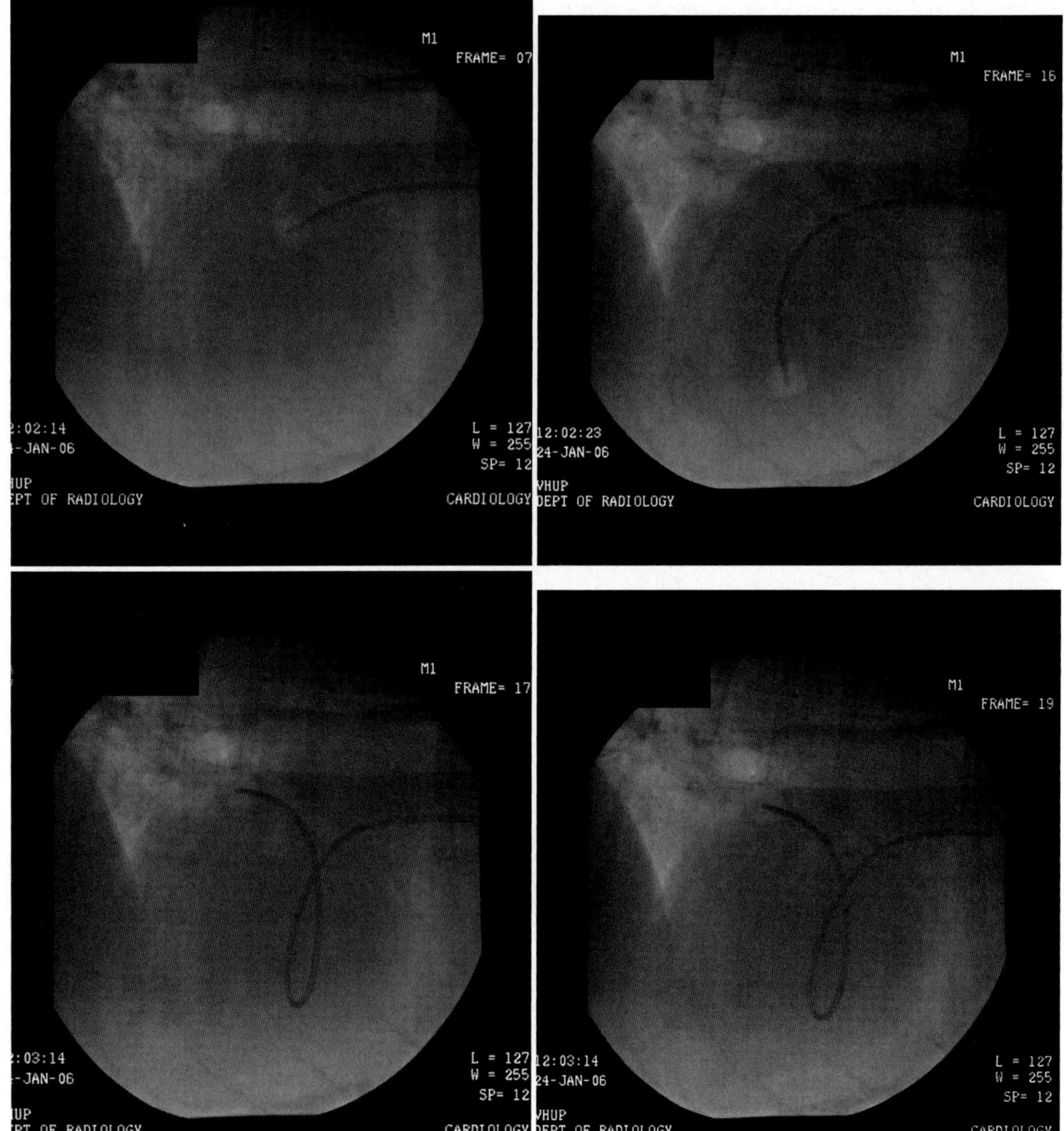

Figure 5-3. Fluoroscopically obtained images of a balloon-tipped cardiac catheter being placed into the right heart. The catheter is advanced to the heart via the jugular vein. The balloon on the tip of the catheter facilitates traversing the tricuspid valve because it will tend to follow blood flow.

Clinical Utility

- Angiocardiography is valuable to diagnose cases of complex heart disease and to guide therapeutic interventions such as balloon valvuloplasty or patent ductus arteriosus occlusion. The approach provides useful morphologic and physiologic information regarding interventional responses to therapy.

Limitations, Risks, and Costs

- Cardiac catheterization requires specialized equipment and training and is typically limited to tertiary care facilities.
- The technique can be time consuming.
- Contrast solutions can result in hemodynamic abnormalities. Patients with severe heart disease or renal disease are at a relatively higher risk.
- Infection, cardiac arrhythmias, air embolism, vascular thromboembolism or perforation are possible complications. With appropriate experience and case selection, mortality rate is low.

SEROLOGIC TESTING

Indications

Animals with clinical signs suggestive of myocardial dysfunction resulting from infectious or immune-mediated etiologies and animals at risk of

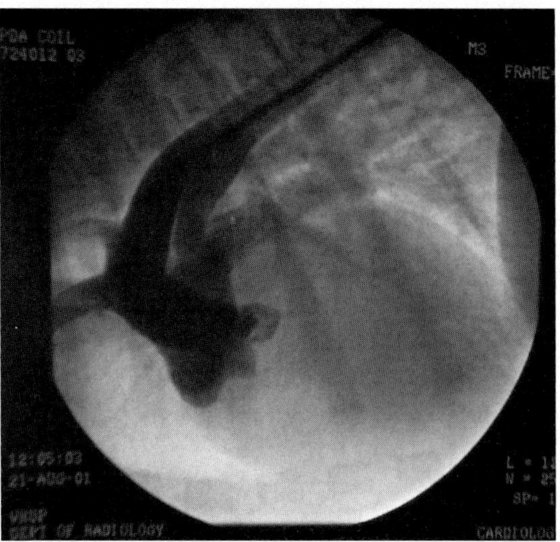

Figure 5-4. Selective aortogram demonstrating a patent ductus arteriosus with radiographic contrast material crossing the ductus and entering the pulmonary artery (left to right flow).

myocardial toxicity from chemotherapeutic agents are candidates.

- Trypanosoma titer. Animals from Mexico, southern Texas, or other regions where Chagas disease is endemic, with right-heart failure.
- Antinuclear antibody titer. Animals with heart failure or arrhythmias in addition to other clinical signs suggestive of immune-mediated disease.
- Toxoplasmosis titer. Cats with myocardial dysfunction, fever, pneumonia, neurologic disease, chorioretinitis or other signs compatible with toxoplasmosis.

Technique

- Serum or plasma should be submitted to a laboratory that has the appropriate facilities to perform the indicated serologic testing.

Clinical Utility

- In selected cases, these tests can be very useful in establishing an etiologic agent and in monitoring patients at risk for myocardial toxicity. Results must be interpreted in concert with the patient's clinical signs.

Limitations, Risks, and Costs

- These tests are only limited by correct interpretation. Otherwise, there are no particular risks. Costs are dependent on the laboratory.

CARDIAC NEUROHORMONES AND BIOMARKERS

Cardiac Troponins

Indications

- Cardiac troponin I and T are specific markers of myocyte injury, ischemia, and necrosis. Cardiac troponin I is more sensitive than cardiac troponin T. Specific indications include cases of suspected myocardial infarction, toxic myocardial disease (e.g., secondary to doxorubicin), myocarditis, or blunt myocardial trauma (e.g., vehicular injury).

Technique

- A variety of human cardiac troponin I assays that cross-react with canine and feline cardiac troponin I are available, but standardization is lacking, making it difficult to compare results from different machines. Most cardiac troponin assays accept either serum or heparinized or ethylenediaminetetra acetic acid (EDTA) plasma. Some use whole blood. If testing is not performed within 12 hours after collection, then the samples should be frozen until testing is done.

Clinical Utility

- Elevated cardiac troponin I has been demonstrated in a wide range of cardiac and extracardiac diseases. Concrete diagnostic, prognostic and therapeutic recommendations based on assay results are not yet available; however, cardiac troponin I results may give useful supportive information to the electrocardiographic, radiographic, and echocardiographic findings in some patients. Serial testing of individual patients is more likely to be useful than one measurement at a single point in time.

Limitations

- Since cardiac troponin I can be elevated with both cardiac and extracardiac disease, the test does not appear to be a useful screening tool for cardiac disease.

NATRIURETIC PEPTIDES (ATRIAL AND B-TYPE)

Indications

Atrial natriuretic peptide (ANP) and B-type natriuretic peptide (BNP) are produced by myocardial tissue in response to increased pressure and wall stress and are markers for cardiac dysfunction and heart failure.

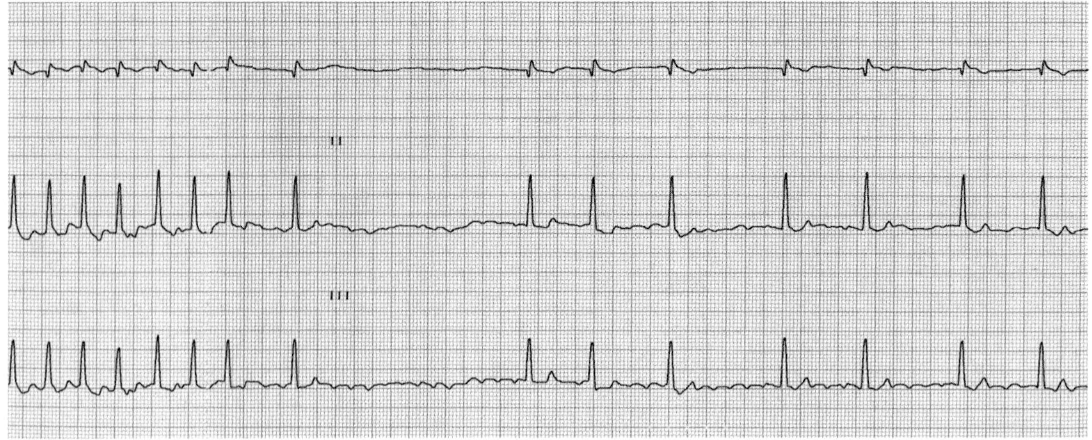

Figure 5-5. Simultaneous lead I, II, and III ECG showing the effect of a vagal maneuver on a supraventricular tachycardia (atrial fibrillation in this example). Note the dramatic slowing of the heart rate which results in clearer demonstration of the hallmarks of atrial fibrillation (irregularly irregular rhythm, lack of P waves and fibrillation waves). 50 mm/sec; 10 mm/mV.

Technique

- Mature ANP and BNP have short half-lives, and clinical assays that target prohormones (proANP and NT-proBNP) are more useful. Depending on the assay being used, heparinized or EDTA plasma or serum is submitted to the appropriate laboratory. Samples should be centrifuged and separated after collection. If analysis is delayed more than a day, samples should be frozen.

Clinical Utility

- These assays have the potential to differentiate between cardiac and extracardiac causes of dyspnea, allow prognostication, and monitor response to cardiac disease therapy. The following guidelines have been established for canine proANP (Vetsign proANP, Guildhay Ltd, UK): proANP > 1700 fmol/ml is consistent with congestive heart failure; proANP < 1350 fmol/ml is considered normal; proANP 1351 to 1700 fmol/ml is suggestive for heart failure, but results are not conclusive. In dogs presenting to emergency services with dyspnea, EDTA plasma proANP concentrations >1350 fmol/ml were consistent with dyspnea due to congestive heart failure (as opposed to dyspnea caused by primary respiratory disease). The following guidelines appear useful for canine NT-proBNP (Canine CardioCare, Veterinary Diagnostics Institute, Irvine, CA): NT-proBNP > 450 pmol/L is consistent with heart disease (but not necessarily congestive heart failure), NT-proBNP > 1000 pmol/L accompanied by clinical signs of dyspnea is consistent with congestive heart failure.

Limitations, Risks, and Costs

- Natriuretic testing in veterinary medicine is a relatively recent phenomenon and caution should be exercised when using new diagnostic tests until they are more fully validated. Further studies are necessary to better characterize the utility of these tests for prognostic and therapeutic monitoring.

NEWER CARDIAC IMAGING TECHNIQUES

- Although these techniques are not widely available, familiarity with their potential applications is helpful for identifying referral candidates. Computed tomography and magnetic resonance imaging are useful adjunctive techniques that are less invasive than angiocardiography, and may be advantageous over echocardiography for certain diseases such as cardiac neoplasia and pericardial disease. Nuclear scintigraphy is particularly useful for quantitative assessment of intracardiac shunts.

Computed Tomography

- An x-ray technique that displays cross-sectional images of the body.
- Assessment of cardiac function and precise definition of intracardiac anatomy requires either electrocardiographic gating or a millisecond computed tomography (CT) scanner.
- An intravenous injection of iodinated contrast is used to define the blood pool.

Magnetic Resonance Imaging

- A high natural contrast exists between blood and cardiovascular structures; therefore, contrast medium is not required to discriminate the blood pool.
- Physiologic gating of the imaging sequence is necessary for cardiac imaging.
- Magnetic resonance images give useful information on cardiovascular morphology, function, and tissue character.

Nuclear Cardiology

- Gamma ray–emitting radiopharmaceuticals (radionuclides) are injected intravenously and are either extracted by the myocardium or remain in the blood pool. A scintillation (gamma) camera interfaced with a computer analyzes and stores the data.
- The direction and severity of congenital intracardiac shunts can be determined. Regional distribution of myocardial perfusion can also be visualized.

Limitations

The required technical expertise and expense of equipment limit their use in general veterinary cardiology.

Frequently Asked Questions

How is a vagal maneuver helpful when assessing a dog with a suspected supraventricular tachycardia?
An effective vagal maneuver will transiently increase vagal tone. The technique can be helpful to differentiate between sinus tachycardia, as during a normal physiologic response to pain, fever, and so on, and a pathologic ectopic supraventricular tachycardia (SVT), such as paroxysmal atrial tachycardia. A gradual slowing of the heart rate (over several seconds) suggests the focus is sinus because the sinus node accelerates and decelerates gradually. An abrupt cessation of the tachycardia is suggestive of a pathologic focus (ie., SVT). Lack of response to a vagal maneuver can occur with either condition and is nondiagnostic. Occasionally an SVT will respond to a vagal maneuver with slowed AV nodal conduction resulting in second degree AV block with an underlying rapid P-wave rate.

SUGGESTED READINGS

Daniel MD, Bright JM: Nuclear imaging, computed tomography, and magnetic resonance imaging of the heart. In Fox PR, Sisson DD, Moise NS, eds: Textbook of canine and feline cardiology, Philadelphia, 1999, WB Saunders.

Kittleson MD: Syncope. In Kittleson MD, Kienle RD, eds: Small animal cardiovascular medicine, St Louis, 1999, Mosby.

Miller MS, Calvert CA: Special methods for analyzing arrhythmias. In Tilley LP, ed: Essentials of canine and feline electrocardiography, ed 3, Malvern, Penn, 1992, Lea & Febiger.

Rush JE: Syncope and episodic weakness. In Fox PR, Sisson DD, Moise NS, eds: Textbook of canine and feline cardiology, Philadelphia, 1999, WB Saunders.

Thomas WP, Sisson D: Cardiac catheterization and angiography. In Fox PR, Sisson DD, Moise NS, eds: Textbook of canine and feline cardiology, Philadelphia, 1999, WB Saunders.

SECTION II

Cardiovascular Disease

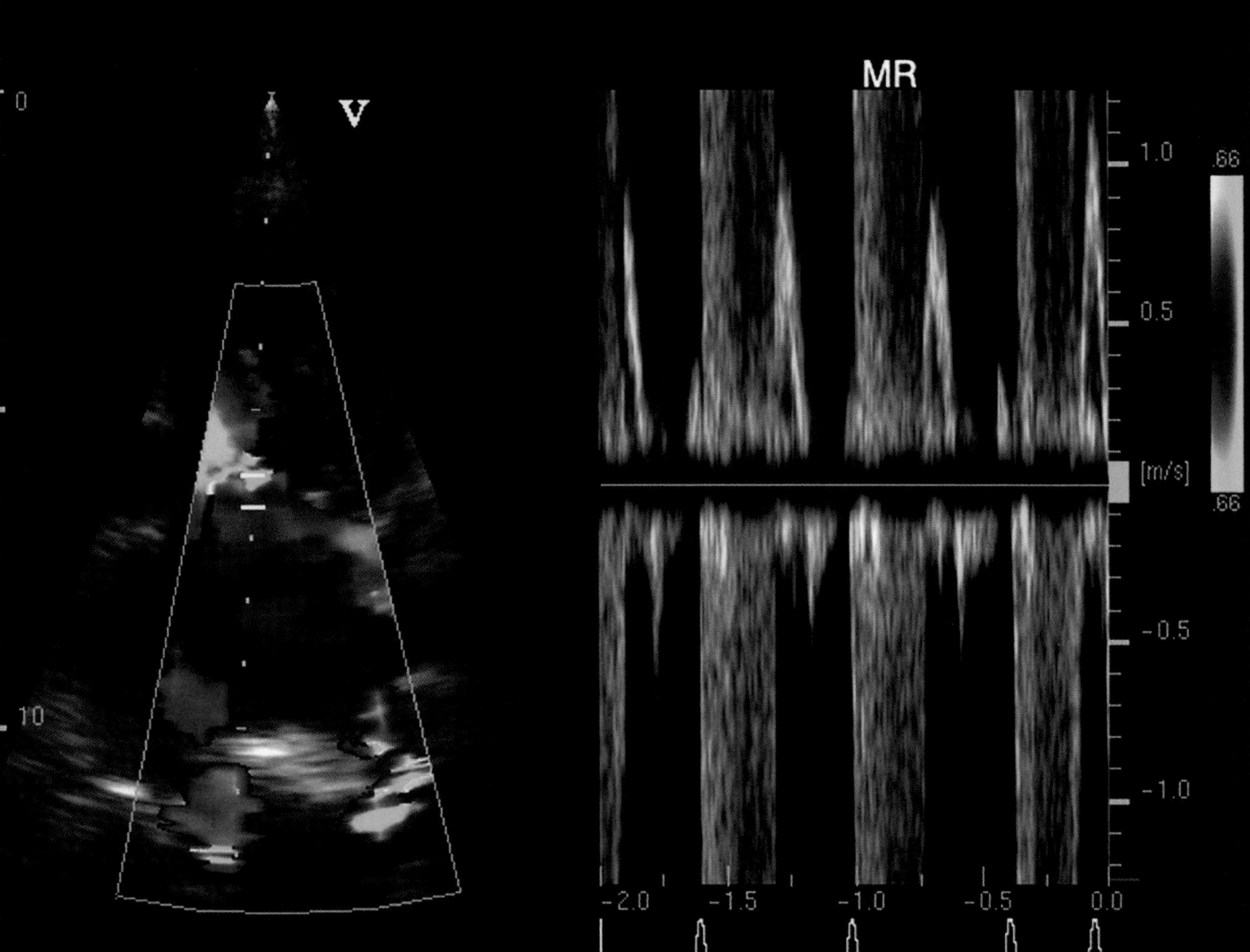

CHAPTER 6

Acquired Valvular Disease

Jonathan A. Abbott

INTRODUCTION

Acquired primary valvular disease in dogs and cats generally is degenerative or less commonly, infective. Other pathologic processes, such as neoplasia, rarely affect the cardiac valves. Myxomatous degeneration of the mitral valve is the most common cardiac disease in the dog. Mitral valve incompetence due to valvular degeneration can result in progressive cardiac enlargement and, in some cases, congestive heart failure (CHF). Clinical signs, particularly cough due to compression of the mainstem bronchi by an enlarged left atrium, may precede the development of CHF. The clinical consequences of degenerative valvular disease are observed primarily in elderly, small-breed dogs.

Infective endocarditis (IE) is an uncommon form of acquired valvular disease that is observed occasionally in dogs and rarely in cats. Middle-aged medium- and large-breed dogs are affected most often. The clinical signs of IE relate to sepsis, thromboembolism, and CHF.

DEGENERATIVE MITRAL VALVE DISEASE

Based on its clinical and pathologic features, numerous designations for degenerative mitral value disease (MVD) have been proposed. The terms *myxomatous valvular degeneration, myxomatous transformation, mucoid degeneration, endocardiosis, chronic valvular disease,* and *degenerative valvular disease* all refer to the same disorder.

Prevalence and Incidence

- Degenerative MVD is the most common cardiac disease in the dog; it is an acquired disease, and the prevalence is greatest in the geriatric population.
- Clinical evidence of degenerative valvular disease is detected in approximately 30% of dogs aged 13 years and older.
- MVD is a progressive disease, and subtle changes in valve structure precede the development of clinically evident valvular dysfunction. Consequently, the prevalence of MVD detected by postmortem examination is higher than that reported in clinical studies.
- Postmortem evidence of advanced degenerative valvular disease was found in 58% of dogs older than 9 years; when mild degenerative changes are included, the postmortem prevalence exceeds 90% in dogs older than 13 years.
- MVD may affect any breed of dog, but clinical consequences of MVD are observed most often in small-breed dogs. Miniature Poodles, Pomeranians, Yorkshire Terriers, Chihuahuas, and other small dogs are commonly affected. The prevalence of MVD in Cavalier King Charles Spaniels is particularly high, and in dogs of this breed, the disease is sometimes clinically evident at a young age.
- Male dogs are affected somewhat more often than females.
- Degenerative valvular disease is uncommon in cats, and when it occurs it seldom results in clinical consequences.

KEY POINT

Degenerative MVD is the most common cardiac disease in the dog; it is an acquired disease, and the prevalence is greatest in the geriatric population.

Pathology

- Grossly, MVD is characterized by nodular distortion of the valve leaflets as well as by thickening and, sometimes, lengthening of the chordae tendineae. The appearance of a small number of nodules at the free edge of the valve leaflet is the initial pathology. As the disease progresses, these nodules increase in number and size and coalesce. In severe cases, the leaflets are contracted, and the free edge of the leaflet rolls inward toward the ventricular endocardium (Figure 6-1). When severe, these abnormalities prevent coaptation of the valve leaflets, resulting in mitral valve incompetence.
- MVD is histologically characterized by the deposition of mucopolysaccharides primarily within the spongiosa layer of the valve leaflet. Fibrosis of the valve is also present, but is not the dominant histologic feature. Inflammatory infiltrates are absent; MVD is a sterile, degenerative disease that bears no known relationship to endocarditis.

KEY POINT

The prevalence of endocarditis is no greater in dogs affected by MVD than in other dogs.

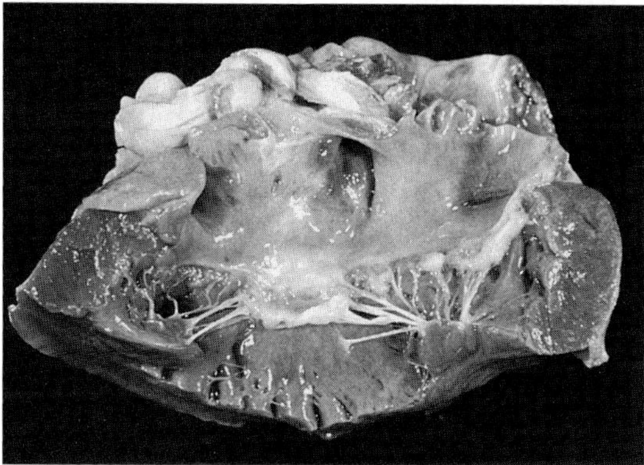

Figure 6-1. A specimen that demonstrates the gross features of severe mitral valve degeneration. The mitral valve leaflets are abnormally thick and nodular. (The author acknowledges the Department of Veterinary Pathology, Western College of Veterinary Medicine, University of Saskatchewan, Saskatoon, SK, Canada S7N 5B4, for providing this photograph.)

Etiopathogenesis

- The cause of MVD is unknown.
- MVD is often observed in chondrodysplastic dog breeds. Because MVD has been associated with concurrent disorders such as bronchomalacia and intervertebral disc disease, it has been suggested that MVD is but one expression of a systemic connective tissue disease.
- Recent evidence suggests a possible role for the vasoactive peptide endothelin in the pathogenesis of MVD. Relative to mitral valve tissue obtained from healthy young dogs, degenerative mitral leaflets had a greater density of endothelin receptors. Furthermore, the density of endothelin receptors was related to the severity of MVD.
- Because distinct breed predispositions are recognized, it is likely that there is a genetic predisposition for the development of MVD. Available evidence suggests that the tendency to develop MVD is not subject to simple Mendelian inheritance but rather is a polygenic trait.
- In Cavalier King Charles Spaniels, parental status with respect to age and murmur intensity is an important determinant of the prevalence of murmurs in 5-year-old offspring. Based on this, it appears that the age at which MVD develops is inherited.

KEY POINT

The cause of MVD is not known but genetic factors are likely important.

Pathophysiology

- The mitral valve apparatus consists of the mitral valve leaflets, the fibrous valve annulus, the chordae tendineae, and the left ventricular papillary muscles.
- The two mitral leaflets are known as the septal (anterior) and the caudal (posterior) leaflets. In health, the mitral leaflets are thin, translucent structures that are tethered to the left ventricular papillary muscles by the chordae tendineae. The two left ventricular papillary muscles arise from the caudal (free) wall of the left ventricle. The basilar attachment of the mitral leaflets is to the fibrous left atrioventricular valve ring, known as the mitral annulus.
- The initiation of valve closure is a passive process; in early systole, when left ventricular pressure exceeds left atrial pressure, the mitral valve leaflets are forced into apposition. In normal individuals, the tethering effect of the chordae

tendineae prevents prolapse, or bowing, of the leaflets into the left atrium.

- Coaptation of the normal mitral leaflets is complete, and there is little or no regurgitation through the valve orifice. The normal mitral valve ensures that the entirety of the left ventricular stroke volume is ejected through the aorta. When the mitral valve is incompetent, a fraction of the left ventricular stroke volume is ejected through the mitral valve regurgitant orifice into the left atrium.
- Mitral valve regurgitation (MR) may be mild and have minimal consequences, or it can be severe. The severity of MR is determined principally by the size of the regurgitant orifice and the relationship between left atrial and left ventricular systolic pressure. Potentially, both of these determinants can be pharmacologically manipulated by administration of vasodilators.
- MR increases left atrial pressure which potentially results in left atrial dilation. When the mitral valve leaks, the pulmonary venous return is augmented by the regurgitant volume; in consequence, the ventricle is filled in diastole not only by blood that has returned from the lungs, but also by blood that has been regurgitated into the atrium. Therefore, MR imposes a volume load on the left ventricle and the left atrium.
- High end-diastolic pressures and volumes result in ventricular dilation and hypertrophy. Hypertrophy of this type, in which the ratio of wall thickness and chamber size remains roughly unchanged, is known as eccentric hypertrophy.
- Severe MR may increase left ventricular filling pressures. High filling pressures are reflected backward, raising pulmonary vein pressure and potentially initiating the development of pulmonary edema.
- The syndrome of clinical signs and neuroendocrine activation that results from cardiac dysfunction is known as heart failure. Because veterinary patients cannot offer subjective observations—the perception of breathlessness during exertion for example—the presence of congestive signs is generally used as an objective criterion for the diagnosis.
- CHF is the syndrome of clinical signs caused by venous pressure elevations that result from cardiac dysfunction. Left-sided CHF is defined by the presence of cardiogenic pulmonary edema. Right-sided CHF refers to clinical signs that result from systemic congestion; in dogs, ascites is the most common manifestation of right-sided CHF.
- Due to maladaptive neuroendocrine responses associated with heart failure, cardiac dysfunction tends to be progressive. Because of this, the elimination of congestive signs does not signify resolution of the heart failure state. When the disorder responsible cannot be definitively corrected, heart failure is a terminal syndrome.
- The imposition of a chronic volume load on the heart can result in deterioration of systolic myocardial function, a state sometimes known as cardiomyopathy of overload. In general, MR is relatively well tolerated by the myocardium because the left atrium represents a low-pressure reservoir into which the ventricle can eject blood. In fact, dogs that develop CHF due to MR often do so at a time when systolic myocardial function (contractility) is, based on echocardiographic indices, normal or only mildly diminished.
- MR may remain clinically silent until it is advanced. When CHF results from MR, clinical signs may include weakness, syncope, cough, and dyspnea.
- Cough is a centrally mediated reflex, and most cough receptors are located in the large airways. The etiology of cough associated with MR in small-breed dogs is probably multifactorial and may result from any of the following:
  - Pulmonary edema when fluid floods the alveoli
  - Compression of the mainstem bronchi by an enlarged left atrium
  - Reflexes mediated through stimulation of the juxtapulmonary (J) receptors; these receptors are associated with the pulmonary capillaries and are sensitive to increases in pulmonary venous pressure.

KEY POINT

It is important to recognize that cough can be associated with MVD in the absence of pulmonary edema. When this is the case, the cough is a sign of heart disease but not a sign of heart failure; this distinction is important because a diagnosis of CHF carries important prognostic and therapeutic implications.

Clinical Presentation

History

- MVD exhibits a broad spectrum of severity. In most affected dogs, MVD does not cause clinical signs, and the disease is detected when a cardiac murmur is incidentally identified in patients presented for routine health care or for management of noncardiac disease.

- In cases in which MVD does become clinically apparent, cough is usually the clinical sign that is first observed by the dog owner. Coughing due to bronchial compression is often dry and harsh. When coughing is due to pulmonary edema or congestion, other signs, such as exercise intolerance and tachypnea, are usually present. The cough associated with pulmonary edema may be moist and productive. The expectoration of pink froth is sometimes observed in patients with fulminant pulmonary edema.
- Occasionally, syncope is the clinical sign that is seen first in dogs with MVD. Syncope is a transient loss of consciousness that is usually related to a sudden and precipitous decline in cerebral perfusion. MVD can be responsible for syncope when cardiac enlargement predisposes to arrhythmias. Additionally, exertional syncope may result when MR limits stroke volume so that cardiac output does not adequately increase to meet the physiologic demands of exercise. Alternatively, syncope on exercise or excitement or associated with paroxysmal cough can result from sudden onset of reflex-mediated bradycardia.
- Other clinical signs related to reduced cardiac performance, including tachypnea, exercise intolerance, and abdominal distention caused by ascites, occasionally prompt owners of affected dogs to seek veterinary attention.

Physical Findings

- The most notable feature of the physical examination is a systolic murmur that is usually heard best over the left cardiac apex. The murmur of MVD is indistinguishable from the murmur caused by other disorders, such as IE or dilated cardiomyopathy (DCM), which also can result in MR. Importantly, however, an acquired, left apical, systolic murmur in an older, small-breed dog is almost always due to MVD. The intensity of the murmur depends on a number of factors, but severe MR usually causes a loud murmur. Severe MR associated with a nonrestrictive regurgitant orifice can result in a soft murmur but this is extremely uncommon in MVD. Phonocardiographically, the murmur of MR typically has a plateau-shaped configuration meaning that the murmur has a similar intensity throughout systole; when the murmur is loud, the second heart sound may be obscured (Figure 6-2).
- An exaggerated apical impulse is often evident on precordial palpation of patients with moderate or severe MR. By definition, a precordial thrill is present when the murmur intensity is grade V/VI or greater.

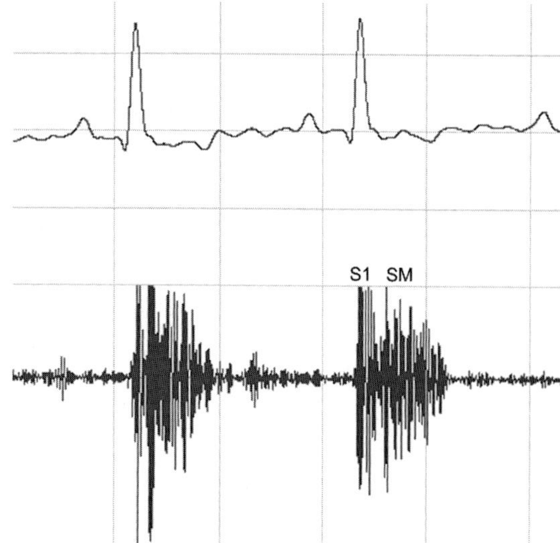

Figure 6-2. A phonocardiogram recorded from a 13-year-old female spayed mixed-breed dog with a grade 4/6 systolic murmur. The systolic murmur *(SM)* begins at the first heart sound *(S1)*, is evident throughout systole and obscures the second heart sound.

- A high-frequency, mid-systolic click (Figure 6-3) is sometimes heard in older, small-breed dogs. These clicks may be associated with prolapse of the mitral valve. In many dogs, clicks are a precursor of MR. Often, a soft systolic murmur of MR can also be heard in patients that have systolic clicks.
- When MR is severe, the third heart sound sometimes is audible and results in an S3 gallop. Care must be taken to distinguish a mid-systolic click from a gallop. In general, a systolic click is louder than is the third heart sound, and in patients with MVD, a click typically is heard in association with findings that suggest mild MR. In contrast, an S3 gallop usually reflects severe MR and generally is heard in patients with loud murmurs. Note that S3 is sometimes audible in patients with DCM. However, DCM is typically a disorder of large and giant breed dogs.
- The femoral arterial pulse is usually of normal strength when MR is present, but the pulse may have a rapid rise. Very severe MR can be associated with diminished pulse strength.
- Crackles may be heard in patients with pulmonary edema. It should be recognized that the prevalence of primary respiratory diseases such as chronic bronchitis in the patients most often affected by MVD is relatively high. Primary respiratory tract diseases can explain adventitious pulmonary sounds, such as crackles, in the absence of pulmonary edema.

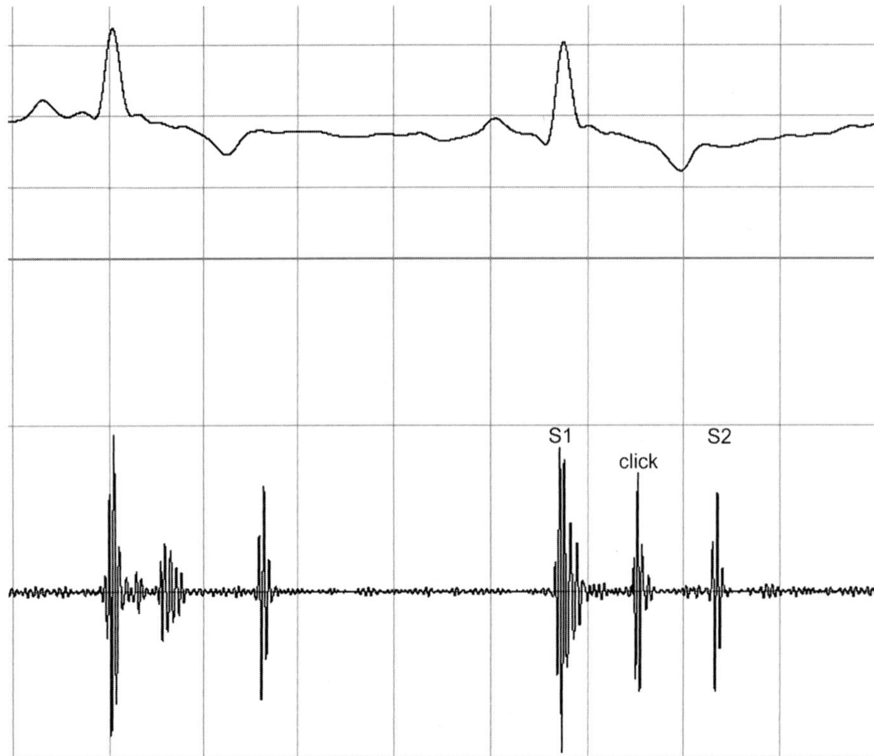

Figure 6-3. A phonocardiogram recorded from an 11-year-old male castrated Shih-Tzu. A mid-systolic click *(click)* is shown.

- Abdominal palpation is usually normal in patients with MVD, but hepatic enlargement or even ascites may be present when there is severe tricuspid valve disease, or when pulmonary hypertension complicates the presentation of MVD.

KEY POINT

Patients with clinically evident MVD have cardiac murmurs. The intensity of the murmur roughly parallels disease severity so that severe MR usually results in a loud murmur.

Patients with Mitral Regurgitation and Concurrent Respiratory Tract Disease

- Primary diseases of the respiratory tract, such as collapsing trachea and chronic bronchitis, are common in the patient group that is affected by MVD. In an individual patient, it can be difficult to determine whether cardiac disease or respiratory disease bears the greatest responsibility for the development of clinical signs.
- In general, patients that have severe MR are more likely than patients with respiratory disease to have poor body condition.
- Although loud murmurs of MR are sometimes clinically inconsequential, it is extremely uncommon for soft murmurs to indicate severe MR with cardiac enlargement.
- The presence of respiratory sinus arrhythmia (RSA) can also be of diagnostic value. Much of the moment-to-moment heart rate variability observed in healthy dogs is due to the effect of vagal discharge. In patients with severe cardiac disease, there is little vagal influence on heart rate and rhythm and as a result, RSA is not prominent. In contrast, sinus arrhythmia is often preserved or even accentuated when primary respiratory tract disease is responsible for clinical signs. The physical finding of RSA is virtually incompatible with a diagnosis of CHF.
- Although exceptions occur, clinical signs are usually related to respiratory tract disease in patients that are overweight, have sinus arrhythmia and a soft cardiac murmur.
- In contrast, the clinical signs of thin patients with loud murmurs and tachycardia are more likely to result from cardiac disease or CHF.

KEY POINT

Primary respiratory tract disease is relatively common in the patient group affected by MVD. The patient history and physical findings are helpful in distinguishing clinical signs caused by cardiac disease from signs caused by respiratory disease.

Table 6-1 Guidelines for Clinical Assessment of Elderly Small-Breed Dogs With Cough and Cardiac Murmur*

	Cardiac Disease	Respiratory Disease
Body condition	Thin	Obese
Cardiac murmur	Loud	Often soft, occasionally loud
Heart rate	Rapid	Normal or slow
Rhythm	Regular, unless pathologic arrhythmias are present	Exaggerated respiratory arrhythmia may be present

*It is important to recognize that exceptions to these generalities certainly occur. However, when a patient exhibits all of the findings in the left-hand column, it is likely that cardiac disease or, perhaps, congestive heart failure, is responsible for the cough. It must be recognized that some patients have both respiratory tract disease and cardiac disease. Ultimately, the distinction between respiratory tract disease and cardiac is made through diagnostic imaging; thoracic radiographs are indispensable, and echocardiography often provides useful, complementary data.

- Coughing in elderly, small-breed dogs that do not have cardiac murmurs is almost always due to primary respiratory tract disease (Table 6-1).

Large-Breed Dogs with Mitral Valve Disease

- A syndrome of severe MR and concurrent myocardial dysfunction is recognized in medium- and large-breed dogs. The fact that this observation was made relatively recently is probably explained by the increasing availability of echocardiography and not by a change in the epidemiology of MVD. Before widespread availability of this technology, large-breed dogs with heart failure generally were assumed to have primary myocardial disease.
- For reasons that are not known but may relate to the geometry or pattern of contraction of inherently larger ventricles, large-breed dogs with MR are more apt to develop echocardiographically evident myocardial dysfunction than are small-breed dogs.
- The gross appearance of the valvular lesions in large dogs tends to be less impressive than it is in small breed dogs.
- Perhaps because myocardial dysfunction complicates MVD in large dogs more often than it does in small dogs, the prognosis may be worse than in smaller dogs.

Diagnostic Findings

Thoracic Radiography

In most cases, thoracic radiography is the most important element of the diagnostic approach to MVD. MVD is extremely common but progresses at a rate that varies greatly among individuals. Many patients with MVD are subclinical ("asymptomatic") and never develop clinical signs related to MR. Early in the course of MVD, the cardiac silhouette is normal. If clinically consequential MR develops, then there is enlargement of the cardiac silhouette. It should be recognized that the ability of thoracic radiographs to delineate specific cardiac chambers is limited. In general, the left atrium can be assessed with the greatest certainty. This is fortunate because, in the overwhelming majority of cases, left atrial enlargement precedes the development of CHF. A diagnosis of left-sided CHF secondary to MVD rarely can be supported in the absence of radiographic left atrial enlargement.

Radiographic Appearance of Left Atrial Enlargement

- The left atrium is left of, and caudal to, the right atrium. Radiographically, it occupies the caudodorsal area of the cardiac silhouette in the lateral projection.
- In the absence of left atrial enlargement, the caudal portion of the trachea curves ventrally over the caudal aspect of the cardiac silhouette.
- When the left atrium is enlarged, the caudal border of the cardiac silhouette straightens, and the trachea is forced dorsally to varying degrees. With marked left atrial enlargement, the left mainstem bronchus is narrowed, and the trachea adopts a path that is parallel to the thoracic vertebrae. Occasionally, severe left atrial enlargement has the appearance of a mass that splits the mainstem bronchi.
- In the ventrodorsal projection, the left atrium is located near the center of the cardiac silhouette. When enlarged, the left atrium splits the mainstem bronchi to varying degrees. This is apparent in well-penetrated radiographs and results in an appearance that is sometimes known as the "crab sign" or the "bowlegged cowboy" (Figures 6-4 and 6-5).
- Additionally, in the ventrodorsal view, enlargement of the left atrium may cause a bulge which represents the atrial appendage at the 3 o'clock position.

Radiographic Findings of Pulmonary Congestion and Edema

- The radiographic finding of pulmonary venous distention reflects increases in pulmonary venous pressure. Pulmonary venous distention suggests

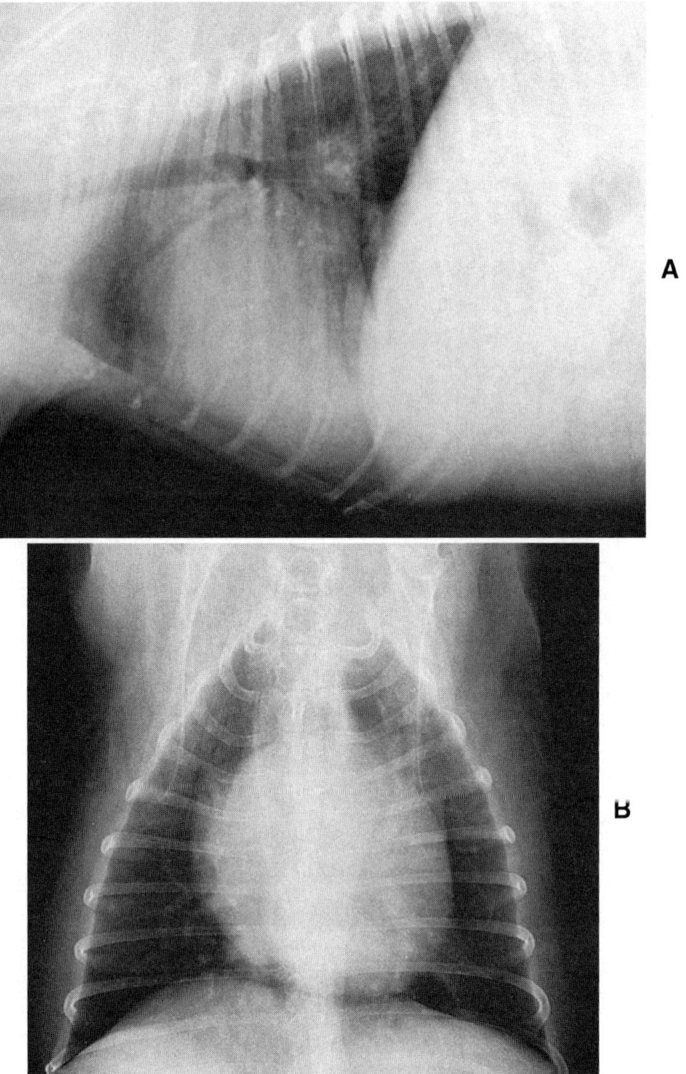

Figure 6-4. Lateral **(A)** and ventrodorsal **(B)** thoracic radiographs obtained from a 10-year-old mixed-breed dog with degenerative mitral valve disease. There is relatively mild but distinct left atrial enlargement, as evidenced by elevation of the trachea and loss of the caudal waist in the lateral film.

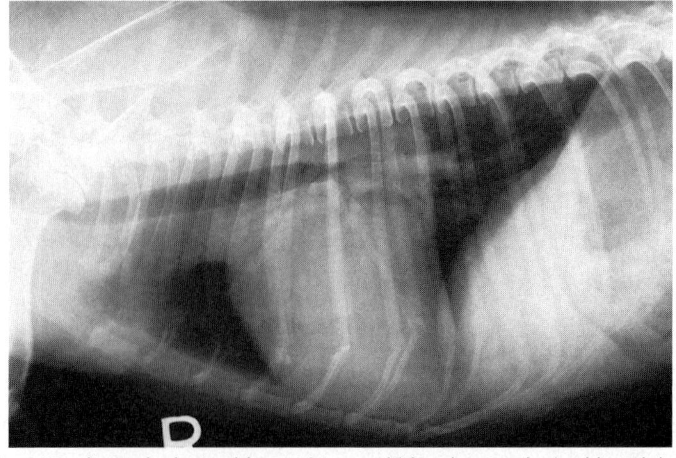

Figure 6-5. A lateral thoracic radiograph obtained from a 14-year-old female spayed mixed-breed dog with severe mitral valve incompetence due to degenerative disease. The left atrium is markedly enlarged, and the left mainstem bronchus is compressed.

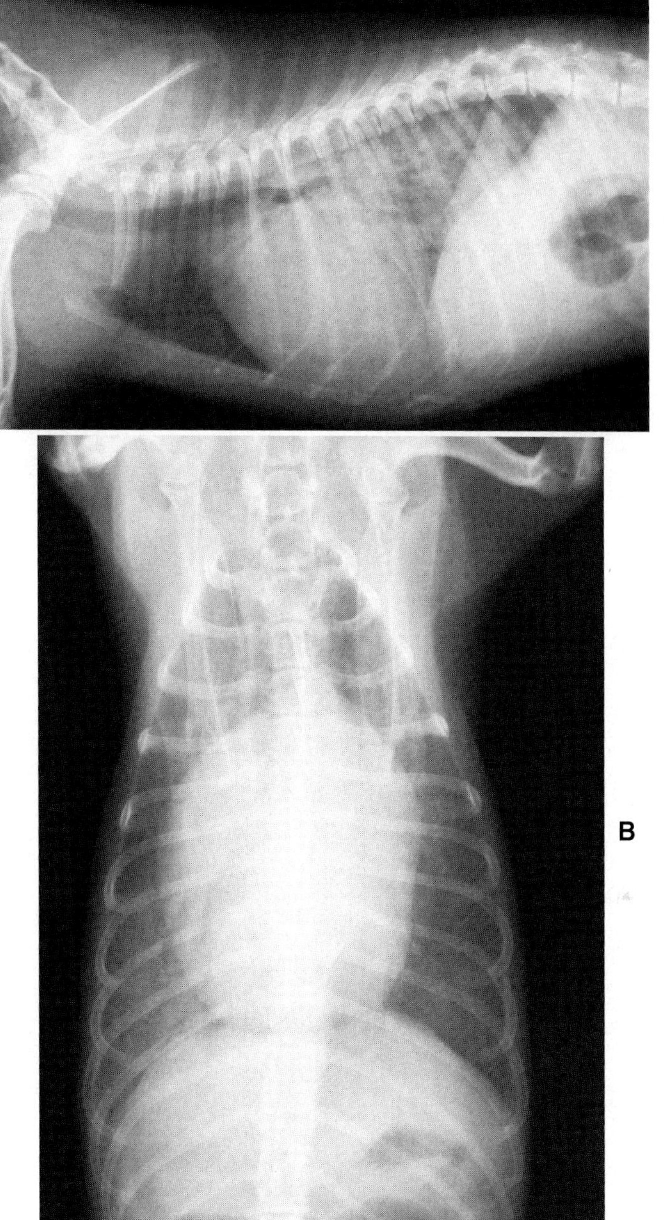

Figure 6-6. Lateral (**A**) and ventrodorsal (**B**) thoracic radiographs obtained from an 11-year-old female spayed Miniature Poodle with degenerative mitral valve disease. The cardiac silhouette is markedly enlarged, and there is evidence of left atrial enlargement. Pulmonary opacities compatible with edema are distributed throughout the lung; the edema is most noticeable in the caudodorsal lung field.

pulmonary congestion and may precede the development of pulmonary edema.

- A central, or perihilar, distribution often characterizes cardiogenic pulmonary edema in dogs.
- The development of interstitial pulmonary edema precedes the appearance of alveolar edema.
- Blurring of vascular detail in the presence of left atrial enlargement and, sometimes, concurrent pulmonary venous distention characterizes the radiographic appearance of interstitial pulmonary edema.
- When tissue fluid weeps into the pulmonary alveoli, it provides contrast with air-filled structures such as the bronchi, resulting in air bronchograms. Alveolar pulmonary opacities together with radiographic evidence of left atrial enlargement are diagnostic of left-sided CHF (Figure 6-6). The presence of alveolar pulmonary edema indicates severe CHF that is almost invariably associated with noticeable respiratory distress.

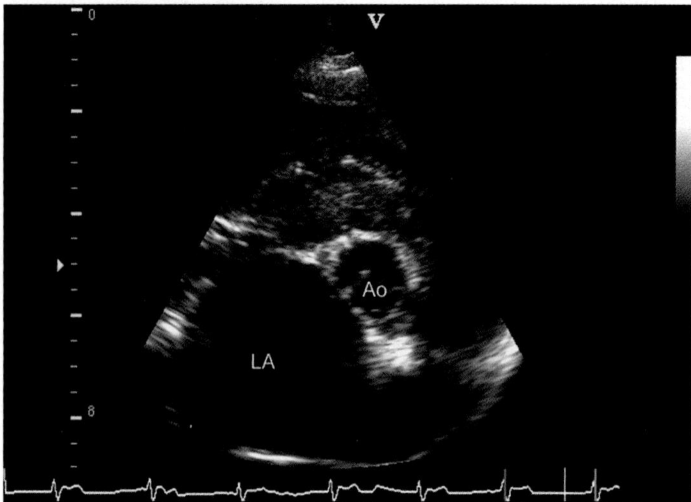

Figure 6-7. A right parasternal short-axis echocardiographic image obtained from an 11-year-old male castrated Cocker Spaniel with severe mitral valve regurgitation. The left atrium *(LA)* is markedly enlarged; the dimension of the body of the atrium is more than twice the diameter of the aorta *(Ao)*.

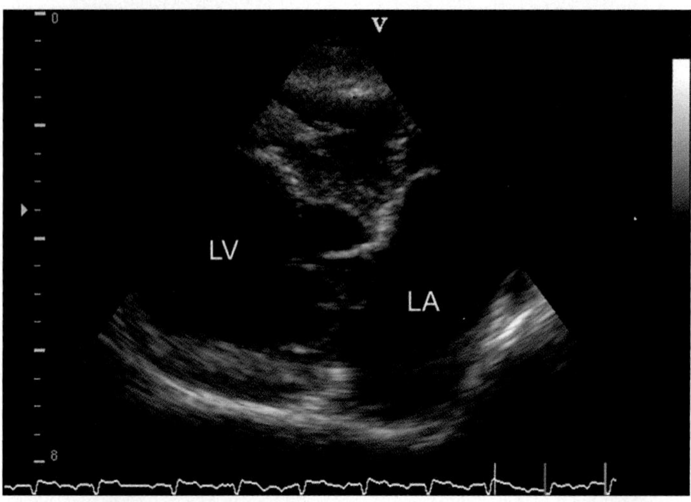

Figure 6-8. A right parasternal long-axis echocardiographic image obtained from a 15-year-old male castrated Cavalier King Charles Spaniel with mitral regurgitation due to degenerative disease. The image was obtained during systole. The left atrium is enlarged and there is distinct prolapse of the mitral valve leaflets. *LV*, Left ventricle; *LA*, left atrium.

KEY POINT

In most cases, thoracic radiography is the most important aspect of the diagnostic approach to MVD.

Echocardiography

- Echocardiographic examination of patients with MVD demonstrates variable degrees of left atrial (Figure 6-7) and left ventricular dilation. Hypertrophy is usually adequate to preserve a near-normal relationship between the diastolic luminal dimension and wall thickness.
- The mitral leaflets may be noticeably thicker than normal, and prolapse of the leaflets into the left atrium in systole is commonly observed (Figure 6-8).
- The echogenicity of affected leaflets is generally uniform and nodular thickening is diffuse. In contrast, infective vegetations typically are localized, may exhibit motion that is independent of the valve leaflet and are more, or less, echogenic than the valve leaflet.
- Often, the tricuspid leaflets are affected, although seldom as markedly as the mitral valve.
- Evaluation of myocardial function in patients with MR is difficult. When MR is moderate or severe, loading conditions imposed on the left ventricle are altered and left ventricular performance is hyperdynamic (Figure 6-9)

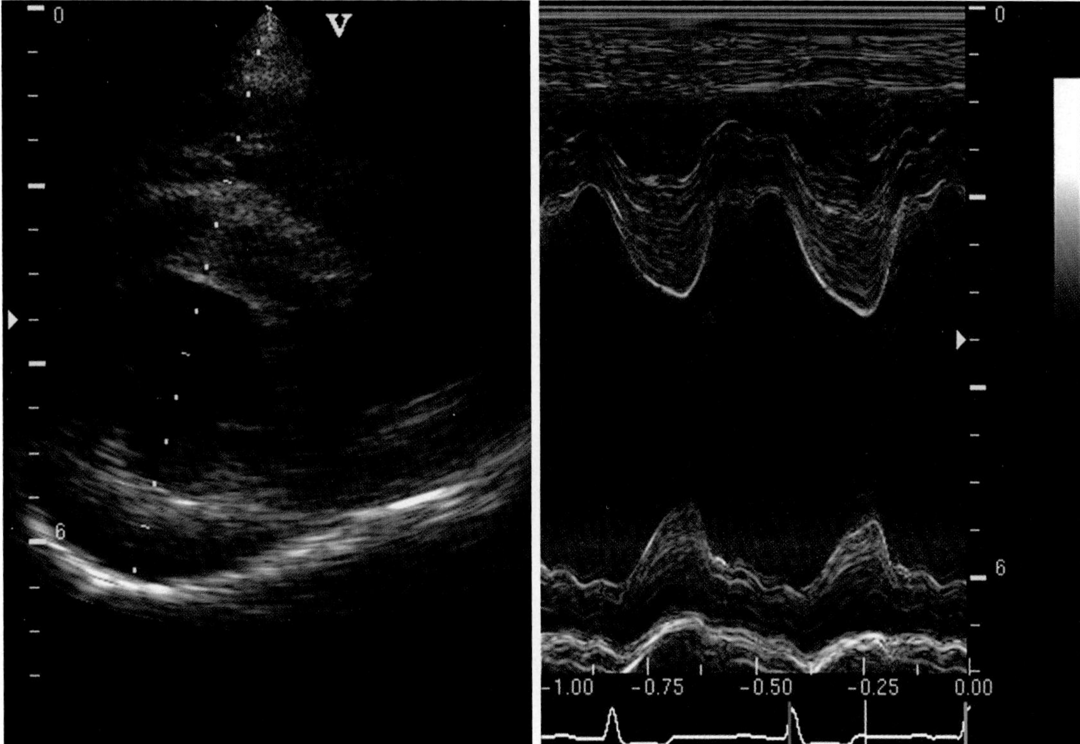

Figure 6-9. M-mode echocardiogram obtained at the level of the left ventricular papillary muscles from an 11-year-old female spayed Cavalier King Charles Spaniel. Left ventricular dilation and hypertrophy are evident. Left ventricular systolic performance is hyperdynamic; the fractional shortening is 46%.

provided myocardial function (contractility) is preserved.

- Ejection phase indices of systolic performance such as fractional shortening are elevated because these variables are highly load-dependent. When MR is present, impedance to ventricular emptying is reduced because the ventricle is able to eject blood into the low-pressure reservoir of the left atrium. Additionally, end-diastolic ventricular stretch associated with MR increases the force of contraction and contributes to the finding of hyperdynamic ventricular performance. A normal or subnormal fractional shortening in the setting of moderate or severe MR suggests systolic myocardial dysfunction (Figures 6-10 and 6-11).
- Because the end-systolic left ventricular dimension is determined by relatively few factors, it is likely a better index of myocardial function but, because cardiac dimensions are related to body size, end-systolic left ventricular dimension has the disadvantage that it must be interpreted in the context of body weight or perhaps more appropriately, the cube root of body weight. Recently a method of echocardiographic mensuration in which cardiac dimensions are indexed to aortic diameter or the aortic diameter predicted based on body weight was proposed. Both allometric scaling, in which echocardiographic dimensions are related to the cube root of body weight, and the use of aorta-based ratio indices overcome some of the theoretical and practical limitations of comparing cardiac dimensions to body weight.
- The end-systolic volume index calculated as $LVIDs^3/BSA$, where *LVIDs* is the end-systolic left ventricular dimension and *BSA* is body surface area has been used in the assessment of myocardial function in dogs with MR. An index greater than 30 ml/m^2 suggests myocardial dysfunction.
- Doppler echocardiography is used to evaluate velocity, direction, and character of blood flow.
- Doppler evidence of disturbed flow within the left atrium during systole is noninvasive confirmation of the presence of MR (see Figure 6-8). When stroke volume is severely affected by MR or systolic failure, reductions in aortic outflow velocities may be apparent.
- Assessment of the severity of MR can be evaluated quantitatively or more often, semi-quantitatively by Doppler echocardiography.
- Quantitative methods include evaluation of the radius of color Doppler proximal flow convergence and the calculation of regurgitant fractions through volumetric flow analysis; however, these

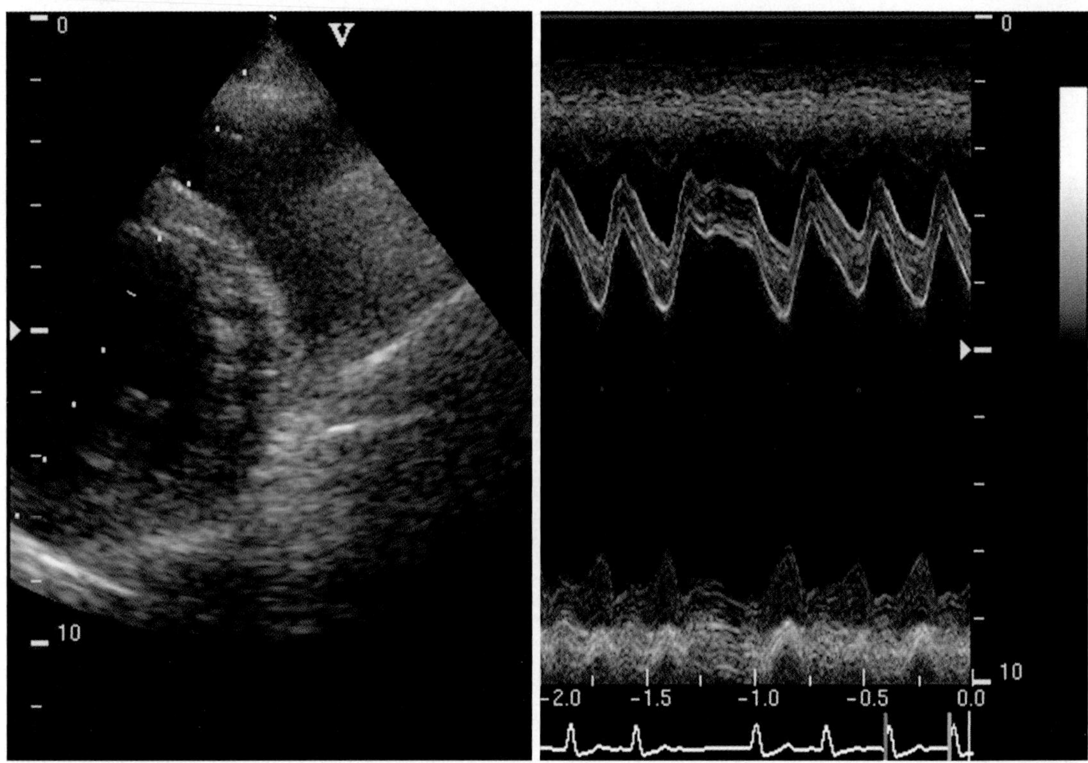

Figure 6-10. M-mode echocardiogram obtained at the level of the left ventricular papillary muscles from 12-year-old male castrated Keeshond weighing 18 kg. There was Doppler evidence of severe mitral regurgitation due to degenerative valve disease. Left ventricular systolic performance evaluated by fractional shortening is normal (38%) but the end-systolic left ventricular dimension is markedly enlarged which provides evidence of systolic myocardial dysfunction. The cardiac rhythm is atrial fibrillation.

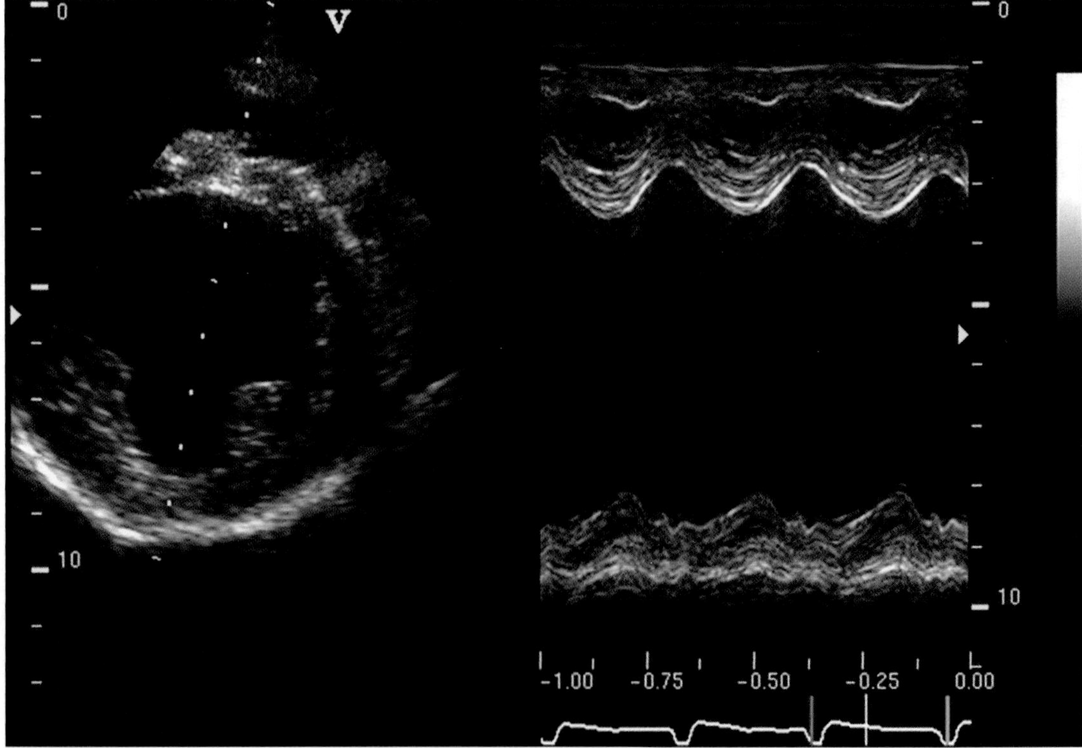

Figure 6-11. M-mode echocardiogram obtained at the level of the left ventricular papillary muscles from 12-year-old male castrated Dalmatian. There was Doppler evidence of severe mitral regurgitation due to degenerative valve disease. Left ventricular systolic performance evaluated by fractional shortening is subnormal (22%) and the end-systolic left ventricular dimension is markedly enlarged. These findings provide evidence of systolic myocardial dysfunction. An examination recorded three years before this one had demonstrated mitral valve regurgitation and mildly hyperdynamic systolic performance. In the interim, the end-diastolic and end-systolic left ventricular dimensions had enlarged. Large dogs are more apt to develop systolic myocardial dysfunction as a consequence of mitral valve disease than are small dogs.

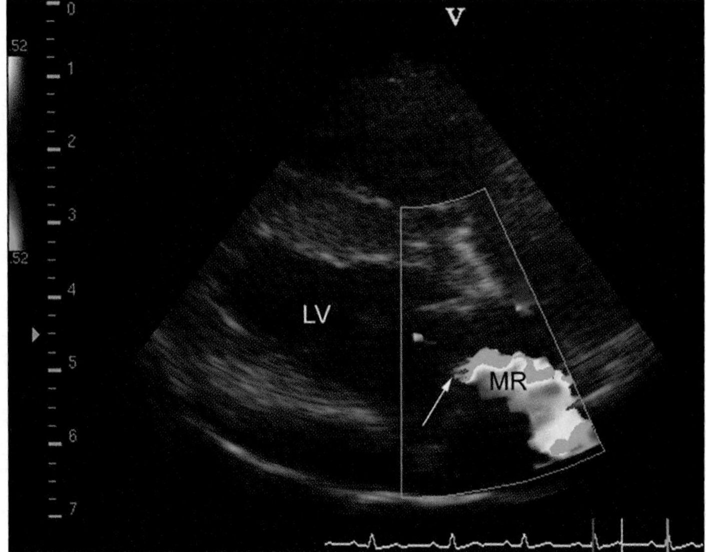

Figure 6-12. A right parasternal long-axis echocardiographic image obtained from a 5-year-old female spayed Cavalier King Charles Spaniel with mitral regurgitation due to early onset degenerative disease. Color-flow Doppler mapping demonstrates mild mitral valve regurgitation *(MR)*. The color mosaic occupies less than 50% of the area of the left atrium and the jet is relatively narrow at its origin *(arrow)*. *LV*, Left ventricle.

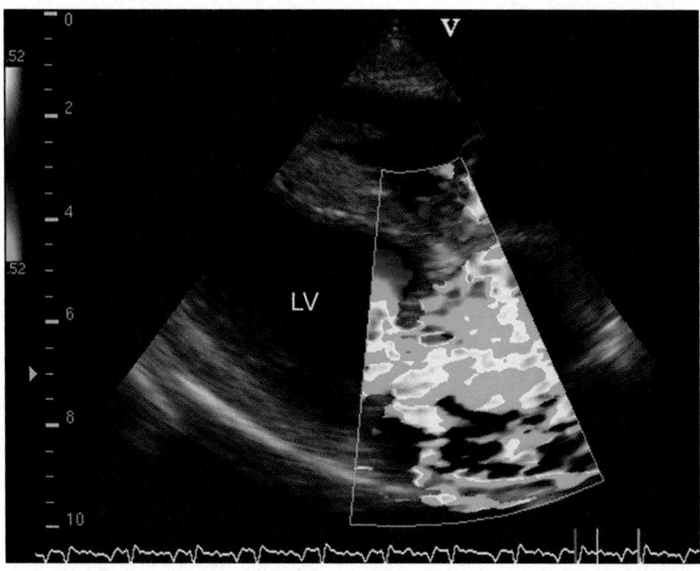

Figure 6-13. A right parasternal long-axis echocardiographic image obtained from a 12-year-old female spayed Whippet with mitral regurgitation due to degenerative disease. Color-flow Doppler mapping demonstrates marked mitral valve regurgitation. The color mosaic nearly fills the enlarged left atrium and more importantly with respect to evaluation of the severity of regurgitation, the jet is very broad at its origin. *LV*, Left ventricle.

methods are time consuming and have not found widespread clinical application.

- The area of the color Doppler regurgitant jet relative to that of the receiving chamber is one means of semi-quantitatively evaluating the severity of valvular regurgitation; however, many physiologic and technical factors influence the size of the jet and this intuitively simple method has limitations. The *width* of the regurgitant jet at its origin is another, perhaps more accurate, means of evaluating the severity of regurgitation; a greater width indicates a larger orifice and, more severe regurgitation (Figures 6-12 and 6-13). The appearance of proximal flow convergence—the color Doppler appearance of acceleration through the regurgitant orifice—suggests that MR is at least of moderate severity (Figure 6-14).
- The density of the regurgitant continuous wave spectral Doppler signal is roughly proportional

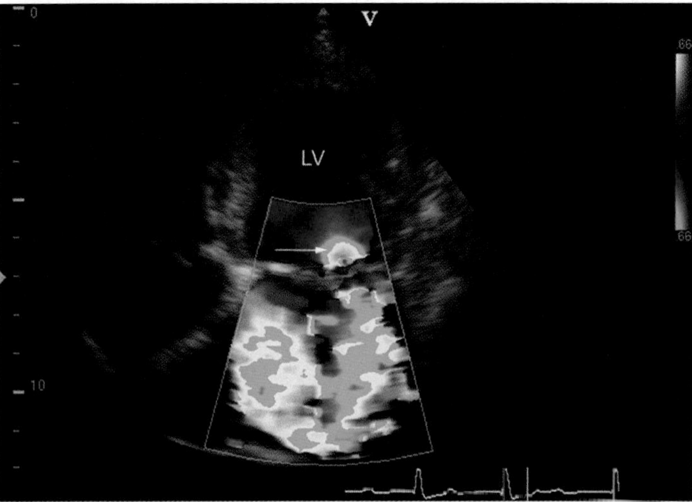

Figure 6-14. A left parasternal apical echocardiographic image from a 13-year-old male castrated mixed-breed dog with mitral regurgitation due to degenerative disease. Color-flow Doppler mapping demonstrates marked mitral valve regurgitation. The region of proximal flow acceleration *(arrow)* is evident within the left ventricle *(LV)*.

to the number of cells that move into the receiving chamber and is an alternative means of semiquantitatively evaluating regurgitant severity (Figure 6-15).

- Ultimately, it is important that the echocardiographic assessment is clinically relevant: in veterinary patients in whom valvular repair is seldom performed, the effect of valvular regurgitation might be of greater importance than its magnitude—information regarding chamber size and myocardial function is essential in placing Doppler findings in the appropriate clinical context.

Relative Merits of Radiography and Echocardiography in Mitral Valve Regurgitation

It should be emphasized that MVD exhibits a broad spectrum of severity. Often, the presence of MR is incidental to the presentation, and clinical signs such as cough are not the result of CHF or even heart disease, but, rather, result from primary respiratory disease. Therefore, in most cases, the thoracic radiograph provides the most useful diagnostic and prognostic information in patients with MVD. Thoracic radiography not only provides an assessment of cardiac size but also allows visualization of the pulmonary vessels and parenchyma. Thus, thoracic radiography provides an indirect assessment of cardiac performance, and currently it is the only widely available noninvasive route to a diagnosis of CHF.

Echocardiography provides a noninvasive means by which to evaluate valvular structure, assess cardiac dimensions, evaluate left ventricular systolic performance, and, with Doppler studies, confirm the clinical diagnosis of MR. However, echocardiography cannot provide a diagnosis of CHF; it can only demonstrate that cardiac disease is sufficiently severe that a diagnosis of CHF is plausible. Although the clinical signs associated with MVD may have a sudden onset, the disease process itself is chronic. Therefore, left atrial dilation and, usually, concurrent left ventricular dilation are expected prior to the onset of clinical signs. Echocardiographic evidence of MR in the absence of left atrial and left ventricular dilation is seldom of clinical importance. In most cases, then, echocardiography is not essential for the clinical management of patients with MR. In patients with suspected MR, echocardiography is likely to provide clinically useful information in the following scenarios:

- When the cause of a cardiac murmur is uncertain (for example, patients in which the signalment is atypical or there is the possibility that the murmur is congenital)
- When it is difficult to discern from thoracic radiographs whether or not the left atrium is enlarged
- When sudden deterioration has occurred, and rupture of the chordae tendineae or left atrium is suspected
- When it is important to evaluate systolic myocardial function
- When pulmonary hypertension is suspected

KEY POINT

Echocardiography is not essential to the management of most cases of MVD but often provides useful, noninvasively acquired, ancillary information.

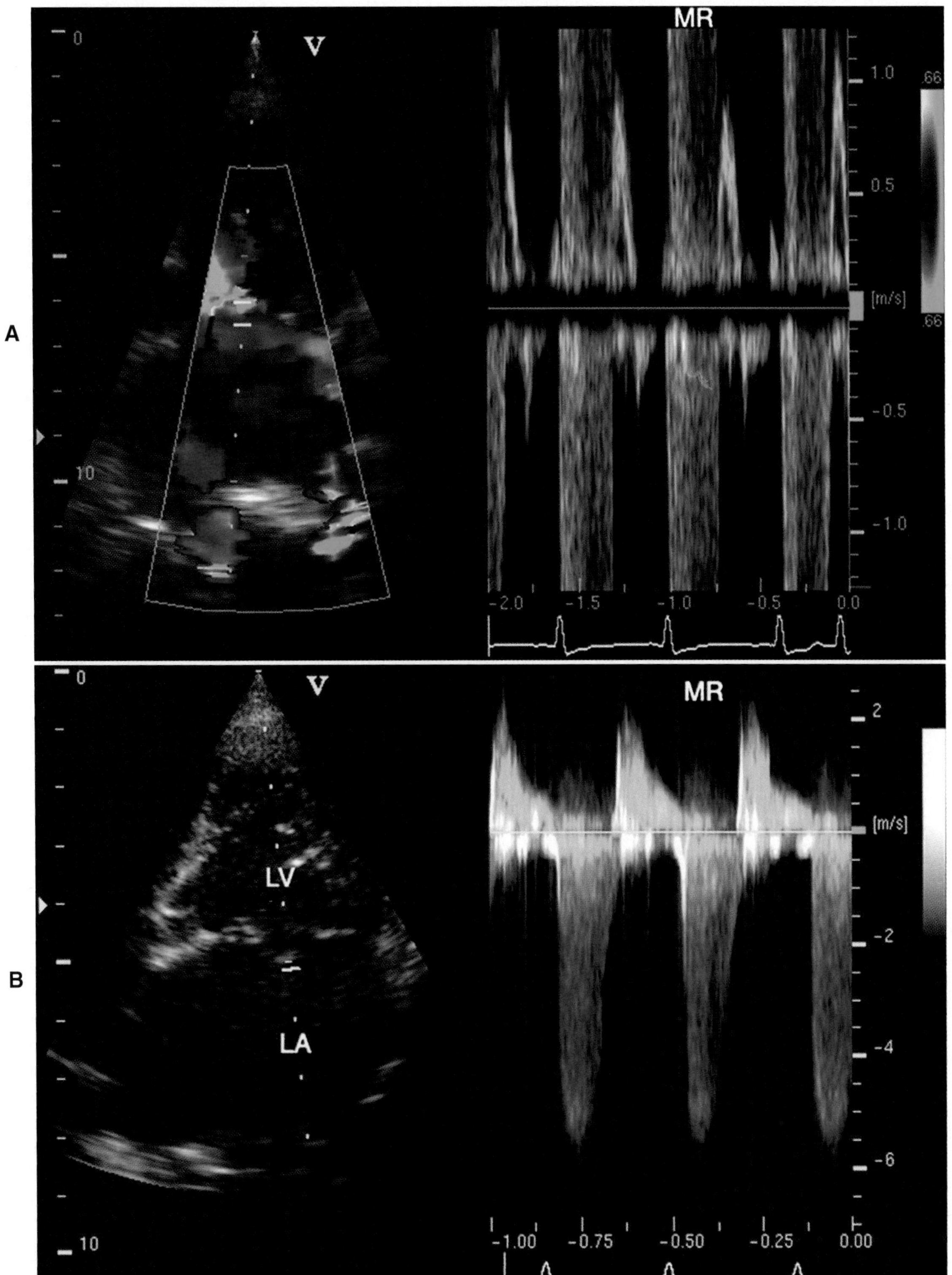

Figure 6-15. **A,** Pulsed wave Doppler echocardiogram obtained from a dog with mitral valve incompetence due to degenerative mitral valve disease. The pulsed wave sample volume was placed within the left atrium; during systole there is a dense, aliasing multifrequency signal. **B,** Continuous wave Doppler study of the left atrium of a dog with severe mitral valve incompetence due to degenerative mitral valve disease. The signal is quite dense, suggesting severe regurgitation.

Electrocardiography

- Electrocardiography is useful primarily for the diagnosis of arrhythmias but also can provide indirect evidence of chamber enlargement.
- The electrocardiogram is an insensitive gauge of cardiac chamber size. Nevertheless, it is likely that findings such as P mitrale are relatively specific; that is, when P waves in the caudal frontal leads (i.e., II, III, and aVF) are wide, the left atrium is usually enlarged (Figure 6-16).
- Arrhythmias can complicate the presentation of MVD. Most often, arrhythmias in MVD take the form of supraventricular tachyarrhythmias that reflect atrial stretch. Atrial premature complexes and paroxysms of atrial tachycardia are relatively common in patients with MVD. Atrial fibrillation develops occasionally and generally indicates advanced disease with marked atrial dilation. Ventricular arrhythmias (ventricular premature complexes) may develop in association with left ventricular dilation and myocardial fibrosis.

Therapy

Subclinical ("Asymptomatic") Mitral Valve Disease

- Definitive published evidence that medical therapy slows the progression of subclinical ("asymptomatic") MVD is lacking.
- A theoretical, ideal treatment for MVD could be used to prevent or reverse myxomatous degeneration. Unfortunately, drug therapy that affects this pathologic process has not been identified.
- In the absence of evidence that medical therapy can alter the progression of valvular degeneration, interest has been directed toward the possibility that drug therapy might improve prognosis in subclinical MVD by decreasing MR or by modifying the process of ventricular remodeling.
- Unfortunately, despite evidence that angiotensi-converting enzyme (ACE) inhibitors favorably affect prognosis in people with asymptomatic ventricular dysfunction, only limited efficacy of ACE inhibitors in subclinical MVD has been demonstrated.
- The possibility that enalapril might delay the onset of heart failure in subclinical MVD has been addressed by two separate clinical trials. In both the Scandinavian Veterinary Enalapril Prevention (SVEP) Trial and the Veterinary Enalapril Trial to Prove Reduction in Onset of Heart Failure (VETPROOF), dogs with subclinical MR were randomized to receive placebo or **enalapril**. Neither trial demonstrated a statistically significant effect of enalapril on time to development of CHF. Although the result of the VETPROOF trial was not statistically significant with respect to the primary end point, the data did show a tendency toward a favorable treatment effect. Atrial enlargement was an inclusion criterion for VETPROOF but not for SVEP; however, it is worthy of consideration that both trials included patients with relatively mild MR. Patients with mild and slowly progressive disease tend to experience few events of interest—death or occurrence of heart failure, for example—even during relatively long periods of follow-up. The inclusion of mildly affected patients in a clinical trial might mask a treatment effect that is evident only for patients with severe disease. It is therefore possible that a subpopulation of preclinical patients with severe MR and cardiomegaly would benefit from ACE inhibition. Although this hypothesis has not been specifically tested, it is partly refuted by the results of SVEP; in that trial, a treatment effect was not observed in the subset of dogs that had radiographic cardiomegaly at study entry.
- The reason that ACE inhibitors do not appear to improve prognosis in subclinical MVD is not

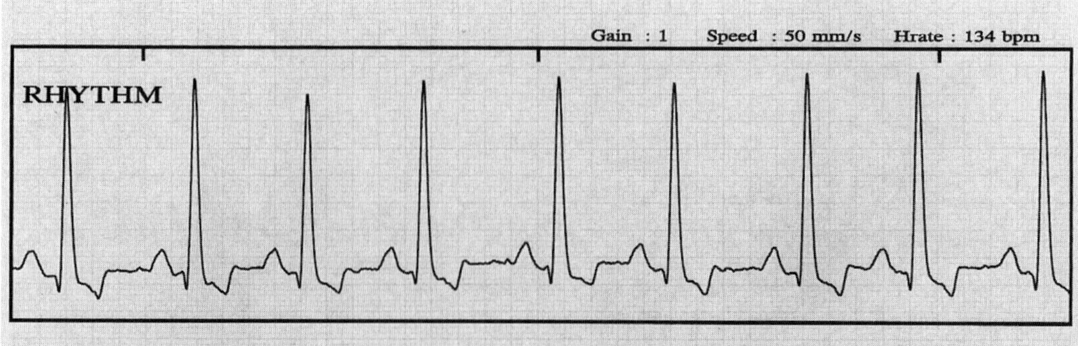

Figure 6-16. An electrocardiogram recorded from a 13-year-old Beagle with physical findings of mitral valve regurgitation. There is P-mitrale, and the R amplitude exceeds 3 mV, suggesting left atrial enlargement and left ventricular hypertrophy, respectively. (Lead II, 50 mm/s, 1 mV = 1 cm.)

known; however, it should be recognized that the widely cited clinical trials of ACE inhibition in people with heart disease generally have enrolled people with past myocardial infarction or idiopathic DCM. MVD in people is generally treated surgically, and, indeed, medical therapy is not recommended for asymptomatic people with MR.

- Pathophysiologic differences between people with ventricular myocardial dysfunction and dogs with MVD might also be relevant. In contrast to the effect of renin-angiotensin-aldosterone system (RAS) suppression in dogs with experimentally induced, primary myocardial disease, neither ACE inhibitors nor angiotensin II antagonists favorably affect ventricular remodeling in dogs with experimentally induced MR. However, the syndrome that results from acute disruption of the mitral valve in the laboratory may differ markedly from spontaneous valvular degeneration associated with chronic, progressive MR. Therefore, the clinical relevance of these research findings is uncertain.
- Theoretical considerations aside, definitive evidence that ACE inhibitors improve prognosis in subclinical MVD is lacking. Although it might be argued that trials to date have had inadequate statistical power, it is likely that a favorable effect of ACE inhibition, if one exists, is modest; the results of VETPROOF suggest that 2 years of therapy with enalapril may delay the onset of pulmonary edema by approximately 4 months. Based on available data, the author generally does not treat dogs with subclinical MVD. On a pragmatic level, the practitioner is sometimes presented with subclinical patients for which radiographic findings suggest that the development of frank heart failure is imminent. In cases where there is marked left atrial enlargement and pulmonary venous distension, the author prescribes an ACE inhibitor. It is noteworthy that long-term ACE inhibition has not been associated with detrimental effects. Furthermore, it is possible that these drugs have benefits that relate to effects on other geriatric disorders such as hypertension or renal disease. Based on this and the suggestion of a favorable effect in the VETPROOF trial, ACE inhibition may be a therapeutic consideration for some patients with cardiac enlargement and subclinical MR; however, the evidence to support this approach is neither direct nor strong.

KEY POINT

Medical therapy that slows the progression of MVD has not been identified.

Cough caused by Airway Compression

- Some dogs with MVD develop a cough that appears to result from compression of the mainstem bronchi by an enlarged left atrium. This type of cough can develop prior to the development of pulmonary edema.
- Radiographically, there is an enlarged cardiac silhouette with distinct evidence of left atrial enlargement. The mainstem bronchi may be noticeably narrowed. The pulmonary veins are sometimes distended, but the pulmonary interstitium and parenchyma have a normal appearance.
- It is important to recognize that primary respiratory tract diseases such as tracheal collapse and chronic bronchitis are common in the same patient group that develops MVD. With very few exceptions, clinical signs related to MVD do not occur in the absence of radiographic left atrial enlargement.
- When radiographic findings suggest that the cause of cough is airway compression but not pulmonary edema, the use of an antitussive such as **hydrocodone** or **butorphanol** is rational.
- Vasodilation causes a decrease in systemic vascular resistance and, in the setting of MR, can increase stroke volume through a decrease in the regurgitant fraction. Potentially these effects can decrease left atrial and pulmonary venous pressures and perhaps, reduce left atrial size.
- Cough due to compression of the airways generally is associated with considerable chamber enlargement and this latter finding is a risk factor for the ultimate development of heart failure. Because of the proven favorable effect of ACE inhibition in patients with heart failure due to MVD, it is reasonable to administer an ACE inhibitor in addition to an antitussive, when cough results from bronchial compression.
- Some of the benefits of ACE inhibition likely relate to their neuroendocrine effects. Because of this and because the ACE inhibitors are not potent vasodilators, a case might be made for the use of **hydralazine** or perhaps **amlodipine** for dogs with MVD and cough due to bronchial compression. Caution must be exercised if these drugs are used and patients should be monitored for the development of systemic hypotension.
- Diuretic administration effectively reduces cardiac volumes and may also be efficacious. The argument can be advanced that this may result in harmful activation of the renin-angiotensin axis. Therefore, in this clinical situation, add furosemide to the drug regimen only when ACE inhibition in combination with an antitussive, fails to result in clinical improvement.

Table 6-2 Suggested Strategies for Diagnostic and Therapeutic Management of Canine Degenerative Valvular Disease

	Subclinical MR	Cough caused by Airway Compression	CHF	Advanced CHF
Diagnostic approach	X-rays as indicated by clinical circumstances (i.e., prior to elective anesthesia, loud murmurs particularly if associated with tachycardia) EKG when auscultation suggests pathologic arrhythmia	X-rays Echocardiography recommended when radiographic evidence of left atrial enlargement is equivocal EKG when auscultation suggests pathologic arrhythmia	X-rays Echocardiography not usually necessary but provides potentially useful ancillary information in most cases EKG when auscultation suggests pathologic arrhythmia	X-rays Echocardiography EKG when auscultation suggests pathologic arrhythmia
Therapeutic approach	Generally none indicated although in some circumstances, the use of an ACE inhibitor might be considered for patients with distinct cardiac enlargement (see text)	Antitussive agent and an ACE inhibitor Short-term anti-inflammatory dose corticosteroids or therapeutic diuretic trial considered for refractory cases	Standard therapy for CHF due to MR consists of furosemide, an ACE inhibitor, and moderate dietary salt restriction	The following can be considered in addition to standard therapy—treatment should be tailored to the individual • Triple diuretic therapy • Amlodipine (or Hydralazine) • Carvedilol • Spironolactone • Pimobendan • Nitroglycerin

- When cough fails to respond to ACE inhibition and modest diuresis, it is important to consider the possibility that the cough results not from heart disease but rather from primary respiratory tract disease.

Treatment of Congestive Heart Failure caused by Mitral Valve Disease

- When MR causes clinical signs in people, the disorder is treated surgically. Mitral valve repair with preservation of chordal attachments is generally preferred to replacement of the valve with a prosthesis. Surgical treatment of dogs with MVD has been reported. However, expense and the need for expertise in open-heart surgery performed during cardiopulmonary bypass have limited the availability of this approach.
- Heart failure due to MVD generally is treated medically (Table 6-2). Unless the cause can be definitively treated, heart failure is a terminal syndrome. Therefore, medical management is intended to alleviate clinical signs and to prolong life. Drug therapy of heart failure consists primarily of interventions that manipulate the determinants of cardiac output and others intended to blunt the maladaptive neuroendocrine response to cardiac dysfunction.
- In CHF due to MR, left ventricular filling pressure (preload) is excessive, and the consequent increase in venous pressures causes tissue fluid to weep into the pulmonary interstitium and alveoli. The administration of agents that reduce intravascular volume, such as diuretics, or of agents that increase venous capacitance, such as nitroglycerin, are therefore a mainstay of therapy.
- **Nitroglycerin** is usually administered transdermally and is used most often as short-term therapy in patients with fulminant edema, or occasionally as adjunctive therapy in patients with advanced disease. The efficacy of transdermal nitroglycerin is uncertain, and in dogs with experimentally induced MR, the effect of nitroglycerin on filling pressure did not differ from that of placebo.
- **Furosemide**, a potent agent that acts on the loop of Henle, is the diuretic that is used most often in veterinary practice. It can be administered orally or parenterally; the route of administration

is chosen based upon the clinical status of the patient. The resultant decrease in intravascular volume reduces left ventricular filling pressures, allows lymphatic drainage of tissue fluid and, resolution of edema.

- It should be recognized that diuretics reduce preload; this decrease in ventricular filling pressures is generally well tolerated by patients with ventricular dilation and has obvious benefits when edema is present. However, excessive diuresis can result in hypotension related to low cardiac output, prerenal azotemia, and electrolyte disturbances. It is generally believed that the optimal dose of furosemide is the lowest one that controls signs of congestion.
- Importantly, many dogs with clinically evident MVD cough in the absence of pulmonary edema, and many of these patients have concurrent primary respiratory tract disease. Therefore, aggressive diuresis following radiographically demonstrated resolution of pulmonary edema is to be avoided. In most cases of CHF due to MVD, the administration of furosemide rapidly and effectively resolves signs. Failure of patients with MR and respiratory distress to respond promptly to diuretic administration should cause the practitioner to question the diagnosis of CHF.
- Most patients that develop radiographic pulmonary edema due to MR require lifelong diuretic therapy. Early in the course of the syndrome, a dose of 1 mg/kg PO every 12 hours may be adequate, although the inevitable progression of MR and CHF and renal tubular adaptations ultimately necessitate higher doses.
- Moderate dietary salt restriction is suggested for patients with CHF due to MVD.
- The benefits of ACE inhibition in CHF due to MR have been demonstrated. Thus, the use of an ACE inhibitor together with furosemide has become standard therapy for CHF due to MVD.
- **Pimobendan** has recently been approved by the United States Food and Drug Administration for use in dogs; it is indicated for the management of the signs of mild, moderate, and severe CHF resulting from DCM or atrioventricular valve insufficiency. Previously, pimobendan had been licensed for use in dogs with heart failure in Canada, Europe, and Australasia.
- Pimobendan is an "inodilator" that has complex pharmacologic properties. It inhibits phosphodiesterase and therefore causes vasodilation and an increase in inotropic state. Additionally, pimobendan increases the sensitivity of the contractile apparatus to available calcium, an effect which also contributes to the inotropic effect. This latter property may be favorable because the increase in inotropic state is associated with a relatively low cost in terms of myocardial oxygen consumption.
- Two recent clinical trials compared the effects of pimobendan with an ACE inhibitor in dogs with heart failure due to MVD. These trials demonstrated that the clinical effects of pimobendan and furosemide were not inferior to established therapy consisting of furosemide and an ACE inhibitor. For some clinical variables, pimobendan was superior to the ACE inhibitor. The effect of pimobendan when used together with an ACE inhibitor in dogs with valvular disease has not been addressed in published trials to date. Therefore, the stage of disease at which pimobendan is most appropriately added to conventional therapy can be debated. It is reasonable to add pimobendan to the therapeutic regimen when there is clinical deterioration despite administration of furosemide and an ACE inhibitor. The concurrent use of pimobendan, an ACE inhibitor, and furosemide as initial therapy can probably be justified when MVD results in severe heart failure. When pet owners are constrained financially, and it is possible to prescribe only pimobendan or an ACE inhibitor, the available data suggest that the use of either drug likely is appropriate.
- In Beagles with mild MVD, chronic, oral administration of pimobendan was associated with histologic valvular lesions that were more severe than those in a similar group of Beagles that received benazepril. These data and a clinical case report suggest that in some circumstances, pimobendan might accelerate the development of degenerative valvular lesions. Pimobendan is not indicated for the management of subclinical MVD.
- When atrial tachyarrhythmias, particularly atrial fibrillation, complicate MVD, the use of digoxin (0.22 mg/m^2 PO every 12 hours) is generally accepted. However, the role of digoxin in the management of patients with CHF who are in normal sinus rhythm remains a point of controversy.
- **Digoxin** has two principal effects; it acts as a positive inotrope and as a negative chronotrope. The latter property is related to the autonomic effects of the drug, which include a central vagomimetic effect and effects that may serve to normalize the baroreceptor dysfunction associated with CHF. There is evidence to suggest that chronic activation

of the adrenergic nervous system is detrimental, and that this abnormality may be partly reversed by the administration of digoxin.

- The need for digoxin in the patient with CHF due to MVD is difficult to assess. Because the commonly used echocardiographic indices of contractility depend on preload and afterload as well as myocardial function, they are difficult to interpret when MR is severe. Furthermore, the results of clinical trials that enrolled people with heart failure cast doubt on the intuitive notion that chronic inotropic therapy is beneficial.
- The effect of digoxin on dogs with heart failure and sinus rhythm has not been evaluated. However, based on the results of a clinical trial that addressed the role of digoxin in people with heart failure, it seems likely that the magnitude of effect in dogs—whether it is positive or negative—is probably small.
- In patients with MVD and sinus rhythm, it seems most reasonable to reserve the use of digoxin for patients with advanced CHF and preserved renal function as digoxin is excreted almost entirely through the kidneys. When administering digoxin to dogs in sinus rhythm, aim for a blood concentration of 0.5 to 1 ng/mg on a sample obtained 8 to 10 hours postdose. Higher concentrations likely are necessary and appropriate when atrial fibrillation is present.

Neuroendocrine Modulation

- ACE inhibitors are part of the standard therapeutic approach to heart failure caused by MR. It is likely that the favorable effect of ACE inhibition is not simply the result of vasodilation. In addition to this mechanical effect, ACE inhibition serves to protect the heart from the apparently detrimental effects of RAS activation.
- Pharmacologic ACE inhibition generally is not complete, and because aldosterone may contribute to the development of myocardial fibrosis, more complete suppression of the RAS may yield positive results. Accordingly, the use of **spironolactone**—a weak diuretic that antagonizes the effect of aldosterone—is considered as adjunctive therapy for patients with severe CHF due to MVD. In humans with CHF, the use of subdiuretic doses of spironolactone prolongs survival.
- Beta blockers decrease mortality in people with heart failure. Because these drugs have a potent negative inotropic effect, the mechanism by which beta blockers improve survival is not intuitively obvious. However, it is now recognized that seemingly compensatory activation of the adrenergic nervous system and RAS is ultimately maladaptive and contributes to the progressive nature of heart failure. The use of beta blockers in this setting is consistent with this paradigm.
- Acutely, beta blockers have a negative effect on cardiac performance and should be used in canines with heart failure only with caution. Beta blockers must be initiated at very low doses and titrated to effect or target dose over the course of weeks.
- The use of beta blockers in patients with systolic failure is predicated on the belief that these agents preserve myocardial function. Although invasive measures may disclose myocardial function in dogs with MR, the primary cause of clinical signs in patients with MVD is likely the mechanical effect of the volume load. Nevertheless, studies of dogs with experimentally induced MR suggest that beta blockade may have a role in the management of MVD.
- **Carvedilol** is a third-generation beta blocker that is also an alpha adrenergic antagonist. Because of this latter property, carvedilol is a weak vasodilator, which might make this beta blocker particularly well suited to the management of MVD.
- The author considers the use of carvedilol, or a less expensive alternative such as **metoprolol** or **atenolol**, when echocardiographic findings suggest incipient or patent myocardial dysfunction.

Therapy of Severe Congestive Heart Failure caused by Advanced Mitral Valve Regurgitation

- The use of triple diuretic therapy—combining **furosemide** with a **thiazide** and a potassium-sparing diuretic such as **spironolactone**—can be considered for patients that require high doses of furosemide to remain free of congestive signs. The use of three different diuretic agents interferes with nephron function at anatomically and functionally distinct sites; together, the drugs may have synergistic effects, allowing the use of lower doses of the individual agents. Additionally, the use of a potassium-sparing agent such as spironolactone serves to limit some of the adverse effects that are associated with the use of high doses of loop diuretics such as furosemide.
- Despite proven efficacy in the management of heart failure due to MVD, the ACE inhibitors are not potent vasodilators. In some patients with CHF due to severe MVD, the use of **hydralazine** or perhaps the vasoselective calcium channel blocker, **amlodipine**, in addition to an ACE inhibitor may be helpful. When vasodilators are used in addition to ACE inhibitors, the initial dose should be low; ideally, the dose is titrated to effect based on serial blood pressure determinations.

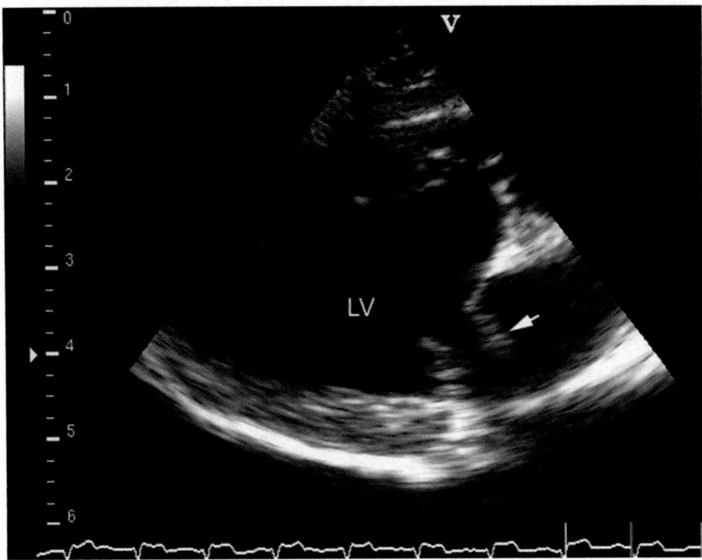

Figure 6-17. An early systolic, right parasternal long-axis echocardiographic image obtained from an 8-year-old, female spayed Papillion. The anterior mitral valve leaflet *(arrow)* was flail—the leaflet is perpendicular to plane of the mitral annulus—because of rupture of a chorda tendineae. *LV,* Left ventricle.

KEY POINT

The author's standard medical therapy for heart failure due to MVD consists of furosemide, an ACE inhibitor, and in some cases, digoxin. Pimobendan has been approved for the treatment of mild, moderate, and severe CHF due to MVD. Spironolactone and beta blockers may have roles as adjunctive therapy.

Complications of Mitral Valve Disease and Its Treatment

Development of Azotemia Associated with Diuretic and Angiotensin-Converting Enzyme Inhibitor Administration

- Monitoring of renal function is suggested for patients that are treated with diuretics and ACE inhibitors. ACE inhibitors are not generally thought to be directly nephrotoxic; however, ACE inhibition results in relatively selective dilation of the efferent arteriole of the nephron, a hemodynamic effect that can predispose to the development of prerenal azotemia. Those patients with preexisting renal disease and those receiving overly aggressive doses of diuretics are most likely to develop azotemia. In addition, patients with severe cardiac dysfunction that are critically dependent upon the effects of angiotensin II to maintain glomerular filtration fraction may also develop azotemia when ACE inhibitors are administered.
- It should be recalled that there are essentially no circumstances under which diuresis will increase stroke volume and renal blood flow. In contrast, judicious vasodilation in the setting of MR can do exactly that. Thus, the development of azotemia is usually managed first by a cautious reduction in the diuretic dose. Should creatinine values fail to decrease, the diuretic can be discontinued; the patient's respiratory rate and character should be carefully monitored. If azotemia persists after discontinuation of diuretic therapy, the ACE inhibitor can be discontinued, and cautious intravenous infusion of fluid can be initiated.

Rupture of Chordae Tendineae

- Rupture of chordae tendineae is a relatively common complication of MVD. When a primary chorda ruptures, the attached mitral leaflet becomes suddenly flail (Figure 6-17), potentially resulting in catastrophic MR, marked elevations in ventricular filling pressures, and fulminant pulmonary edema. Rupture of minor chordae may result in less impressive clinical signs or may be subclinical.
- Rupture of a primary chorda tendinea may occur in patients that have substantial, preexisting MR and cardiac enlargement and result in clinical decompensation the severity of which varies. However, the development of acute pulmonary edema in patients with normal cardiac dimensions is uncommon.

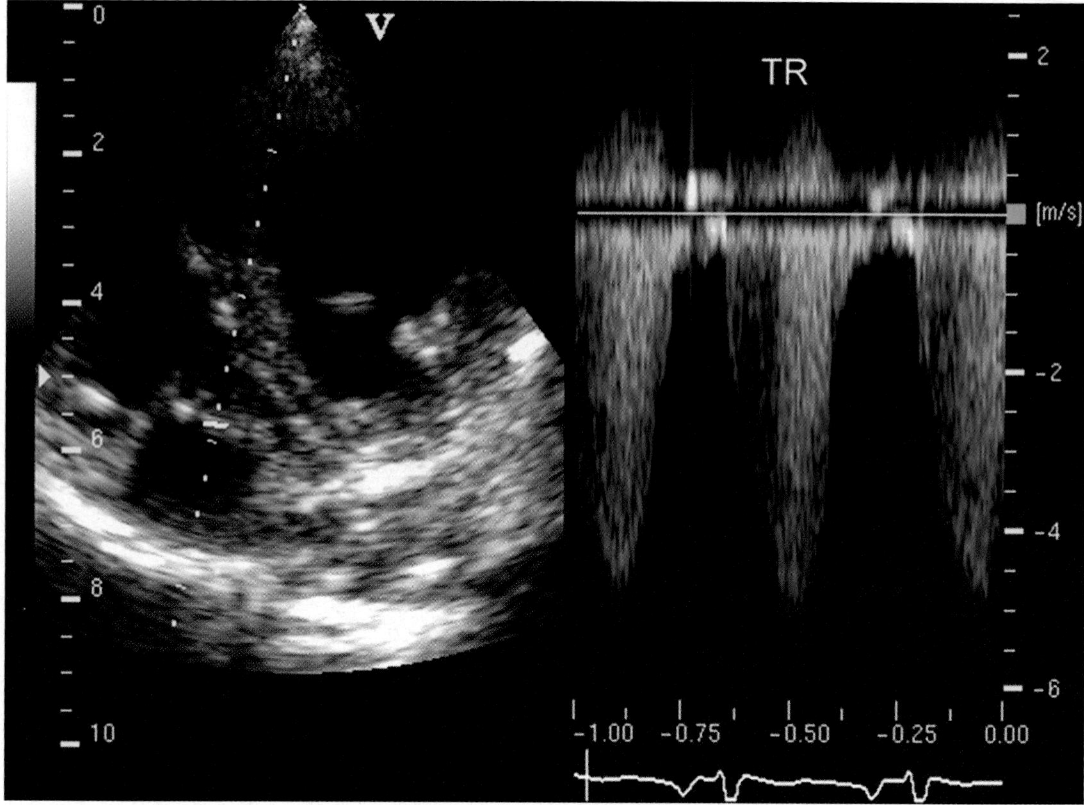

Figure 6-18. Continuous wave Doppler study performed with the Doppler cursor through the right atrium of a dog with severe endocardiosis. There is tricuspid valve regurgitation *(TR);* the peak velocity of the TR jet was nearly 5 m/s. This corresponds to a systolic right atrial–right ventricular pressure difference that is close to 100 mm Hg and provides evidence of severe pulmonary hypertension. In this case, elevated left atrial pressure was partly responsible for pulmonary hypertension but the predicted pulmonary artery pressure was out of proportion to any credible estimate of left atrial pressure. Reactive vasoconstriction of the pulmonary arterioles may have contributed to the development of pulmonary hypertension.

- Acute CHF due to chordal rupture is treated similarly to acute or decompensated heart failure caused by other disorders although there may be a particular role for the intravenous administration of nitroprusside in addition to parenteral diuretic administration.
- The prognosis depends on numerous factors of which response to therapy is probably most important.

Pulmonary Hypertension

- Pulmonary hypertension occasionally complicates the clinical presentation of MVD in the dog. Doppler studies can provide noninvasive estimates of pulmonary artery pressure. Doppler echocardiographic evidence of tricuspid valve regurgitation (TR) is commonly observed in patients with MVD. The velocity of the TR jet is related to the systolic pressure difference between the right atrium and the right ventricle by the modified Bernoulli equation ($\Delta P = 4v^2$, where ΔP is the pressure difference and v is the velocity of the regurgitant jet). The right atrial pressure is approximated based on clinical findings; in the absence of right-sided CHF, the right atrial pressure is likely less than 10 mm Hg. Provided pulmonary stenosis (PS) is excluded by Doppler evaluation of the right ventricular outflow tract, right ventricular and pulmonary artery pressures are equal during systole. Thus, measurement of the velocity of the TR jet can provide noninvasive estimates of systolic pulmonary artery pressure (Figure 6-18).
- The cause of pulmonary hypertension associated with MVD is probably multifactorial. The primary function of the right ventricle is to propel the stroke volume through the pulmonary vascular tree to the left atrium. Elevations in left atrial pressure cause commensurate increases in right ventricular systolic pressure; if mean pulmonary artery pressure does not exceed mean left atrial pressure, there is no impetus for forward flow. The tendency for left atrial hypertension to cause pulmonary hypertension is probably the primary explanation for high pulmonary artery pressures in most cases; however, in some patients, the

increase in estimated pulmonary artery pressure is disproportionate to any credible estimate of left atrial pressure. In these cases, pulmonary arterial constriction—sometimes known as "reactive vasoconstriction" probably contributes. Alternatively, pulmonary hypertension may be also related to the presence of concurrent pulmonary or airway disease.

- There is no established therapy for patients with pulmonary hypertension associated with MVD. Most vasodilators have a relatively predictable effect on the systemic vasculature; however, the pulmonary arterioles respond inconsistently to the commonly used vasodilator agents, and, in consequence, it should be recognized that the use of vasodilators in patients with pulmonary hypertension due to severe pulmonary vascular disease is not without risk. If a vasodilator with potent peripheral effects fails to decrease pulmonary vascular resistance, systemic hypotension or detrimental increases in right ventricular pressure and myocardial oxygen demand may result.
- As initial therapy, interventions that reduce left atrial pressure are reasonable. Diuretic therapy should be tailored to rid the patient of radiographic evidence of pulmonary congestion or edema. Alveolar hypoxia is a stimulus for constriction of the pulmonary arterioles. If bronchoconstriction associated with primary respiratory disease has contributed to the development of pulmonary hypertension, the administration of bronchodilators may be helpful.
- When effective control of pulmonary congestion or therapy of primary respiratory tract disease fails to lower pulmonary artery pressure, and clinical signs such as weakness can plausibly be related to pulmonary hypertension, the use of sildenafil in addition to an ACE inhibitor can be considered. Sildenafil is an inhibitor of phosphodiesterase-V that appears to have a relatively selective effect on pulmonary arterioles. When possible, systemic blood pressure should be monitored when therapy with this drug is initiated (see Chapter 9).

Prognosis

- The prognosis associated with the development of MVD depends on numerous factors. The majority of patients with MR due to MVD succumb to noncardiac disease. In the absence of noncardiac disease, patients with cough or syncope and distinct radiographic evidence of left atrial enlargement often go on to develop CHF. When CHF develops, the disease is generally terminal. Even with palliative medical therapy, survival is usually measured in months, with 8 to 14 months being typical.

INFECTIVE ENDOCARDITIS

IE occurs occasionally in dogs and rarely in cats. The prognosis is generally grave, and most cases are terminal even with aggressive medical therapy. This latter point emphasizes the importance of detecting IE, a disease that sometimes poses a considerable diagnostic challenge.

Prevalence and Incidence

- IE is a relatively uncommon disease that is observed occasionally in dogs but rarely in cats. Mural endocarditis and infection of the tricuspid valve are observed occasionally, as is infection of endocardial pacing leads; however, bacterial infection of the aortic or mitral valve leaflets is most common.
- Middle-aged, large-breed male dogs, including German Shepherds and Boxers, are affected most often.
- In people, the presence of a congenital cardiac malformation is a risk factor for the development of IE. An association between congenital subvalvular aortic stenosis and IE of the aortic valve has been demonstrated, and it is likely that subvalvular aortic stenosis and, perhaps, other congenital malformations, are important factors in the epidemiology of IE in dogs.

Etiopathogenesis

- Based on experimental studies, it is likely that the following factors are important in the pathogenesis of infective valvular endocarditis:
  - Endocardial damage (which may result from valvular insufficiency, stenosis, or a shunting lesion)
  - Activation of clotting factors
  - Bacteremia and colonization of a noninfective thrombus
- The development of a noninfective thrombus precedes valvular infection. Episodes of bacteremia can result in infection of the thrombus and the initiation of a variably aggressive inflammatory process that results in distortion and destruction of the valve leaflets and their associated structures.
- In clinical cases of canine IE, a congenital cardiac malformation may represent a predisposition for the development of the disease. Prostatitis,

pyelonephritis, or even dental disease can provide a source for the development of bacteremia; often, however, the site of bacterial entry into the bloodstream remains undiscovered.
- Degenerative valvular disease has no known association with IE. Interestingly, despite the prevalence of dental disease in patients with MR due to MVD, IE is extremely uncommon in this patient group.
- Gram-positive bacteria such as the streptococci and staphylococci are most often implicated in the development of IE. Valvular infection with gram-negative organisms such as *Escherichia coli* is less common.
- With regards to the etiology of IE, there has been recent interest in the fastidious, intracellular organisms of the genus *Bartonella*. Four species of *Bartonella* have been documented to cause canine IE. Although geographical distribution of *Bartonella* IE may not be uniform, *Bartonella* is an important cause of IE in northern California and probably elsewhere. Patients with *Bartonella* infection are often concomitantly seropositive for tick-borne diseases and *Bartonella* itself may be arthropod borne. *Bartonella* spp. are difficult to culture using standard microbiological techniques. The diagnosis depends on documentation of serum antibodies to *Bartonella* or more specifically, demonstration of *Bartonella* antigens through polymerase chain reaction testing performed on bacterial isolates or valve tissue.

Pathophysiology

- The clinical signs of IE relate to sepsis, thromboembolism, and cardiac dysfunction. IE results in intermittent shedding of bacterial organisms into the bloodstream, resulting in episodes of bacteremia. Signs of sepsis, including pyrexia and, rarely, circulatory collapse, may be observed.
- Sequelae of sepsis related to chronic antigenic stimulation and the consequent development of immune complex disease are observed fairly commonly in IE. Polyarthritis is observed often, and glomerulonephritis can also develop.
- In canine IE, it is often the destruction of the valve leaflets and associated structures that is of greatest clinical importance. The development of infected thrombi results in failure of the valve leaflets to coapt. Occasionally, perforation of the valve leaflets contributes to valvular incompetence. The hemodynamic consequences of MR have been discussed previously.
- IE of the aortic valve typically results in aortic valve incompetence, which is a potentially catastrophic hemodynamic lesion. When the aortic valve becomes incompetent, the left ventricle is filled during diastole by the pulmonary venous return and by the blood that enters through the regurgitant orifice. When severe, the increase in ventricular filling pressures (diastolic ventricular pressures) is reflected back upon the pulmonary venous circulation, resulting in pulmonary congestion and edema. In contrast to MR, aortic valve insufficiency (AI) causes a substantial increase in left ventricular afterload and therefore, myocardial oxygen demand. As a result, myocardial dysfunction (cardiomyopathy of overload) is observed commonly and early in the course of aortic valve IE.
- Embolization of fragments from the endocarditis lesion occurs commonly. Sites where infected thrombi lodge include the spleen, the kidney, and occasionally the brain. Most often, embolization of the spleen is clinically silent; infarction of the kidneys or central nervous system can be catastrophic, resulting in renal failure and nervous system signs such as head tilt. Embolization of joints, resulting in bacterial arthritis, can also occur.

Clinical Presentation

History

- IE in dogs is observed most commonly in a subacute form. In these cases, historical evidence of prior illness or of infectious disease may be lacking. A congenital cardiac murmur may or may not have been detected. IE is also observed in an acute form.
- Clinical signs in subacute IE are often vague; lameness, inappetence, dyspnea, syncope, and exercise intolerance are observed most commonly. The lameness is often mild and may be difficult to localize. The embolization of infected thrombi to joints contributes to lameness, although immune complex arthropathy may be of equal etiologic importance.
- Clinical signs of sepsis may be more prominent in patients that develop acute IE. The sudden onset of fever and the development of a new cardiac murmur in the critically ill suggest the presence of IE.

Physical Findings

- Fever is a common but not necessarily a consistent finding in patients with IE. Published cases series of canine IE reflect the experience of referral centers and are therefore biased. At some point in the natural history of the disease it is likely that most patients are pyrexic; however, fever associated with IE can be intermittent and may resolve before clinical presentation.

- The pulse rate is often elevated, as some degree of cardiac dysfunction is commonly present at the time of presentation.
- The respiratory rate is elevated, and respiratory distress is usually apparent, in patients that have developed CHF.
- A cardiac murmur is present in the majority of patients with established valvular infection. MR results in a systolic murmur that is most easily heard over the left cardiac apex. Aortic valve IE usually results in a diastolic decrescendo murmur that is typically heard most easily over the left cardiac base. A concurrent systolic murmur related to the increase in left ventricular stroke volume associated with AI results in a murmur known as "to-and-fro" or "bellows" murmur.
- Diastolic murmurs are uncommon in veterinary patients and are usually soft; consequently, they may escape detection. Despite this, they are of considerable diagnostic and prognostic importance; acquired diastolic murmurs in dogs most often result from aortic valve IE.
- When moderate or severe AI is present, the arterial pulses are hyperkinetic, or bounding, a physical finding that should prompt consideration of IE whenever signalment and other clinical findings are suggestive.

Diagnostic Findings

Thoracic Radiography

- Radiographic findings in IE are variable. Cardiac enlargement is apparent when valvular lesions have imposed a chronic volume overload on the heart. Pulmonary congestion or edema is commonly observed (Figure 6-19). Occasionally, IE results in severe and acute AI; this is one of the few clinical scenarios in which cardiogenic pulmonary edema is observed in association with a normal or minimally enlarged cardiac silhouette.

Electrocardiography

- There are no electrocardiographic findings that are diagnostic of IE. However, all manner of cardiac arrhythmias can be observed in association with this disease. Ventricular tachyarrhythmias, including ventricular tachycardia, are relatively common, and supraventricular tachyarrhythmias, including atrial fibrillation, are also observed.
- The association of third-degree atrioventricular block with IE deserves mention. Occasionally an aggressive aortic lesion will invade the interventricular septum or, alternatively, embolize the nodal coronary artery, resulting in destruction of the atrioventricular node or AV bundle. This catastrophic complication is relatively uncommon, but lesser degrees of atrioventricular block or intraventricular conduction delays, such as left bundle branch block, are observed fairly often.
- Electrocardiographic evidence of cardiac chamber enlargement is observed in patients that survive long enough for the volume overload associated with IE to result in chamber dilation and hypertrophy.

Echocardiographic Findings

- The term vegetative endocarditis is generally used to refer to cases in which there is a macroscopic, infected thrombus associated with a valve leaflet.
- The echocardiographic findings in vegetative IE are distinctive. In most cases, nodular distortion of the valve leaflets is readily apparent (Figure 6-20). Often the valvular abnormality is discrete and the lesion may oscillate independently of valve motion.
- When these abnormalities are associated with the aortic valve leaflets, the diagnosis is usually assured.
- Nodules affecting the mitral valve leaflets are of lesser diagnostic specificity (Figure 6-21), as it can be difficult to distinguish severe MVD from infection of the mitral valve leaflets. To some extent, this distinction is made based upon the patient's signalment. As stated previously, IE is very uncommon in elderly small-breed dogs which are, of course, the patients most likely to develop severe MVD.
- The interpretation of subtle valvular abnormalities detected by echocardiography poses a difficult clinical problem, and other, ancillary clinical data, including the results of blood cultures, must be considered.
- The absence of a readily detectable valvular nodule on echocardiographic examination does not eliminate IE from the differential diagnosis.
- When vegetative IE of the aortic or mitral valve is present, there is often echocardiographic evidence of left atrial and left ventricular enlargement. Premature diastolic closure of the mitral valve and diastolic flutter of the anterior mitral valve leaflet indicate severe AI (Figure 6-22). Some degree of systolic myocardial dysfunction is typically present when cardiac enlargement results from AI. Doppler echocardiography is used to confirm the presence of valvular incompetence.

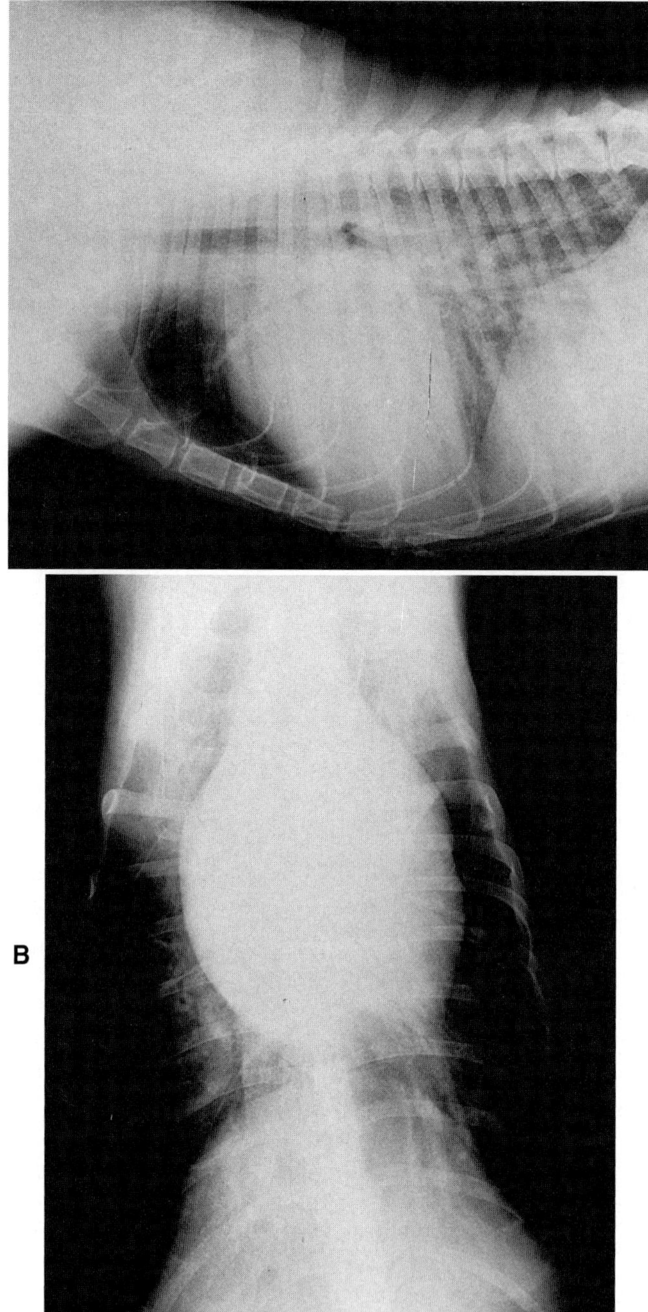

Figure 6-19. Lateral **(A)** and ventrodorsal **(B)** thoracic radiographs obtained from a 1-year-old German Shepherd with aortic valve endocarditis. The cardiac silhouette is enlarged and there is evidence of left atrial enlargement. Pulmonary opacities indicate the presence of pulmonary edema.

Laboratory Data

- In many cases of IE, the hemogram reveals leukocytosis, but this finding is not consistently present. In subacute cases of IE, the leukocytosis is relatively mild, and evidence of acute inflammation may or may not be present.
- Abnormalities in the serum chemistries are not specific and, when present, are secondary to the disease process. Azotemia is relatively common and can be pre-renal, as a result of poor renal perfusion, or it can result from renal infarction. Hypoalbuminemia, hyperglobulinemia, and elevations in serum alkaline phosphatase may also be observed.
- Bacteria are cultivated from whole blood samples in 60% to 80% of IE cases. When possible, three whole-blood samples are obtained over a 12- to 24-hour period from a central vein after aseptic preparation of the overlying skin. When clinical circumstances

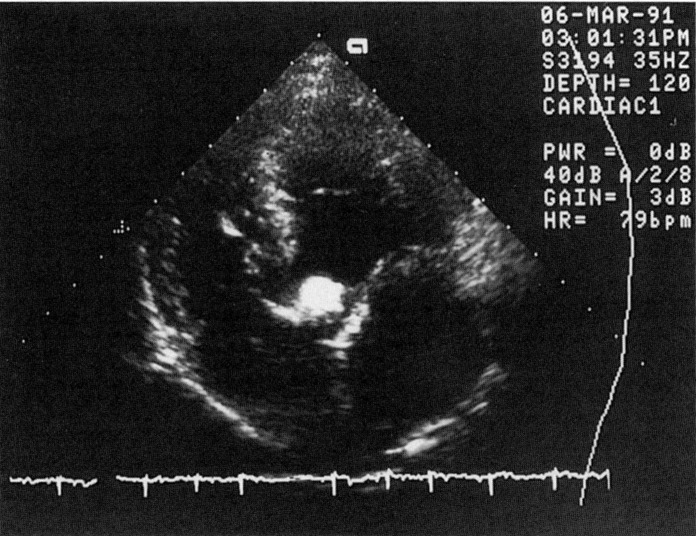

Figure 6-20. Two-dimensional echocardiographic image obtained from a Boxer with aortic valve endocarditis. This left apical five-chamber view demonstrates the presence of a large, highly echogenic nodule attached to one of the aortic valve leaflets.

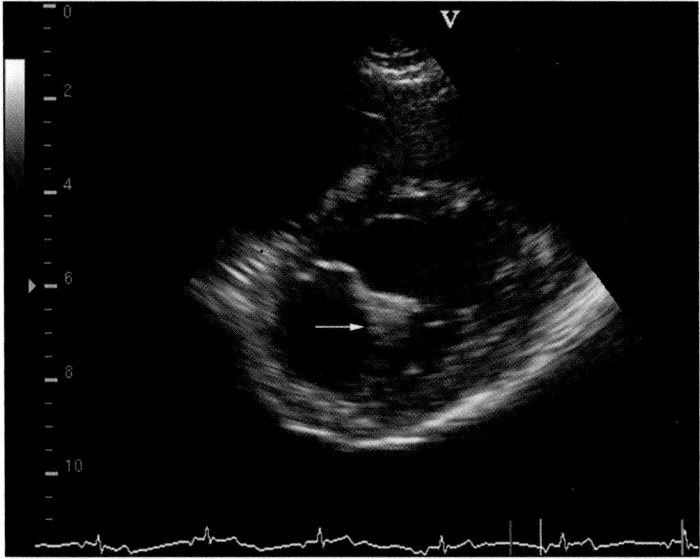

Figure 6-21. Two-dimensional echocardiographic short axis image obtained from a 5-year-old female spayed Doberman Pinscher with mitral valve endocarditis. There is a discrete nodule attached to anterior mitral valve leaflet *(arrow)*.

allow, blood samples are obtained prior to the institution of antibacterial therapy, and the results are used to guide treatment. Taking samples over a shorter time period, say 1 to 3 hours, likely is reasonable when the clinical findings suggest that institution of antibiotic therapy should not be delayed.

Therapy

- Therapy of IE is directed toward the control of sepsis, the prevention of thromboembolism, and the management of cardiac dysfunction that results from valvular incompetence.
- Antibacterial therapy is best guided by the results of bacterial culture and sensitivity testing of whole blood samples. When culture results are unavailable, or when attempts to isolate bacteria from blood are unsuccessful, antibiotics are chosen on an empirical basis.
- Most often, IE in dogs results from gram-positive organisms, and agents such as the clavulanate potentiated penicillins or the cephalosporins are appropriate. **Azithromycin** may have a role in the management of IE due to *Bartonella* spp. In general, bactericidal agents are preferred. A long course of therapy, 6 to 8 weeks, is generally

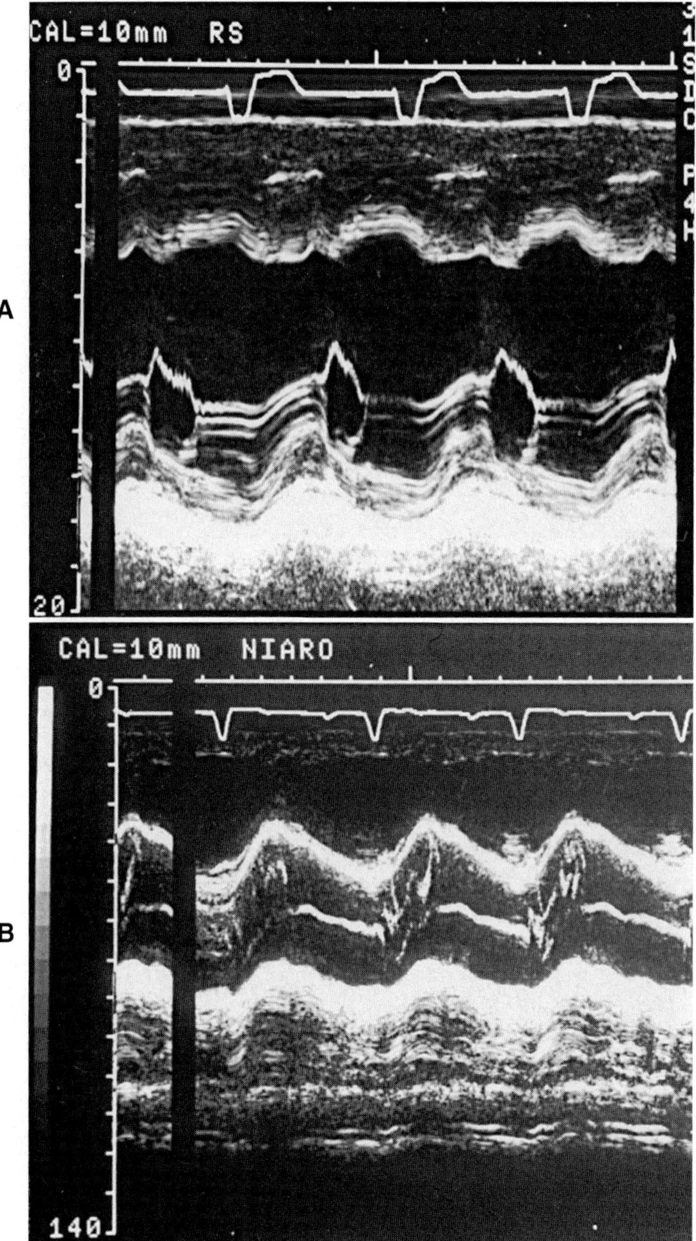

Figure 6-22. M-mode echocardiograms obtained from dogs with severe aortic valve incompetence due to bacterial endocarditis. **A,** An M-mode echocardiogram obtained at the mitral valve level. There is diastolic flutter of the anterior mitral valve leaflet and premature closure of the mitral valve—indirect echocardiographic evidence of severe aortic valve incompetence. **B,** An M-mode echocardiogram obtained at the aortic level. The motion of the visible aortic valve leaflet is chaotic because it is flail, having been all but destroyed by an aggressive endocarditis lesion.

recommended. There may be some advantage to initiating antibiotic therapy using the intravenous route because high serum levels of drugs are achieved quickly and with certainty.

- When clinical signs of sepsis are prominent and blood culture results are negative, initial therapy using a combination of intravenous **gentamicin** (or **amikacin**) and **ampicillin** (or a **cephalosporin**) is justified. When patients are free of gastrointestinal signs such as vomiting or diarrhea, oral antibiotic therapy is probably appropriate.
- Cardioactive agents are chosen based on the results of radiographic and echocardiographic examinations. When there is left atrial and left ventricular enlargement due to AI, therapy with ACE inhibitors is generally employed. **Furosemide** (1 to 2 mg/kg PO every 12 hours) is used together with an ACE inhibitor in cases where there is radiographic

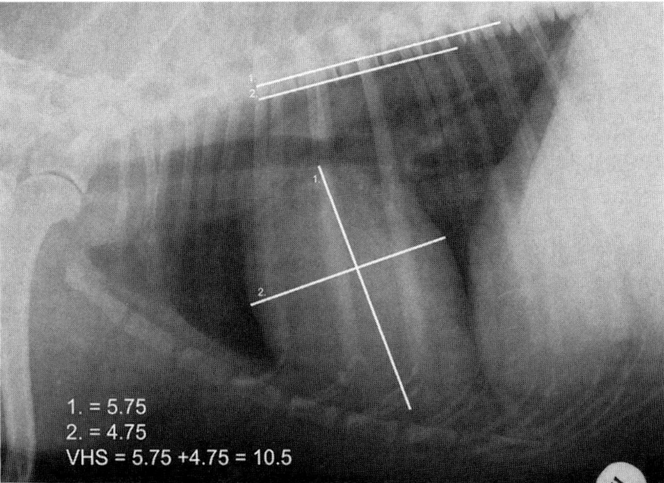

Figure 6-23. Lateral radiographic projection of a clinically normal Cocker Spaniel. The dimensions used to calculate the vertebral heart sum *(VHS)* are shown. The vertebral bodies, beginning at the fourth thoracic vertebra are used as a scale.

evidence of CHF. Digoxin may have a role in the management of patients with severe CHF. Careful attention to renal function must be paid when digoxin is used in patients with IE. In addition to the presence of CHF and the use of ACE inhibitors, which are themselves risk factors for the development of azotemia, patients with IE may develop renal dysfunction related to renal infarction.

Monitoring of Therapy

- As with other patients with CHF, it is prudent to monitor serum electrolytes and renal function. Further monitoring of patients with IE may include serial blood cultures and follow-up echocardiographic studies.
- It is tempting to believe that appropriate antibiotic therapy will result in resolution of echocardiographically detected valvular lesions. The valvular lesions of dogs with the more common form of IE, in which the presentation is subacute and there is echocardiographic evidence of severe valvular incompetence, do not generally resolve. Serial echocardiographic studies in these cases usually demonstrate progressive valvular incompetence and myocardial dysfunction.

Prognosis

- The long-term prognosis for patients with echocardiographic evidence of vegetative, subacute IE is grave. By the time the disease is detected, most cases of IE have progressed to the extent that there is irreversible damage to the valve. Failing surgical valve replacement, which is rarely practical in veterinary patients, the clinical picture of IE is one of progressive cardiac dysfunction. A few dogs die of renal failure related to renal infarction or are euthanized after septic thrombi have embolized to the central nervous system. However, in most cases, death occurs as a result of medically refractory CHF, or suddenly from malignant arrhythmia even when antibiotic therapy is successful in controlling signs related to sepsis. In general, when an echocardiographic diagnosis of IE is made in a dog, survival is usually measured in weeks or months. With aggressive medical therapy, survival of 4 to 8 months is occasionally observed. The prognosis associated with more acute forms of IE that are treated early and aggressively is likely better.

Frequently Asked Questions

Subjective evaluation of cardiac size from thoracic radiographs is difficult. Are there objective criteria that define radiographic cardiac enlargement?

Thoracic radiographs are indispensable in the diagnostic evaluation of dogs with MVD, but it is likely that the accuracy of subjective evaluation of radiographic cardiac size is dependent on observer experience. It is relevant that the patients that most often develop clinically important MVD are small dogs that that have roughly cylindrical thoraces. In the lateral projection particularly, patients with this conformation tend to have a large cardiothoracic ratio even when the heart is, in fact, normal.

One method that can be used to overcome some of the limitations inherent in the subjective evaluation of radiographic cardiac size is the use of the vertebral heart scale. Beginning at the fourth thoracic vertebra and using the vertebral bodies as a scale, the craniocaudal and dorsoventral dimensions of the cardiac silhouette are summed (Figure 6-23). This index of cardiac size is less than 10.5 in most healthy dogs. Higher values suggest cardiac enlargement.

There is current interest in the use of spironolactone as adjunctive therapy for heart failure in dogs. What are the indications for spironolactone in MVD?
Spironolactone is an antagonist of the mineralocorticoid aldosterone. It is not a potent diuretic and interest in the use of this drug primarily relates to its presumed extrarenal effects. Cardiac dysfunction is associated with neuroendocrine responses that result in supraphysiologic aldosterone activity. Aldosterone is a ligand for specific renal receptors that mediate retention of sodium and excretion of potassium. Additionally, there are data that support a role for aldosterone in the development of myocardial fibrosis in animals with experimentally induced cardiovascular disease. Inhibition of aldosterone activity by spironolactone reduced mortality in people with severe heart failure and this effect was evident at a dose that did not have a diuretic effect. Although invasive studies may disclose systolic myocardial dysfunction in dogs with mild but experimentally induced MR, contractility is apparently preserved until late in the natural history of MVD. Based on this, it seems reasonable to reserve spironolactone for patients with heart failure due to MVD. Additionally, the use of spironolactone is apparently safe but not entirely benign. Because this drug generally is used in conjunction with ACE inhibitors, there is potentially a danger of hyperkalemia resulting from excessively diminished aldosterone activity. Indeed, after publication of the major study which documented the favorable effect of spironolactone in people, a number of reports of adverse effects appeared in the literature. Based on retrospective evaluation of clinicopathologic data, the use of spironolactone together with ACE inhibitors and furosemide is apparently safe in dogs; however, it is prudent to monitor serum electrolytes and renal function.

SUGGESTED READINGS

Anderson CA, Dubielzig RR: Vegetative endocarditis in dogs, J Am Anim Hosp Assoc 20:149, 1984.

Atkins CD, Keene BW, Brown WA, et al: Results of the veterinary enalapril trial to prove reduction in onset of heart failure in dogs chronically treated with enalapril alone for compensated, naturally occurring mitral valve insufficiency, J Am Vet Med Assoc 231: 1061-1069, 2007.

Buchanan JW: Chronic valvular disease (endocardiosis) in dogs, Adv Vet Med 21:75, 1979.

Buchanan JW, Bucheler J: Vertebral scale system to measure canine heart size in radiographs, J Am Ved Med Assoc 206:194, 1995.

Bulmer BJ, Sisson DD: Therapy of heart failure. In Ettinger SJ, Feldman EC, eds: Textbook of veterinary internal medicine, ed 6, Philadelphia, 2005, WB Saunders.

Calvert CA: Valvular bacterial endocarditis in the dog, J Am Vet Med Assoc 180:1080, 1982.

Chetboul V, Lefebvre HP, Sampedrano CC, et al: Comparative adverse cardiac effects of pimobendan and benazepril monotherapy in dogs with mild degenerative mitral valve disease: a prospective, controlled, blinded, and randomized study, J Vet Intern Med 21:742-753, 2007.

Dell'Italia LJ: The renin-angiotensin system in mitral regurgitation: a typical example of tissue activation. Curr Cardiol Rep 4:97, 2002.

Ettinger SJ, Benitz AM, Ericsson GF, et al: Effects of enalapril maleate on survival of dogs with naturally acquired heart failure, J Am Ved Med Assoc 213: 1573-1577, 1998.

Griffiths LG, Orton EC, Boon JA: Evaluation of techniques and outcomes of mitral valve repair in dogs, J Am Ved Med Assoc 224:1941, 2004.

Haggstrom J, Hansson K, Kvart C, Swenson L: Chronic valvular disease in the cavalier King Charles spaniel in Sweden, Vet Rec 131:549-553, 1992.

Haggstrom J, Kvart C, Pedersen HD: Acquired valvular disease. In Ettinger SJ, Feldman EC, eds: Textbook of Veterinary internal medicine, ed 6, Philadelphia, 2005, WB Saunders.

Haggstrom J, Pedersen HD, Kvart C: New insights into degenerative valve disease in dogs, Vet Clin North Am Sm Anim Pract 34:1209-1226, 2004.

Kvart C, Haggstrom J, Pedersen HD, et al: Efficacy of enalapril for prevention of congestive heart failure in dogs with myxomatous valve disease and asymptomatic mitral regurgitation, J Vet Intern Med 16(1): 80-88, 2002.

MacDonald KA, Chomel BB, Kittleson MD, et al: A prospective study of canine infective endocarditis in northern california (1999-2001): emergence of *Bartonella* as a prevalent etiologic agent, J Vet Intern Med 18:56, 2004.

Sisson D, Thomas WP: Endocarditis of the aortic valve in the dog, J Am Ved Med Assoc 184:570, 1984.

Sisson D, Kvart C, Darke PG: Acquired valvular heart disease in dogs and cats. In Fox PR, Sisson D, Moise NS, eds: Textbook of canine and feline cardiology: principles and clinical practice, ed 2, Philadelphia, 1999, WB Saunders.

CHAPTER 7

Canine Cardiomyopathy

Mark A. Oyama

INTRODUCTION

Cardiomyopathy is defined as a primary disease of the heart muscle of unknown etiology. Disease of the heart muscle secondary to toxins, nutritional deficiencies, endocrinopathies, and infectious agents is often regarded as a "secondary cardiomyopathy." The most common form of canine cardiomyopathy is dilated cardiomyopathy (DCM), which is characterized by progressive ventricular dilation and loss of myocardial contractility. Other forms of cardiomyopathy, such as hypertrophic cardiomyopathy (HCM), are rare in dogs. DCM is most common in adult large breed dogs, and in particular the Doberman Pinscher, Irish Wolfhound, Scottish Deerhound, and Great Dane. The important features of canine DCM include (1) the presence of an asymptomatic or occult phase during which diagnosis of disease is difficult, (2) the high prevalence of congestive heart failure, and sudden death in severely affected dogs, and (3) the need for aggressive and comprehensive medical therapy to help alleviate clinical signs. Boxers with cardiomyopathy possess a unique pathophysiology, clinical presentation, and natural history, such that disease is best described as arrhythmogenic right ventricular cardiomyopathy (ARVC). Sudden death from ventricular arrhythmias is very common in Boxers with ARVC, much more so than chronic congestive heart failure. Secondary cardiomyopathies due to nutritional deficiencies appear in breeds of small and medium size, most notably in the American Cocker Spaniel. A highly fatal juvenile form of DCM is seen in the Portuguese Water Dog.

DILATED CARDIOMYOPATHY

Prevalence and Signalment

Surveys indicate that between two and six dogs are diagnosed with DCM per 600 case referrals. In certain breeds, the prevalence of DCM is remarkably high. Approximately 25% of Irish Wolfhounds, 50% of male Doberman Pinschers, and 33% of female Doberman Pinschers develop DCM. The typical age at diagnosis is between 6 and 8 years; however, it is not uncommon to diagnose DCM in dogs as young as 3 years and as old as 12 years. Male dogs appear to be more frequently affected, especially in the Doberman Pinscher breed.

Natural History

The clinical progression of DCM is best described as occurring in two distinct phases.

Asymptomatic Occult Phase

- No clinical signs are evident; however, myocardial or electrical abnormalities are present and may include:
  - Increased left ventricular and atrial dimensions
  - Decreased myocardial contractility
  - Ventricular premature beats
- The duration of the occult phase is highly variable and thought to last for months to years.
- During this phase, progressive heart enlargement and worsening arrhythmias occur.
- Occult phase ends with the appearance of the first clinical signs of disease.

- Approximately 40% of Doberman Pinschers experience sudden cardiac death as the first clinical sign.

Overt Clinical Phase

- Clinical signs develop
  - Congestive heart failure
  - Syncope
  - Exercise and activity intolerance
- Arrhythmias in the form of ventricular premature beats, ventricular tachycardia, and atrial fibrillation are common.
- Death is due either to advanced congestive heart failure that is refractory to medical therapy or sudden death.
  - Between 30% and 50% of Doberman Pinschers die suddenly
  - Many dogs with advanced heart failure are euthanized due to chronic respiratory distress, severe activity intolerance, anorexia, and weight loss.

History and Physical Examination Findings

Asymptomatic Occult Phase

- Common findings include:
  - Soft systolic heart murmur
  - Irregular heart rhythm with pulse deficits
- Occasional findings include:
  - Diastolic gallop rhythm
  - Decreased intensity of heart sounds
  - Weak femoral pulse quality
  - Jugular vein distension or pulses

Overt Clinical Phase

- History may include exercise intolerance, syncope, lethargy, anorexia, difficulty breathing, coughing, abdominal distension
- Common findings include:
  - Moderate intensity systolic heart murmur
  - Irregular heart rhythm with pulse deficits
  - Increased respiratory rate and effort
  - Increased bronchovesicular sounds
  - Decreased intensity of heart sounds
  - Weakness
- Occasional findings include:
  - Jugular vein distension or pulses
  - Hepatomegaly
  - Ascites
  - Pale mucous membranes
  - Hypothermia
  - Pulmonary crackles
  - Depressed mentation

Diagnostic Tests

Ideally, all dogs should receive an electrocardiogram (ECG), chest radiographs, echocardiogram, urinalysis, and serum chemistry. In many cases, additional diagnostics, such as 24-hour ambulatory ECG (Holter) monitoring, are performed.

Electrocardiography

- Electrocardiography is the test of choice for detecting arrhythmias and may provide evidence of heart enlargement; however a normal ECG does not rule out the presence of cardiomyopathy.
  - Asymptomatic occult phase
    - Arrhythmias are often the first indication of disease and screening is recommended in breeds at high risk for DCM.
    - Routine ECG detects frequent arrhythmias but may have limited sensitivity in dogs with infrequent or intermittent arrhythmias.
    - Detection of the following ECG signs is associated with a high index of suspicion for occult cardiomyopathy:
      - One or more ventricular premature beats in a Doberman Pinscher or Boxer. In Boxers, ventricular premature beats with a left bundle branch block morphology (upright QRS complex in lead II) are highly suggestive of ARVC (Figure 7-1).
      - Criteria for left ventricular or atrial enlargement (QRS duration > 0.06 sec, R wave amplitude > 3.0 mV, P wave duration > 0.04 sec)

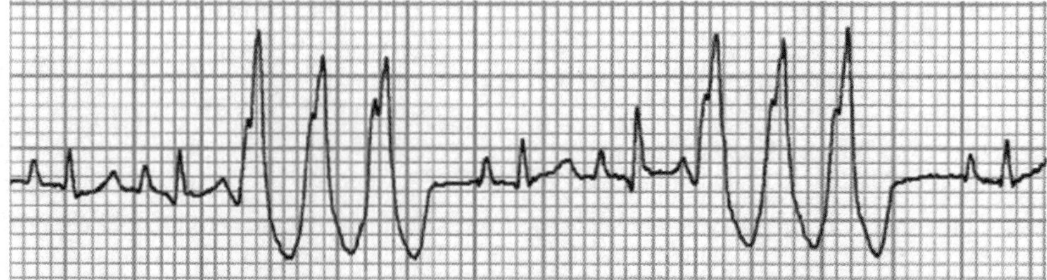

Figure 7-1. Lead II ECG tracing from a 7-year-old male, castrated Boxer with arrhythmogenic right ventricular cardiomyopathy. Ventricular premature beats with left bundle branch block morphology are a common finding in dogs with this condition. 25 mm/sec; 0.5 cm/mV.

- In Irish Wolfhounds, atrial fibrillation is often an early sign of disease as opposed to other breeds where atrial fibrillation is associated with advanced stages of disease.
- Holter monitoring detects arrhythmias with greater sensitivity and is recommended in dogs at high risk (i.e., dogs with a familial history of disease).
  - Greater than 100 ventricular premature beats in a 24-hour period is highly suggestive of occult DCM or ARVC.
  - A total of 50 to 100 ventricular premature beats in a 24 hour period is suspicious for disease and should be followed by another Holter examination in 2 to 6 months.
  - Day-to-day variability in the frequency of arrhythmia can produce false-negative results, and if the initial Holter examination is inconclusive, multiple Holter examinations may be indicated, especially in dogs with a family history of disease or in those that have experienced syncope.
- During the overt clinical phase, the following may be detected:
  - Occasional to frequent ventricular or supraventricular premature beats
  - Ventricular tachycardia
  - Criteria for left ventricular or atrial enlargement (see previous section)
  - Left bundle branch block
  - Atrial fibrillation (Figure 7-2)

KEY POINTS

The author regards Holter monitoring as the current gold standard for detection of occult DCM in Doberman Pinschers. Holter monitoring is relatively easy to perform and equipment is readily available to the general practitioner through human and veterinary medical suppliers. Many veterinary telemedicine or remote consulting practices lease Holter units and assist in result analysis.

Chest Radiography

- Chest radiographs are relatively insensitive to mild increases in the heart size. A single set performed in the asymptomatic occult phase contributes relatively little to the immediate diagnosis; however, serial radiographs are well suited to monitor progressive heart enlargement and progression of disease. In the overt clinical phase, radiographs are invaluable in helping to diagnose congestive failure and to monitor response to treatment.
  - The chest radiographs in Doberman Pinschers are often misleading in that heart enlargement is less striking than in other breeds with similar clinical signs. In these instances, cardiac ultrasound helps to determine the magnitude of left-sided heart enlargement and systolic dysfunction.
  - The chest radiographs in Boxers with ARVC are usually normal.

Echocardiography

- Echocardiography is widely used to quantify heart enlargement and systolic function. Routine echocardiography is not particularly sensitive in detecting early changes in occult disease, nor is it particularly helpful after a diagnosis of end-stage disease is made. As such, the utility of echocardiography increases as disease moves out of the occult phase to the overt clinical phase then declines again as the patient advances into end-stage disease. Early in the course of disease, many dogs possess normal echocardiographic examinations, despite having a significant numbers of ventricular arrhythmias.
  - Echocardiographic criteria are used to help diagnose occult DCM.
    - In Doberman Pinschers, a left ventricular end-diastolic diameter (LVIDd) > 46 mm or a left ventricular end-systolic diameter (LVIDs) > 38 mm is highly suggestive of early disease. These values may not be applicable to Dobermans with very large body weights, and LVIDd > 49 mm or LVIDs > 42 mm may be better guides in this population.
    - In Doberman Pinschers, fractional shortening is an unreliable index for occult DCM, as this breed typically has fractional shortening values in the mid or low 20% range. Similarly, large-breed dogs with athletic lifestyles commonly display fractional shortening values in the mid 20% range, and longitudinal echocardiographic studies or Holter monitoring is required to determine whether disease is truly present.
    - In Irish Wolfhounds, occult disease is defined as LVIDd > 61.2 mm, LVIDs > 41 mm, fractional shortening < 25%, end-systolic volume index > 41 ml/m^2, or E-point to septal separation > 10 mm.
    - Newer ultrasound modalities such as Doppler tissue imaging may be more sensitive in detecting early abnormalities of myocardial contractility.

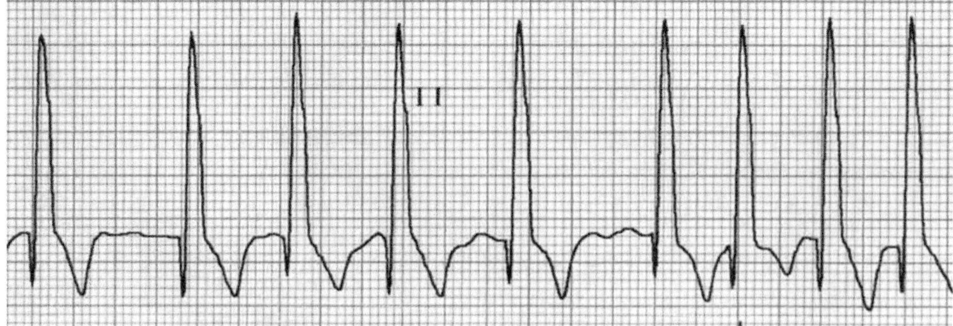

Figure 7-2. Lead II ECG tracing from a dog indicating atrial fibrillation and left ventricular enlargement. Note the irregular rhythm, lack of P waves, and widened QRS complex. 50 mm/sec; 10 mm/mV.

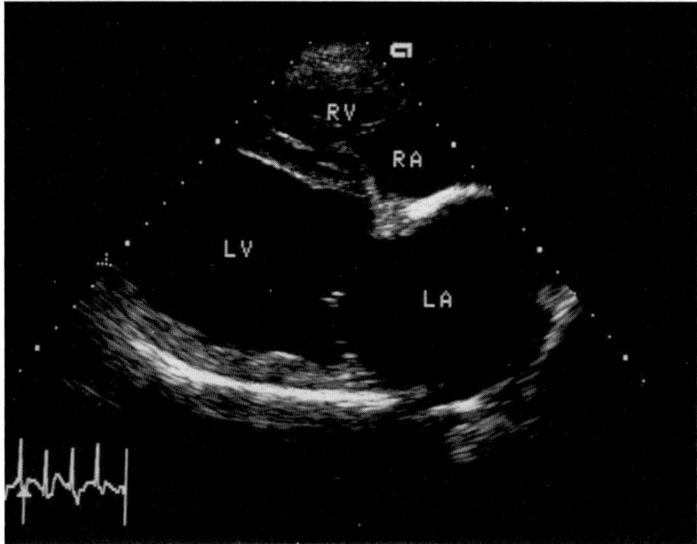

Figure 7-3. 2-dimensional echocardiogram of the left ventricle *(LV)* and atrium *(LA)* of a Great Dane with dilated cardiomyopathy. Note the dilated ventricular and atrial chambers. *RV,* Right ventricle; *RA,* right atrium.

- As disease progresses from occult to overt, echocardiography helps monitor heart enlargement, assess contractility, and evaluate secondary mitral regurgitation. Echocardiography is used in conjunction with chest radiographs to help decide when to initiate therapy.
- Common echocardiographic findings in dogs with advanced occult or overt clinical disease include the following:
  - Moderate to severe left ventricular and atrial enlargement (Figure 7-3).
  - Reduced systolic motion of the left ventricular wall and interventricular septum (Figure 7-4).
  - Mild to moderate mitral regurgitation secondary to mitral annulus dilation.
  - Incomplete systolic opening of the aortic valves.
  - Decreased aortic blood flow velocity.
  - Increased mitral valve E-point to septal separation (normal < 6 mm) (Figure 7-5).
  - Decreased systolic thickening of the left ventricular wall and interventricular septum.
- The echocardiogram in Boxers with ARVC is usually normal. Subtle right ventricular dilation or wall motion abnormalities may be noted.

Concomitant Abnormalities in Moderate or Severe Dilated Cardiomyopathy

- Azotemia is commonly detected in dogs that are receiving diuretic therapy and is typically prerenal in nature.
  - Mild azotemia (blood urea nitrogen < 60 mg/dl and creatinine < 2.5 mg/dl) usually does not require specific treatment or cessation or reduction of diuretic therapy.
  - More severe azotemia (blood urea nitrogen > 80 mg/dl and creatine > 3.0 mg/dl) can contribute to patient morbidity and may require reduction of angiotensin-converting enzyme

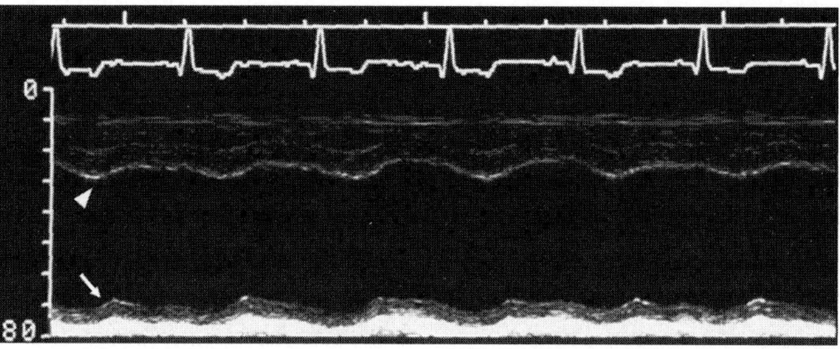

Figure 7-4. M-mode echocardiogram of the left ventricle of a Cocker Spaniel with dilated cardiomyopathy. Note the decreased systolic motion of the interventricular septum *(arrow)* and left ventricular free wall *(arrowhead).*

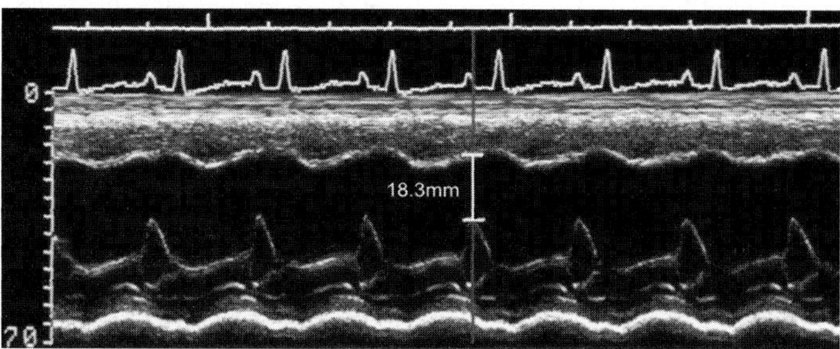

Figure 7-5. M-mode echocardiogram of the left ventricle and mitral valve of a Brittany Spaniel with dilated cardiomyopathy. Electronic calipers are being used to measure the E-point to septal separation (EPSS), which is markedly increased over normal.

(ACE) inhibitor and diuretic dose or parenteral fluid supplementation.

- If fluids are administered, then administering half-strength saline or Ringer's solution will reduce the sodium load to the patient.
- ACE inhibitor therapy can be temporarily discontinued or the dosage reduced. Initiation of the ACE inhibitor therapy should be delayed or done with caution.
- Aggressive parenteral fluid therapy can aggravate congestive heart failure and should be used with caution.
- Many instances can be treated by reduction of diuretics and allowing the patient to drink enough water to reestablish hydration on their own.

- Azotemia reduces renal clearance of digoxin and predisposes to toxicity. Serum digoxin levels should be determined especially if the patient displays anorexia, vomiting, diarrhea, or frequent arrhythmias.

- Electrolyte abnormalities are common in dogs with congestive heart failure due to DCM. Most changes are mild and do not require specific treatment.
  - Potassium levels may be either increased or decreased. Mild hypokalemia (K^+ = 2.5 to 3.0 mEq/l) is commonly associated with high doses of diuretics and usually does not require specific treatment. Severe hypokalemia (K^+ < 2.5 mEq/l) can cause cardiac arrhythmias and contribute to muscle weakness. Reduction of potassium-wasting diuretics (e.g., furosemide) or institution of potassium-sparing agents (e.g., ACE inhibitors, spironolactone) is performed. Clinically important hyperkalemia is uncommon and usually associated with reduced cardiac output, poor renal perfusion, and renal failure.
  - Mild hyponatremia is common and is dilutional in nature. Serum concentration of sodium is decreased secondary to water retention and expansion of the plasma volume despite elevated total body sodium content. Mild hyponatremia does not require specific treatment. In the author's experience, profound hyponatremia (Na^+ < 130 mEq/l) signals a poor prognosis. Treatment requires reduction of diuretic dose, water restriction, and dietary sodium supplementation.
- Hypothyroidism is a common concurrent disease in middle-aged to older dogs, especially in Doberman Pinschers. A causal relationship between hypothyroidism and DCM is doubtful. Supplementation does not improve survival.
- Natriuretic peptides are produced by the atrial and ventricular tissues in response to increased

wall stress. Their biologic actions counter those of the renin-angiotensin-aldosterone system. Atrial and B-type natriuretic peptide are elevated in dogs with symptomatic DCM and reflect severity of disease. Atrial and B-type natriuretic peptide are able to distinguish between cardiogenic and noncardiogenic causes of dyspnea in dogs. In humans, natriuretic peptides provide information regarding diagnosis, prognosis, and efficacy of treatment. A similar utility is likely to exist for dogs.

- Cardiac troponin-I forms part of the actin-myosin contractile apparatus and is released into circulation following myocyte injury or necrosis. Cardiac troponin-I is elevated in dogs with DCM and modestly correlates with degree of left ventricular hypertrophy. One study indicated that dogs with plasma cardiac troponin-I > 0.20 ng/ml have shorter survival times versus those with lower values.

Nutritional Deficiencies

- Taurine deficiency is a contributing cause of DCM in the American Cocker Spaniel, and a potential contributing factor in Dalmatians, Labrador Retrievers, and Golden Retrievers. In contrast, the incidence of taurine-responsive disease is virtually nonexistent in the traditional breeds of dogs with DCM. Recognition of taurine deficiency is important in that heart function may be substantially improved following supplementation. In any nontraditional breed of dog, that is, in any dog that is *not* a Doberman Pinscher, Boxer, Great Dane, Irish Wolfhound, or Scottish Deerhound, the author recommends plasma taurine assay. Interestingly, most taurine-deficient dogs are receiving an adequate meat-based diet, and abnormalities of taurine absorption, metabolism, or excretion are the likely cause of disease.
  - Most dogs with taurine deficient DCM have plasma taurine < 25 nmol/ml.
- L-Carnitine deficiency is not a primary cause of canine DCM; however, some dogs that are taurine deficient require both L-carnitine and taurine in order to improve.
  - Plasma L-carnitine concentration is not reflective of myocardial tissue concentration and plasma assays are of little clinical utility. As such, diagnosis of myocardial L-carnitine deficiency requires myocardial biopsy. A presumptive diagnosis of deficiency is often considered when dogs are concurrently taurine deficient.

Treatment

Standard treatment involves the use of diuretics, positive inotropes, and ACE inhibitors. Ventricular arrhythmias and atrial fibrillation requires use of specific antiarrhythmics. More recently, beta adrenergic blocking agents and combined positive inotropic-vasodilator drugs have been used. Treatment depends on the breed, stage of disease, and presence of congestive heart failure or arrhythmias.

Drug Classes Used for Treatment

- Diuretic therapy alleviates signs of congestion. As disease worsens, use of multiple diuretics helps achieve increased diuresis. Diuretic monotherapy increases activity of the renin-angiotensin-aldosterone system and concomitant ACE inhibition should be used. Diuretic therapy is commonly accompanied by mild azotemia and hypokalemia. The potent loop diuretic, **furosemide,** is routinely used in symptomatic patients. Thiazide diuretics, though less potent, have a longer half-life, act at a site separate from furosemide, and provide additional diuresis in patients already receiving high doses of furosemide. **Spironolactone** is a weak potassium-sparing diuretic that is typically administered in conjunction with a thiazide. Spironolactone's beneficial effects are probably due to its anti-proliferative actions and subsequent reduction of ventricular remodeling and fibrosis, rather than its very weak diuretic action.
- Positive inotropic therapy is used to improve contractility. Drugs include digoxin, beta adrenergic agonists (e.g., **dopamine, dobutamine**), phosphodiesterase inhibitors (e.g., **milrinone**), and calcium sensitizers (e.g., **pimobendan**). As a positive inotrope, digoxin is a relatively weak and not useful in the emergency setting. Digoxin is, however, useful as an antiarrhythmic used to control the ventricular rate in patients with atrial fibrillation. The beta adrenergic agonists and phosphodiesterase inhibitors are administered using constant rate infusion and are useful in the emergency setting. Pimobendan is a unique drug due to its combined inotropic and vasodilatory properties. Survival and quality of life is likely improved by this drug.
- Venous vasodilators reduce preload and arterial vasodilators reduce afterload.
  - ACE inhibitors blunt activity of the renin-angiotensin-aldosterone system, reduce salt and water retention, and elicit mild arterial

vasodilation. ACE inhibitors improve survival and quality of life in dogs with DCM. Dogs with severe heart failure and poor renal perfusion may become uremic while taking ACE inhibitors, especially when high doses of diuretics are being concurrently used.

- **Sodium nitroprusside** elicits potent arterial and venous vasodilation and is very effective in cases of life-threatening heart failure. Due to the risk for hypotension, arterial blood pressure monitoring is required during its use. Sodium nitroprusside is administered as a constant-rate infusion (CRI).
- Topical **nitroglycerin** produces minimal venous vasodilation in dogs due to poor absorption and low plasma concentrations.

- Antiarrhythmic agents suppress life-threatening ventricular arrhythmias and control the ventricular rate during atrial fibrillation. For ventricular arrhythmias, drugs in classes I (e.g., **lidocaine** and **mexiletine**), II (beta blockers), and III (e.g., **sotalol**) can be used alone or in certain combinations. Drugs in class II and IV (calcium channel blockers) and digoxin are used for atrial fibrillation.
- Beta-adrenergic blocking agents are extensively used in humans with DCM. In dogs, little clinical data exists. Beta-blocking agents blunt the effects of chronic sympathetic nervous system activity (i.e., tachycardia, arrhythmias, myocyte death, ventricular remodeling, elevated activity of the renin-angiotensin-aldosterone system). Overly aggressive use may exacerbate congestive heart failure, and patients should be clinically stable before being titrated onto this class of drug.
- Inodilators are drugs that improve cardiac contractility and elicit vasodilation. **Pimobendan** is a calcium-sensitizing inodilator that increases the myocardial response to calcium. Pimobendan should be used in dogs with symptomatic disease that are already receiving conventional therapy. Pimobendan improves quality of life and is likely to improve survival.

Treatment of Asymptomatic Occult Disease

Treatment in the occult phase represents both an opportunity and a challenge. Clearly, treatments that slow progression in this phase would help delay or prevent symptomatic disease, yet the discovery of effective drugs is hindered by the difficulty in performing large-scale prospective clinical trials with sufficient statistical power. There are no known treatments that definitively slow progression of disease in the occult state. Insofar as gradual derangement of neurohormonal activity is associated with worsening cardiac function, use of ACE inhibitors, beta blockers, and spironolactone has been suggested. Current recommendations are based on small veterinary trials and extrapolation from human medicine. Three drug classes are typically considered during the occult phase.

- Use of beta blockade is scientifically supported in virtually all human patients with left ventricular systolic dysfunction with current or prior symptoms, and consensus opinion extends this recommendation to use in asymptomatic patients. In dogs, sympathetic tone is increased during the occult phase, thus providing rationale for administration of beta blockers in dogs with early disease.
- Use of ACE inhibition is scientifically supported in virtually all human patients with left ventricular systolic dysfunction regardless of symptoms. In dogs, the time course of ACE activation is uncertain. Although several studies indicate that heightened activity of the renin-angiotensin-aldosterone is not present in early disease, there is a need to distinguish between circulating and local tissue ACE activity. Though circulating ACE activity is not upregulated until later in disease, evidence suggests that a locally contained myocardial ACE system contributes much earlier in disease. Thus, tissue-penetrating ACE inhibitors, such as benazepril or ramipril, may be beneficial.
- **Spironolactone** is primarily used in humans with symptomatic DCM; however, the benefit in preventing aldosterone-mediated remodeling may begin in earlier stages of disease.
- Due to the high incidence of sudden death in Boxers and Doberman Pinschers, antiarrhythmic therapy is often initiated in asymptomatic dogs based on Holter monitor findings. Dogs with runs

KEY POINTS

The natural history of cardiomyopathy is substantially influenced by breed. Large- or giant-breed dogs commonly develop atrial fibrillation and congestive heart failure, while Doberman Pinschers and Boxers with ARVC commonly exhibit syncope, ventricular arrhythmias, and sudden death. Thus, in Great Danes, Irish Wolfhounds, and similar affected breeds, treatment efforts should focus on the resolution of heart failure, whereas in Doberman Pinschers and Boxers, antiarrhythmic therapy is commonly prescribed.

of ventricular tachycardia or R-on-T phenomenon are started on **sotalol** (1.5 to 2.0 mg/kg every 12 hours) or the combination of **mexiletine** (5 to 8 mg/kg every 8 hours) and **atenolol** (0.3 to 0.4 mg/kg every 12 hours). The efficacy of this treatment in preventing sudden death is unproven.

Treatment of Overt Clinical Disease

Treatment of Severe Life-Threatening Congestive Heart Failure

Congestive heart failure is relieved through aggressive diuretic, vasodilator, and positive inotropic therapy.

- Manual removal of heart failure fluid should be performed in all patients with clinically significant pleural or abdominal effusion, as this will rapidly improve respiratory effort and alleviate distress.
- Intravenous or intramuscular **furosemide** (3 to 8 mg/kg) is administered. When given parenterally, duration of effect is approximately 2 hours; therefore, additional doses should be administered if the patient's respiratory rate and effort have not improved within this time period. Patient recovery can be significantly hindered due to insufficient dosing of furosemide during the first 12 hours of treatment.
  - Efficacy of diuretic therapy is assessed by monitoring patient respiratory rate and effort, urine output, and body weight. To confirm the resolution of pulmonary edema or to reassess patients that are not responding to therapy, chest radiographs are performed 12 to 24 hours after initiation of therapy.
  - The presence of severe underlying renal dysfunction may necessitate lower doses and less frequent dosing.
- **Sodium nitroprusside** (2 to 5 mcg/kg/min CRI) is a very effective vasodilator. Nitroprusside can produce profound hypotension, and arterial blood pressure monitoring is required when using it. The infusion rate is adjusted to elicit a 15 mm Hg decrease in mean blood pressure as long as the mean value does not fall below 70 mm Hg.
- Intravenous positive inotropes such as **dopamine** (2 to 10 mcg/kg/min CRI) or **dobutamine** (5 to 15 mcg/kg/min CRI) help improve cardiac output. High doses may aggravate ventricular arrhythmias or cause sinus tachycardia.
- **Milrinone** is a potent positive inotrope that acts downstream of the myocardial beta adrenergic receptor. It increases contractility in patients receiving beta blockers or in patients that are not responding to dopamine or dobutamine therapy. Milrinone is administered as a 30 to 50 mcg/kg loading bolus given intravenously over 10 minutes then CRI of 1 to 8 mcg/kg/min.
- Oral **pimobendan** (0.25 mg/kg every 12 hours) may be useful if intravenous positive inotrope therapy is not available.
- When given orally, **digoxin** requires several days to reach effective concentration, and as such, has little role as an emergency positive inotrope. Intravenous digoxin commonly produces toxicity and is not recommended.
- Supplemental oxygen therapy is administered either in an oxygen cage (fraction of inspired oxygen = 40%) or given nasally (50 to 100 ml/kg/min).
- One of the most difficult clinical decisions is whether or not to specifically treat ventricular arrhythmias. Overly aggressive treatment may cause hypotension or predispose to even more malignant arrhythmias.
  - Ventricular premature beats and short runs of ventricular tachycardia that occur at relatively slow heart rates (< 160 bpm) typically do not require treatment. Often, resolution occurs spontaneously once congestive heart failure and hypoxia are successfully treated.
  - Rapid ventricular arrhythmias that are life-threatening are accompanied by clinical signs (i.e., weakness, syncope, hypotension, blanching of mucous membranes). Intravenous **lidocaine** (2 mg/kg IV bolus followed by CRI of 40 to 80 mcg/kg/min) or **procainamide** (6 to 8 mg/kg IV bolus followed by CRI of 20 to 40 mcg/kg/min) is often effective.
  - Due to the high incidence of sudden death in Boxers and Doberman Pinschers, aggressive antiarrhythmic therapy in these species is more commonly warranted, and especially in dogs that have previously experienced syncope. Once stabilized, either oral sotalol or combination of mexiletine and atenolol are prescribed (see next section).

Transitioning the Improved Emergency Patient to Chronic Oral Treatment

Aggressive emergency therapy successfully resolves acute heart failure in approximately 75% of dogs. In most dogs, significant improvement in clinical signs will be apparent within 48 hours. Patients refractory to therapy beyond this point have a grave prognosis. As the patient becomes increasingly stable, intravenous medications are gradually reduced and replaced with oral medications. During this time, patient hydration status, body weight, appetite, respiratory effort, electrolytes, and renal function continue to be monitored.

- Once the patient's respiratory rate and effort has improved, parenteral **furosemide** is discontinued in favor of oral furosemide (typical oral dose: 1 to 2 mg/kg every 8 to 12 hours). **Nitroprusside** and **dopamine** or **dobutamine** are gradually reduced over 12 to 24

hours and replaced by an ACE inhibitor (**enalapril** 0.5 mg/kg every 12 hours or **benazepril** 0.5 mg/kg every 24 hours) and digoxin (0.003 mg/kg every 12 hours) or **pimobendan** (0.25 mg/kg every 12 hours). Due to the potential for side effects (i.e., anorexia, vomiting) some clinicians stagger the initiation of digoxin and ACE inhibitor. In these cases, digoxin is withheld for 3 to 5 days until the patient is known to be tolerating the ACE inhibitor. In patients with atrial fibrillation, the urgency for digoxin treatment is more acute, and **digoxin** can be started first, followed by an ACE inhibitor in 5 to 7 days.
- **Lidocaine** or **procainamide** is gradually reduced over 12 to 24 hours and replaced by **sotalol** (1.5 to 2.5 mg/kg every 12 hours) or a combination of **mexiletine** (5 mg/kg every 8 hours) and **atenolol** (0.3 to 0.4 mg/kg every 12 hours).
- Aggressive use of beta adrenergic blocking antiarrhythmics, such as sotalol or atenolol, may exacerbate heart failure (see next section). Gradual titration of these agents may be required.
- Dietary sodium restriction (40 to 70 mg Na/100 kcal).

Treatment of Refractory Heart Failure

- Patients that are already receiving high doses of loop diuretics may benefit from additional diuretics that target areas of the nephron other than the loop of Henle.
  - **Hydrochlorothiazide** (1 to 4 mg/kg every 12 to 48 hours) is a moderately potent diuretic that acts in the distal convoluted tubule and has a longer half-life than furosemide. Initially, it is given in conjunction with furosemide and gradually increased as needed to control congestion. Hydrochlorothiazide is also supplied as a tablet combined with equal amounts of spironolactone (**hydrochlorothiazide-spironolactone**; 2 to 4 mg/kg every12 to 24 hours).
- In patients with right heart failure or severely decreased cardiac output, absorption and renal delivery of oral furosemide may be decreased. In these cases, substituting subcutaneous injections of furosemide often restores effectiveness. Usually, the total daily dose of furosemide can be modestly decreased when administered in this fashion.
- End-stage DCM is often accompanied by inappetence and weight loss. The author has occasionally prescribed anabolic steroids (**stanozolol** 1 to 2 mg per dog every 12 hours) to counteract this catabolic state. The long-term safety of this treatment is questionable.
- **Pimobendan** (0.25 mg/kg every 12 hours), when added to conventional therapy often helps control heart failure and improves appetite and demeanor of patients with refractory disease

Treatment of Dilated Cardiomyopathy Accompanied by Atrial Fibrillation

Atrial fibrillation commonly occurs in dogs with advanced DCM. The incidence of atrial fibrillation is higher in giant-breed dogs (e.g., Great Danes, Irish Wolfhounds) than in Doberman Pinschers and Boxers. Atrial fibrillation with rapid ventricular rates (> 180 bpm) exacerbates congestive heart failure and low cardiac output. Conversion of atrial fibrillation back to normal sinus rhythm is usually futile, and management is targeted at slowing the ventricular rate. One of three drugs can be administered for this purpose.
- **Digoxin** (0.003 mg/kg every 12 hours)
- **Diltiazem** (0.5 to 2.0 mg/kg every 8 hours) or **Diltiazem XR** (1.5 to 4.0 mg/kg every 12 to 24 hours)
- **Atenolol** (0.25 to 1.0 mg/kg every 12 hours)

In most instances, digoxin is preferred due to its concomitant positive inotropic effects. If rate control is not achieved by digoxin alone, then the addition of diltiazem or atenolol is warranted. Overly aggressive dosing of atenolol or atenolol co-administered with diltiazem can produce bradycardia, heart block, and hypotension. Intravenous administration of digoxin is not recommended due to the high likelihood of toxicity. In patients that require immediate rate control due to extremely rapid ventricular rates, oral loading of digoxin (0.006 mg/kg for the first one or two doses) or intravenous diltiazem (0.1 to 0.2 mg/kg IV bolus then 2 to 6 mcg/kg/min CRI) can be attempted.
- The ideal heart rate for dogs with DCM and atrial fibrillation is not known; however, most clinicians use a value of 150 bpm as their threshold between an acceptable rate and need for more aggressive treatment.
- 24-hour ambulatory ECG (Holter) monitoring is the preferred method to determine mean heart rate and efficacy of long-term oral treatment.

Additional Oral Medications

In addition to the combination of diuretics, ACE inhibitor, and pimobendan, other medications are likely beneficial in DCM. The use of these medications is based on beneficial effects demonstrated in human or animal model studies. As clinical data become increasingly available in dogs, the use of these medications will continue to grow. The following recommendations are based on a limited number of reports in dogs and the author's own experience.
- In addition to their antiarrhythmic use, beta adrenergic blockers such as **metoprolol** and **carvedilol** are used to slow progression of heart enlargement and systolic dysfunction. Initiation of these drugs

is done in patients with clinically stable heart disease, and as such, beta blocking agents should not be used in patient with active signs of congestion (the exception would be emergency beta blocker use to control rapid atrial fibrillation). Initiation of beta blockade can acutely worsen contractility; thus patients are gradually titrated onto the medications over 4 to 8 weeks. Adverse side effects include bradycardia, hypotension, and exacerbation of congestive heart failure. Clinicians who prescribe beta blockers must be prepared to manage acute heart failure secondary to drug initiation. In humans, beta blockers slow progression of disease and improve survival but do not dramatically improve quality of life. Beneficial effects require several months of continuous treatment, and in dogs with end-stage disease, treatment may not be practical. Accordingly, both the maximum benefit and the minimum risk of beta blocker use are probably early in the course of disease.

- **Metoprolol** (initial dose of 0.1 to 0.2 mg/kg PO every 12 hours followed by gradual titration to 0.4 to 0.8 mg/kg PO every 12 hours over 4 to 8 weeks).
- **Carvedilol** (initial dose of 0.1 mg/kg PO every 12 hours followed by gradual titration to 0.5 mg/kg PO every 12 hours over 4 to 8 weeks).

- Calcium-sensitizing agents purportedly increase cardiac contractility while reducing cellular calcium overload, myocardial oxygen demand, and arrhythmia formation. Agents with combined vasodilatory properties may offer additional advantages in patients with severe DCM.
  - **Pimobendan** (0.25 mg/kg PO every 12 hours) results in substantial improvement in quality of life. Pimobendan is typically used in patients with severe disease, and as such, is used in conjunction with diuretics, ACE inhibitors, and occasionally, digoxin. Benefit from pimobendan during occult disease is possible, but requires additional study.
- Aldosterone antagonists, such as spironolactone, act as mild diuretics but even more importantly, reduce the proliferative effects of aldosterone within the myocardium and vasculature. Other beneficial properties include blunting of sympathetic nervous activity and normalization of baroreceptor function. In the presence of severe heart disease, ACE inhibition alone may not be sufficient in suppressing aldosterone production, and in humans with heart failure, spironolactone improves survival.
  - **Spironolactone** (1 to 2 mg/kg PO every 12 hours) is commonly prescribed with hydrochlorothiazide in dogs with severe heart disease. Due to its anti-proliferative effects, spironolactone may also be beneficial in the occult and early symptomatic stages of disease.
- Amino acid deficiency is present in some breeds with DCM (e.g., American Cocker Spaniels).
  - **Taurine** supplementation (500 mg PO every 12 hours for Cocker Spaniels) is recommended in dogs with low plasma taurine concentration.
  - Concurrent **L-carnitine** supplementation (1 g every 12 hours for Cocker Spaniels) is recommended in dogs with taurine deficiency. Alternatively, due to the relative expense of L-carnitine compared to taurine, L-carnitine is withheld during the initial three months of taurine treatment and administered only to those dogs that have not responded to taurine alone.
  - **L-Carnitine** deficiency was detected in a family of Boxers with left ventricular dilation and systolic dysfunction. Supplementation (50 mg/kg PO every 8 to 12 hours) should be considered in dogs with this presentation. The value of supplementation in Boxers with arrhythmias and no left ventricular dilation (which is the most common presentation) is doubtful.
  - Dogs that respond to amino acid supplementation can often reduce or discontinue conventional heart failure medications (i.e., furosemide, ACE inhibitors, digoxin); however, **taurine** and/or

KEY POINTS

Beta blockade represents one of the cornerstones of treatment in human patients with DCM. In these patients, beta blockers slow progression of disease, improve systolic function, and prolong survival. These benefits are dose dependent and aggressive therapy yields the greatest results. In canine patients, little is known about the ideal timing, dose, and drug that should be used. In healthy dogs, oral carvedilol doses ranging from 0.5 to 1.5 mg/kg PO every 12 hours blunt response to sympathetic stimulation with isoproterenol. The appropriate dose for dogs with heart disease is unknown, but it is likely to be lower than that used in healthy dogs. In dogs with experimental mitral valve disease, oral carvedilol at 0.4 mg/kg PO every 24 hours reduced heart rate, whereas in a small study of dogs with advanced naturally occurring DCM, oral carvedilol at 0.3mg/kg PO every 12 hours did not result in any measurable improvement in echocardiographic heart size or systolic function. Thus, the effective dose of carvedilol in affected dogs is likely to be > 0.3mg/kg PO every 12 hours.

carnitine supplementation should continue indefinitely.

- Heart disease is accompanied by elevations of circulating cytokines and alterations of energy production, both of which may contribute to the heart failure syndrome of weight loss, muscle wasting, and poor appetite.
  - Fish oil supplements can reduce interleukin concentrations and help improve cardiac cachexia.
  - Coenzyme Q_{10} is part of the mitochondrial respiratory transport chain and supplementation may improve quality of life.
  - The benefit of supplementary antioxidant vitamins E, A, or C is unknown.

Prognosis

The time course from occult to symptomatic DCM is highly variable and can be years. During this phase, serial echocardiographic and electrocardiographic exams are recommended. Sudden death can occur during the occult phase, especially in Boxers and Doberman Pinschers. Once clinical signs such as congestive heart failure develop, the long-term prognosis is poor. Survival times derived from clinical studies are difficult to assess due to nonstandardized treatment, lack of ACE inhibitor use, and statistical issues surrounding euthanasia. Median survival time is likely 3 to 4 months in Doberman Pinschers and 5 to 6 months in other breeds. Dogs that survive greater than 7 months may do well for an extended period of time. One-year survival is approximately 10% to 15%. The presence of atrial fibrillation, biventricular congestive failure, and young age at time of presentation (< 5 years) are associated with worse prognosis. Although the overall survival rate is disheartening, it is difficult to assess how any individual dog may fare. The author suggests aggressive intravenous management of dogs with fulminant heart failure and reevaluation after 24 to 72 hours of therapy.

HYPERTROPHIC CARDIOMYOPATHY

Hypertrophic cardiomyopathy (HCM) is an uncommon myocardial disease of dogs. HCM is characterized by idiopathic concentric left ventricular hypertrophy, and can lead to heart failure or sudden death. HCM, if accompanied by systolic anterior motion of the mitral valve and left ventricular outflow tract obstruction, is specifically referred to as hypertrophic obstructive cardiomyopathy. The majority of dogs reported to have HCM are male and of young age (typically < 3 yrs), suggesting a heritable etiology. The left ventricular hypertrophy associated with HCM can be symmetrical (i.e., affecting both the interventricular septum and left ventricular posterior wall equally) or asymmetric (in humans, the septum is typically more affected than the posterior wall). In the author's experience, most cases of canine HCM involve symmetric LV hypertrophy. Significant left ventricular hypertrophy causes diastolic dysfunction, left atrial enlargement, heart failure, and arrhythmias. Most dogs with HCM are asymptomatic and the diagnosis is made during evaluation of a heart murmur or arrhythmia. Echocardiography is the diagnostic method of choice. Treatment is aimed at abolishing the obstructive component of disease with beta-blocking agents (atenolol 0.5 to 1.0 mg/kg every 12 to 24 hours), alleviating heart failure with diuretics, and suppressing arrhythmias. Sudden death appears to be more common than congestive heart failure. Many dogs with HCM remain asymptomatic for years.

Frequently Asked Questions

What Causes DCM?

The etiology of primary DCM is unknown. DCM is a description of the heart's response to injury (i.e., dilation and systolic dysfunction), and as such, may be the end result of multiple causes. In fact, given the forms of DCM that are unique to different breeds, it is likely that more than one etiology exists. Possible causes include genetic/familial, immune-mediated, infectious, toxic, or nutritional. DCM in Doberman Pinschers may involve specific components of the cytoskeleton or extracellular matrix. Cellular energy production is markedly reduced in affected Doberman Pinschers, but whether these changes are primary abnormalities or secondary changes has yet to be determined. Boxers with ARVC are thought to possess abnormal calcium cycling, which is detected in certain forms of ARVC in humans.

Combination Therapy with Beta Blockers and Pimobendan

There is a wealth of data supporting use of beta blockers in humans with DCM. Although these agents are effective at slowing pathologic ventricular remodeling and improving survival, they do relatively little to improve quality of life or exercise tolerance. In contrast, pimobendan, though not proven to improve survival in humans, has a marked benefit on quality of life in dogs. A practice adopted by some cardiologists is to combine pimobendan and beta blocker use in dogs with symptomatic DCM. The positive inotropic effect of pimobendan may increase the likelihood of successful titration and tolerance of beta blockers, and thereby achieve both increased quality and quantity of life.

SUGGESTED READINGS

Borgarelli M, Tarducci A, Tidholm A, Haggstrom J: Canine idiopathic dilated cardiomyopathy. Part II: Pathophysiology and therapy, Vet J 162(3):182-195, 2001.

Calvert CA, Pickus CW, Jacobs GJ, Brown J: Signalment, survival, and prognostic factors in Doberman pinschers with end-stage cardiomyopathy, J Vet Int Med 11(6):323-326, 1997.

Fuentes VL, Corcoran B, French A, et al: A double-blind, randomized, placebo-controlled study of pimobendan in dogs with dilated cardiomyopathy, J Vet Int Med 16(3):255-261, 2002.

Kittleson MD, Keene B, Pion PD, Loyer CG: Results of the multicenter spaniel trial (MUST): taurine- and carnitine-responsive dilated cardiomyopathy in American cocker spaniels with decreased plasma taurine concentration, J Vet Int Med 11(4):204-211, 1997.

Monnet E, Orton EC, Salman M, Boon J: Idiopathic dilated cardiomyopathy in dogs: survival and prognostic indicators, J Vet Int Med 9(1):12-17, 1995.

O'Grady MR, O'Sullivan ML: Dilated cardiomyopathy: an update, Vet Clin North Am Small Anim Pract 34(5):1187-1207, 2004.

Tidholm A, Svensson H, Sylven C: Survival and prognostic factors in 189 dogs with dilated cardiomyopathy, J Am Anim Hosp Assoc 33(4):364-368, 1997.

Tidholm A, Haggstrom J, Borgarelli M, Tarducci A: Canine idiopathic dilated cardiomyopathy. I. Aetiology,clinical characteristics, epidemiology and pathology, Vet J 162(2):92-107, 2001.

CHAPTER 8

Feline Cardiomyopathy

Richard D. Kienle

INTRODUCTION

The term *cardiomyopathy* literally means "heart muscle disease" and designates a disorder of the heart in which the primary abnormality lies within the muscle tissue (myocardium). Primary indicates the myocardial disease is not secondary to valvular disease, pericardial disease, coronary vascular disease, systemic or pulmonary hypertension, congenital abnormalities, or systemic disease. Most primary cardiomyopathies are of unknown etiology (idiopathic). A secondary cardiomyopathy is a disease that affects the myocardium secondary to infectious, toxic, metabolic, or other disease processes. The World Health Organization has categorized the types of cardiomyopathies and based the categorization scheme primarily on the dominant pathophysiology produced by the myocardial disease.

FELINE CARDIOMYOPATHIES

General Comments

- The majority of cardiomyopathies diagnosed in cats are idiopathic (primary). Only one etiology, taurine deficiency in dilated cardiomyopathy, has been identified for a feline cardiomyopathy.
- Intermediate (or intergrade) cardiomyopathy and restrictive cardiomyopathy are poorly defined clinical entities in cats. These "diagnoses" have been assigned to many feline patients with presumed primary myocardial disease that do not meet the criteria for making a diagnosis of hypertrophic or dilated cardiomyopathy.
- The widespread use of echocardiography in veterinary practice allows for more frequent and accurate recognition of myocardial disease in cats.

KEY POINT

In domestic cats, cardiomyopathies are the dominant form of cardiac disease.

Classification

- Cardiomyopathies are classified according to their morphologic appearance. Within each classification, a wide range of morphologic and clinical presentations may be seen. In some cats it may be difficult to comfortably place a cat's myocardial disease into one of these categories. Also, since cardiomyopathies are so common in cats it is common for other forms of cardiac disease to be misidentified as one of the forms of cardiomyopathy.

Primary Cardiomyopathies

- Hypertrophic cardiomyopathy (HCM)
- Idiopathic dilated cardiomyopathy (DCM)
- Restrictive cardiomyopathy (RCM)
- Unclassified cardiomyopathies (UCM)
- Arrhythmogenic right ventricular cardiomyopathy

KEY POINT

In this chapter, I chose not to perpetuate the pretense that what have been called RCM and intermediate cardiomyopathy represent distinct and well-known disease processes for which substantiated recommendations regarding treatment and prognosis can be made. The term ***unclassified cardiomyopathy*** has been used as a reminder that the only conclusions that can be drawn about these cats' hearts is that they have myocardial disease.

Specific/Secondary Cardiomyopathies

- Nutritional (taurine deficiency)
- Metabolic (hyperthyroidism, acromegaly)
- Infiltrative (neoplasia, amyloidosis)
- Inflammatory (toxins, immune reactions, infectious agents)
- Genetic (HCM, DCM)
- Toxic (doxorubicin, heavy metals)

Clinical Classification and Pathophysiology

- Abnormalities in myocardial function during systole or diastole can underlie or influence the clinical signs observed. Systolic dysfunction is present when the ability of the ventricle to eject blood is impaired and may result in signs of low output and possibly congestive heart failure (CHF). Diastolic dysfunction is present when the ability of the ventricle to relax is impaired and may result in signs of CHF.

KEY POINT

Ideally an understanding of the underlying etiology of a disease dictates specific therapy to reverse the condition; however, in most cases, treatment of cardiac disease is palliative. Therefore, when tailoring rational therapy for a patient with cardiac disease, the clinical status of the patient is the primary consideration.

- Right-sided CHF is present when elevated systemic venous, and therefore capillary, pressures resulting from cardiac disease manifest as ascites or peripheral edema.
- Left-sided CHF is present when elevated pulmonary venous, and therefore capillary, pressures resulting from cardiac disease manifest as pulmonary edema (and likely also as pleural effusion in cats).
- Biventricular CHF is present when elevated systemic and pulmonary venous, and therefore capillary, pressures manifest as any combination of the previously mentioned signs, or as pleural effusion.
- Low-output heart failure, or cardiogenic shock, is inadequate cardiac output, often a result of myocardial failure.
- High-output heart failure is CHF, left or right sided, resulting from excessive flow through a capillary bed.
- Myocardial failure is a reduction in myocardial contractility characterized by a reduced shortening fraction and an increased end-systolic dimension on the echocardiogram.

KEY POINT

It is important to realize that heart failure and myocardial failure represent heart disease, and that heart failure, either congestive or low-output, may, in some cases, be a result of myocardial failure; however, heart failure can be, and often is, present in the absence of myocardial failure. Similarly, myocardial failure may be present in association with or in the absence of heart failure (Figure 8-1).

Signalment and Presenting Complaints

KEY POINT

The clinical presentation, physical exam findings, radiographic findings, and electrocardiographic (ECG) findings are similar for all forms of myocardial disease and generally cannot be used to differentiate among them. Echocardiography is necessary to determine the specific disorder that is present.

- The typical clinical presentation, physical exam findings, radiographic findings, and ECG findings will be discussed in this section. The echocardiographic findings will be discussed with the specific disease later.
- The most common historical clues in cats with myocardial disease include:
  - Dyspnea/tachypnea
  - Poor general condition, weakness, lethargy, or, rarely, exercise intolerance
  - Anorexia
  - Acute posterior paresis or paralysis
  - Coughing and abdominal distention, common findings in dogs with cardiac disease, are rare findings in cats with cardiac disease.

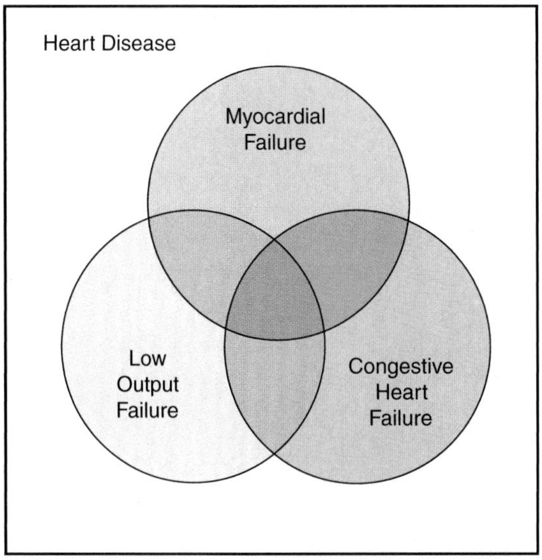

Heart Disease

Myocardial Failure

Low Output Failure

Congestive Heart Failure

Figure 8-1. Venn diagram illustrates the various potential combinations of congestive heart (backward) failure, low-output (forward) heart failure, and myocardial failure (each represented by a circle) that may be detected in patients with heart disease (the box). As all the circles reside in the box, each represents a form of heart disease, and the overlapping portions of the circles illustrate how the conditions may coexist.

Physical Examination

- Early detection of disease should be a primary goal. A thorough physical examination, with careful attention to auscultation, should be performed. Many patients present with acute onset of dyspnea, paresis, lethargy, or anorexia; however, the majority of patients is asymptomatic and will be identified after a murmur, gallop sound, or other abnormality is identified during a routine physical examination. The most common physical clues suggesting myocardial disease include:
- Systolic murmur (commonly heard along the sternal border). This murmur may relate to either mitral regurgitation or outflow tract obstruction or both.
- Gallop sound, At normally rapid heart rates these gallop sounds often represent a summation of the third and fourth sounds.
  - Dysrhythmia
  - Tachypnea/dyspnea
  - Muffled or harsh lung sounds
  - Hypothermia
  - Jugular pulses/distention
  - Acute paresis associated with pain in regions with evidence of reduced peripheral perfusion

Ancillary Tests

- Thoracic radiography and electrocardiography may direct or reinforce suspicion that a cardiac disorder is present. They may also further characterize the disorder and alert the clinician to secondary ramifications that may require attention; however, neither electrocardiography nor thoracic radiography provides adequate evidence for ruling out, confirming, or classifying feline cardiac disease. Contrast radiography or, preferably, echocardiography, is required to confirm or rule out and categorize myocardial disease.
- Electrocardiography often shows:
  - Intraventricular conduction abnormalities (left bundle branch block, left anterior fascicular block pattern, pre-excitation syndrome)
  - Increased amplitude of R waves
  - Ventricular arrhythmias are common but are generally mild with relatively infrequent single premature ventricular contractions.

KEY POINTS

- A normal thoracic radiograph does not preclude the diagnosis of a cardiomyopathy. Many asymptomatic cats with mild changes and normal LA size will have a normal thoracic radiograph.
- Echocardiography, including Doppler echocardiography, is essential for noninvasive determination of a functional and anatomic diagnosis. Before assigning a diagnosis of cardiomyopathy based solely upon morphologic/functional appearance, a concerted effort should be made to rule out cardiac and extracardiac diseases that might mimic the echocardiography of primary myocardial diseases.
- Other diagnostic tests do not usually contribute to the diagnosis of myocardial disease but are important for determining the overall status of the patient, identifying concomitant disorders, and assessing the efficacy or untoward effects of therapy. When possible, routine biochemistries, urinalysis, and hemogram should be performed prior to pharmacologic intervention to establish baseline values for the patient and to rule out concurrent or secondary metabolic or hematologic disturbances.
- Chemical and cytologic evaluation of pleural fluid with respect to protein concentration and cellularity can help determine whether CHF underlies the production of pleural fluid. Cats with CHF can develop true chylous effusion.
- Plasma and whole blood taurine concentrations should be measured in all cats with echocardiographically documented myocardial failure (see Taurine Deficiency–Induced Myocardial Failure).

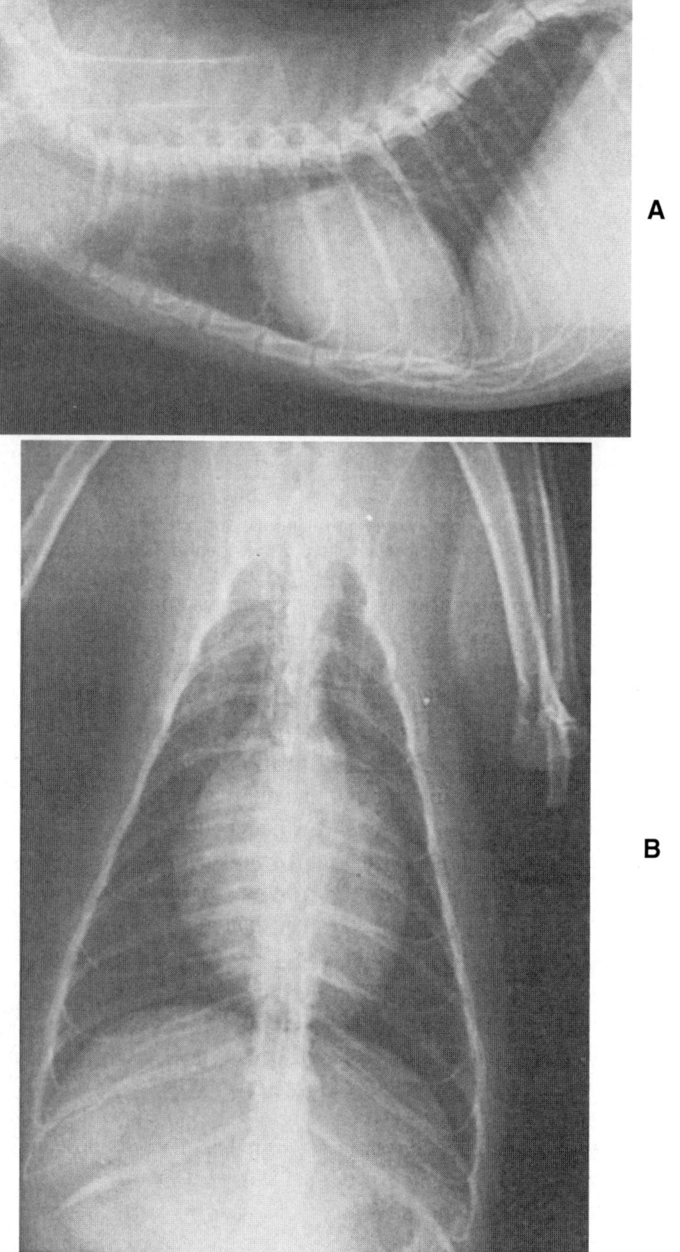

Figure 8-2. **A,** Lateral thoracic radiograph from a cat with dilated cardiomyopathy demonstrates severe generalized cardiomegaly. **B,** Dorsoventral thoracic radiograph from the same cat as in **A.**

- Occasionally cats will have more complex arrhythmias. Some cats with severe LA enlargement will develop atrial fibrillation.
- Thoracic radiography is most useful for detecting gross cardiac enlargement and clinical sequelae to cardiac dysfunction (e.g., pulmonary venous congestion, pulmonary edema, enlarged great veins, pleural effusion) (Figures 8-2 and 8-3). Restraint for radiographic procedures can be life threatening to dyspneic cats. Extreme caution should be taken before proceeding with radiography. The author often delays radiography until after stabilizing the patient (Figure 8-4). Diagnostic and potentially therapeutic thoracocentesis should precede radiography in dyspneic cats.

Therapy

- Therapy should be based upon the clinical and functional classification of the disease process in the individual patient and not by

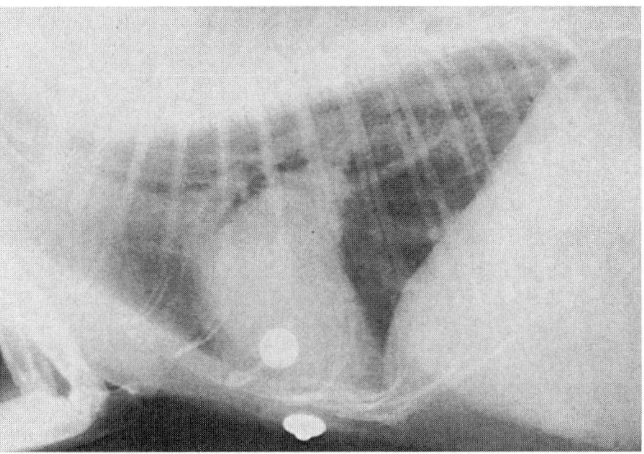

Figure 8-3. Lateral thoracic radiograph from a cat with hypertrophic cardiomyopathy demonstrates marked left atrial enlargement, pulmonary venous engorgement, and pulmonary edema.

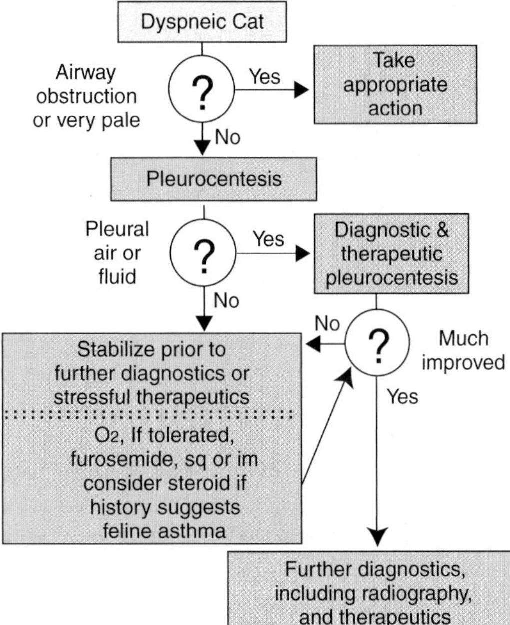

Figure 8-4. Algorithm outlining choices and decisions encountered in the management of life-threatening dyspnea in the cat. The most important point illustrated is not to proceed with stressful diagnostic or therapeutic procedures until the patient is stable. Stressed cats die.

following a standard approach based solely upon the diagnosis.

- With only two exceptions, the indications for and benefits of therapeutic intervention in asymptomatic cats with myocardial disease are controversial. These exceptions are:
  - Myocardial failure secondary to taurine deficiency
  - Thyrotoxic heart disease
- Dyspneic cats are easily stressed and may acutely deteriorate and die if stressful diagnostic or therapeutic interventions are initiated too early. An algorithm for management of the dyspneic cat is presented in Figure 8-4.
- All patients with evidence of significant and life-threatening CHF (pulmonary edema, pleural effusion) require immediate therapy (i.e., appropriate combinations of pleurocentesis, diuretics, oxygen).
  - **Furosemide** is the diuretic of choice in cats. Furosemide should be administered intravenously (1 to 2 mg/kg every 1 to 2 hours as needed) or intramuscularly (1 to 2 mg/kg every 2 hours as needed) depending upon the stress level of the cat. Dosing must be dramatically reduced once the respiratory rate begins to reduce. Generally, aggressive diuretic therapy is continued until the respiratory rate is below 40 breaths per minute.
  - Not all cats respond well to being placed in an oxygen cage. Carefully observe patients after placing in a closed oxygen cage and opt for a quiet, unoxygenated environment if the patient appears more distressed in the oxygen cage.
  - Tranquilization with an agent such as **acepromazine** may be indicated to calm distressed patients.
  - The use of topical **nitroglycerin** as a preload reducing agent in acute and chronic situations is recommended by some, but evidence of efficacy is lacking.
- Cats with significant pleural effusion will benefit most from immediate pleurocentesis. Patients with significant pericardial effusion and cardiac tamponade require pericardiocentesis and should not receive diuretics prior to pericardiocentesis.
- Maintenance therapy is generally aimed at minimizing signs and prevent acute crisis. Lower doses of **furosemide** (6.25 mg twice a day to 12.5 mg three times a day PO) are indicated for chronic maintenance control of CHF. Angiotensin-converting enzyme (ACE) inhibitors (**enalapril** 0.25 to 0.50 mg/kg PO every 24 to 48 hours or **benazepril** 0.25

to 0.50 mg/kg PO every 24 hours) are also quite effective in cats with CHF. Antiarrhythmic drugs may be indicated to control significant arrhythmias. Inotropic agents may be indicated in patients with myocardial failure or low-output heart failure.

- The judicious use of intravenous fluids may infrequently be indicated in patients with signs of low-output heart failure, primarily in situations where the patient has stopped taking in oral fluids, has received excessive treatment with diuretics, or has concurrent renal dysfunction and there is concern about maintaining adequate renal perfusion.
- Specific therapies designed to alter the natural history of disease should be instituted concurrently and may, in some cases, in time, eliminate the need for drugs to control heart failure (see specific conditions discussed later).
- All cats with myocardial failure should be supplemented with **taurine** (see section on Taurine Deficiency–Induced Myocardial Failure) until proven to be not taurine deficient and not taurine responsive.
- Several strategies to prevent an initial thromboembolic event or to avoid recurrence of aortic thromboembolism in cats with cardiomyopathy have been devised and recommended. None of these strategies has been evaluated by controlled studies.
  - Low-dose **aspirin** (25 mg/kg PO every 2 to 3 days) is the most widely employed prophylactic measure. Although aspirin is known to exert antithrombotic effects, there is no objective evidence of its efficacy for the prophylaxis of systemic aortic thromboembolism in cats. Recurrence of thromboembolic events in aspirin-treated cats were as high as 75% in one study.
  - **Lovenox (enoxaparin),** a low molecular weight heparin, has shown promise in anecdotal clinical settings. No large clinical trials have been completed. The most commonly used dose is 1 mg/kg SQ every 12 to 24 hours.
- Left untreated, the outcome of arterial occlusion will depend upon the extent of occlusion and time to spontaneous reperfusion, either via the primary vessel or the collateral circulation. Cats may lose the affected leg(s) because of ischemic necrosis, die of toxemia, remain paralyzed from peripheral nerve damage, or regain full or partial function of the leg. Overall, response to presently available conservative or aggressive clinical intervention has been poor.
- Therapeutic options include:
  - Surgical removal of emboli
  - Catheter embolectomy
  - Medical therapies—most are untested and unproven
- Anticoagulation with **heparin** (220 units/kg IV followed 3 hours later by maintenance dose of 66 to 200 U/kg SQ four times a day) is used to prevent further thrombosis. Adjust dose to maintain the activated partial thromboplastin time at or slightly above the upper limit of the normal reference range.
- Vasodilation with **acepromazine** (0.2 to 0.4 mg/kg SQ three times a day) or **hydralazine** (0.5 to 0.8 mg/kg PO three times a day) is used to promote collateral blood flow.
- **Streptokinase** and **urokinase** are significantly less expensive than newer fibrinolytic agents (e.g., tissue plasminogen activator), but little clinical experience has been reported. Tissue plasminogen activator: Though clinically effective thrombolysis has been documented in the cat, expense, morbidity associated with rapid reperfusion, and inability to prevent recurrence make this option impractical in most cases.

Prognosis

- Inadequate information is available to make broad generalizations regarding prognosis for cats with myocardial diseases. Although echocardiography provides the basis for diagnosis, clinical and radiographic data should be strongly considered for prognostication.
- Cats with severe myocardial disease and no evidence of heart failure may survive for long periods of time. Conversely, cats with much less severe echocardiographic evidence of disease presenting with significant and difficult to control signs of heart failure may survive for very short periods under the best of situations.
- The long-term prognosis for cats with thromboembolic disease is grave because mortality associated with individual episodes is high, and recurrence is common despite prophylaxis.

Pathology

- Gross examination of the heart provides useful anatomic information and should be performed when possible to confirm antemortem findings.
- In most cases histopathologic evaluation adds little useful information and, unless readily available at low cost, is not recommended unless specific indications are present (see the section Specific Diseases).

HYPERTROPHIC CARDIOMYOPATHY

HCM is a disease of the ventricular (primarily left ventricular [LV]) myocardium characterized by mild to severe thickening (concentric hypertrophy) of the papillary muscles and ventricular walls. The word *primary* in this context means that the hypertrophy is due to an inherent problem in the myocardium and is not secondary to a pressure overload or to hormonal stimulation.

General Comments

- When any other disease process that may lead to concentric hypertrophy is present, the diagnosis of HCM is excluded. Secondary disorders typically produce symmetric concentric hypertrophy and typically produce a maximum increase in wall thickness of 50% or less, even with severe disease. If severe or asymmetric concentric hypertrophy is present in a patient with one of these disorders, then concomitant HCM should be considered.
- HCM is the most commonly diagnosed cardiac disease in cats and its prevalence appears to be increasing; however, echocardiographic screening for the disease has also become more prevalent over the past ten years so increased awareness and ease of diagnosis may be a major contributing factor to this increase.
- In most cases the etiology is unknown (idiopathic). The disease is known to be inherited in some breeds of cats. The first "family" of cats with an inherited form of HCM was identified in Maine coon cats in 1992 and reported in 1999. The disease is inherited as a simple autosomal dominant trait in this breed and 100% expressed in experimental cats housed in a colony. A family of American shorthair cats, primarily with systolic anterior motion (SAM) of the mitral valve, but with other evidence of HCM as well has also been identified. The disease in this breed also appears to be inherited as an autosomal dominant trait. In addition to these breeds, there is anecdotal evidence of HCM being inherited in numerous other breeds, including Persian, British shorthair, Norwegian forest, Ragdoll, Turkish van, and Scottish fold cats, along with others.
- HCM is most likely inherited when it is identified in a specific breed; however, HCM is most commonly identified in domestic (mixed-breed) cats. Whether the disease is inherited in these cats, is due to a de novo mutation in these cats, or is associated with a completely different disease process is unknown although suspicion of inheritance has been reported in mixed breed cats.

Clinical Classification and Pathophysiology

- HCM is characterized by enlarged papillary muscles and a thick LV myocardium with a normal to small LV chamber. These changes may be mild, moderate, or severe and may be symmetrical or asymmetric. When it is severe, the concentric hypertrophy by itself increases chamber stiffness. In addition, blood flow and especially blood flow reserve to severely thickened myocardium is compromised, which may cause myocardial ischemia, cell death, and replacement fibrosis. Increased concentrations of circulating neurohormones may also stimulate interstitial fibrosis. These also increase chamber stiffness and are probably the primary reasons for the marked diastolic dysfunction seen in this disease. The stiff chamber causes an increase in diastolic intraventricular and LA pressures, LA enlargement, and may lead to CHF. The concentric hypertrophy may also result in a decrease in afterload because of the increase in wall thickness which may result in a decrease in end-systolic volume, often to zero (cavity obliteration).
- Abnormal papillary muscle orientation and other unexplained factors commonly produce SAM of the mitral valve. In one survey of 46 cats, SAM was present in 67% of cases. Cats with HCM and SAM are commonly said to have the obstructive type of HCM or to have hypertrophic obstructive cardiomyopathy. SAM of the mitral valve produces a dynamic subaortic stenosis that increases systolic intraventricular pressure in mid to late systole. The dynamic subaortic stenosis increases the velocity of blood flow through the subaortic region and often produces turbulence. Simultaneously, when the septal leaflet is pulled toward the interventricular septum, this leaves a gap in the mitral valve creating mitral regurgitation which is typically only mild to moderate in degree. These abnormalities are by far the most common cause of the heart murmur heard in cats with HCM. The degree to which SAM and mitral insufficiency contribute to the development of left-heart failure in cats with HCM is unknown and deserves further study.
- Sudden death may occur in any individual and may be unrelated to disease severity. The incidence of sudden death in cats with HCM is unknown.

- Pleural effusion is common in cats with heart failure. It can be a modified transudate, pseudochylous, or true chylous in nature. The exact pathophysiology of pleural effusion secondary to heart failure is unknown. The most likely possibility is that feline visceral pleural veins drain into the pulmonary veins such that elevated pulmonary vein pressure causes the formation of pleural effusion.
- Thrombi in cats with HCM may form in the left atrium or left auricle. LA thrombi commonly break loose (become emboli) and are carried by blood flow most commonly to the terminal aorta where they lodge. These thromboemboli occlude aortic blood flow and elaborate vasoactive substances that constrict collateral vessels. The net result is cessation of blood flow to the caudal legs resulting in acute paresis/paralysis and pain.

Signalment and Presenting Complaints

- In cats the disease has been observed as young as 6 months of age and as old as 16 years of age. In Maine coon cats that are going to develop severe disease, HCM most commonly develops to its most severe stage in males by around 2 years of age. Females are more variable but most frequently develop to an end-stage of wall thickening by three years of age. The average age of onset and rate of progression in mixed breed cats is unknown.
- Males are affected more commonly than females.
- Cats with HCM may be completely asymptomatic, may be presented to a veterinarian with subtle signs of heart failure, may have moderate to severe heart failure, or may be presented because of thromboembolic disease. Sudden death is also a common "presentation."
- Asymptomatic cats can have mild to severe LV thickening; however, those with severe thickening usually go on to develop heart failure. Cats with severe disease that appear to have no clinical signs may show subtle signs of heart failure (e.g., tachypnea) that may be detected by an observant owner. The respiratory rate is often increased in these cats at rest and they may become more tachypneic or even dyspneic if stressed. Stressed cats with severe HCM may recover quickly following stress or may go on to develop fulminant heart failure. Cats with mild to moderate thickening may never develop clinical signs referable to their disease and may live normal lives. In others, the LV wall may progressively thicken and complications may develop when they are older.
- Cats with severe HCM and moderate to severe heart failure are usually presented to a veterinarian because of respiratory abnormalities (tachypnea and/or dyspnea) due to pulmonary edema, pleural effusion, or both.
- Cats with HCM may develop systemic thromboembolism.
- Cats with HCM may die suddenly, often with no prior clinical signs referable to heart disease or failure. The cause of the sudden death in these cats is unknown.
- In humans, sudden death appears to be either due to an arrhythmia, acute worsening of the outflow tract obstruction associated with stress or exercise, or a large thrombus occluding flow in the left.
- The incidence of sudden death in feline HCM is probably under represented in the veterinary literature because cats that die suddenly are not presented or reported to veterinarians.

Echocardiography

- Cats with severe HCM have papillary muscle hypertrophy, markedly thickened LV walls (7 to 10 mm), and usually an enlarged left atrium (Figure 8-5). The hypertrophy can be global, affecting all areas of the LV wall or can be more regional or segmental. Segmental forms can have the entire or a region of the interventricular septum or free wall primarily affected, the apex primarily affected, or the papillary muscles (and often the adjacent free wall) primarily affected. Papillary muscle hypertrophy may be the only manifestation of the disease.
- Because of these forms, HCM is a diagnosis that should be made by examining several different two-dimensional echocardiographic views and measuring wall thicknesses in diastole from the thickest region or regions on the two-dimensional images. M-mode echocardiography may miss regional thickening unless it is guided by the two-dimensional view. The LV end-diastolic or end-systolic dimension may be normal or decreased and end-systolic cavity obliteration may occur. An enlarged left atrium indicates increased LV end-diastolic pressure. Occasionally, a thrombus is imaged in the LA or its appendage.
- SAM of the mitral valve may be identified by two-dimensional or, more commonly, by M-mode examination (Figure 8-6). Color flow Doppler echocardiography can be used to demonstrate the hemodynamic abnormalities associated with

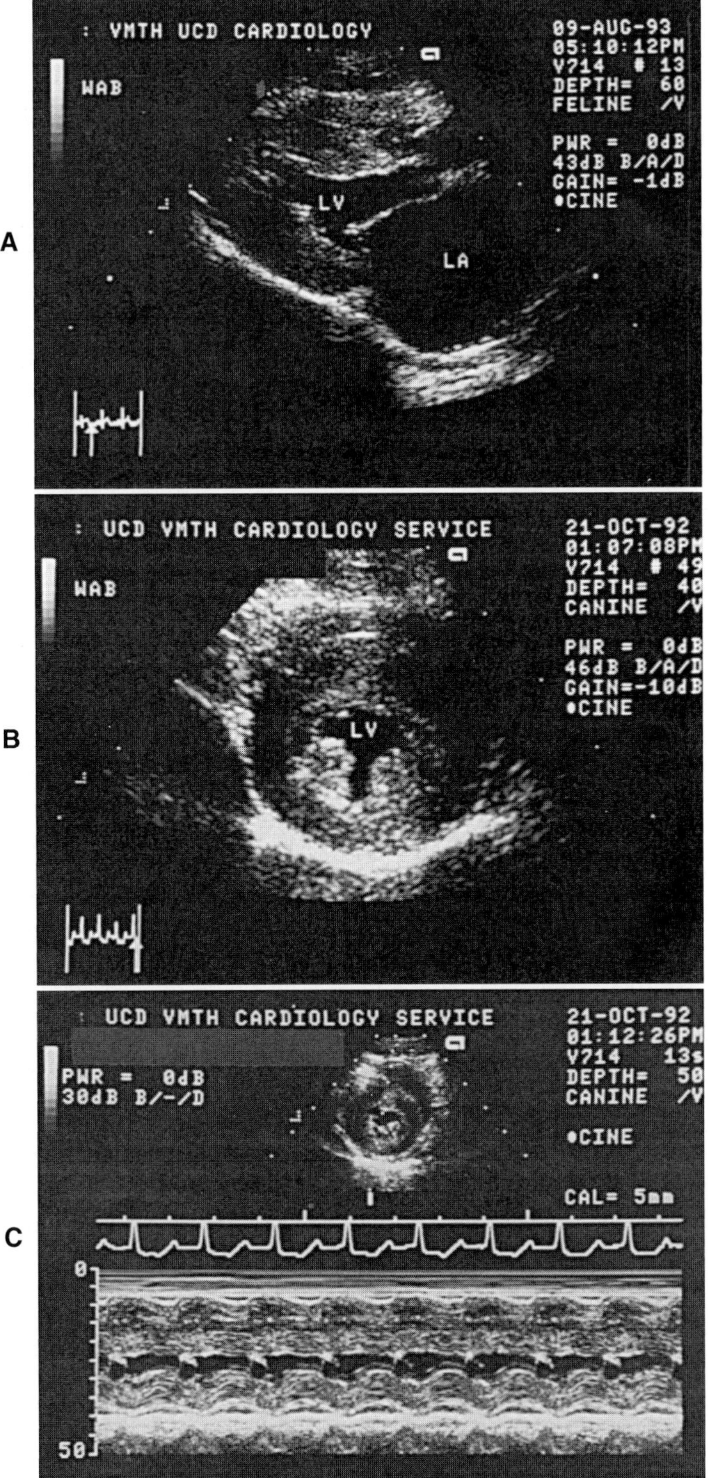

Figure 8-5. Echocardiograms from a cat with hypertrophic cardiomyopathy. **A,** Right parasternal long-axis view shows concentric hypertrophy of the left ventricle *(LV)* and left atrial *(LA)* dilation. **B,** Right parasternal short-axis view shows the thick interventricular septum and left ventricular wall and a comparatively small left ventricular chamber. **C,** M-mode echocardiogram at the level of the left ventricle, showing the thickened myocardium and small LV cavity.

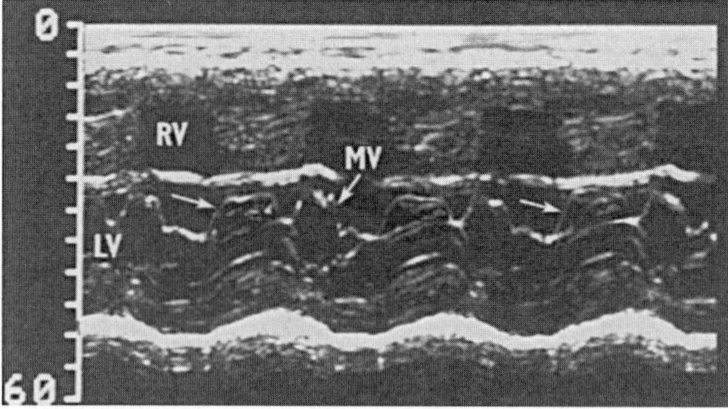

Figure 8-6. M-mode echocardiogram of the mitral valve from a cat with hypertrophic cardiomyopathy demonstrates systolic anterior motion of the mitral valve. The mitral valve moves toward the interventricular septum in early systole *(unlabeled arrows)* and returns to normal position shortly before the beginning of diastole. *LV*, Left ventricle; *RV*, right ventricle; *MV*, mitral valve. (Courtesy Mark D. Kittleson, D.V.M., Ph.D.)

SAM. Two turbulent jets originating from the LV outflow tract are seen—one regurgitating back into the left atrium and the other projecting into the aorta. Spectral Doppler can be used to determine the pressure gradient across the region of dynamic subaortic stenosis produced by the SAM. The pressure gradient roughly correlates with the severity of the SAM although it can be quite labile, changing with the cat's level of excitement. SAM is not present in all cats with HCM. The majority of cats with severe HCM have SAM. However, on the other end of the spectrum, some cats develop SAM before they have any evidence of wall thickening, when their papillary muscles are thickened or long. Although the basilar region of the interventricular septum is often thickened in diastole in cats with HCM, the basilar LV outflow tract does not need to be narrowed for SAM to occur.

- Diastolic dysfunction in cats with severe HCM has been documented using Doppler tissue imaging and measures of transmitral flow and relaxation time. Cats with severe HCM routinely have a decrease in early diastolic wall motion of the LV free wall and mitral valve annulus using Doppler tissue imaging. In addition, peak E wave velocity is reduced, peak A wave velocity is increased, isovolumic relaxation time is prolonged, and rate of deceleration of early inflow is reduced.

Therapy

- There currently is no evidence that any drug alters the natural history of HCM in domestic cats until they are in heart failure. Diltiazem, atenolol, benazepril, and enalapril are commonly administered to cats with mild to severe HCM that are not in heart failure on an empirical basis. Because there are likely many cats with mild to moderate HCM in the cat population that never progress to a more severe form of the disease, condemning owners to pill their cat twice or even once a day for the rest of the cat's life is questionable, given the lack of data. Many veterinarians feel compelled to treat a patient with a disease, and some owners demand treatment for their pet, even if there is only a theoretical case for using a drug. Consequently, whenever HCM is diagnosed in a cat the veterinarian must explain the situation to each owner and try to let the owner make an informed decision based on their wishes and life style. Because no intervention is known to change the course of the disease, there is no mandate to treat at this stage.
- Two classes of agents, oral beta blockers and oral calcium channel blockers, have been advocated to improve LV filling and cardiac performance in cats with HCM. Although there is no clear evidence as to which therapy is more beneficial in *symptomatic* individuals, many cardiologists believe patients with documented HCM should receive one or the other as part of their chronic management. Whatever the initial choice, response to therapy should dictate whether dose adjustment, changing drug class, or discontinuation of therapy is warranted.

Adrenergic Beta Blockers

- **Atenolol**: 6.25 to 12.5 mg/cat every 12 hours. Atenolol is supplied as 25 mg tablets.

Calcium Channel Blockers

- **Diltiazem** is currently the preferred calcium channel blocker. Beneficial effects include lessened edema formation and decreased wall thickness in some cats. Exactly how these beneficial effects occur is open to debate. Only a few cats experience a clinically significant decrease in wall thickness in my experience.

- **Cardizem** 7.5 mg PO every 8 hours. This product is supplied as 30 mg tablets. One-quarter tablet is given every 8 hours.
- **Dilacor XR:** 30 mg PO every 12 hours. This product is supplied as 120, 180, and 240 mg capsules. Each large capsule can be opened to yield two, three, or four 60 mg tablets, which are then halved to achieve a 30 mg dose.
- **Cardizem CD:** 45 mg PO every 24 hours. Cardizem CD is supplied as 180 mg capsules that contain many smaller capsules. The larger capsule can be opened and the smaller capsules divided into a number that produces an appropriate dose. The smaller capsules can be divided into groups of four (45 mg each) and placed in smaller gelatin capsules for administration. One capsule is then administered once per day.

KEY POINT

The authors generally use diltiazem first in cats without outflow tract obstruction, tachycardia or arrhythmias. The authors generally use atenolol first in cats with outflow tract obstruction, tachycardia or arrhythmias. The authors may switch to the alternate therapy if the response is suboptimal or becomes suboptimal.

Prognosis

- Prognosis is generally based upon clinical presentation, echocardiographic evidence of elevated intracardiac pressures, and response to therapy. Inadequate data has been published to reach definitive conclusions; therefore, statements on prognosis are largely based upon clinical experience and conjecture.
- Asymptomatic cats with mild to moderate hypertrophy and no LA enlargement are believed to have a good long-term prognosis. Reported average survival times are generally in the range of 4 to 6 years. Asymptomatic cats with obvious wall thickening and LA enlargement are likely at higher risk for developing heart failure. These cats are also believed to be at risk for developing thromboembolic disease. Asymptomatic cats with severe wall thickening and normal LA size are occasionally observed. Although it is tempting to predict that these cats are at greater risk for progressive disease, inadequate data are available.
- In general, cats that present with heart failure have a poor prognosis. A median survival time after diagnosis of about 3 months is reported. Cats that present in heart failure and respond favorably to therapy may do well for prolonged periods of time.
- In general, cats presenting with aortic thromboembolism have a poor prognosis. A median survival, after diagnosis, of about 2 months is reported. Cats that survive the thromboembolic episode may do well for extended periods; however, these cats are generally at high risk for recurrence of thromboembolism.
- Owners should always be warned of the potential for sudden death. The exact incidence of sudden death in cats with HCM is unknown. It is in some cats, it is the first and only clinical sign.

Pathology

- In severe cases the entire LV wall may be impressively thick. Papillary muscle hypertrophy is usually prominent, and the LV cavity is usually decreased in size owing to encroachment. Both symmetric and asymmetric (asymmetric septal hypertrophy) forms of hypertrophy are recognized in cats. The left atrium is often enlarged, and, occasionally, a thrombus is present within the left atrium.
- Cats with milder forms have less dramatic wall thickening and normal or near-normal LV chamber size. The LA may be normal or only mildly enlarged. Occasionally, the disease is manifested only by papillary muscle hypertrophy with normal LV free wall and septal thickness. There is considerable variability in the degree and location of the hypertrophy.
- Myocyte hypertrophy is the hallmark of histopathologic examination with approximately 30% of the cases also having myocardial fiber disarray involving at least 5% of the septal myocardium.

FELINE (IDIOPATHIC) DILATED CARDIOMYOPATHY

DCM is a disease of the ventricular myocardium (predominantly left) characterized by *primary* myocardial failure.

General Comments

- Prior to 1987, DCM was one of the most commonly diagnosed heart diseases in cats. Most cases at that time were likely a secondary cardiomyopathy associated with nutritional taurine deficiency. Primary idiopathic DCM is currently not a common cardiac condition in cats. Because there are no published reports defining differences between cats with myocardial failure associated with taurine deficiency and with idiopathic DCM, there is very little, if anything, known about idiopathic DCM in cats.

- There is no reason to expect that clinical findings and results of ancillary tests (other than blood taurine concentration and funduscopic examination) should be dramatically different between these disorders.
- Myocardial failure secondary to other causes (e.g., long-standing congenital or acquired LV volume overload or toxic, ischemic, nutritional, or metabolic problems that may underlie myocardial failure) must be ruled out to definitively assign a diagnosis of idiopathic DCM.
- The underlying etiology remains unknown and may represent a common endpoint to many processes.

KEY POINT

Although myocardial failure secondary to taurine deficiency is now quite rare in cats, all cats with myocardial failure should be assumed to be taurine deficient until shown not to be taurine responsive.

Pathophysiology

- The underlying abnormality leading to clinical manifestations in cats with idiopathic DCM is primary systolic myocardial failure. End-systolic LV volume increases owing to a reduction in myocardial pump function. As a result, stroke volume and cardiac output decrease. Neurohumoral compensatory mechanisms promote an increase in intravascular volume and end-diastolic pressures, stimulating eccentric hypertrophy (dilation). At these larger LV end-diastolic volumes, the geometry of the ventricle is such that small changes in chamber dimension during systole provide adequate stroke volume and cardiac output; however, working at these larger volumes is energetically inefficient for the ventricle. At any point in this degenerative process that end-diastolic pressures rise too high or cardiac output drops too low, the patient may present with signs of CHF or low-output heart failure, respectively (Figure 8-7).
- The factors that contribute to patients going from asymptomatic, well-compensated myocardial failure, to a symptomatic, uncompensated state are poorly understood.
- The degree to which alterations in diastolic function contribute to decompensation of patients with DCM is likely larger than previously appreciated.

Signalment and Presenting Complaints

- The reported age at diagnosis ranges from 5 months to 14 years (mean age 7 to 8 years).
- No sex predilection is evident.
- Cats with DCM may have a variable period of lethargy, anorexia, and malaise prior to overt signs of CHF.
- Cats may present with no prior signs and an acute onset of CHF or systemic thromboembolism.

Physical Examination

- Physical examination is similar to that of other forms of myocardial disease.

Ancillary Tests

- Ancillary tests are similar to taurine deficiency myocardial failure (see next section); however, one must rule out taurine deficiency using whole blood and plasma taurine assays.

Therapy

- For acute CHF, see the earlier section on treatment of CHF in the Therapy section of General Information.
- Cats with DCM and signs of low-output heart failure (cardiogenic shock) represent a therapeutic challenge. Suggestions based upon clinical experience with cats with myocardial failure associated with taurine deficiency are presented in the section on this disorder.

Prognosis

- There are no reports documenting the clinical characteristics of cats with idiopathic DCM that do not respond to taurine supplementation. There is no evidence that clinical intervention alters the progression of myocardial failure in patients that do not respond to taurine supplementation. The expected survival time for patients is more a function of their clinical condition at the time of diagnosis than of the treatment they receive.
- Asymptomatic cats diagnosed because a murmur or gallop is identified during a routine physical examination may survive for years with myocardial failure before developing signs of CHF or low-output heart failure.

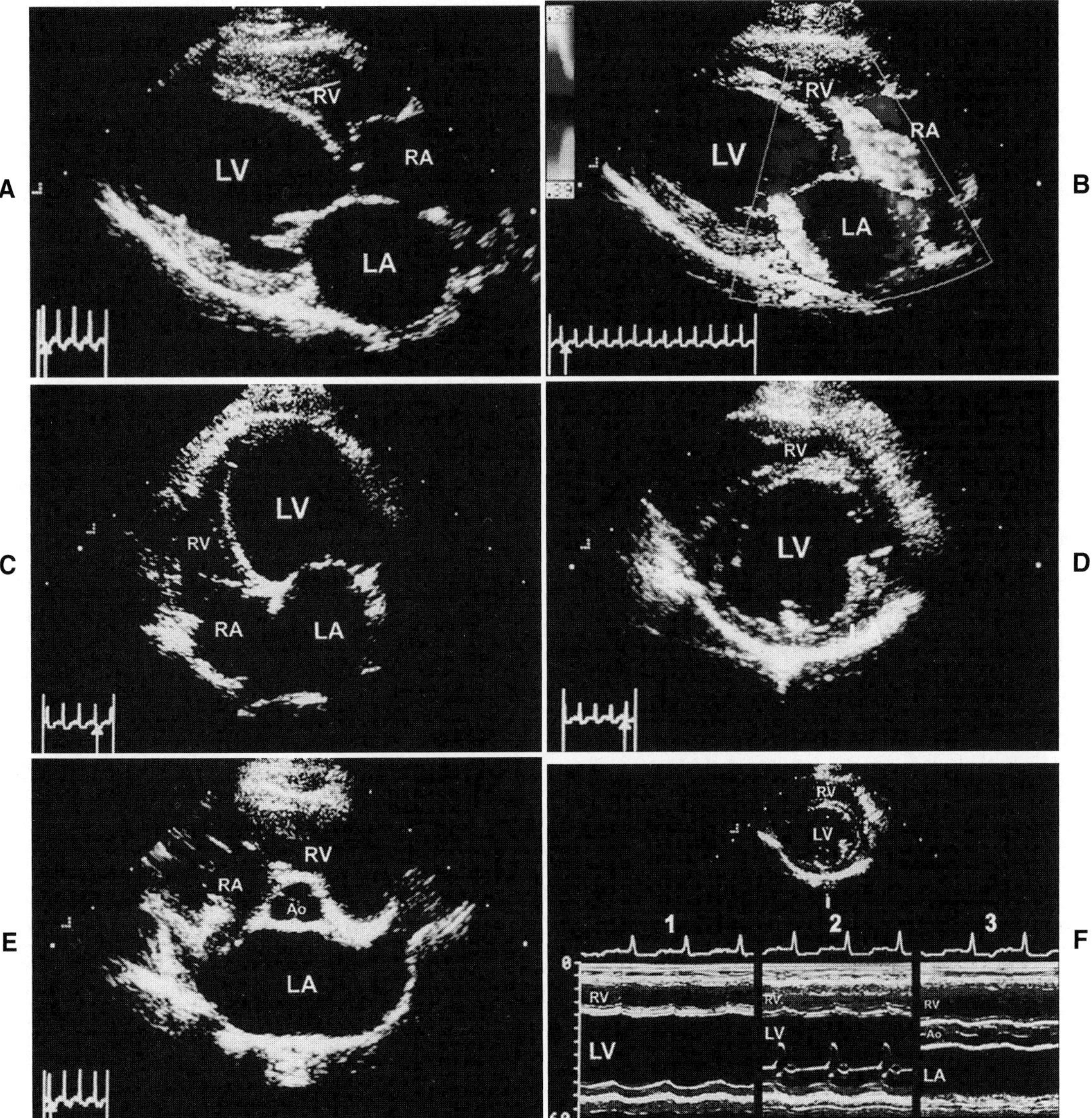

Figure 8-7. Dilated cardiomyopathy in a cat. **A,** Right parasternal long-axis view showing dilation of the left atrium *(LA)* and left ventricle *(LV)*. **B,** Systolic color Doppler image of the same view as in A showing modest secondary mitral and tricuspid valve regurgitation. **C,** Left apical four-chamber view showing the dilated left atrium and ventricle. **D,** Right parasternal short-axis view showing left ventricular dilation. **E,** Right parasternal short-axis view at the heart base showing moderately severe left atrial dilation. **F,** M-mode recordings at the level of the ventricles [1], mitral valve [2], and aortic valve [3]. There is marked dilation of the left atrium and left ventricle and decreased left ventricular systolic motion. In addition, the opening motion of the mitral valve is decreased, and the distance between the open mitral valve and ventricular septum (EPSS) is markedly increased (10 mm). *RA,* Right atrium; *RV,* right ventricle. (From Nyland TG, Mattoon JS: Small animal diagnostic ultrasound, ed 2, Philadelphia, 2002, WB Saunders.)

- Cats presenting with signs of CHF or low-output heart failure have a very guarded prognosis. These cats usually either die soon after admission from cardiogenic shock or succumb to refractory CHF or thromboembolism. Based upon a small number of documented cases, expected survival is 1 to 2 months after diagnosis.

Pathology

- There is currently no information available, but there is no reason to suspect that findings should be different from taurine-deficient cats with myocardial failure or patients with DCM in other species in which there are no specific or pathognomonic changes found.

FELINE RESTRICTIVE CARDIOMYOPATHY

RCM is a diverse group of conditions characterized by restriction of diastolic filling. Specific clinical and morphologic criteria for this diagnosis in the cat have not been as clearly defined as they have in humans.

General Comments

- Without the use of invasive diagnostic procedures or necropsy examination, it is not possible to distinguish this disorder from infiltrative diseases of the myocardium and UCM.
- This disorder is uncommon in the author's experience. Much of what follows is summarized from the literature and not from direct clinical experience.

Pathophysiology

- In the most widely recognized form in cats, endocardial, subendocardial, or myocardial fibrosis or infiltration results in diastolic dysfunction.
- LV pathology predominates. In most cases systolic function is preserved. Papillary muscle fibrosis, distortion of the mitral valve apparatus, and changes in LV geometry may contribute to the development of mitral regurgitation and left-sided CHF.
- Similar pathophysiology may result from pericardial fibrosis (restrictive pericarditis) or infiltrative neoplastic and inflammatory diseases of the epicardium or myocardium. Signs referable to biventricular restriction predominate in pericardial disease.

Signalment and Presenting Complaints

- Signalment is difficult to report accurately because there is little agreement among cardiologists as to which cases fall within this classification. Presenting complaints are similar to those of other forms of myocardial disease.

Physical Examination

- Physical examination findings are similar to that of other forms of cardiomyopathy.

Ancillary Tests

- As with other forms of myocardial disease, ancillary tests rarely help discriminate the diagnosis. In general the findings are similar to what is discussed earlier in the chapter.
- Although not reported, in my experience cats with RCM are more likely to have intraventricular conduction abnormalities (left bundle branch block, left anterior fascicular block pattern, pre-excitation syndrome) on electrocardiograms and seem to have a higher frequency of ventricular arrhythmias.
- There is often very dramatic LA enlargement on thoracic radiographs and pulmonary veins are often enlarged and tortuous. When CHF is present, pulmonary edema is more common than pleural effusion.
- The echocardiographic findings in RCM (Figure 8-8) are quite variable. Severe LA dilation is a common feature. The LV internal dimensions are normal or mildly reduced and LV systolic function is generally normal. Two-dimensional echocardiography may demonstrate loss of normal LV symmetry and distorted or fused papillary muscles. Some authors report increased endocardial echogenicity. Mitral regurgitation is detectable with spectral and color-flow Doppler in most affected cats. Intracardiac thrombus (most commonly left atrium) may be present.

Therapy

- For acute CHF, see the earlier section on treatment of CHF in the Therapy section of General Information.
- No specific therapy for controlling the fibrous tissue reaction is available.
- Beta blockers or calcium channel blockers are not effective for improving diastolic function due to fibrosis. Negative chronotropic, dromotropic, and antiarrhythmic effects of these drugs may be beneficial in cats with ventricular or supraventricular tachyarrhythmias.

Prognosis

- As with other forms of cardiomyopathy, prognosis is difficult to predict for individual cases prior to observing the initial response to therapy; however, in general the prognosis is relatively poor even when initial response to therapy is good. Average survival time in the authors' experience is usually only 4 to 6 months.
- A high incidence of serious arrhythmias, systemic thromboembolism, and refractory CHF has been reported by some authors.

Pathology

- The postmortem changes are unique to this form of cardiomyopathy and may be used to differentiate it from other disorders.

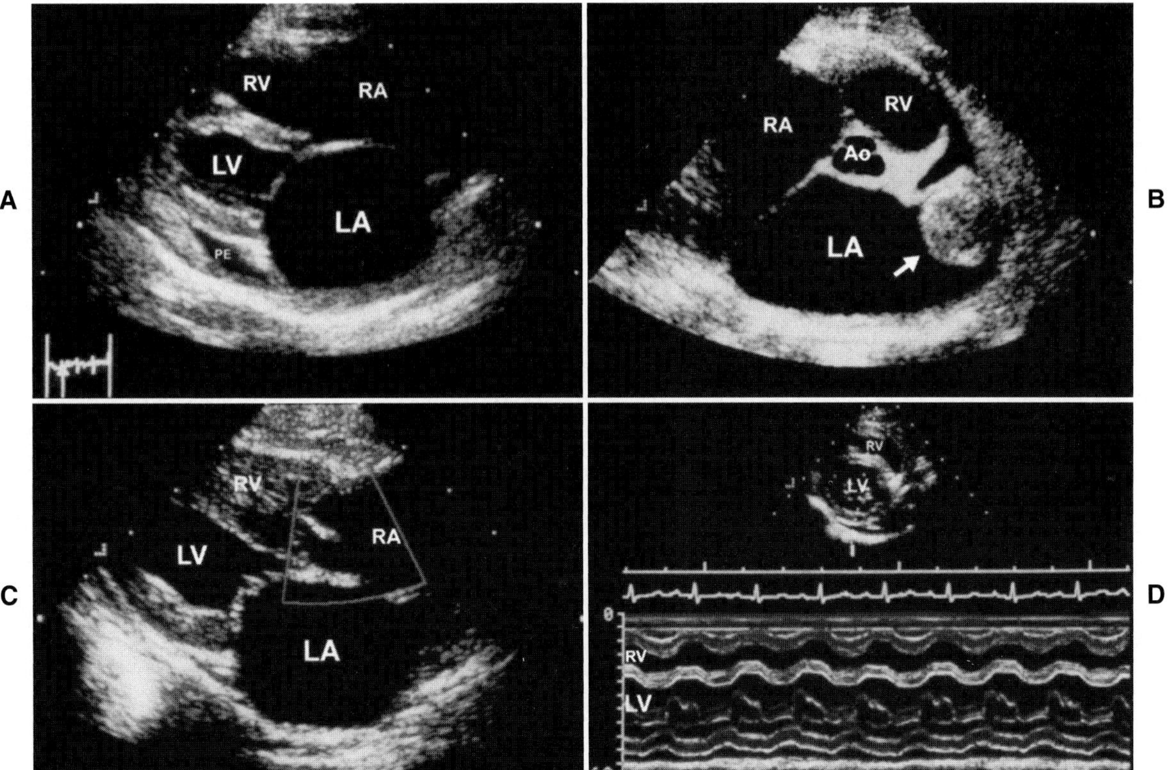

Figure 8-8. Atypical (restrictive?) cardiomyopathy in the cat. **A,** Right parasternal long-axis view showing marked dilation of the left atrium *(LA),* right atrium *(RA),* and right ventricle *(RV).* Note that the left ventricle *(LV)* is neither dilated nor thickened. **B,** Right parasternal short-axis view from the same cat as in **A** showing marked right and left atrial dilation. In addition, a ball-like thrombus is visible within the dilated left auricle *(arrow).* **C,** Right parasternal long-axis view of another cat with biatrial dilation, a nonhypertrophied and nondilated left ventricle, and mild secondary tricuspid valve regurgitation. **D,** M-mode recording at the mitral valve level from the same cat as in **A** and **B.** The right ventricular wall, septal, and left ventricular wall thicknesses are normal, but all show mildly hyperdynamic systolic motion. The mitral-septal distance (EPSS) is normal. (From Nyland TG, Mattoon JS: Small animal diagnostic ultrasound, ed 2, Philadelphia, 2002, WB Saunders.)

- Patchy or diffuse endocardial, subendocardial, or myocardial deposition of fibrous tissue is characteristic. Fibrosis without eosinophilia is the most common form reported in the cat. Fibrous adhesions between papillary muscles and the myocardium, with distortion and fusion of the chordae tendineae and mitral valve leaflets, may be noted. As with most cardiomyopathies, the LV appears to be most severely affected.
- Extreme LA and left auricular enlargements are common.

UNCLASSIFIED FELINE CARDIOMYOPATHIES

The author (and other colleagues) has chosen to apply the term *unclassified cardiomyopathies* to a diverse set of cardiac presentations in cats. They are unclassified because the lesions do not conform to expectations for HCM or DCM, or to other known cardiac disorders. What follows is intended to describe the spectrum of lesions that are labeled UCM.

General Comments

- In recent years, increasing numbers of cats have been recognized with obviously abnormal hearts, many presenting in heart failure, but not fitting into any recognized disease classification. It is not known whether these cases represent a single disease category. It is not known whether these cases represent a congenital or acquired disease. It is not known whether these cats are afflicted by a primary myocardial disease or by a secondary condition.
- Although no controlled studies have been performed, taurine deficiency or metabolic abnormalities (e.g., hyperthyroidism) have not been consistent findings in affected cats.

Pathophysiology

- The pathophysiology is unknown; however, clinical observations suggest diastolic dysfunction, similar to that described for RCM, is the predominant functional abnormality in these cats.

Signalment and Presenting Complaints

- No sex, breed, or age predispositions are known.
- Cats in this category are generally older adults.
- Presenting complaints are believed to be similar to other forms of myocardial disease.

Physical Examination

- Physical examination is similar to that of other forms of myocardial disease.

Ancillary Tests

- Common thoracic radiographic findings include often severe left or bi-atrial enlargement. When CHF is present, pulmonary edema is more common than pleural effusion although both may be observed.
- By nature of the definition the echocardiographic findings are extremely variable. In my opinion, the most consistent echocardiographic finding is severe dilation of the left atrium (see Figure 8-7). The left ventricle is usually normal sized or only mildly dilated; however, severe LV dilation may be observed along with normal wall thickness (eccentric hypertrophy). Various patterns of mild regional myocardial hypertrophy are observed in the septum or LV free wall of some cats. Enlargement of the right heart is variable but may be marked in some cases. Systolic contractile indices may be normal or mildly depressed. Mitral, and on occasion tricuspid, regurgitation can be detected with spectral and color-flow Doppler in most affected cats. It is generally mild but may be moderate in some cases. A thrombus may be observed within the LA (Figure 8-9).

Therapy

- For acute CHF, see the earlier section on treatment of CHF in the Therapy section under General Information.
- As the underlying etiology and pathophysiology have not been defined, no specific therapy can be recommended for these disorders.
- With the presumed pathophysiology of this group of disorders, the use of calcium channel blockers to support or improve diastolic dysfunction makes sense; however, no studies have confirmed that this therapy has any benefit for supporting CHF or improving survival in cats with UCM. I generally use diltiazem in these cats (see earlier HCM section) unless there is a direct contraindication or untoward effects of the medication.
- For cats with chronic CHF, diuretics and ACE inhibitors are recommended (see previous section)

Prognosis

- The prognosis is generally based upon clinical presentation, echocardiographic and radiographic evidence of elevated diastolic pressures, and response to therapy.
- Asymptomatic cats with mild LA enlargement are believed to have a good long-term prognosis. Asymptomatic cats with marked LA enlargement are likely to be at higher risk for developing heart failure.
- In general, cats that present in heart failure have a poor prognosis. Although cats that present in heart failure and respond favorably to therapy may do well for prolonged periods of time.
- In general, cats with aortic thromboembolism have a poor prognosis. Cats that survive the thromboembolic episode may do well for extended periods; however, these cats are generally at high risk for recurrence of thromboembolism.

TAURINE DEFICIENCY–INDUCED MYOCARDIAL FAILURE

Taurine deficiency–induced myocardial failure is associated with low plasma, whole blood, and tissue taurine concentrations that and may be reversible after taurine supplementation. In 1987 it was determined that many cats presenting with DCM were taurine deficient and that supplementation with taurine reversed the myocardial failure.

Therefore, much of the literature published before 1987 referring to idiopathic DCM in cats should be considered to be referring to this condition, not to idiopathic DCM.

General Comments

- Supplementation of commercial cat foods with additional taurine has greatly reduced the prevalence of this near-uniformly fatal condition.
- Not all taurine-deficient cats develop myocardial failure. The other factor(s) required for taurine deficiency to lead to the development of myocardial failure are unknown. A genetic predisposition has been proposed.
- It is reasonable to assume that nutritional taurine deficiency combined with other causes of myocardial failure (e.g., long-standing congenital or acquired LV volume overload or toxic, ischemic, nutritional, endocrine, or metabolic problems) may lead to synergistic complicating effects.

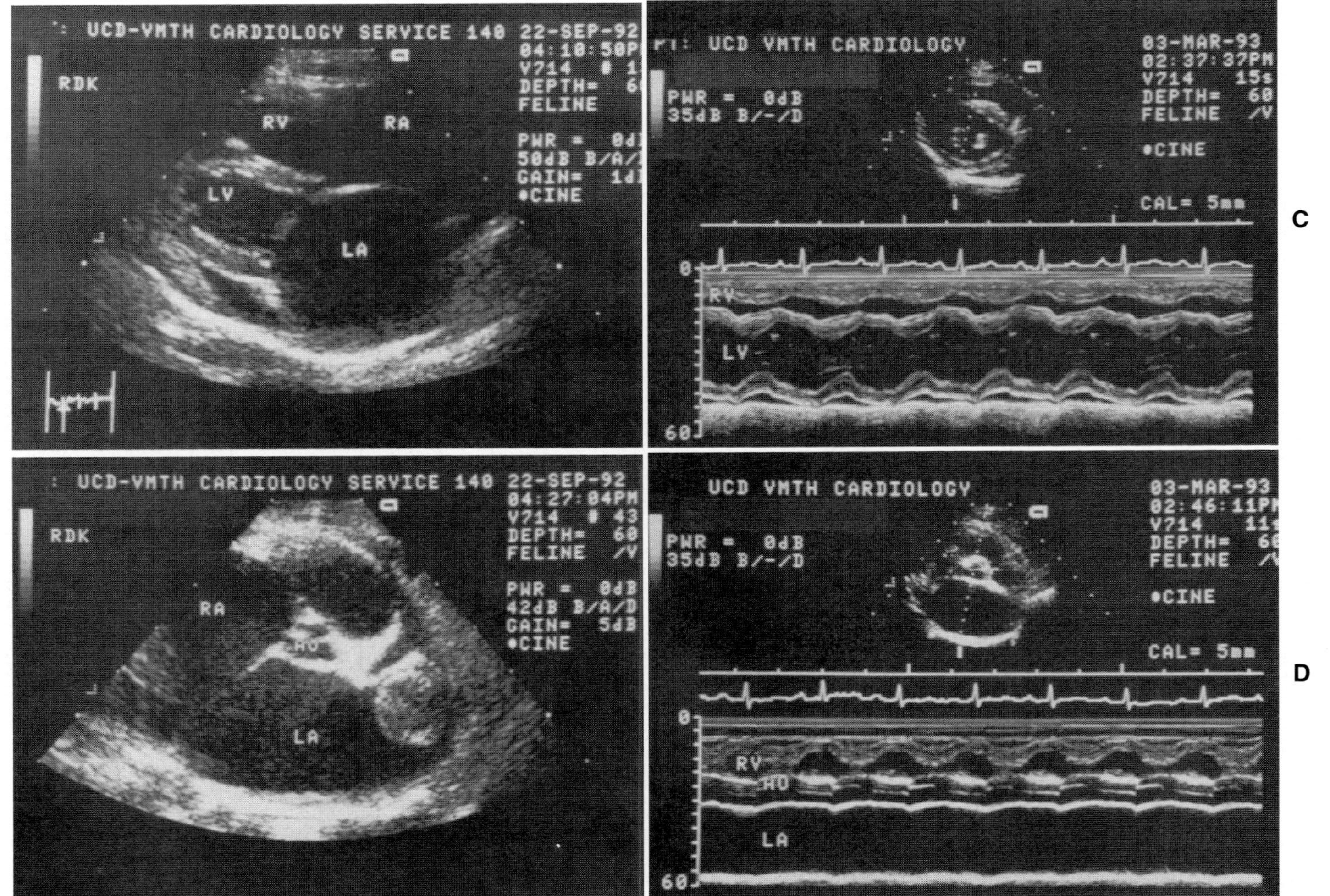

Figure 8-9. Echocardiograms from a cat with an unclassified form of cardiomyopathy. **A,** Right parasternal long-axis view. There is marked dilation of both left and right atria and mild dilation of the right ventricle. *LV,* Left ventricle; *LA,* left atrium; *RV,* right ventricle; *RA,* right atrium. **B,** Right parasternal short-axis view shows the marked right and left atrial dilation. In addition, a thrombus is visible within the dilated left auricle. *AO,* Aorta. **C** and **D,** M-mode recordings at the ventricular level and aortic level, respectively. The right ventricular wall, septal, and left ventricular wall thickness are normal. The left ventricular chamber is only mildly dilated, and the left ventricular shortening fraction is in the low normal range (30%). The left atrium is markedly dilated.

- A precise requirement for taurine cannot be determined for all foods because the requirement is dependent upon many factors. No commercial diet should be assumed to be taurine sufficient until the manufacturer has provided feeding trial data documenting that the food maintains normal taurine concentrations in blood and tissue during a trial of at least 6 months.

Pathophysiology

- The hemodynamics and pathophysiology are believed to be similar to idiopathic DCM as previously outlined.
- In most cases, taurine deficiency is believed to be nutritionally derived, as a result of inadequate amounts of taurine in the diet. The role that taurine, an essential amino acid in the cat, plays in the maintenance of myocardial function remains unknown.

Signalment and Presenting Complaints

- Signalment and presenting complaints are similar to those of other forms of cardiomyopathy.

Physical Examination

- The physical examination is similar to that of other forms of cardiomyopathy.
- Funduscopic evaluation may reveal the presence of taurine deficiency–induced central retinal degeneration.

Ancillary Tests

- Ancillary tests do not provide a definitive diagnosis. The results of electrocardiography and thoracic radiographs are similar to other forms of myocardial disease. The echocardiographic findings are similar to those for idiopathic DCM.
- The primary echocardiographic abnormality is an increase in end-systolic diameter (more than 12 mm) with a reduced shortening fraction (less than 35%). The end-diastolic dimension is also often enlarged (more than 17 mm) (Figures 8-10 and 8-11). Significant LA enlargement is common. The E-point to septal separation (EPSS) is often increased (> 2 mm). The right ventricle and right atrium are variably affected. Mitral regurgitation may be detected with spectral and color-flow Doppler. In some cases, a thrombus is observed within the body of the left atrium or in the left auricular appendage.
- Diet history should be accurately ascertained during the initial workup of any cat with *myocardial failure*. Many owners have managed to formulate diets with inadequate amounts of taurine and need to be educated to prevent recurrence. In addition, it is likely that a small number of cases will continue to be the result of commercial cat foods containing inadequate amounts of taurine, and the veterinary profession, to whom these cats will present for diagnosis and treatment, remains the most effective sentinel for detecting patterns with regard to diet and disease occurrence.
- Cats diagnosed with any form of myocardial failure should have plasma and whole blood taurine concentrations determined from blood samples obtained prior to supplementation. Even a single dose of taurine may make interpretation difficult and proper sample handling is critical for accurate results.
- The following guidelines should be used in handling samples for taurine analysis:
  - Submit both heparinized plasma and heparinized whole blood.
  - Place the sample on wet ice or centrifuge the sample and separate plasma immediately.
  - Make sure the sample contains no clots or hemolysis.
  - Store and ship samples frozen (dry ice or ice packs).
- Normal values:
  - Plasma: taurine greater than 60 nmol/ml (at risk when less than 30 nmol/ml). Note: Plasma taurine concentration is very labile; 24 hours of fasting can cause plasma concentrations to fall below 30 nmol/ml.
  - Whole blood: taurine greater than 200 nmol/ml (at risk when less than 100 nmol/ml). Whole blood taurine concentration is not as labile. Fasting does not significantly affect values.

Therapy

- During the initial phase of therapy, proper supportive and symptomatic care for CHF (as described previously under general comments on therapy) is essential if CHF is present. Cats with documented taurine deficiency should be supplemented with 250 mg every 12 hours until echocardiographically determined LV dimensions normalize. This usually occurs within 4 to 6 months. Clinical improvement is usually evident within about 2 weeks.

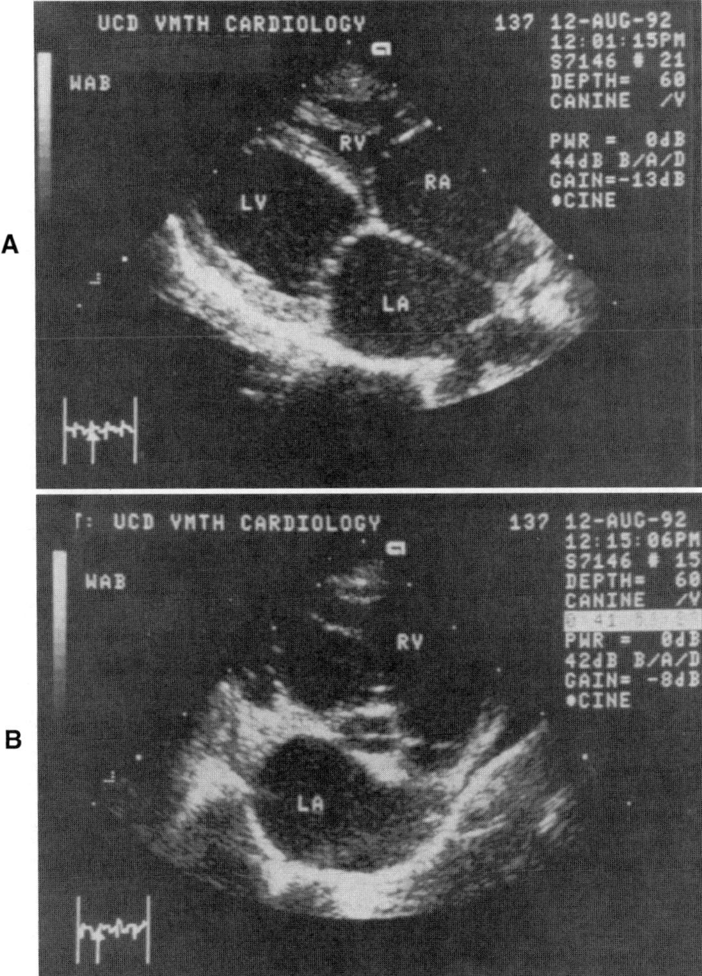

Figure 8-10. Two-dimensional echocardiograms from a cat with myocardial failure associated with taurine deficiency. Right parasternal long-axis **(A)** and short-axis **(B)** views, respectively, demonstrate marked dilation of all four cardiac chambers. *LV,* Left ventricle; *LA,* left atrium; *RV,* right ventricle; *RA,* right atrium.

- Diuretics and ACE inhibitors can be discontinued when signs of CHF resolve, and radiographic improvement in cardiac size is noted. The ACE inhibitor should be removed first and then the diuretic tapered over a period of 2 weeks. The owner should be taught to monitor respiratory rate while withdrawing heart failure medications, and clinical and radiographic evaluation should be repeated 1 week after withdrawing medications to detect any decline in the cat's condition.
- **Digoxin** is not routinely administered as a part of therapy, but there is no contraindication to doing so. When used initial dose should be one fourth of a 0.125 mg tablet PO every 48 hours. Digoxin levels are taken 6 to 8 hours after the seventh dose and are used to adjust therapy. I rarely increase the dose to more than one fourth of a 0.125 mg tablet PO every 24 hours.
- The diet should be altered to maintain normal plasma taurine concentrations (greater than 60 nmol/ml). Taurine supplementation can be discontinued once echocardiographic values return to within normal limits, and the cat is eating a diet with adequate amounts of taurine.
- Taurine concentration in plasma and whole blood should be monitored periodically to be certain that the diet fed is maintaining concentrations within acceptable limits. If taurine concentrations are depleted again, then many cats will again develop myocardial failure.

Prognosis

- Because results of taurine analysis are not immediately known and a recent dietary change may normalize taurine values, all cats with myocardial failure should be supplemented with taurine and given an initially guarded-to-grave prognosis. In one large study, 30% of cats with myocardial

failure died within the first week after diagnosis. Hypothermia and thromboembolic disease were associated with a poor prognosis. Taurine supplementation did not provide benefit with regard to survival until 2 weeks after treatment is begun. Cats that survive 1 week and respond to treatment for CHF can be upgraded to a fair prognosis. Cats that survive 2 weeks and are shown to be taurine deficient can be upgraded to a good prognosis.
- Most taurine-responsive cats have complete reversal of echocardiographic and clinical evidence of myocardial failure after supplementation with taurine (see Figure 8-11). Occasionally cats may have residual mild myocardial failure (LV shortening fraction 25% to 30%); however, these cats are generally asymptomatic and rarely require any form of therapy other than maintaining normal plasma taurine concentrations.

Pathology

- The most predominant pathologic features are severe LV and LA enlargement. The LV walls may appear thin and the papillary muscles and trabeculations are less prominent than normal. The right ventricle and right atrium may also be enlarged. There are no specific histologic or electron microscopic lesions.
- In the past, many of these cases were classified as RCM or intermediate cardiomyopathy. The echocardiographic appearance in many cases suggests that the hemodynamics resemble those of RCM; however, few cases have documented characteristic histopathologic lesions. The term intermediate suggests a combination of or transition between states. There is no evidence that this represents a combination of or a transitional state between two forms of cardiomyopathy. In fact, as stated previously, there is no evidence that these cases represent a single disease entity or are proven to be a cardiomyopathy.
- The whole blood analysis is most important.

THYROTOXIC HEART DISEASE

Thyrotoxic heart disease is cardiac changes resulting from direct and indirect effects of elevations in circulating thyroid hormone (hyperthyroidism).

General Comments

- A frequently recognized secondary cardiomyopathy that may be confused with primary myocardial diseases in older cats

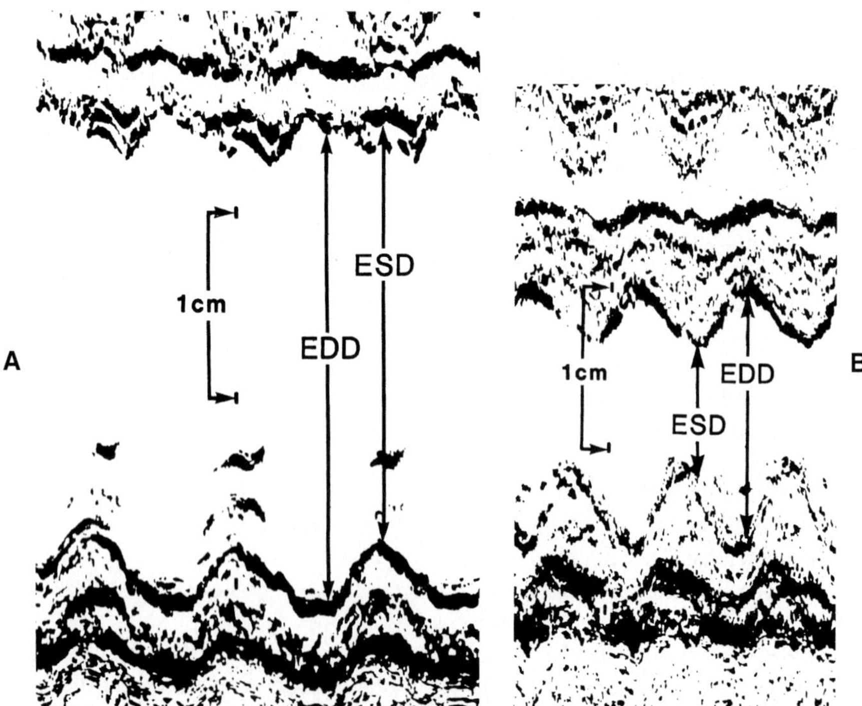

Figure 8-11. M-mode echocardiograms from a cat with myocardial failure associated with taurine deficiency before **(A)** and after **(B)** taurine supplementation and diet modification. Before therapy the left ventricle was markedly dilated, and the left ventricular shortening fraction was severely reduced. Those parameters both normalized after taurine supplementation. *EDD*, Left ventricular dimension at end-diastole; *ESD*, left ventricular dimension at end-systole.

- Thyrotoxic heart disease or hyperthyroidism does not cause HCM.
- The prevalence and severity of thyrotoxic heart disease has been decreasing in recent years, likely as a result of increased awareness and therefore early diagnosis and treatment of hyperthyroidism.

Pathophysiology

- The effects of thyroid hormone on the heart are believed to be both direct and indirect.
  - Direct actions
    - Increased protein synthesis (mitochondrial, ion pump, and contractile proteins)
    - Alteration of myosin subtype ("slow" to "fast" type myosin; V3 to > V1)
    - Less economical energy conversion from chemical (adenosine triphosphate) to mechanical (force) by the myocardium
    - Increased rate of calcium cycling by the sarcoplasmic reticulum
    - Up-regulation of cardiac beta receptors
    - Enhanced rate of spontaneous depolarization by sinoatrial node cells
    - Shortened action potential duration
  - Indirect actions
    - Enhanced metabolic demand by other tissues results in a "high-output state;" the heart must increase its throughput to meet the increased demands of the peripheral tissues that are similarly stimulated to a higher metabolic state by the excess circulating thyroid hormone.
    - Reduced systemic vascular resistance (not the same as hypotension) plays an important role in the overall cardiac status of patients with hyperthyroidism. Afterload is reduced while preload is increased in the presence of an increased intravascular volume.
    - In some, hypertension is a predominant finding and leads to:
      - Significant concentric hypertrophy of the left ventricle
      - Risk of retinal detachment or hemorrhage
- The sum of these effects when there is excess thyroid hormone (hyperthyroidism) is a heart that operates at a faster rate (tachycardia), is hypertrophied, can contract faster and more powerfully (enhanced contractility), and has a propensity to abnormal electrical depolarizations (arrhythmias).
- Although these might at first glance sound like beneficial changes (bigger, faster, stronger, more excitable), the thyrotoxic state greatly strains the energy economy of the heart and increases the overall work of the heart. Additionally, the thyrotoxic heart, although hyperkinetic when the patient is at rest, has less "reserve capacity" available for when increased cardiac work is necessary (e.g., exercise). This situation, placed on top of preexisting cardiac disease (e.g., HCM, RCM, or DCM, valvular disease) can lead to decompensation of a previously well-compensated cardiac disease.
- Reduced systemic vascular resistance in the presence of an increased intravascular volume (not documented in cats) associated with significant increases in cardiac output are what define the high-output state of the cardiovascular system in hyperthyroid cats. This high-output state can (especially in the presence of underlying primary cardiac pathology, such as valvular insufficiency) progress to result in clinically apparent signs of CHF in hyperthyroid cats.
- Despite the reduced systemic vascular resistance that is part of the high-output, hyperthyroid state, hypertension, rather than hypotension, is observed in many (87% of 39 cats in one study) hyperthyroid cats. Hypertension resolves in most treated cases once a euthyroid state is reached.

Signalment and Present Complaints

- Cats are generally older, with no gender or breed predispositions.
- Most cats present for routine examination or because of signs or symptoms of hyperthyroidism (e.g., polyphagia, polyuria/polydipsia, weight loss).
- Occasionally cats present with CHF or low-output heart failure.

Physical Examination

- Classic signs of hyperthyroidism, including evidence of weight loss, unkempt hair coat
- Systolic heart murmur or gallop rhythm may be present
- Sinus tachycardia is usually present
- A thyroid nodule may be palpable

Ancillary Tests

- Electrocardiography
  - Sinus tachycardia is commonly present
  - Tall R waves suggestive of LV hypertrophy or dilation
  - Variable arrhythmias, including atrial premature complexes and ventricular premature complexes

- Uncommonly, intraventricular conduction disturbances are seen
- Thoracic radiography: Common findings include
  - Generalized cardiomegaly with or without LA enlargement
  - When CHF is present, pulmonary edema and pleural effusion are equally likely to be present.
- Echocardiography
  - Reported echocardiographic changes in cats with hyperthyroidism include increased aortic root dimension, LA enlargement, increased end-diastolic or end-systolic LV dimensions, mild to moderate concentric hypertrophy of the LV free wall or septum, and an increased (or, rarely, decreased) LV shortening fraction.
  - In the author's experience the typical echocardiographic changes in cats with hyperthyroidism *without CHF* include hyperkinetic LV wall and septal motion with mild LV dilation (eccentric hypertrophy) and varying degrees of LA enlargement. In general the LV wall and septal thicknesses are not excessive in relation to the chamber dimensions and *do not* resemble the typical changes associated with HCM.
  - There are reports of cats with myocardial failure demonstrating marked increases in LV end-diastolic and end-systolic dimensions, moderate to severe LA enlargement, and a reduction in shortening fraction. The relationship of this presentation to a deficiency of the amino acid taurine is unknown, but may also represent late irreversible changes associated with hyperthyroidism.

Therapy

- For acute CHF, see the section on treatment of CHF in the Therapy section under General Information.
- Signs of CHF may be difficult to control prior to beginning to control the hyperthyroid state. Begin with pharmacologic manipulations; thyroidectomy or the physical isolation required after radioactive iodine therapy present a high risk to uncompensated animals. Once signs of CHF are well controlled and the hyperthyroid state is attenuated, more specific therapy may be pursued.
- In cats with asymptomatic thyrotoxicosis, therapy is generally aimed at controlling the hyperthyroid state (i.e., Tapazole, thyroidectomy, or radioactive iodine therapy).
- Beta-adrenergic blockade is a common recommendation in the literature. There is no contraindication to its use, but benefits have not been documented in most cases. The authors recommend beta-adrenergic blockade in the following situations:
  - To manage significant supraventricular or ventricular tachyarrhythmias
  - In hyperthyroid cats undergoing anesthetic procedures

KEY POINT

We have found beta blockade therapy beneficial in cats with hyperthyroidism that are unable to complete specific antithyroid therapy because of concurrent renal insufficiency. Beta blockers are also helpful in controlling cardiovascular signs of thyrotoxicosis pending a euthyroid state in cats started on methimazole (Tapazole).

Prognosis

- Asymptomatic cats can be managed very well without the use of specific cardiovascular therapy prior to appropriate therapy for the hyperthyroid state, and most evidence indicates that the cardiovascular changes are reversible.
- Most cats with CHF can be managed successfully if the hyperthyroid state is controlled.
- Most cats with severe systolic myocardial failure have a poor prognosis, as the changes appear to be irreversible unless influenced by taurine deficiency.

ACROMEGALIC HEART DISEASE

Acromegalic heart disease is cardiac changes resulting from direct and indirect effects of elevations in circulating growth hormone (hypersomatotropism).

General Comments and Historical Perspective

- A syndrome resembling acromegaly in humans has been reported in a group of middle-aged and older cats with growth hormone–secreting tumors of the pituitary gland.
- In 14 cases all affected cats had insulin-resistant diabetes mellitus and enlargement of the liver, heart, kidneys, or tongue. Various cardiovascular abnormalities were seen in most of the affected cats.
- An increase in serum growth hormone concentration in about 60% of the cats with HCM but without signs of acromegaly. Growth hormone is a known inducer of myocardial hypertrophy, and cats with acromegaly can have quite severe

concentric hypertrophy of the LV myocardium. Whether the increase in serum growth hormone concentration is the cause, is the result, or is unrelated to feline HCM is unknown.

Pathophysiology

- The pathogenesis of heart disease in cats with acromegaly is unclear. The importance of a direct trophic effect of excessive growth hormone on the myocardium as opposed to secondary effects resulting from volume expansion, hypertension, or other secondary effects requires further study.
- The increased plasma growth hormone concentration in some cats with HCM suggests a potentially important role for growth hormone in cats with hypertrophic heart disease.

Signalment and Presenting Complaints

- Cats with acromegaly generally do not present for signs referable to cardiovascular disease.
- Presenting complaints commonly include polyuria/polydipsia and weight loss referable to uncontrolled diabetes.
- Although no breed predilections have been identified, almost all of the reported cases have occurred in older neutered male cats.

Physical Examination

- Systolic murmurs were noted in 9 of the 14 cats described.
- Physical features of acromegaly include prognathia inferior, cranial and abdominal enlargement, organomegaly (especially kidneys and liver), increased body size, and weight gain.
- Signs of CHF may develop late in the course of the disease.

Ancillary Tests

- Electrocardiography: abnormalities were not detected in any of the 14 cats reported.
- Thoracic radiography: radiographic cardiomegaly was identified in 12 of 14 cats.
- Echocardiography: septal and LV wall concentric hypertrophy, resembling HCM, was identified in seven of eight cats examined.
- Other
  - The diagnosis of acromegaly is tentatively based on the presence of insulin-resistant diabetes mellitus or renal failure in a cat with clinical features of acromegaly.
  - Documentation of a pituitary mass on computed tomographic scan or magnetic resonance imaging provides further support.
  - A definitive diagnosis requires demonstration of increased baseline serum growth hormone concentration.

Therapy

- Generally, therapy is aimed at controlling the diabetic state and renal failure. If CHF is present, supportive care (diuretics and vasodilators) may also be beneficial.
- Successful therapy for feline acromegaly has not been reported. Potential therapeutic modalities include radiation therapy, medical therapy, and hypophysectomy.
- Supportive therapy for CHF should be employed in those cats with consistent clinical findings. (See the section on treatment of CHF in the Therapy section under General Information.) Of the six reported cases of CHF, four of these cats died, three of which had concurrent renal failure.

Prognosis

- The short-term prognosis is good. Pituitary tumors grow slowly, and neurologic signs are uncommon; the diabetes can be relatively well controlled with high doses of insulin.
- Mild to moderate CHF responds fairly well to symptomatic therapy.
- Most cats eventually died or were euthanized owing to refractory CHF or renal failure. Reported survival ranged from 4 to 24 months after diagnosis.

Pathology

- LV hypertrophy is the hallmark pathologic feature. Myocardial histologic lesions include myofiber hypertrophy, multifocal myocytolysis, interstitial fibrosis, and intramural arteriosclerosis.

NEOPLASTIC INFILTRATION OF THE HEART

General Comments and Historical Perspective

- Rare in cats
- Echocardiography is generally required for nonsurgical detection.

- Cardiac tumors reported in cats include:
  - Lymphoma
  - Chemodectoma
  - Hemangiosarcoma
  - Metastatic pulmonary carcinoma
  - Metastatic mammary gland carcinoma.
- Lymphoma is the most common tumor of the feline myocardium. Reported cardiac abnormalities in cats with lymphoma include complete heart block, pericardial effusion, and CHF.
- Echocardiographic findings in cats with diffuse neoplastic infiltration of the myocardium can mimic those of HCM.
- Regression of neoplastic infiltration was reported in one cat with lymphoma following treatment with combination chemotherapy.

Drugs, Toxins, and Physical Injury

- A large number of drugs and toxins are reported to cause myocardial injury in domestic animals, but very few are likely to be encountered in clinical small animal practice. Of these, doxorubicin has received the most attention in cats.
- Decreased fractional shortening and increased LV end-systolic dimensions were reported in four of six experimental cats given cumulative doses of doxorubicin of 170 to 240 mg/m^2. However, clinical signs of heart failure were not observed even after a cumulative dose of 300 mg/m^2, and no cat showed electrocardiographic abnormalities during the study. As in other species, pathologic studies revealed extensive areas of myocyte vacuolization and myocytolysis. Similar clinical observations have been reported in cats with malignancies treated with doxorubicin. None developed overt heart failure, and arrhythmias were only rarely observed.
- With the possible exception of heat stroke and hypothermia, physical causes of myocardial damage are infrequently recognized in cats. Traumatic myocarditis appears to be either uncommon or unrecognized in most cats that experience thoracic trauma.

INFECTIOUS MYOCARDITIS

- Infectious myocarditis is infrequently recognized in cats. Liu and associates described a syndrome of acute nonsuppurative myocarditis in 25 young cats (mean age 2.6 years). Most cats died unexpectedly, and necropsy revealed focal or diffuse infiltration of the endocardium and myocardium with mononuclear cells and a few neutrophils. A viral etiology was suspected but never identified.
- One report describes a transmissible myocarditis/diaphragmitis in cats. No organism has been isolated, but transmission between cats by injecting blood from infected cats into other cats does reliably reproduce the disease. All cats developed high fever (103.8° to 105.7° F), were lethargic, and were partially anorexic. Complete blood counts and chemistries were normal in all cats for 6 weeks except for an elevation of creatine phosphokinase in three of seven cats. The disease resolved on its own in these cats. Necropsy revealed pale 1 to 3 mm discrete foci surrounded by hemorrhage on ventricular myocardium and on the diaphragm. No clinical signs referable to the cardiovascular system were noticed.
- The relationship of endomyocarditis to the other cardiomyopathies of cats is unknown. Other reported causes of myocarditis in cats include toxoplasmosis and metastatic infection from sepsis or bacterial endocarditis.

SUMMARY

- HCM is very common and probably represents the largest percentage of cardiac diseases currently diagnosed in the cat.
- Presumed myocardial diseases that cannot be classified into one of the known primary disorders, but that also lack common features allowing classification as a single clinical entity, are increasing in frequency. Little is known about the etiology, pathophysiology, therapy, and prognosis associated with these UCMs.
- Of the secondary cardiomyopathies discussed, only nutritional (taurine-responsive) DCM and thyrotoxic heart disease are encountered with any frequency. Both of these disorders have been well classified, and both respond dramatically to appropriate specific therapy. The other secondary cardiomyopathies occur infrequently and are generally poorly understood. The general approach, diagnosis, and therapy for these disorders are similar to those for other feline cardiomyopathies.
- One must recognize that the associated clinical and diagnostic findings frequently overlap, often making a definitive diagnosis difficult. Echocardiography is the one diagnostic aid that reliably allows differentiation among the different cardiomyopathies encountered in cats; however, even with a thorough ultrasound examination, distinctions are still often unclear.

Frequently Asked Questions

There was a young male cat that was admitted for routine orchiectomy. His pre-operative complete blood count, chemistry screen and urinalysis were normal. His pre-operative thoracic radiographs also appeared normal. Physical examination was within normal limits, except the cat appeared small for his age.

The lightly sedated cat was subjected to mask induction with isoflurane because the attending veterinarian sometimes used this approach in quiet healthy cats. They were able to intubate, but not resuscitate this patient. Why did this cat die during this induction?

In this case, post-mortem confirmed cardiomyopathy—it was not a laryngospasm. Key points to consider:

1. HCM can be present, and the thoracic radiographs still be normal.
2. Many cats with cardiomyopathy are asymptomatic.
3. Sudden death may occur in otherwise healthy appearing cats.
4. As per the anesthesia chapter, caution is needed as follows, quoted, "Mask induction with isoflurane or sevoflurane is not recommended in cardiac patients. Most animals become very excited during mask induction, even with adequate preanesthetic medication, which could predispose to arrhythmias and increased myocardial work secondary to the stress response."

Cats are not good candidates for mask induction. Safe combination anesthetic regimens are available that make the technique of inhalant induction by mask unnecessary today. In the past, many of these anesthetic accidents were attributed to rare adverse primary anesthetic reactions if cause of death was not determined by testing.

What is the significance of SAM in a cat with cardiomyopathy? Key points to consider:

1. Key point is the pressure gradient across the region of dynamic subaortic stenosis produced by the SAM. The pressure gradient roughly correlates with the severity of the SAM although it can be quite labile, changing with the cat's level of excitement.
2. SAM is not present in all cats with HCM. The majority of cats with severe HCM have SAM.
3. SAM can develop in advance of chamber wall changes, so it may be an early finding in some cats.

A cat is diagnosed with DCM—and you have not seen a case since changes in food formulations 20 years ago? Key points to consider:

1. Taurine is not processed as efficiently in some dog breeds when compared with others—this may happen in certain lines/breeds of cats perhaps too? (conjecture—not yet confirmed in published studies)
2. It is known that the commercial processing of tinned cat foods results in the destruction of some of the taurine due to presumed damage from high temperature processing. The owner is using a high temperature pressure cooker to make her home-made diet (she is not simmering constituents as per nutritionist instructions) so perhaps heat is damaging the taurine in the home-made food. Commercial manufacturers put in higher levels of taurine into canned food recipes to allow for this intraprocessing destruction of taurine.
3. Though most DCM cases are taurine deficiency–associated, some DCMs are not clearly associated with low blood levels.
4. It is important to test taurine levels before any taurine supplementation is started.

In cats, what do the UCMs represent? Key points to consider:

1. Cats do not always fall into clear categories of heart disease.
2. Even with echocardiography the parameters may not clearly fit into one specific type, but rather share features of more than one type.
3. Most cases of cardiomyopathy in cats are idiopathic.
4. These UCMs only allow one to assume cardiac disease is present—no more.

SUGGESTED READINGS

Atkins CE: The role of noncardiac disease in the development and precipitation of heart failure, Vet Clin North Am Small Anim Pract 21:1035, 1991.

Fox PR: Feline myocardial disease. In Fox PR, ed: Canine and feline cardiology, New York, 1988, Churchill Livingstone.

Fox PR: Myocardial diseases. In Ettinger SJ, ed: Textbook of veterinary internal medicine, ed 2, Philadelphia, 1989, WB Saunders.

Harpster NK: Feline myocardial diseases. In Kirk RW, ed: Current veterinary therapy IX, Philadelphia, 1986, WB Saunders.

Jacobs G, Panciera DL: Cardiovascular complications of feline hyperthyroidism. In Kirk RW, Bonagura JD, eds: Kirk's current veterinary therapy XI, Philadelphia, 1992, WB Saunders.

Kittleson MD: Management of heart failure: concepts, therapeutic strategies, and drug pharmacology. In Fox PR, ed: Canine and feline cardiology, New York, 1988, Churchill Livingstone.

Kittleson MD, Kienle RD: Small animal cardiovascular medicine, St Louis, 1998, Mosby.

Liu SK, Tilley LP: Animal models of primary myocardial disease, Yale J Biol Med 53:191-211, 1980.

Liu SK, Maron FJ, Tilley LP: Feline hypertrophic cardiomyopathy, Am J Path 102:388-395, 1981.

Pion PD, Kittleson MD, Rogers QR: Cardiomyopathy in the cat and its relation to taurine deficiency. In Kirk RW, ed: Current veterinary therapy X, Philadelphia, 1989, WB Saunders.

Pion PD, Kittleson MD: Therapy for feline aortic thromboembolism. In Kirk RW, ed: Current veterinary therapy X, Philadelphia, 1989, WB Saunders.

CHAPTER 9

Cor Pulmonale and Pulmonary Thromboembolism

Lynelle R. Johnson

INTRODUCTION

Cor pulmonale is defined as right-heart failure caused by pulmonary or thoracic disease. It may be characterized by clinical signs of fluid accumulation or by radiographic or echocardiographic evidence of right ventricular overload. By definition, pulmonary hypertension (PH) must be present in cor pulmonale in order for the right heart to fail. Heartworm disease with pulmonary vascular obstruction is the most common cause of cor pulmonale in the canine population, although any pulmonary vascular obstruction has the potential to result in PH and cor pulmonale. Pulmonary arterial obstruction can result from lodging of clot material (pulmonary thromboembolism [PTE]) or from embolization of fat, septic material, neoplastic cells, or heartworms in the pulmonary arteries or capillary bed.

COR PULMONALE AND PULMONARY THROMBOEMBOLISM

Physiology

- Pulmonary circulatory pressures are maintained at a level much lower than systemic pressures in order to reduce the workload on the thin-walled right ventricle. Normal pressures in the dog and cat are reported as a systolic pulmonary artery pressure of 15 to 25 mm Hg, end-diastolic pulmonary artery pressure of 5 to 10 mm Hg, and a mean pulmonary artery pressure of 10 to 15 mm Hg. The pulmonary circulation maintains low right ventricular pressure in the face of increases in cardiac output through recruitment of closed capillaries and distension of existing capillaries.
- Distribution of pulmonary blood flow is altered by hypoxic pulmonary vasoconstriction and is also modulated by endothelial release of vasoconstrictors and vasodilators. Hypoxic pulmonary vasoconstriction is a protective mechanism that prevents de-oxygenated blood from entering the circulation by preferentially constricting vascular supply to poorly ventilated lung regions. Thus, local alveolar hypoxia results in local vascular constriction that preserves gas exchange. However, global hypoxia or diseases that disrupt the normal response to hypoxia can result in a deleterious rise in pulmonary artery pressure. Alterations in endothelium-derived mediators can also impact pulmonary artery pressures. The most potent vasoconstrictor is endothelin-1; thromboxane A2 and superoxide also mediate vasoconstriction. Vasodilators produced by the endothelium include nitric oxide and prostacyclin. Release and activity of these vasoreactive mediators can be altered in disease states, and imbalance among the various mediators can result in a rise in pulmonary artery pressure.
- PTE results in abnormal gas exchange, altered vascular control, changes in pulmonary mechanics, and loss of ventilatory control. Physical obstruction of large pulmonary arteries leads to increased vascular pressure and reactive pulmonary vasoconstriction from release of clot associated factors

such as thromboxane that increase vascular resistance. Secondary alterations in pulmonary physiology worsen and perpetuate derangements in gas exchange. Release of humoral mediators such as serotonin from platelets results in bronchoconstriction and increased airway resistance. Surfactant function is altered leading to loss of elastic recoil and atelectasis, decreased pulmonary compliance, and increased right-to-left shunting. Work of breathing increases because of augmented alveolar dead space from nonperfused lung regions.

Etiology

- Cor pulmonale can result from disorders that impact the pulmonary vasculature, such as obstructive or obliterative diseases of the pulmonary circulation, or sustained hypoxic vasoconstriction associated with chronic parenchymal or tracheobronchial disease. Rarely, an increase in pulmonary blood flow will result in PH. Not all animals with associated disorders will develop PH and cor pulmonale, and it is likely that genetic or other influences will determine the vascular response. PH and cor pulmonale appear to be encountered more commonly in dogs than in cats. Primary PH is relatively uncommon; however, various pulmonary conditions can lead to secondary PH in the dog or cat, including chronic tracheobronchial disorders, pneumonia, or interstitial lung disease (Box 9-1). A minority of these animals will develop overt clinical signs of right-heart failure.
- PTE is a secondary condition that occurs in association with diseases that cause blood stasis, alter endothelial integrity, or increase coagulability. PTE has been linked most commonly with immune-mediated hemolytic anemia, neoplasia, sepsis, protein losing nephropathy, cardiac disease, and hyperadrenocorticism (Box 9-2). Clinically silent pulmonary embolism occurs in a majority of dogs (82%) undergoing total hip replacement surgery. Small pulmonary thromboemboli are rapidly lysed and removed by the local fibrinolytic system; however, occlusion of larger pulmonary arteries or massive showering of emboli to a large circulatory volume can lead to acute right ventricular overload.

Box 9-1 Causes of Cor Pulmonale

Pulmonary vascular disease
Heartworm disease
Chronic pulmonary thromboembolism
Chronic pulmonary disease
Tracheobronchial disease or collapse
Pulmonary fibrosis/interstitial pneumonia
Pneumonia
Primary pulmonary hypertension

Box 9-2 Predisposing Conditions for Pulmonary Thromboembolism

Immune mediated hemolytic anemia
Neoplasia
Sepsis
Protein-losing nephropathy/enteropathy
Cardiac disease
Hyperadrenocorticism
Central catheter use
Hemodialysis
Total parenteral nutrition
Hip replacement surgery
Trauma

Clinical Presentation

History and Clinical Signs

- Dogs or cats with PH and cor pulmonale can be of any age, depending on the underlying etiology of elevated pulmonary artery pressures. Generally there is a history of signs referable to the pulmonary system or to congestive failure. Animals can display any combination of signs including lethargy, weakness, cough, respiratory distress, tachypnea, abdominal distention, and syncope. Historical features and clinical signs are not specific for PH or cor pulmonale but instead reflect the underlying cardiopulmonary disease.
- PTE is generally a disorder of older animals, and history and clinical signs reflect the underlying disease process. Difficulty in clinical recognition of this disorder is high, and animals with PTE are often presented for signs of weight loss, lethargy, and anorexia rather than for respiratory signs, although tachypnea is often present on admission. Secondary PTE should be suspected in an animal with a predisposing condition that develops an acute onset of tachypnea, cyanosis, and/or hypoxemia that is refractory to oxygen therapy.

KEY POINT

PTE occurs secondary to a variety of underlying conditions. Affected animals may present for signs reflecting the primary condition or for refractory respiratory distress.

Physical Examination

- Animals with cor pulmonale will generally display tachypnea or respiratory distress due to fluid accumulation (ascites or pleural effusion) or because of underlying pulmonary disease. A systolic heart murmur due to mitral or tricuspid regurgitation is found in the majority of dogs with PH. Animals that develop clinical signs of overt right-heart failure will display jugular venous distention, ascites, or subcutaneous edema.
- Dogs and cats with PTE have tachypnea and hyperpnea that is not alleviated by oxygen administration. Cough is relatively uncommon. Harsh lung sounds or loud bronchovesicular sounds can be detected; however, crackles or wheezes are less common. Physical examination abnormalities will reflect the underlying disease, such as pale mucous membranes in the case of immune mediated hemolytic anemia or a pot-bellied appearance due to Cushing's disease.

Diagnostic Testing

Laboratory Testing

- Basic laboratory tests generally reflect the underlying disease and do not add to the diagnosis of PH, cor pulmonale, or PTE. The diagnosis of PTE is particularly problematic. Testing for plasma D-dimer, a breakdown product resulting from the action of plasmin on cross-linked fibrin, has been shown in human medicine to have high sensitivity but low specificity in the diagnosis of PTE. In veterinary medicine, several diseases can result in a positive D-dimer test, although the magnitude of the elevation may enhance the suspicion of pulmonary embolization. It is unclear whether a negative test excludes the possibility of PTE.
- Pulse oximetry and arterial blood gas analysis are useful for detecting abnormal gas exchange. Hemoglobin saturation (S_pO_2) is related to arterial oxygen partial pressure by a sigmoidal relationship, with values above 95% indicating normoxemia. Below 95%, values for S_pO_2 lie on the exponential part of the curve, and small changes in S_pO_2 reflect very large changes in arterial oxygen. Thus, pulse oximetry provides only a crude estimate of lung function. Arterial blood gas analysis provides more precise assessment of oxygenation and can be used to follow response to therapy. Arterial blood gas analysis often reveals hypoxemia, hypocapnia, and increased alveolar-to-arterial gradient in dogs with PTE; however, normal arterial oxygenation does not exclude the diagnosis of PTE. Some but not all animals with PTE will respond to supplemental oxygen administration with normalization of arterial oxygen. Animals with additional cardiac or pulmonary pathology that increases shunt fraction will not necessarily have a complete response to exogenous oxygen supplementation.

Radiographs

- Radiographic evidence of right-heart enlargement in an animal with lung or pulmonary vascular disease is supportive of cor pulmonale. (Figure 9-1) Retrospective review of radiographs in animals with PTE may allow the detection of regional oligemia, lack of normal vascular tapering, or enlarged central pulmonary arteries; however, in the clinical setting, radiographic changes appear less obvious, because PTE is often not suspected in the large proportion of dogs that die with PTE.
- Thoracic radiographic abnormalities are common in PTE but are rarely specific. Pulmonary infiltrates may be interstitial, alveolar, or lobar in dogs and cats. Alveolar infiltrates may represent hemorrhage, edema, or infarction. Cardiomegaly and mild to moderate pleural effusion are common in dogs and cats. Importantly, normal chest radiographs are reported in 7% to 27% of dogs and cats with necropsy confirmed PTE, and PTE should be a top differential diagnosis in an animal with marked respiratory distress and normal thoracic radiographs.

KEY POINT

Normal chest radiographs in a tachypneic animal that fails to respond to oxygen administration should be considered suggestive of pulmonary embolism.

Electrocardiography

- Reported abnormalities with right ventricular enlargement due to PH or PTE include deep S waves in leads II and aVF and a right axis deviation. Right atrial enlargement is supported by tall or peaked P waves; however, electrocardiographic evaluation of right heart enlargement is insensitive, and abnormalities have been reported in < 15% of dogs with PH. The electrocardiogram should be closely examined for rhythm disturbances, which may be found in up to 25% of dogs with PH.

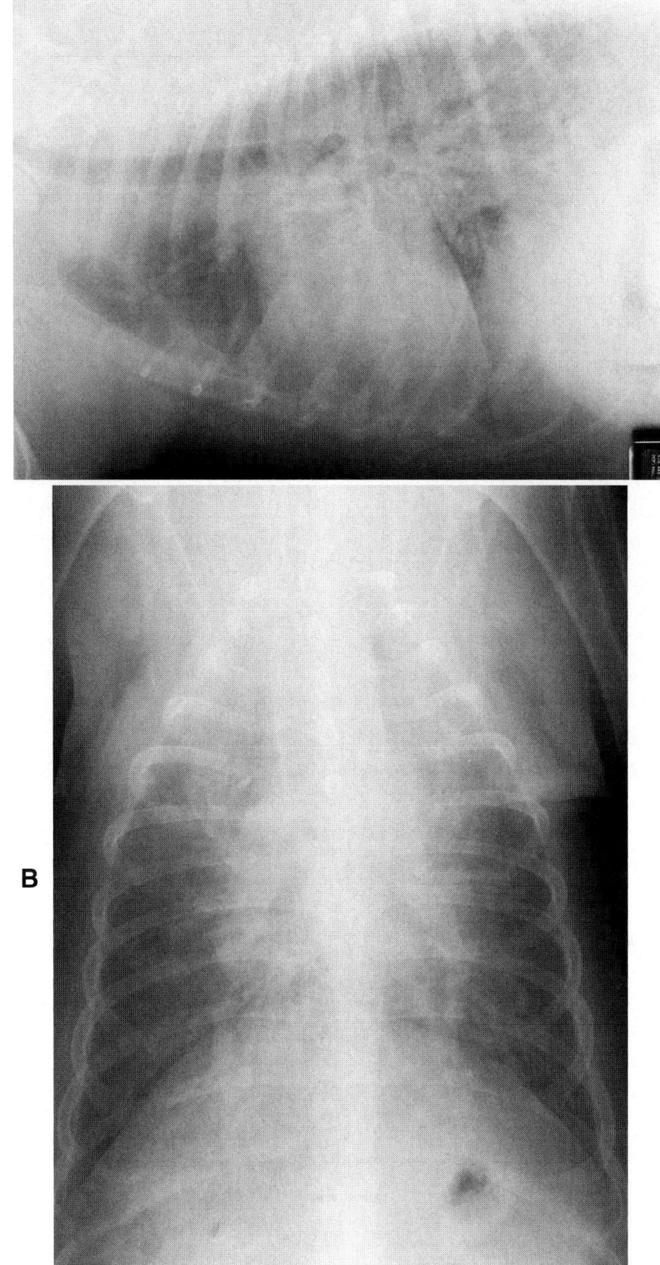

Figure 9-1. There is generalized enlargement of cardiac silhouette on the right lateral **(A)** and dorsoventral **(B)** views. Pulmonary arteries are enlarged and appear to taper slowly. Numerous pleural fissure lines are identified, and there is a diffuse heavy interstitial and peribronchial pattern identified within the lung.

Echocardiography

- Two-dimensional echocardiography can provide subjective evidence of PH leading to cor pulmonale (when pulmonic stenosis has been ruled out). Supportive evidence of right ventricular overload includes right ventricular concentric hypertrophy and dilation, dilation of the main pulmonary artery, systolic flattening of the interventricular septum, and paradoxical septal motion.

Doppler echocardiography can be used to estimate pulmonary artery pressure when tricuspid regurgitation or pulmonic insufficiency is present. (Figure 9-2) Using the modified Bernoulli equation (Pressure gradient = $4 \times \text{velocity}^2$), spectral Doppler allows reasonably accurate estimation of right ventricular systolic pressure via measurement of tricuspid regurgitation velocity, and estimation of pulmonary artery diastolic

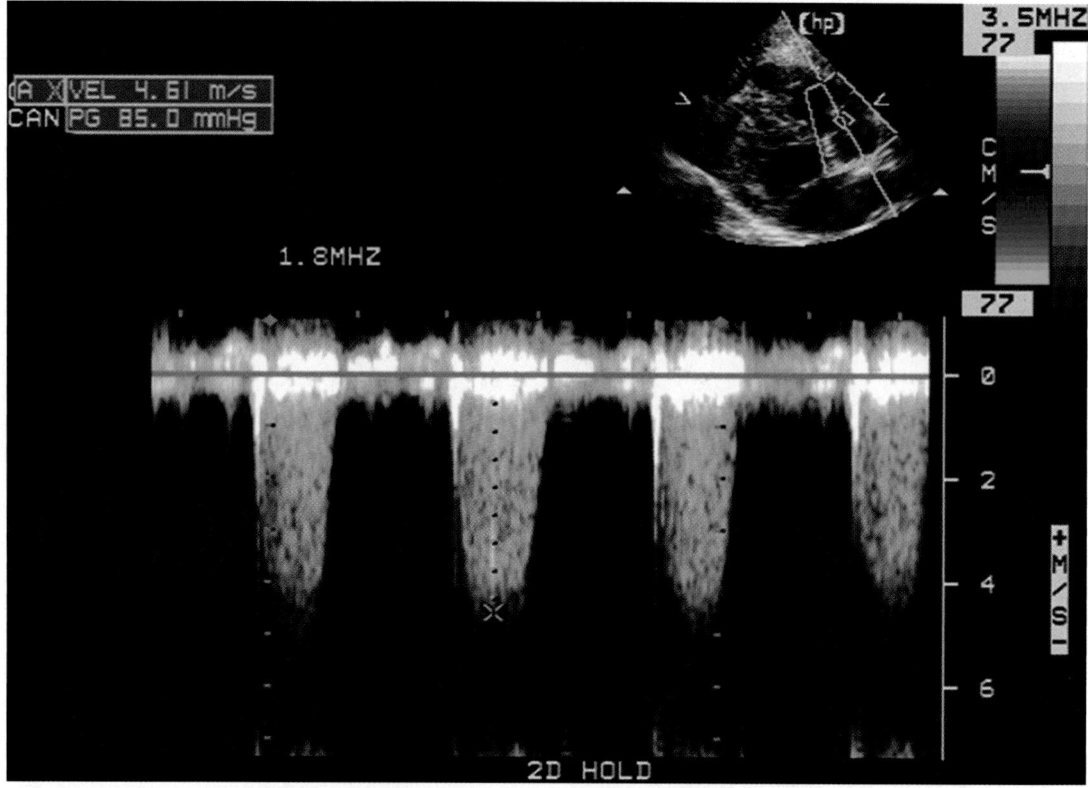

Figure 9-2. Tricuspid regurgitant jet in a dog with pulmonary hypertension. Based on the modified Bernoulli equation, the right ventricular-to-right atrial pressure gradient is 85 mm Hg. (Courtesy Dr. Fiona Campbell, University of California, Davis)

pressure via measurement of pulmonic insufficiency velocity. PH is documented by a tricuspid regurgitant jet > 2.8 m/sec or a pulmonic insufficiency jet > 2.2 m/sec.

- Echocardiographic features consistent with pulmonary embolization overlap with those found in PH. In addition, a thrombus can occasionally be visualized within the heart or great vessels. Therefore, animals with predisposing conditions that develop an acute onset of respiratory distress could benefit from echocardiographic assessment for right ventricular dilatation, pulmonary artery enlargement, or septal flattening that might suggest pulmonary embolization.

KEY POINT

Echocardiography should be considered in dogs suspected of PTE.

Catheterization and Advanced Imaging

- Direct measurement of pulmonary artery pressure through right heart catheterization is the gold standard for diagnosing PH. Cardiac catheterization also allows performance of acute pharmacologic testing of vasodilators to identify reversible vasoconstriction. Lowering of the pressure gradient in response to intervention would suggest a potential response to medical therapy. Unfortunately, sedation or general anesthesia is required for catheterization, and animals with PH are at increased risk for anesthetic complications. Therefore, this procedure is rarely performed in the clinical situation.
- Pulmonary angiography has been considered the gold standard for diagnosis of PTE in humans; although contrast helical computed tomography is being used increasingly more often. Neither imaging modality is used commonly in veterinary medicine because anesthesia is required, and patients with severe PH or PTE are high-risk anesthetic candidates. Definitive angiographic diagnosis of PTE depends on visualization of an intraluminal filling defect in a pulmonary artery or loss of visualization of an artery.
- Ventilation:perfusion scanning uses technetium-99m–labeled macroaggregated albumin as a vascular marker and technetium-99m–labeled diethylenetriaminepentacetic acid as a ventilatory marker to define segmental or lobar perfusion defects in areas of normal ventilation. Ventilation

scans are rarely performed on nonanesthetized animals; however, perfusion scanning alone can be completed without anesthesia and can assist in documentation of perfusion deficits. This is a safe, noninvasive technique for evaluation of PTE, although it is somewhat nonspecific because perfusion deficits can reflect true regions of thrombosis or simply a lung region experiencing hypoxic pulmonary vasoconstriction.

Therapy

- Currently, little is known about the optimal therapy for either PH or PTE. In animals with cor pulmonale, cautious diuretic therapy is warranted to reduce fluid accumulation, and judicious use of thoracocentesis or abdominocentesis can be used to improve respiration. Excessive removal of fluid is to be avoided since animals may develop volume contraction or systemic hypotension.
- Therapy of PH has not been well defined in veterinary medicine. Systemic vasodilators are not generally effective in lowering pulmonary artery pressures and can cause deleterious side effects because of excessive hypotension. Standard treatment of the underlying cardiopulmonary condition should be employed and may lessen PH. Anticoagulant therapy is recommended in human patients with PH associated with PTE or to limit in situ thrombosis that can result in progressive vascular obstruction. Low molecular weight heparin therapy is often used because of reduced risk of bleeding due to its favorable factor X: factor II activity. However specific information on pharmacokinetics and pharmacodynamics of the available products is currently lacking in veterinary medicine. Ultra-low-dose **aspirin** (< 1 mg/kg every 24 [dog] to 72 [cat] hours) can be used also in an attempt to inhibit platelet aggregation. Newer antiplatelet drugs are currently under investigation.
- Insight into various therapies for PH has been gained by reviewing treatment of primary PH in humans, which is partially mediated by alterations in endothelium-derived vasodilators and constrictors and by vascular proliferation. Drugs that have been employed include intravenous or inhaled prostacyclin (a breakdown product of arachidonic acid metabolism) and inhaled nitric oxide. These vasodilators are selective for the pulmonary circulation and have more pronounced impact on pulmonary pressures than systemic pressures. However, these drugs require sophisticated or complicated delivery and result in only minimal reductions in pulmonary artery pressures. Although these reductions are statistically significant and provide some clinical benefit in human patients, it is unclear whether these small changes in pulmonary arterial pressures would be beneficial in veterinary patients.
- An orally available nitric oxide donor **sildenafil** (Viagra), which causes accumulation of cyclic guanosine monophosphate in vascular smooth muscle and resultant vasodilation, has some efficacy in reducing pulmonary artery pressures in both humans and experimental animals. Occasional reports in dogs suggest that it might also be beneficial in some veterinary patients. Supplementation with arginine has been investigated for use in human medicine since arginine is converted into nitric oxide through combination with molecular oxygen. A nonselective endothelin antagonist **(Bosentan)** has been shown to be efficacious in lowering pulmonary artery pressures in patients with PH, although again, the reduction in pressure was quite modest. Endothelin antagonists have not been evaluated in veterinary patients. Anticoagulants may be beneficial by reducing in situ thrombosis, progressive vascular occlusion, and continued proliferative vascular disease.

Frequently Asked Questions

What clinical findings would support the diagnosis of cor pulmonale and how could this be confirmed?
Animals with clinical signs relative to cor pulmonale generally display respiratory abnormalities (tachypnea, hyperpnea, and/or cough) and may also exhibit signs of right-heart failure (ascites, jugular venous distention, and/or subcutaneous edema). Radiographically, cor pulmonale is evident as right-sided heart enlargement. Right atrial enlargement and dilation of the caudal vena cava support the diagnosis. Two-dimensional echocardiography reveals eccentric dilation of the right ventricle. With chronic PH or PH in a young animal, right ventricular hypertrophy can be found. In the presence of tricuspid regurgitation or pulmonic insufficiency, Doppler echocardiography can confirm PH by detection of a velocity jet greater than 2.8 or 2.2 m/sec, respectively.

What tests confirm the diagnosis of PTE and provide support for institution of anticoagulant therapy?
Unfortunately, ante-mortem diagnosis of PTE remains challenging, and definitive diagnosis is often not achieved in the clinical setting. Suspicion for PTE should be present in an animal with a recognized predisposing condition (see Box 9-2) that develops an acute onset of respiratory distress. Normal chest radiographs do not preclude the diagnosis. Supportive evidence of PTE would include a positive D-dimer test, echocardiographic evidence of right ventricular overload, and perfusion deficits on pulmonary scintigraphy in an animal with refractory respiratory distress. Anticoagulant therapy with low molecular weight heparin would often be instituted in a patient with these findings. Thrombolytic therapy is rarely employed because of the risk of generating a systemic fibrinolytic state or creating ischemia-reperfusion injury. Because of the difficulty in establishing a diagnosis of PTE and the morbidity and mortality associated with this secondary complication, prophylactic anticoagulant therapy should be considered in animals with recognized predisposing conditions.

What type of treatment can be considered for PH?
Aggressive management of underlying cardiopulmonary conditions should be instituted. Animals with chronic bronchitis or small airway collapse often require steroids (oral or inhaled) and extended-release theophylline (10 mg/kg PO every 12 hours [dog] or 15 to 19 mg/kg PO in the evening [cat]). Interstitial lung diseases are less likely to respond to medical therapy. In either group of animals with respiratory dysfunction, supplemental oxygen therapy either at home or in the hospital setting can improve clinical presentation. Use of sildenafil (0.5 to 2.0 mg/kg every 8 to 12 hours) can be considered for animals with severe PH. Blood pressure and echocardiographic monitoring for side effects and efficacy are recommended.

SUGGESTED READINGS

Bach JF, Rozanski EA, MacGregor J, et al: Retrospective evaluation of sildenafil citrate as a therapy for pulmonary hypertension in dogs, J Vet Intern Med 20(5):1132-1135, 2006.

Berger M, Haimowitz A, Van Tosh A, et al: Quantitative assessment of pulmonary hypertension in patients with tricuspid regurgitation using continuous wave Doppler ultrasound, J Am Coll Cardiol 6:359, 1985.

Fluckiger MA, Gomez JA: Radiographic findings in dogs with spontaneous pulmonary thrombosis or embolism, Vet Rad 23:124, 1984.

Glaus TM, et al: Clinical and pathological characterisation of primary pulmonary hypertension in a dog, Vet Rec 154:786, 2004.

Johnson L, Boon J, Orton EC: Clinical characteristics of 53 dogs with Doppler derived evidence of pulmonary hypertension: 1992-1996, J Vet Intern Med 13:440, 1999.

Johnson LR, Lappin MR, Baker DC: Pulmonary thromboembolism in 29 dogs: 1985-1995, Vet Intern Med 13:338, 1999.

Koblik PD, Hornoff W, Harnagel SH, et al: A comparison of pulmonary angiography, digital subtraction angiography, and ^{99m}Tc-DTPA/MAA ventilation-perfusion scintigraphy for detection of experimental pulmonary emboli in the dog, Vet Radiol Ultrasound 30:159, 1989.

La Rue MG, Murtaugh RJ: Pulmonary thromboembolism in dogs: 47 cases (1986-1987), J Am Vet Med Assoc 197:1369, 1990.

Liska WD, Poteet BA: Pulmonary embolism associated with canine total hip replacement, Vet Surg 32:178, 2003.

Michelakis ED, et al: Long-term treatment with oral sildenafil is safe and improves functional capacity and hemodynamics in patients with pulmonary arterial hypertension, Circulation 108(17):2066, 2003.

Nelson OL, Andreason C: The utility of plasma D-dimer to identify thromboembolic disease in the dog, J Vet Int Med 17:830, 2003.

Norris CR, Griffey SM, Samii VF: Pulmonary thromboembolism in cats: 29 cases (1987-1997), J Am Vet Med Assoc 215:1650, 1999.

Pyle RL, Abbott J, MacLean H: Pulmonary hypertension and cardiovascular sequelae in 54 dogs, Intern J Appl Res Vet Med 2:99, 2004.

Schermerhorn T, Pembleton-Corbett JR, Kornreich B: Pulmonary thromboembolism in cats, J Vet Int Med 18:533, 2004.

Schober K, Baade H, Ludewig E, et al: Cor pulmonale in terrier breed dogs with chronic-progressive, idiopathic pulmonary fibrosis: 19 cases (1996-2001), Tierarztliche Praxis Ausgabe K, Kleintiere/Heimtiere 30:180, 2002.

Thomas D, Steiz M, Rtanabe G, et al: Mechanism of bronchoconstriction produced by thromboemboil in dogs, Am J Phys 206:1207, 1964.

Uehara Y: An attempt to estimate the pulmonary artery pressure in dogs by means of pulsed Doppler echocardiography, J Vet Med Sci 55:307, 1993.

CHAPTER 10

Heartworm Disease

Clay A. Calvert and Justin David Thomason

INTRODUCTION

Heartworm disease is a common problem in tropical and subtropical regions. Heartworm infection has spread throughout most areas of the United States, but the prevalence is still low at high elevations and in most northern states. Endemic foci frequently occur in regions with otherwise low prevalence and it is difficult to eliminate heartworms from a region once they have been established. Wild animal reservoirs include wolves, coyotes, foxes, California gray seals, sea lions, raccoons, and ferrets.

HEARTWORM DISEASE

Etiology and Life Cycle

Heartworm infection is produced by the parasite *Dirofilaria immitis* and is transmitted to dogs mostly by 10 to 15 species of mosquitoes. Mosquitoes can transmit infective larvae (L_3) 2 to 3 weeks after ingesting a blood meal. Infection rates vary among cats in endemic regions but are usually 10% to 20% of that of dogs within the same enzootic region. Being male, a large breed, and outdoors increases the risk of infection in dogs.

Canine Infection Life Cycle

- Female mosquitoes are the intermediate hosts and acquire the first-stage larvae (microfilaria) by feeding on infected dogs. Two molts then occur to produce the infective L_3 stage.
- Larvae development to the third stage usually requires 1 to 2.5 weeks, depending on the ambient temperatures. Mosquitoes can survive the development of only low numbers (< 10) of larvae. Larvae development within the mosquito requires an average daily temperature of at least 57° Fahrenheit. The cooler the temperature, the longer the time required for L_3 to develop and vice versa. Transmission is unlikely to occur during the cold months of the year, even in most southern regions of the United States. This is because when the temperatures are moderately low, the time required for development from L_1 to L_3 may exceed the life-span (30 days) of the mosquito. Third-stage larvae (L_3) infect the dog via the bite wound created during feeding.
- Larvae migrate through the subcutaneous tissues and vascular adventitial tissues for about 100 days. During this time, two molts occur. Young adults (L_5 larvae) enter the vascular system at 3 to 3.5 months post-infection and are in the small pulmonary arteries after 5 to 6 months.
- In the dog, adult worms and microfilaria are thought to have a natural life-span of 3 to 5 years and 1 to 2 years, respectively.

KEY POINT

Adult worms are present in the pulmonary arteries approximately 6 months after transmission from the mosquito.

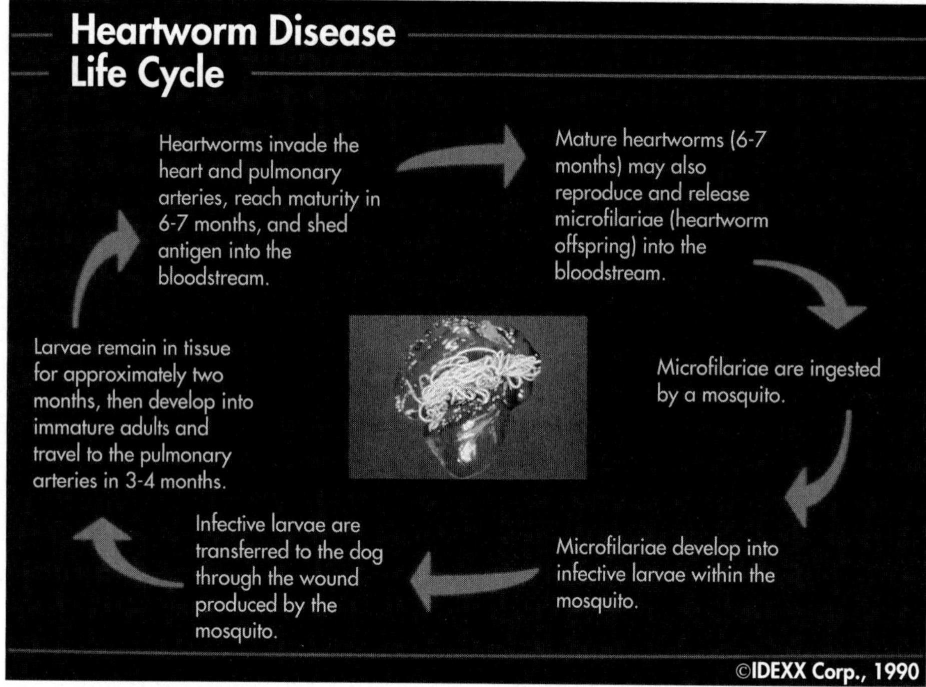

Figure 10-1. Life cycle of *Dirofilaria immitis*. (Courtesy Idexx Corp., Westbrook, Maine.)

- See Figure 10-1.
- Microfilaria can appear after 6 months, increase in concentration for 6 months, plateau for several months, and then decrease in concentration as long as super-infection does not occur.
- Microfilaria-specific antibody-mediated, occult infections occur in the presence of persistent host antibody excess. Antibody-dependent leukocyte adhesions entrap microfilaria in the pulmonary microcirculation. Between 10% and 67% of all heartworm infections are occult, and some of these are due to immune-mediated host reaction. In most endemic regions, the incidence of occult infections is approximately 20% to 25% of all infections. Dogs administered macrolide prophylaxis that are, or become, infected will not have microfilaremia.
- Microfilaria-leukocyte (neutrophils and eosinophils) complexes are engulfed by phagocytic cells of the mononuclear phagocyte system, resulting in granulomatous inflammation.
- Predominately eosinophilic inflammation, with minimal granulomatous inflammation, produces allergic pneumonitis.
- Progressive granulomatous inflammation occasionally occurs and leads to lethal pulmonary eosinophilic granulomatosis.

Feline Infection Life Cycle

- Some mosquito species do not like to feed on cats and cats are relatively resistant to infection, requiring a greater L_3 inoculation. Therefore, the infection rate in unprotected cats is at least 80% lower than that of unprotected dogs. The numbers of infective larvae that mature are fewer than in dogs, and the pre-patent period is usually 1 to 2 months longer. The natural survival time of adult worms in the cat is thought to be no more than 2 years.

Prevalence

Heartworm infection is most common in tropical and subtropical climates. Infection is inevitable in chronically unprotected dogs along the southern Atlantic and Gulf coasts and other highly endemic regions. The prevalence in cats varies by geographic region. It is much lower than dogs in some areas, similar to dogs in some areas, and the incidence is probably underestimated. Dogs housed outdoors have a four- to five-fold increased risk compared to those housed indoors. Infection is most common in dogs 4 to 7 years of age, but in highly endemic regions infection is common in younger dogs.

Pathogenesis

Disease onset and severity largely reflect the number of adult heartworms. In infected cats, the average number of adult worms is 3 to 6, depending on the concentration of infected mosquitoes and the ambient temperature in any given region.

Worm Location

- Until the adult worm burden exceeds 50 in a 25 kg dog, nearly all worms are located in the pulmonary arteries. Worm burdens of approximately 75 are associated with worms located in the right atrium. Caval syndrome typically is associated with worm burdens of 100 or greater.

Response to Live Worms in Dogs

- Pulmonary pathology is produced beginning with the young adults. Even if infection is identified 7 months post-infection, the L_5 have already been in the pulmonary arteries for a few months and some pathology has occurred. Pulmonary arterial endothelial damage and subsequent myointimal proliferation most severely affects the caudal and intermediate lung lobes, which are those receiving the highest blood flow.
- Pulmonary lobar arterial enlargement, tortuosity, and obstruction of smaller branches begin within a few weeks of worm arrival. Intrapulmonary blood flow is obstructed as the disease progresses, and blood is diverted to less severely affected lobes. Small downstream arterioles become damaged and leak plasma and inflammatory cells into the surrounding lung parenchyma. This causes interstitial and alveolar lung infiltrates and granulomatous inflammation.
- Pulmonary arterial obstruction and lung inflammation cause fever, coughing, dyspnea, hemoptysis, leukocytosis, and thrombocytopenia. Pathology is more severe and accelerated in active dogs, relative to inactive dogs, for any given worm burden. Small dogs do not tolerate heartworm infection as well as large dogs.

Response to Live Worms in Cats

- The response in cats and ferrets is similar to that of dogs but there is more pulmonary arterial muscular hypertrophy and the barrier to oxygen diffusion is more severe than in the dog. Mortality in cats and ferrets is higher than in dogs.

Response to Dead Worms

- The most severe disease is seen in response to dead worm fragments that are swept into small arterioles. Pulmonary vascular compliance and blood flow become impaired to varying degrees and severe arterial disease results in pulmonary hypertension, increased right ventricular afterload, and eventually right-sided congestive heart failure (CHF). Parenchymal lung disease (infarction and consolidation) develops secondary to pulmonary arterial thromboembolism and increased vascular permeability.

History

Dogs

- The history in dogs with heartworm infection varies considerably. Many infections are discovered in asymptomatic dogs by immunodiagnostic screening. Some dogs are totally without signs; others have unexplained tachypnea, exercise intolerance, or cough. Signs consistent with pulmonary hypertension, with or without overt right-sided CHF, are associated with severe heartworm disease.

Cats

- The history in cats also varies considerably. Lethargy and decreased appetite may be reported by the owners. Coughing, emesis, and sudden or episodic dyspnea are typical signs in cats. However, sudden death may be the first sign of infection. CHF is uncommon.

Clinical Signs

The clinical signs associated with heartworm infection reflect the adult worm burden, duration of infection, and host-parasite interaction. Respiratory signs are most prominent.

Dogs

- Exercise intolerance, coughing, dyspnea, and respiratory crackles occur in dogs with moderate and advanced heartworm disease. Hemoptysis occurs with severe disease and is caused by pulmonary thromboembolism. It can be seen before, but occurs more often after adulticide treatment. Acute dyspnea and increased pulmonary radiographic infiltrates may develop secondary to spontaneous worm death. Syncope is associated with severe pulmonary arterial disease and pulmonary hypertension. Signs of elevated central venous pressure indicate severe pulmonary hypertension with incipient or overt right-sided CHF. Physical findings include prominent jugular pulse, distended jugular veins, hepatomegaly, and ascites.
- Hemoglobinuria commonly occurs in association with caval syndrome (i.e., acute hemolytic

crisis caused by obstruction of the vena cava with adult worms) and occasionally when severe pulmonary arterial disease results in hemolysis due to fibrin-thrombus related RBC trauma. Thrombocytopenia is usually a consequence of these complications.
- Nephrotic syndrome occasionally occurs as the result of severe glomerular disease (amyloidosis or immune complex glomerulonephritis). Manifestations include proteinuria, hypoalbuminemia, hypercholesterolemia, ascites and occasionally peripheral edema and azotemia.

Cats

- Clinical signs in cats are different than in dogs. The common signs are vomiting, collapse or syncope, asthma-like syndrome, coughing, sudden death, and occasionally central nervous system signs. Signs occur most often early in the infection and again when young adult worms arrive in the pulmonary arteries. Severe pulmonary complications and death are most likely to occur whenever one or more adult worm dies, either spontaneously or as a result of Immiticide administration.
- Asthmatic signs are a common manifestation and often occur about 3 to 4 months post-infection. A strong antibody response at this time may destroy the developing larvae. If not, then a period of quiescence occurs only to have asthma-like signs recur in some cats 7 to 8 months post-infection.
- Vomiting is a common, sporadic sign. It often is not associated with eating, may include food, but mucus and bile are often the major components. Vomiting and coughing in a cat should increase the index of suspicion.
- Sudden death related to spontaneous worm death and thromboembolism is more common in cats than in dogs.
- Neurologic signs, usually seizures, occur occasionally when aberrant worm migration to the brain occurs.
- See Box 10-1.

Box 10-1 Clinical Signs Associated with Feline Heartworm Disease

Acute Signs	Chronic Signs
Sudden death*	PIE† syndrome
Respiratory	Coughing
Pulmonary embolism	Dyspnea
Collapse; shock	Cardiopulmonary
Hemoptysis	Lethargy
Dyspnea; cough	Weakness
Pneumonitis	Right-sided CHF‡
Dyspnea; cough	Anorexia
Neurologic	Gastrointestinal
Blindness	Vomiting
Seizures	
Ataxia	
Coma	
Circling	
Syncope	
Gastrointestinal	
Vomiting	

*From severe pulmonary thromboembolism or heartworm occlusion of main pulmonary artery.
†Pulmonary infiltrates of eosinophilia.
‡Congestive heart failure.
Modified from Calvert C. Feline heartworm disease. In Fox PR, ed: Canine and feline cardiology, New York, 1988, Churchill Livingstone.

KEY POINT

The combination of vomiting, eosinophilia, and hyperglobulinemia warrant a high index of suspicion of heartworm infection in cats.

Diagnosis

The diagnosis of heartworm infection in dogs is based on immunodiagnostic antigen testing. Microfilaria in the peripheral blood can be detected by a direct smear or a concentration test (modified Knott test or millipore filter test) in dogs with or without clinical or radiographic findings consistent with the disease. Testing puppies younger than 6 months of age is not indicated.

Affected cats usually lack circulating microfilaria, may have suggestive radiographic abnormalities, and echocardiography is very useful. A positive enzyme-linked immunosorbent assay (ELISA) test for heartworm antigen, antibody or both may be present.

Laboratory Studies

- The minimum data base varies depending on the patient's age, clinical signs, and preference of individual clinicians. The minimum pretreatment database for all dogs suspected of having heartworm infection includes packed cell volume, blood urea nitrogen, urine specific gravity, urine protein determination, and heartworm antigen test. Thoracic radiographs should always be taken because they reveal more about disease severity than any other single test.
- The minimum data base for cats should include thoracic radiographs. Echocardiography and

fecal studies for lungworms are useful for the differential diagnosis of heartworm infection, feline asthma, cardiomyopathy, bronchitis, pulmonary fibrosis, and lung parasites. A tracheal or bronchial wash may be useful for detecting lung parasitic lesions, such as those produced by *Aelurostrongylus* spp.

Clinical Pathology

No abnormal test results are pathognomonic for heartworm infection.

Complete Blood Count

- Eosinophilia and basophilia are the most common abnormalities in dogs. Eosinophilia is more common and the highest counts tend to occur with occult infections. *Dipetalonema (Acanthocheilonema) reconditum* infections produce eosinophil counts as high as those associated with *D. immitis* infection.
- Neutrophilic leukocytosis with a left shift is usually the result of pulmonary thromboembolism.
- Thrombocytopenia is usually present when there is severe pulmonary arterial disease and thromboembolism.
- Hemoglobinuria, usually accompanied by thrombocytopenia, is seen with caval syndrome and with severe pulmonary thromboembolic disease.

Serum Biochemistry and Urinalysis

- Azotemia may occur in dogs with complicated infections. Prerenal azotemia can be caused by dehydration or right-sided CHF. Primary azotemia can result from glomerulopathies. Increased hepatic enzyme activities may occur; however, increases up to 10-fold do not affect treatment, complications, or survival. Hepatic failure with icterus can occur in dogs with chronic right-sided CHF.
- Proteinuria is common and is most pronounced in patients with severe infections or renal amyloidosis. Mild proteinuria usually resolves after Immiticide treatment.
- Hypoalbuminemia occurs in some dogs with severe infections; hyperglobulinemia is common in dogs and cats with chronic heartworm disease.
- Loss of albumin into the third space occurs with right-sided CHF and is complicated by hepatic insufficiency, intestinal congestion, and free-water retention. Hyponatremia and/or mild hyperkalemia may result.

Screening in Dogs

- Screening in dogs is usually recommended for the late spring in cooler climates to maximize the likelihood of detecting infections acquired in the previous year. In hotter climates, infections may be acquired as late as November or early December and these infections are not detectable until May or June. Run an antigen test 7 months after the end of the previous transmission season (Figure 10-2).

Screening in Cats

- Infections in cats can usually be identified by echocardiography. Combined antibody and antigen testing is recommended for cats. A negative antibody test weighs against the diagnosis. Although a positive antigen test confirms infection in cats, many infected cats are antigen test negative (Figures 10-3 and 10-4).

Immunodiagnostic Testing

- These tests must be performed in strict compliance with the manufacturer's instructions. False-positive test results are usually the result of poor technique. Serodiagnosis of adult heartworm antigens in dogs is accomplished readily by membrane and microwell ELISA tests and membrane immunochromatographic tests. Numerous specific and sensitive tests are available. Test time duration is less than 30 minutes and for some tests is approximately 10 minutes. All of these tests can be performed with plasma or serum samples, and the majority can be run with whole blood.
- Positive antigen test results are the result of the presence of adult female worms. The antigen is associated with the worm's reproductive tract.
- The particular test employed is influenced by the number of tests performed daily, the amount of whole blood or serum required, and the speed of results. Some tests, such as DiroCHEK (Synbiotics), are very efficient for testing multiple samples simultaneously.
- Weakly positive test results should be verified by repeat testing using a different test.
- Most immunodiagnostic tests (ELISA based) are semi-quantitative because rapid and strong positive test results are thought to be related to higher antigen concentrations. Low antigenemia indicates a low adult heartworm burden and reduced risk of post-adulticide thromboembolic complications.
- High-antigenemia may be the result of a heavy worm burden and may indicate increased risk of thromboembolism; however, large quantities of

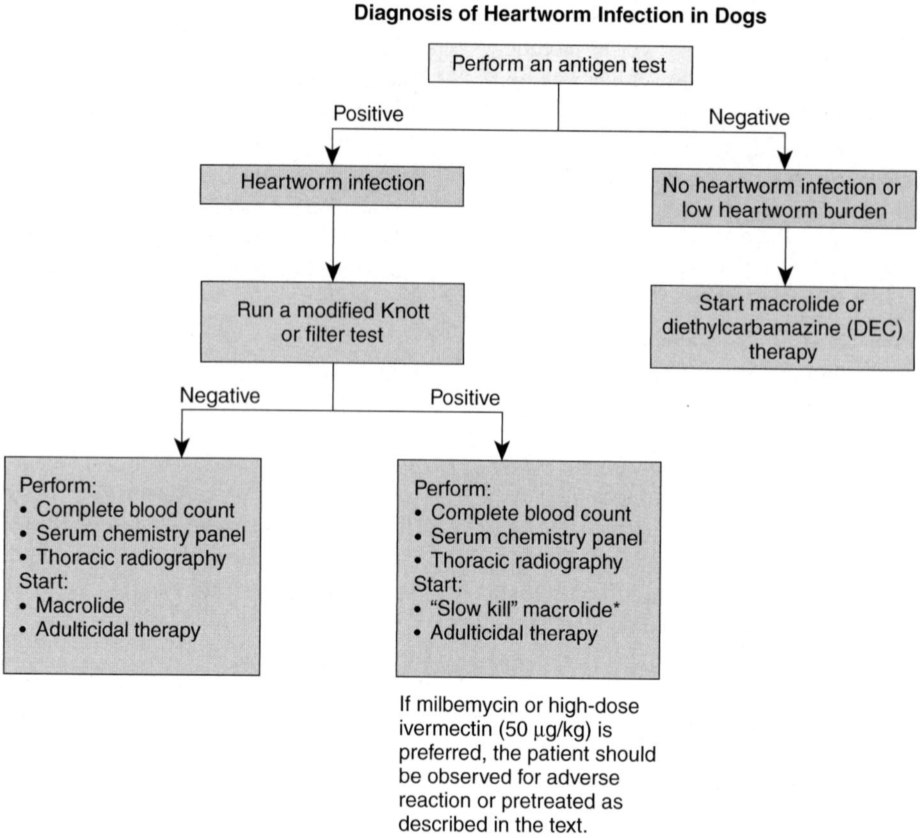

Diagnosis of Heartworm Infection in Dogs
Perform an antigen test
Positive
Negative
Heartworm infection
No heartworm infection or low heartworm burden
Run a modified Knott or filter test
Start macrolide or diethylcarbamazine (DEC) therapy
Negative
Positive
Perform: • Complete blood count • Serum chemistry panel • Thoracic radiography Start: • Macrolide • Adulticidal therapy
Perform: • Complete blood count • Serum chemistry panel • Thoracic radiography Start: • "Slow kill" macrolide* • Adulticidal therapy
If milbemycin or high-dose ivermectin (50 μg/kg) is preferred, the patient should be observed for adverse reaction or pretreated as described in the text.

Figure 10-2. An algorithm approach to the diagnosis of heartworm infection (HWI). (Modified from Ettinger SE, Feldman EC: Textbook of veterinary internal medicine: diseases of the dog and cat, ed 6, St Louis, 2005, WB Saunders.)

Routine Screening for Feline Heartworm Infection
Antibody
Positive
Negative
Antigen
No heartworm infection or low heartworm burden
Positive
Negative
Heartworm infection
Possible heartworm infection
Preventative okay
• Start preventative • Treat symptomatically, as needed
Perform (optional): • Complete blood count • Thoracic radiography • Echocardiography • Microfilaria tests Start: • Preventative

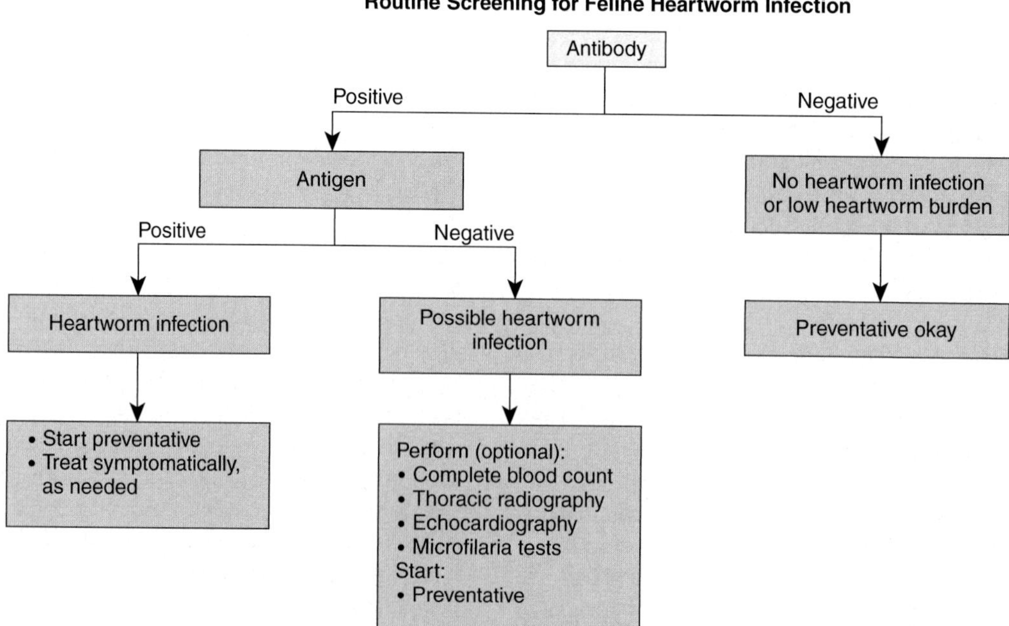

Figure 10-3. An algorithm demonstrating a reasonable approach to screening cats for heartworm infection.

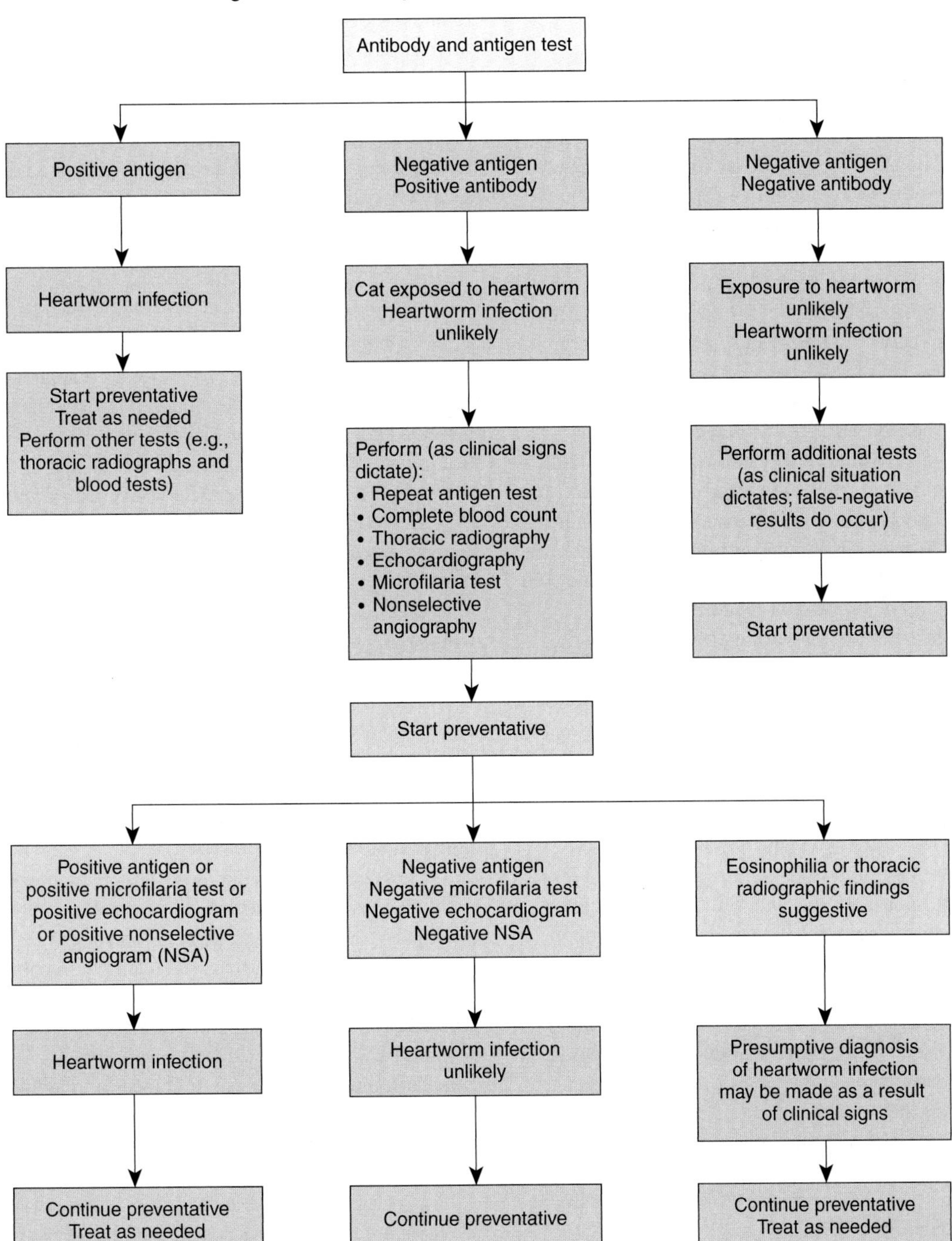

Figure 10.4. An algorithm demonstrating a reasonable approach to diagnose HW in cats in which heartworm infection is suspected. (Modified from Ettinger SE, Feldman EC: Textbook of veterinary internal medicine: diseases of the dog and cat, ed 6, St Louis, 2005, WB Saunders.)

antigen released from dead worms results in a quick, strong test reaction, but does not necessarily mean that the worm burden is high.

- Immunodiagnostic tests are required for diagnosis in dogs receiving monthly macrolide prophylaxis.
- In cats, antigen tests are specific, but false-negative results are common. False-negative test results are explained by low worm burden, male-only infections, and infections with young (< 7 months old) female worms that have immature reproductive

tracts. The antigen test is usually positive if there are 3 or more mature female worms.

Heartworm Antibody Test

- Heartworm-associated antibody tests are useful to rule out infections in cats. Antibodies may appear by 2 to 3 months post-infection and are usually present by 5 months. A positive antibody test indicates exposure but not necessarily active infection. Approximately 10% of infected cats do not produce antibodies.
- Asthma-like signs due to developing larvae often occur months before the antigen test can become positive.
- Larvae induced antibodies can persist after the larvae have been killed by a macrolide drug.
- A strongly positive test result indicates pre-adult infection, live adult infection or persistent (at least 6 months) antibodies after adult heartworm death. Antigen testing and echocardiography are needed to confirm the diagnosis. Intermediate titers should be repeated in 1 month.
- Tests that may support a diagnosis and should be evaluated include: thoracic radiographs, echocardiography, serum globulins (hyperglobulinemia), and CBC (eosinophilia, basophilia).

Microfilaria Detection

- In dogs, the incidence of occult (amicrofilaremic) infections is greater than the incidence of false-negative antigen test results.
- Annual microfilarial detection tests are required for dogs receiving diethylcarbamazine prophylaxis. Otherwise, microfilarial detection tests are mostly indicated if the intent is to kill the microfilaria rapidly using Interceptor. Evaluate a direct blood smear immediately after procurement of a diagnostic blood sample. If the direct smear is negative, then a concentration test is performed. The Knott test (a centrifugal concentration test) or a filter test is at least 25% more sensitive for the detection of microfilaria compared to a direct smear analysis.

Radiography

- A common finding in heartworm infected dogs is dilation of the main pulmonary artery segment at the one o'clock position on the ventrodorsal or dorsoventral projection. The main pulmonary artery segment is not visible in the cat because of its midline position. Next, evaluate the lobar pulmonary arteries. The caudal lobar arteries are the first and most severely effected (Figure 10-5).
- If the lobar arteries are at least 1.5 times the diameters of the ninth ribs, then severe (class 3) arterial pathology has occurred.
- Patchy ill-defined infiltrates around the lobar arteries can result from plasma leakage and inflammation in the lung parenchyma.
- Lobar artery dilation and tortuosity are indicative of severe pathology.
- Abrupt lobar artery branch "pruning" may be visible resulting from obstructed blood flow due to myointimal proliferation and thrombus formation.

Electrocardiography

- The electrocardiogram (ECG) is not a component of the minimum data base although it is sometimes helpful. The ECG is not a sensitive test for identification of mild-to-moderate right ventricular hypertrophy. Even though the ECG will reflect severe hypertrophy, clinical signs and thoracic radiographic analysis provide much more clinical information.
- A right ventricular hypertrophy pattern (S waves in leads I, II, aVF, V2, and V4) is common in dogs with severe pulmonary hypertension and is found in 90% of dogs with overt right-sided CHF (ascites). However, significant pulmonary hypertension may exist in the absence of ECG abnormalities.
- Cardiac rhythm disturbances, including atrial fibrillation, can occur in dogs with severe infections.

Echocardiography

- Evidence of right ventricular and pulmonary artery enlargement can be detected by two-dimensional echocardiography. Occasionally, worms may be detected in the right ventricle, the main pulmonary artery and the right/left lobar arteries (Figure 10-6). Echocardiography is particularly useful in antigen negative cats.
- Echocardiography is the test of choice for diagnosis of caval syndrome (a mass of worms is found in the tricuspid valve orifice and in the vena cava).
- The echocardiographic features of severe heartworm disease include right ventricular eccentric hypertrophy, septal flattening, underloading of the left ventricle and left atrium (Figure 10-7), dilation of the main pulmonary artery segment (Figure 10-8) and main arteries, and high-velocity tricuspid and pulmonic regurgitations (Figure 10-9). The latter two findings are indicative of pulmonary hypertension.

KEY POINT

Thoracic radiography is the most important diagnostic test for determining the severity of heartworm disease.

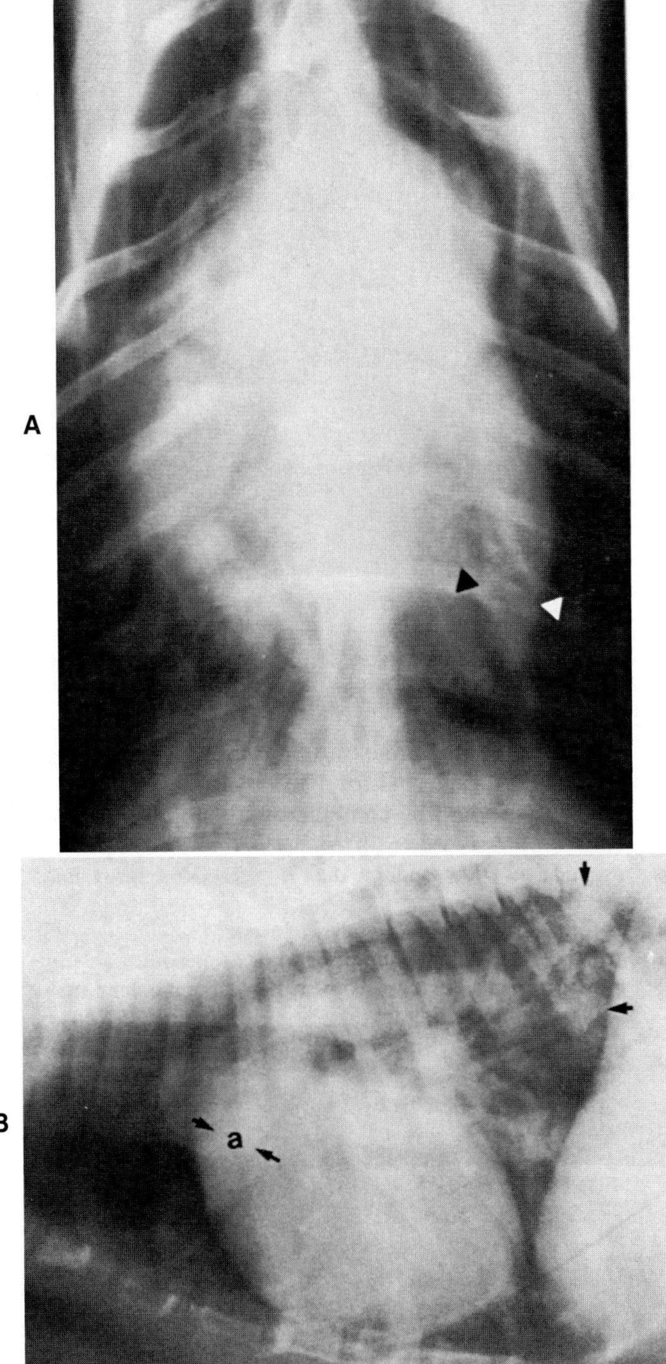

Figure 10-5. Dorsoventral **(A)** and lateral **(B)** radiographic projections of the heart in a dog with class III heartworm disease. On the dorsoventral projection, the caudal lobar arteries are greatly enlarged *(arrowheads)*. These same abnormalities are seen on the lateral projection *(arrows)*, and the right cranial lobar artery *(a)* is enlarged.

> **KEY POINT**
>
> Echocardiography is a sensitive test for heartworm infection in cats.

SEQUELAE OF HEARTWORM INFECTION

Parenchymal Lung Disease

Parenchymal lung disease results from pulmonary arteriolar thromboembolism with leakage of plasma and inflammatory cells into the adjacent

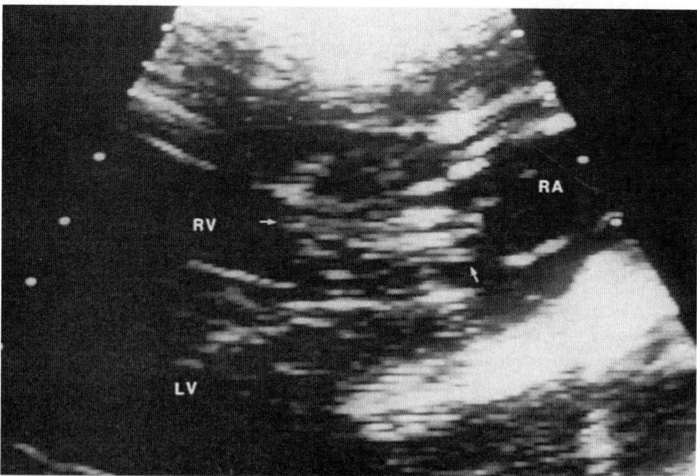

Figure 10-6. Two-dimensional cardiac ultrasound study demonstrating parallel, linear echodensities *(arrows)* produced by heartworms in the right heart. The dog had class III disease. *RA,* Right atrium; *RV,* right ventricle; *LV,* left ventricle.

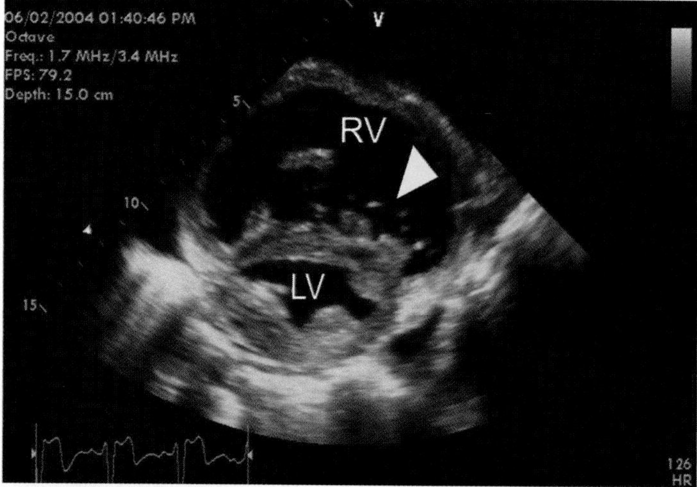

Figure 10-7. Right parasternal, short-axis, two-dimensional cardiac ultrasound of the left and right ventricles. Note the severely enlarged right ventricle. The arrowhead points to echogenic worms within the right ventricle. *RV,* Right ventricle; *LV,* left ventricle.

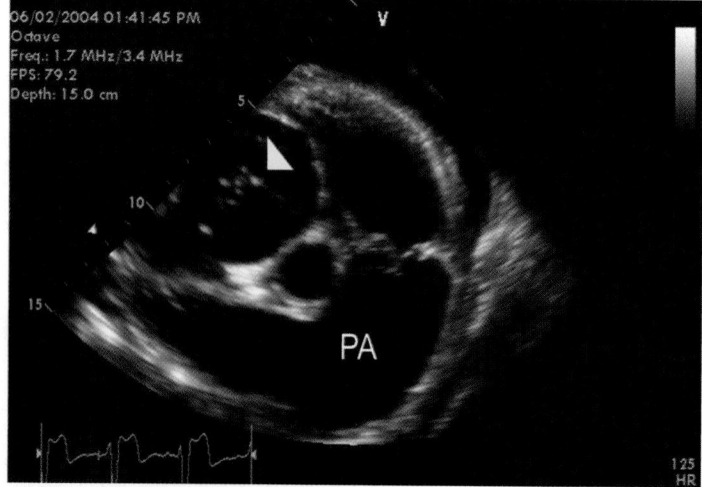

Figure 10-8. Right parasternal, short axis, two-dimensional cardiac ultrasound of the heart base showing the severely dilated main pulmonary artery *(PA).* The arrow head points to echogenic worms within the right atrium.

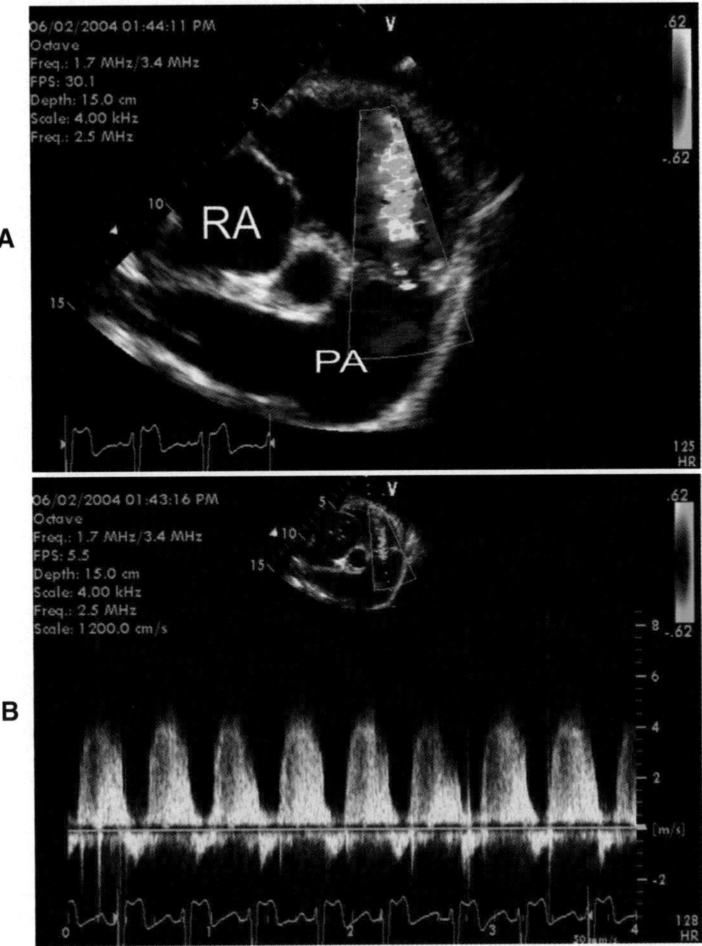

Figure 10-9. **A,** Color flow Doppler echocardiogram obtained from the same position as Figure 10-8. Note the aliasing color flow pattern consistent with significant pulmonary valve regurgitation. *RA,* Right atrium; *PA,* pulmonary artery. **B,** Continuous wave Doppler echocardiogram obtained through the pulmonary valve. Note the high-velocity flow pattern consistent with pulmonary valve regurgitation and pulmonary hypertension.

tissues. Severity varies, disease is most prevalent in the caudal and intermediate lung lobes, and it is most concentrated surrounding the lobar arteries. The degree of caudal lobar arterial disease is best assessed by the dorsoventral radiographic projection. The caudal lobar arteries, especially the right, are the first to enlarge and typically are the most severely diseased. The diameters of the caudal lobar arteries should not exceed that of the ninth rib at the point of their superimposition. Tortuosity and pruning of the arteries (the latter due to thromboembolism) are best seen on the dorsoventral projection; the caudal lobar vessels are the most severely effected. The cranial lobar arteries are best evaluated on the lateral projection; their diameters should not exceed that of the proximal portion of the fourth rib.

Allergic Pneumonitis

The incidence is 10% to 20% of occult infections. It is associated with eosinophilia, coughing, and dyspnea. This mixed diffuse interstitial-alveolar lung disease is best visualized in the caudal lobes. It often occurs with minimal pulmonary arterial enlargement and can be mistaken for left-sided CHF (pulmonary edema) or blastomycosis.

Pulmonary Eosinophilic Granulomatosis

This uncommon complication of occult heartworm disease probably results from the granulomatous inflammation known to be associated with occult infections. The reaction in some cases is progressive and assumes a neoplastic-like behavior.

Table 10-1 Classification of Heartworm Disease Severity Based on Signs, Physical Examination, and Radiographic Findings

Class	Clinical Signs	Examination Findings	Radiographic Findings
1	None to occasional cough	Normal examination	No lesions
2	Occasional cough and mild-to-moderate exercise intolerance	Increased lung sounds Fair general condition	Slight pulmonary arterial enlargement. Circumscribed perivascular density plus mixed alveolar-interstitial lesions
3	Persistent cought, moderate-to-severe exercise intolerance Weight loss, cachexia Respiratory distress Overt right heart failure General loss of condition	Increased lung sounds Accentuated or Split S_2 Right apical gallop Tachypnea, dyspnea	Moderate-to-severe pulmonary arterial enlargement RV enlargement Diffuse and severe pulmonary infiltrates

Feline Asthma–Like Syndrome

Coughing, wheezing, and dyspnea are consistent with feline heartworm infection and the radiographic picture resembles feline asthma. The syndrome first appears about 4 months after infection and tends to be episodic. A quiescent period follows the initial few weeks of clinical signs, but latent relapse of intermittent asthma-like signs may occur.

CLASSIFICATION OF HEARTWORM DISEASE SEVERITY

Severity of heartworm disease is determined by worm burden, duration of infection, and host responses to the worms. Most severe pulmonary complications are associated with occult infections. Three classes are defined which correlate with clinical signs and pulmonary arterial disease. Class assignment may assist in customizing Immiticide treatment (Table 10-1).

- Class 1: Asymptomatic or mild clinical signs.
- Class 2: Moderate clinical and radiographic abnormalities.
- Class 3: Severe clinical and radiographic abnormalities, including right-sided CHF.
- Caval syndrome: This syndrome is sometimes referred to as class 4. However, caval syndrome is not a reflection of the severity of pulmonary arterial disease. Rather it is a syndrome caused by obstruction of blood flow into and through the right heart. Caval syndrome causes mechanical hemolysis and hepatic failure due to acute passive congestion.

The outcome in class 1 and 2 patients is excellent when proper treatment and restriction of activity are accomplished. The outcome for class 3 patients is less encouraging and treatment can be intensive and expensive.

Treatment

The goal of treatment is to kill all adult heartworms with minimal drug toxicity and a tolerable degree of pulmonary thromboembolism caused by the dying worms. Microfilaria should be eliminated, but it is not necessary to administer a rapid-kill microfilaricide such as Interceptor. Gradual elimination of microfilaria over a period of 6 to 8 months with monthly macrolide administration is acceptable.

Patient Selection

Although most heartworm infected dogs can be treated successfully, there are exceptions.

Contraindications to Adulticide Treatment

Immiticide should not be administered to cats because a safe and effective regimen of **melarsomine dihydrochloride** (Immiticide, Merial) has not been developed. Major organ failure such as hepatic failure, nephrotic syndrome, and severe renal failure are contraindications in dogs. The combination of right-sided CHF and icterus is a contraindication to treatment.

Treatment of Old Dogs

Heartworm disease pathology may be nonprogressive in old dogs that have chronic infections with low worm burdens. Adulticide treatment may not be necessary for dogs with class 1 infection that have low-level antigenemia; however, it is recommended by the American Heartworm Society. Monthly administration of **ivermectin** (Heartgard, Merial) at the standard prophylactic dosage will gradually kill adult worms over a period of 16 to 30 months; however, pulmonary damage may continue over this time and resistance may develop in dogs treated in this manner.

Treatment of Cats

Treat asthma-like signs with **prednisolone** (1.0 to 2.0 mg/kg, daily for 10 days; then taper the dose to prevent signs of disease). Do not use aspirin in cats. Immiticide should not be used. Each worm will cause pulmonary thromboembolism when it dies and if multiple worms die simultaneously, severe pulmonary thromboembolism will occur. It is generally believed that 30% to 50% of cats survive their infections.

Wolbachia (Rickettseae): Is It Important?

Wolbachia is a vertically transmitted endosymbiotic, gram-negative, intracellular bacterium that is harbored by *D. immitis* larvae and adults. It is possible that metabolic products and surface proteins from *Wolbachia* can illicit an inflammatory response in the host dog or cat. The host is exposed to *Wolbachia* when larvae or adult worms die or are killed and *Wolbachia* may be expulsed from the uterus of females or the excretory system of either gender of *D. immitis*. Organs most vulnerable to inflammation are the lungs and kidneys. Doxycycline may be lethal to *Wolbachia* and it is postulated that the administration of doxycycline aimed at reducing *Wolbachia* numbers prior to Immiticide treatment might reduce post-Immiticide inflammation. Clinical studies testing this hypothesis have not been reported.

Adulticide Therapy in Dogs

The approved available adulticidal agent is **Immiticide**. The following regimens have proved to be effective. The manufacturer recommends an initial 2 dose, separated by 24 hours, regimen for dogs with class 1 and 2 infections. The authors do not recommend this protocol.

Graded-Kill Immiticide Protocol

- We recommend this protocol for classes 1, 2, and 3 infections. This regimen kills worms gradually and reduces subsequent pulmonary thromboembolism severity.
- 2.5 mg/kg Immiticide injected intramuscularly, once. This dose contains 0.75 mg/kg of total arsenic. The injection is given into the epaxial musculature at the level of the third to fifth lumbar vertebrae.
- The appropriate volume of the reconstituted drug is aspirated into a syringe, and then a new needle is placed on the syringe.
- For dogs weighing more than 10 kg, use a 1½-inch, 22-gauge needle, and for smaller dogs, use a 1-inch, 23-gauge needle.
- The injection should be completed before the needle is withdrawn, and finger pressure should be applied over the needle tract during and for a short time after withdrawal.
- Approximately 50% (most males and some of the females) of adult worms are killed.
- Two follow-up injections (2.5 mg/kg each) at a 24-hour interval are administered after 1 to 3 months. Post-treatment thromboembolism recurs, but the severity is reduced because fewer worms are present.
- Data indicate that 100% of male and 98% of female worms are killed by the 3 doses.

KEY POINT

Use the graded-kill Immiticide protocol.

Treatment of Class 3 Heartworm Disease

- Severe pulmonary arterial disease occurs in 10% of infected dogs in highly endemic regions, and in some patients, the adult worm burden is very great. Extraction of adult worms from the vena cava, right atrium, right ventricle, and main pulmonary arteries is possible. Worm extraction is only for patients with many worms in the right heart and pulmonary arteries. These patients have a high antigen concentration, and the high burden is confirmed by echocardiography. The technique requires fluoroscopy and long, flexible alligator forceps or a horsehair brush that is introduced into the right jugular vein via a surgical approach and manipulated through the heart into the pulmonary arteries. Numerous passages to grasp and remove worms are required, and the procedure is aided by fluoroscopy. This procedure is highly effective in experienced hands.
- After the patient has been stabilized, treat with Immiticide to kill any remaining worms. It is assumed that some worms are not removed. Subsequently, remaining worms can be detected by echocardiography or by a positive antigen test result after 4 to 6 months.

Side Effects and Efficacy of Immiticide Treatment

- Mild myositis of 1 to 3 days, duration often is observed after Immiticide injections. Approximately one third of treated dogs experience some swelling, and a sterile seroma occurs uncommonly.
- If an injection of Immiticide causes a local reaction, then consider administration of an antihistamine and rapid acting corticosteroid before subsequent injections.
- Hepatic and renal toxicity associated with Immiticide is uncommon; excessive dosage can produce noncardiogenic pulmonary edema.
- Confirmation of efficacy can be established after 6 months by antigen testing. Mean antigen concentration is reduced to 1% of pretreatment levels, indicating nearly complete elimination of worms.

Drug Storage

- Immiticide is purchased as a lyophilized powder that does not require refrigeration and has a shelf life of at least 2 years. The reconstituted drug must be kept refrigerated.

Post-Adulticide Complications

- Strict patient confinement is essential for 4 to 6 weeks post-treatment. Reduced blood flow demand through the pulmonary arteries is beneficial to diminish endothelial damage and to promote vascular repair.
- Thromboembolic complications may occur from several days to 4 to 6 weeks post-Immiticide. Most complications occur between 1 to 3 weeks.
- Most severe thromboembolism occurs in dogs with class 3 infections with high antigen concentrations. Coughing, gagging, lethargy, anorexia, tachypnea, dyspnea, syncope, hemoptysis, and fever are common. Thrombocytopenia and an inflammatory leukogram are usual.
- Radiographic evidence of parenchymal lung disease is always present.

Treatment of Caval Syndrome

- Caval syndrome (class 4) is uncommon except in highly endemic regions. It is associated with large numbers of worms in the right heart and vena cava. It is seen most often in the late spring and early summer in young dogs that have received a heavy inoculation over a short time period the previous year. Acute cardiovascular collapse and shock occur and is fatal within hours unless the worms are removed and the obstruction to blood flow is alleviated.
- Clinical signs are variable, including a systolic heart murmur, diastolic gallop, and hemoglobinuria.
- Echocardiography is diagnostic.
- Surgical retrieval of the worms is the only recommended acute treatment.
- Minimal or no sedation is used. Rather local anesthesia is used to perform a surgical cut-down on the right jugular vein. A long, flexible alligator forceps or horsehair brush is introduced and advanced to the heart base in order to retrieve as many worms as possible from the vena cava and right atrium with multiple passages. The procedure is finished when several passages fail to retrieve additional worms. This is highly effective but experience is required for optimal results.
- After a period of stabilization, Immiticide is administered to eliminate remaining worms.

When to Initiate Macrolide Prophylaxis in Infected Dogs

Macrolide prophylaxis should be initiated as soon as infection is confirmed. Heartgard, Revolution, or Advantage Multi can be initiated for prophylaxis in microfilaremic infections. Interceptor should not be administered to microfilaremic dogs unless rapid kill is intended. In fact, in patients that have neither clinical signs nor obvious radiographic abnormalities, it is appropriate to initiate prophylaxis and wait for several months before administering Immiticide. This approach eliminates migrating larvae that might not be killed by Immiticide.

Rapid Microfilaricide Therapy

We recommend against the use of Interceptor or high-dose ivermectin to kill microfilaria rapidly. Eliminating the microfilaria with monthly prophylaxis is acceptable.

KEY POINT

Rapid kill of microfilaria is unnecessary.

Confirmation of Adulticide Efficacy

- Anantigen test should be performed 6 months after the third Immiticide injection. Occasionally, a weakly positive test result may occur. Wait two additional months and retest. Whether to retreat is

controversial. Very few worms are likely to have survived and re-treatment may not be necessary.
- Re-treatment is recommended for class 3 infections, if clinical signs persist, and for performance dogs.

Adjuncts to Adulticide Therapy

KEY POINT

Test for Immiticide efficacy no sooner than 6 months after the last dose.

Heparin
- Recommended for rapidly dropping platelet counts and hemoglobinuria.
- Administer 75 to 100 units/kg SQ every 8 hours, for several days up to 1 week.
- Combine with strict cage confinement.

Corticosteroids
- Reduce parenchymal inflammatory disease in the lungs but promote thrombosis and reduce pulmonary arterial blood flow if used for longer than 10 to 14 consecutive days. Do not use corticosteroids routinely, but only as needed to control sequelae.

Oxygen
- The only effective means of dilating the pulmonary arteries.
- For class 3 infections associated with dyspnea, orthopnea, or CHF.
- Administer intra-nasally or by oxygen cage.

TREATMENT OF SEQUELAE

Pulmonary Thromboembolism

- This common complication of moderate to severe pulmonary arterial disease can occur before adulticide therapy, but is most common 7 to 21 days after adulticide therapy. In dogs, clinical signs include coughing, dyspnea, fever, and hemoptysis.
- A regenerative leukocytosis with thrombocytopenia usually is present.
- Positive d-dimers (>500mg/dl) may be a sensitive indicator. However, in the authors' experience, negative d-dimers do not exclude thromboembolism.
- Thoracic radiographs reveal severe pulmonary arterial disease with periarterial parenchymal disease of variable severity.
- Initiate cage confinement for 5 to 10 days.
- Administer **heparin** at 200 units/kg SQ every 8 hours.
- Administer **prednisone** (1.0 mg/kg PO every 24 hours for 3 to 10 days).
- Use intranasal or cage-administered oxygen for dyspneic patients.

Allergic Pneumonitis

- This complication occurs in 10% to 20% of patients with occult infections. The clinical signs include dyspnea, coughing, respiratory crackles, and exercise intolerance. Thoracic radiographs contain diffuse interstitial-alveolar infiltrates. Eosinophilia is common, and eosinophils predominate in tracheal lavage cytology. The syndrome responds well to oral **prednisone** (1 to 2 mg/kg every 24 hours for several days). Stop prednisone therapy after 3 to 7 days and begin Immiticide therapy as soon as dyspnea, coughing, and pulmonary infiltrates have resolved.

Pulmonary Eosinophilic Granulomatosis

- This uncommon complication of occult heartworm disease probably results from the granulomatous inflammation known to be associated with occult infections. **Prednisone** (2 mg/kg PO every 24 hours for 7 to 14 days; then gradually taper dose) with **azathioprine** (50 mg/m^2 PO every 24 hours for 7 days; then 25 mg/m^2 every 24 hours for 7 days; then 25 mg/m^2 every 48 hours) may induce partial or complete remission. Relapses are common even in the face of medical therapy. The prognosis is guarded, and surgical excision of lobar lesions may be required. Adulticide treatment should be delayed until remission is attained.

Feline Asthma–Like Syndrome

- Treat asthma-like signs in cats with **prednisolone** (1.0 to 2.0 mg/kg PO daily for 10 days; then taper the dose to prevent signs of disease).

PREVENTION

- A microfilarial examination always is indicated before initiation of drugs that can be associated with an acute adverse reaction. These drugs are Interceptor and diethylcarbamazine. Prevention should be in place whenever the average daily temperature exceeds about 57° F. Year-round prevention is practiced in hotter climates, even though transmission is uncommon in December and January in the continental United States.

- Start as early as 6 to 8 weeks of age. In cooler climates, start puppies on prophylaxis as soon after 8 weeks of age as dictated by seasonal risk.
- Heartgard, Interceptor, Revolution, and Advantage Multi should be started within 1 month of the transmission season. These drugs kill migrating larvae during the first 6 to 8 weeks after L_3 inoculation.
- Successful prophylaxis is confirmed by a negative antigen test result one year after initiation.
- Macrolides are safe for collies when prescribed according to the label.
- Macrolide prophylaxis not only interferes with larval embryogenesis, which reduces the circulating levels of microfilaria, but also gradually kills existing microfilaria over a period of 6 to 8 months.

KEY POINT

In all studies to date, owner administration compliance has been poor.

Ivermectin

- Ivermectin (Heartgard), at a dosage of 6 to 12 micrograms/kg given monthly, is an effective preventive drug. A chewable formulation of Ivermectin plus pyrantel pamoate (Heartgard Plus) is an effective heartworm preventive that also controls ascarid and hookworm infestations. Drug reactions are rare at the recommended dosage.
- The reach-back larvacidal action is 100% at 1 month and nearly 100% at 2 months.
- If initiated 4 months following L_3 inoculation and continued for at least 1 year, the likelihood of developing infection is reduced by at least 98%.
- When administration is begun 5.5 months post-L_3 inoculation, the subsequent adult worm burden is reduced by about 50%.
- When administration is begun 6.5 months post-L_3, the subsequent adult worm burden is reduced by about one third.
- Heartgard Plus kills adult heartworms slowly over a 16- to 30-month period and microfilariae over a period of 6 to 8 months.
- A dose of 24 μg/kg administered monthly is an effective heartworm prophylaxis in cats, and it controls hookworms.

Milbemycin

- Milbemycin (Interceptor), at a dosage of 0.5 to 0.99 mg/kg, is an effective once-a-month preventive agent for heartworm disease in dogs and cats.
- It is not as effective as ivermectin at preventing the maturation of larvae when monthly administration is started 4 months post-L_3 inoculation.
- It also controls hookworm, roundworm, and whipworm infestations.
- One dose of Interceptor at the prophylactic dosage will kill most microfilaria within 24 hours. If the microfilaria concentration is high, an adverse reaction is likely.

Moxidectin

- A topical solution formulation (Advantage Multi) is an effective once-a-month heartworm preventative agent for dogs and cats. Advantage Multi also controls fleas, hookworms, roundworms, whipworms, and ear mites.

KEY POINT

All macrolide preventive drugs eliminate microfilaria, either quickly or slowly. For this reason, chronic dosing with Heartgard, Revolution, Interceptor, or Advantage Multi leads to "occult" status in infected dogs. All monthly prophylactic drugs can be administered without prior testing and fear of adverse reactions.

Diethylcarbamazine

- Diethylcarbamazine (2.5 to 3.0 mg/kg, PO) given daily is an effective prophylactic drug. If the owner skips more than a few days of treatment, do not reinstitute preventive treatment before performing a microfilarial concentration test. Diethylcarbamazine has been largely supplanted by the macrolide drugs. The duration of action of diethylcarbamazine is short because the drug affects the L_3-L_4 (larval) molt 9 to 12 days postinfection.
- Begin therapy before mosquito season and continue for 2 months after the first frost (or year-round in regions that have mosquitoes all year).
- Combination diethylcarbamazine and oxibendazole (Filaribits Plus) controls intestinal helminths. An occasional side effect of oxibendazole is increased liver enzyme activity, icterus, and hepatic insufficiency, which is reversible after the drug is discontinued.

KEY POINT

Never initiate diethylcarbamazine treatment in microfilaremic dogs because a severe reaction may occur.

MISSED DOSES OF ORAL MACROLIDE PROPHYLACTIC DRUGS

- One dose of any macrolide will kill all larvae that have infected a dog in the previous month.
- One dose of Heartgard, Interceptor or Revolution will kill virtually all larvae that have infected a dog during the prior two months.
- Heartgard, Interceptor, and Revolution will prevent almost all infections from maturing after three consecutive doses are missed, providing that at least 12 consecutive subsequent monthly doses are administered.

MACROLIDE EFFICACY AGAINST ADULT HEARTWORMS

- Heartgard will kill almost all adult heartworms if administered every month for 30 months.
- We rarely recommend Heartgard for adulticide treatment because progressive pulmonary pathology can occur and resistance is a possibility.

RETESTING DOGS RECEIVING MACROLIDE PROPHYLAXIS

- Macrolide prophylactic drugs are highly efficacious, and therefore annual retesting often is not performed; however, we recommend annual retesting because:
- Owner compliance has been proven to be poor in all regions examined.
- Inadequate dosing is likely in growing puppies.

Frequently Asked Questions

Is Immiticide an effective adulticide in cats and should treatment be attempted?
An Immiticide dosage schedule that is both safe and effective in cats has not been developed. Dying worms, whether the result of Immiticide or natural death, will always cause pulmonary thromboembolism which may be fatal. Immiticide dosages have been investigated but some were too low to kill worms and others were high enough to cause acute pulmonary toxicity (acute respiratory distress syndrome).

How likely is it that a cat will survive heartworm infection?
Estimates are that mortality is about 50% whether or not Immiticide is administered.

What is the most practical method to rule out heartworm infection in cats?
A negative antibody test is associated with a high likelihood that infection is absent. If there is still concern, then echocardiography is indicated.

Why is it unnecessary to kill microfilaria quickly?
Microfilaria will be eliminated in 6 to 8 months with macrolide prophylaxis and the likelihood of the infected dog being responsible for spread during this period is low.

What is the proper course of action if 3 consecutive prophylactic doses are missed?
Administer Heartgard, Interceptor or Revolution for at least 12 consecutive months and the likelihood of maturation of heartworm larvae is extremely low. In fact, if the infection is only about 2 months old, one dose of any of these preventatives will stop almost all infections.

Is Heartgard recommended as an adulticide treatment?
No. Almost all dogs with adult heartworm infection should be treated with Immiticide. The slow kill-rate of Heartgard against adults may allow progressive pulmonary pathology and resistance is possible.

SUGGESTED READINGS

Atkins C: Canine heartworm disease. In Ettinger SJ Feldman EC, eds: Textbook of veterinary internal medicine, Philadelphia, 2005, WB Saunders.

Atkins C: Feline heartworm disease. In Ettinger SJ, Feldman EC, eds: Textbook of veterinary internal medicine, Philadelphia, 2005, WB Saunders.

Heartworm disease. In Kahn CM, ed: The Merck manual. Whitehouse Station, NJ, 2005, Merck and Co.

Heartworm disease, In Birchard SJ, Sherding RG, eds: Saunders manual of small animal practice, St. Louis, 2006, WB Saunders.

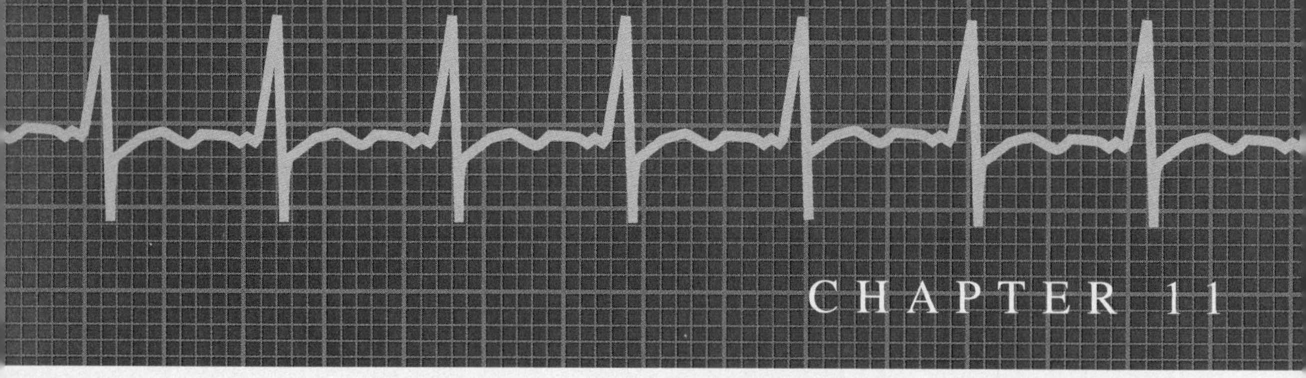

Pericardial Disorders and Cardiac Tumors

Anthony H. Tobias and Elizabeth A. McNiel

INTRODUCTION

- Most pericardial disorders in small animals are associated with pericardial effusions (abnormal accumulations of fluid within the pericardial sac) leading to cardiac tamponade (significant compression of the heart by accumulating pericardial contents).
- Most pericardial effusions in dogs are associated with cardiac tumors. Similarly, most cardiac tumors are associated with pericardial effusions. Consequently, cardiac tamponade typically dominates the clinical presentation in dogs with cardiac tumors.
- Pericardial effusions in cats occur most commonly among cases suffering from congestive heart failure; however, pericardial effusions in this species are usually mild and incidental manifestations of underlying disease, rather than the primary cause for the presenting signs. Consequently, the ensuing discussion pertains primarily to dogs.

PERICARDIAL EFFUSIONS

Incidence and Signalment

- At the University of Minnesota Veterinary Medical Center (UMVMC) from January 1999 to December 2001, pericardial effusions were confirmed as the primary cause for clinical signs in 87 dogs. This represents an incidence of 0.43%, or 1 in every 233 new canine admissions to the UMVMC.
- Symptomatic pericardial effusions most commonly occur in older and larger dogs. In the UMVMC study population, average age among dogs with confirmed pericardial effusions was 9.7 (± 2.2) years and average weight was 31.2 (± 12.6) kg.
- Males and females were nearly equally represented (46 [53%] males to 41 [47%] females).
- Pericardial effusions were most frequently diagnosed in Golden Retrievers (23 [26%] of the 87 cases), and this was the only breed that was overrepresented when compared to the general hospital population (odds ratio = 4.4; 95% confidence interval 2.7 to 7.0).

Chief Complaints and History

In most cases, clinical signs in dogs with pericardial effusions are nonspecific and have an acute onset. Presenting signs in the UMVMC study population included:

- Lethargy (53%)
- Respiratory difficulty (44%)
- Collapse (40%)
- Reduced appetite (38%)
- Vomiting (30%)
- Abdominal distention (23%)

Less common complaints included polydipsia, weakness, and coughing.

Physical Examination Findings

- Dogs with pericardial effusions present with clinical signs ranging from subtle to hemodynamic collapse (severe clinical tamponade).

- In the UMVMC study population, muffled heart sounds were the most common physical examination abnormality, occurring in 71% of the cases.
- Other physical examination findings included:
  - Depression (63%).
  - Weak pulses (62%).
  - Abdominal distention with a fluid wave due to ascites (43%). Ascites, when present, is usually mild, and consequently not recognized by owners in about half of the dogs in which it is detected on physical examination.
- Thorough physical examination usually discloses jugular distention.
- *Pulsus paradoxus*, phasic variations in pulse quality associated with respiration, is occasionally identified.

Diagnostic Procedures

Radiology

- Thoracic radiographic features that support a diagnosis of pericardial effusion are:
  - An enlarged and globoid cardiac silhouette with tracheal elevation and widening of the caudal vena cava
  - Overlap of the cardiac silhouette and diaphragm and bilateral contact between the pericardial sac and the costal margins
  - A sharply delineated edge to the cardiac silhouette because the distended pericardial sac undergoes little, if any, motion during systole and diastole
  - Lung fields that show no evidence of left-sided congestive heart failure (i.e., no cardiogenic pulmonary edema, Figure 11-1)
- However, these "typical" radiographic findings are only present in more chronic cases with large volume pericardial effusions. With smaller pericardial effusions, the cardiac silhouette is variably enlarged, and it is not necessarily globoid. Also, pericardial effusions in dogs are frequently accompanied by pleural effusions that may obscure the cardiac silhouette.
- Despite these limitations, thoracic radiographs are important in the diagnostic evaluation of cases with suspected pericardial effusions. In addition to facilitating a diagnosis of pericardial effusion in many cases, thoracic radiographs may demonstrate the presence of abnormalities such as pulmonary metastases, or radiopaque intrapericardial foreign bodies.

Electrocardiography

- Most dogs with pericardial effusions have either a normal sinus rhythm or a sinus tachycardia.
- Ventricular arrhythmias are fairly common and supraventricular arrhythmias occasionally occur.
- Low voltage QRS complexes (R waves < 1 mV in all limb leads) are present in approximately half of the cases (Figure 11-2, *A, B*).
- Electrical alternans, a beat-to-beat variation in the contour and amplitude of the QRS and ST-T complexes (Figure 11-2, *C*), is strongly suggestive of a pericardial effusion. Electrical alternans is present in up to approximately 20% of dogs with pericardial effusions.

Pericardial Fluid Analysis

- Pericardial effusions in dogs irrespective of cause are virtually always sanguinous or serosanguinous sterile inflammatory exudates.
- Total nucleated cell counts, red cell counts, protein concentrations and pericardial fluid pH overlap extensively between the various neoplastic and non-neoplastic causes.
- Hemangiosarcoma and aortic body tumors, the most common tumors associated with pericardial effusions in dogs, are rarely identified on cytologic evaluation of pericardial fluid. Also, pericardial diseases that lead to effusion result in dramatic mesothelial proliferation, and exfoliated mesothelial cells often have characteristics that mimic malignancy. Cytology must be interpreted very cautiously.
- However, some of the less common causes of pericardial effusion, such as infectious pericarditis and lymphosarcoma, are diagnosed primarily on the basis of pericardial fluid cytology. Consequently, the authors submit pericardial fluid for analysis in all cases with pericardial effusions, despite the generally low diagnostic yield of this test.

KEY POINT

Cytologic examination of pericardial effusates is unreliable in distinguishing neoplastic vs. non-neoplastic (i.e., inflammatory) etiologies in the large majority of cases of pericardial effusion in the dog.

Echocardiography

- Echocardiography is the most sensitive and specific noninvasive method to confirm the presence of pericardial effusion.
- With two-dimensional echocardiography, pericardial effusion appears as an anechoic space surrounding the heart. In cases with concurrent pleural effusion, the pericardium is well visualized with anechoic fluid on either side.
- The heart may show swinging motions within the pericardial fluid.

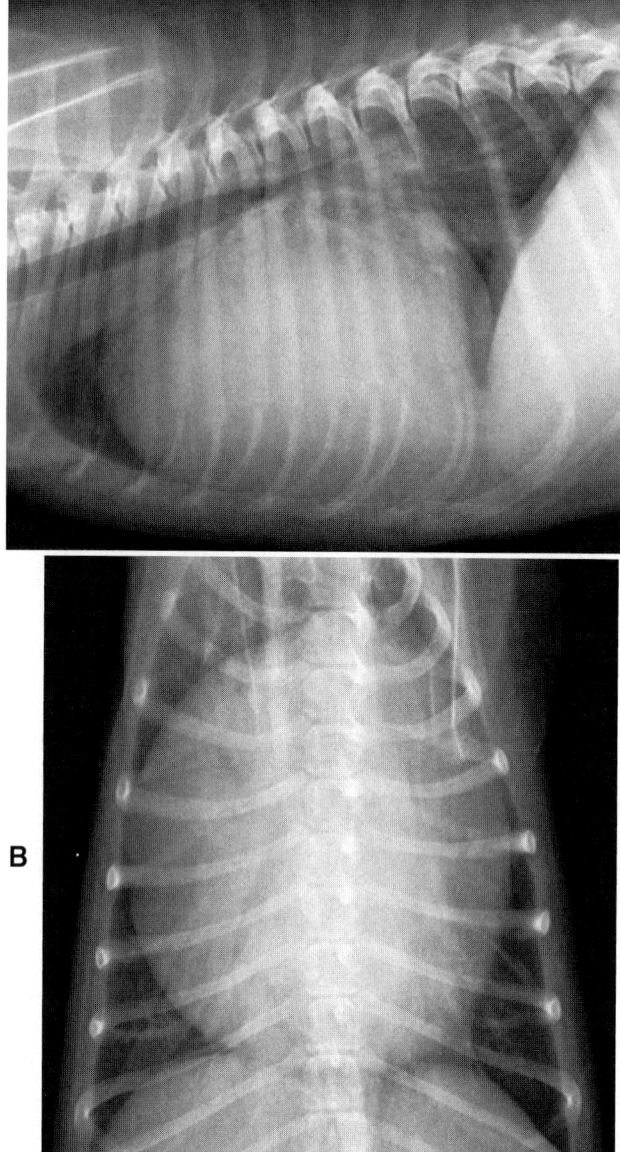

Figure 11-1. Thoracic radiographs from a dog with pericardial effusion. **A,** The lateral projection shows a markedly enlarged cardiac silhouette, tracheal elevation, and overlap of the cardiac silhouette and diaphragm. **B,** The ventrodorsal projection shows bilateral contact between the pericardial sac and the costal margins. The edge of the cardiac silhouette is sharply delineated, and the lung fields are clear of any infiltrate that would indicate the presence of left-sided congestive heart failure.

- The various heart chambers may appear small and the walls may show thickening or pseudohypertrophy due to external compression.
- The right atrial free wall is normally rounded throughout the cardiac cycle, reflecting the normal positive right atrial transmural pressure. Any inversion or collapse of the right atrial free wall provides indirect evidence of elevated intrapericardial pressure and transient reversal of transmural pressure (echocardiographic evidence of cardiac tamponade). Right atrial inversion occurs in late diastole and continues into ventricular systole for a variable period before normalizing (Figure 11-3, *A*).
- Cardiac tamponade leading to right ventricular diastolic collapse is characterized by inward motion of the right ventricular free wall (Figure 11-3, *B*). This may range from transient and localized concavity of the right ventricular free wall, to virtual complete right ventricular chamber obliteration throughout diastole.
- In addition to confirming the presence of pericardial effusion and cardiac tamponade, echocardiography is the noninvasive procedure of choice to

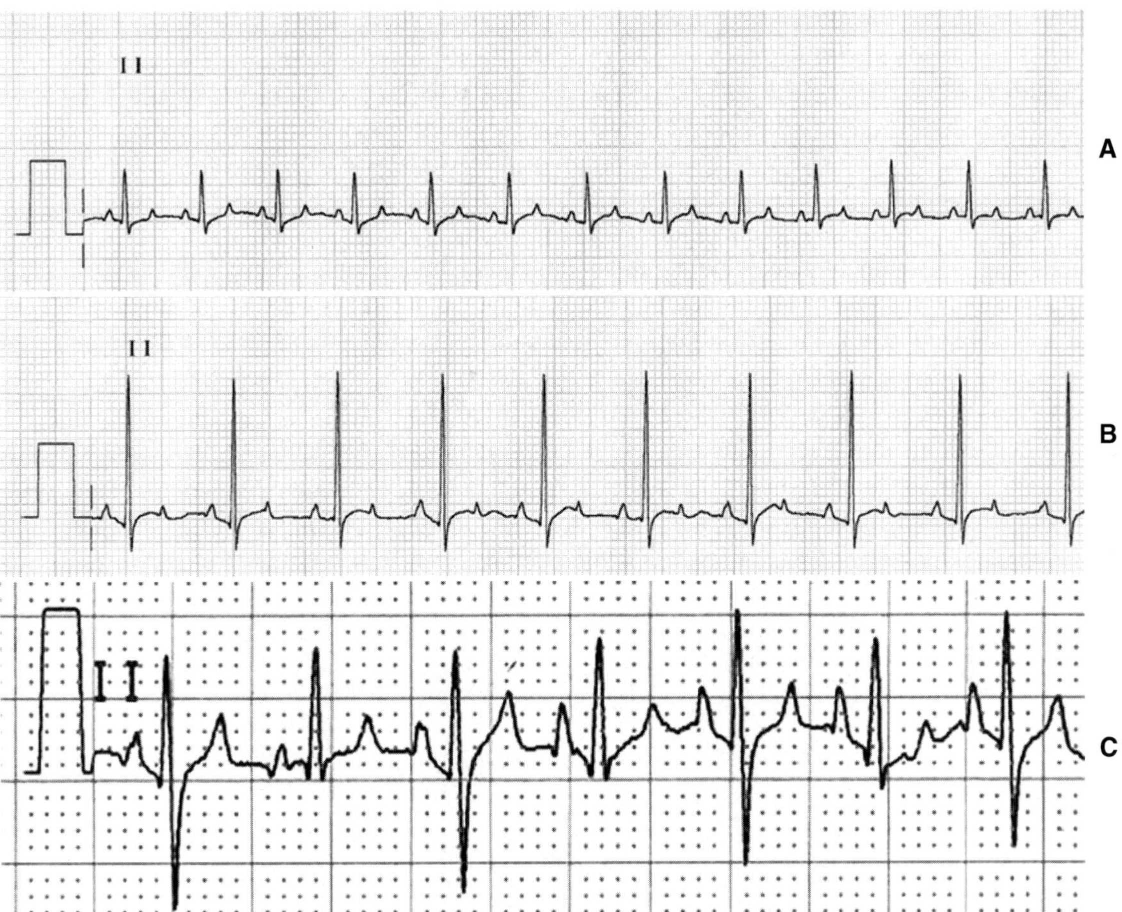

Figure 11-2. Electrocardiograms (lead II) from dogs with pericardial effusion. Calibration square wave is 1 mV in amplitude. **A,** Before pericardiocentesis, the complexes are low voltage (R wave < 1 mV) and heart rate is 140 beats per minute (bpm). **B,** After pericardiocentesis, R wave amplitude is almost 2 mV and heart rate is 100 bpm. **C,** Beat-to-beat variations in amplitude and contour of the QRS and ST-T complexes that characterize electrical alternans. (Modified from Tobias AH: Pericardial disorders. In Ettinger SJ, Feldman EC, eds: Textbook of veterinary internal medicine, ed 6, St Louis, 2005, WB Saunders.)

detect associated intrapericardial masses such as hemangiosarcoma and heart base tumors. Whereas histopathology is necessary to confirm and definitively identify a tumor, the echocardiographic location and characteristics of an intrapericardial or myocardial mass provides important information about the probable tumor type.

- The following echocardiographic features are consistent with a diagnosis of hemangiosarcoma:
  - Hemangiosarcoma most commonly arises from the wall of the right atrium or auricle, protrudes into the pericardial space, and moves with the right auricle or atrium (Figure 11-4).
  - These tumors may also protrude into the right atrial chamber, spread to involve other areas of the heart base and pericardium, and involve the right atrioventricular groove (see Figure 11-3, *A*).
  - Hemangiosarcoma typically contains small hypoechoic spaces, giving the tumor a mottled or cavitary appearance, and the tumors are occasionally cystic (see Figure 11-4).
  - Hemangiosarcoma, when present, is usually demonstrated while imaging from the right parasternal long- and short-axis views. However, these tumors may be small and elusive. Imaging from the left parasternal locations to provide alternate imaging planes, especially of the right auricle, is necessary to demonstrate the presence of hemangiosarcoma in some cases.
  - Hemangiosarcoma involving the wall of the left ventricle has been described.
- The following echocardiographic features are characteristic for heart base tumors:
  - Heart base tumors are usually associated with the ascending aorta (Figure 11-5, *A*).
  - They vary from small ovoid structures attached to the ascending aorta, to very extensive masses that surround the aorta and main pulmonary artery.

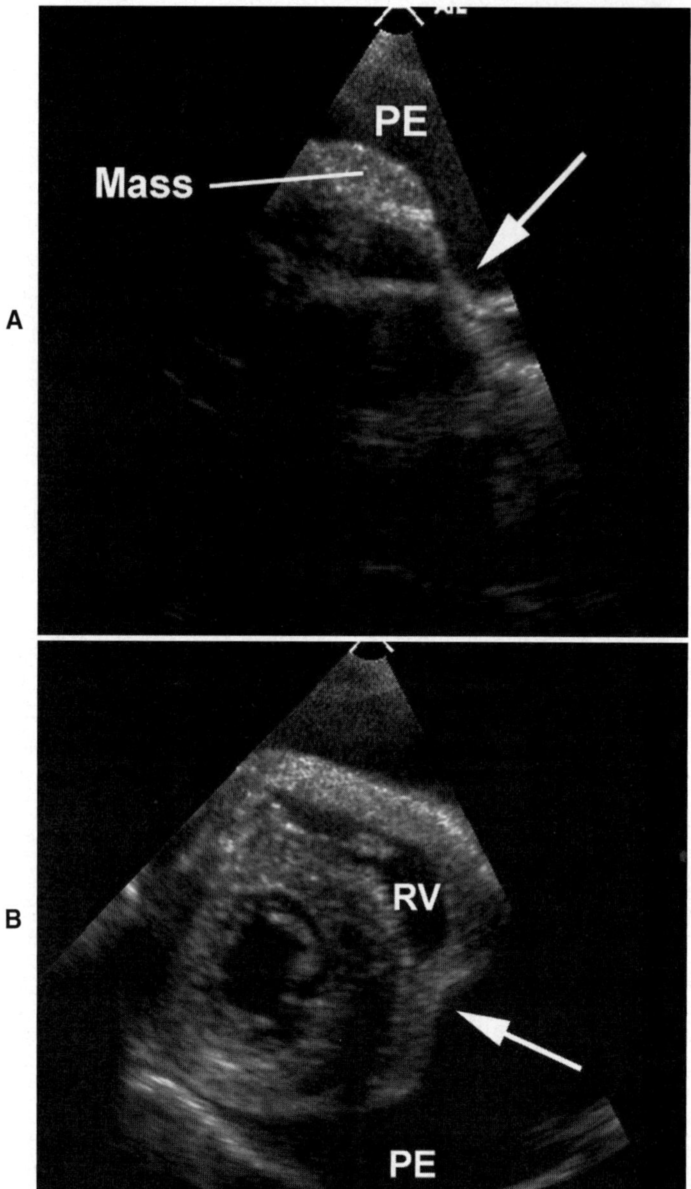

Figure 11-3. Echocardiographic tamponade in a dog with pericardial effusion *(PE)*. The images were recorded from the right parasternal location. **A,** Late diastolic inversion of the right atrium *(arrow)*. The mass at the atrioventricular groove was confirmed as hemangiosarcoma by surgical biopsy. **B,** Diastolic inversion of the right ventricular wall *(arrow)*. *RV,* Right ventricle.

- Tumor indentation or invasion of the atria and major blood vessels may be seen (Figure 11-5, *B*).
- Heart base tumors tend to have a more homogenous appearance than the mottled or cavitary appearance of hemangiosarcoma.
- Heart base tumors are usually, but not invariably, associated with pericardial effusions.
- Echocardiography may also demonstrate:
  - Cardiac tumors other than hemangiosarcoma and heart base tumors.
  - The presence of abdominal viscera within the pericardial sac in cases with peritoneopericardial diaphragmatic hernia.
  - Benign intrapericardial cyst.
  - Intrapericardial thrombi associated with left atrial perforation. Left atrial perforation is suspected when signs of acute tamponade develop in smaller breed dogs with significant mitral regurgitation.

Initial Patient Stabilization: Pericardiocentesis

- Pericardiocentesis to remove as much pericardial fluid as possible is necessary for initial patient stabilization in any case with a pericardial

KEY POINT

The presence of pericardial fluid greatly facilitates the detection of intrapericardial masses, and this is particularly relevant to the diagnosis and delineation of hemangiosarcoma and heart base tumors. Pericardial fluid forms an echolucent zone around the right atrium and auricle and the ascending aorta, the locations at which these tumors most commonly occur. In the absence of pericardial fluid, these locations are obscured by lung interference. Consequently, whenever the clinical condition of the patient permits, pericardiocentesis should be deferred until a thorough echocardiographic examination has been completed.

effusion that is causing significant hemodynamic compromise (clinical cardiac tamponade).

- The authors' preferred approach is to restrain the animal in left lateral recumbency and to approach the pericardium from the right side. This reduces the risk of lacerating a coronary blood vessel during the procedure.
- Dogs usually tolerate the procedure without sedation, but mild sedation is necessary in some cases.
- The authors usually use a 14- or 16-gauge over-the-needle catheter system to perform pericardiocentesis in dogs. Two small side holes are made near the tip of the catheter to avoid any blockages and aspirating the myocardium against a single end hole during the procedure.
- The catheter system is coupled to a large volume syringe via an extension tube and a three-way stopcock.
- The right thorax is shaved and the ideal location to perform the procedure is determined by echocardiography. The location is selected to avoid lung and to approach the pericardium perpendicularly with the catheter system. This usually coincides with the fifth or sixth intercostal space at about the level of the costochondral junction.
- The skin, intercostal muscles, and parietal pleura are infiltrated with local anesthetic, and the area is surgically prepared.
- A small skin incision is made (Figure 11-6, *A*) and the catheter system is advanced towards the pericardium (Figure 11-6, *B*).
- Slight negative pressure is applied and maintained via the syringe and extension tube as the catheter system is advanced.
- Once the needle and catheter enters the pericardium, fluid flows into the extension tube and syringe.
- The catheter is then advanced over the needle into the pericardial space (Figure 11-6, *C*), the needle is removed, the extension tube is connected to the catheter (Figure 11-6, *D*), and a small amount of fluid is aspirated (Figure 11-6, *E*).
- The gross appearance of pericardial fluid is almost invariably indistinguishable from blood. To confirm that the catheter is in the pericardial space, an aliquot of fluid is placed in an activated clotting time tube. Blood will normally clot in an activated clotting time tube within 60 to 90 seconds. In contrast, sanguinous effusions in body cavities are rapidly depleted of clotting factors and thrombocytes, and pericardial fluid will consequently not clot. If no clots form within the activated clotting tube after 3 to 5 minutes, samples are collected for fluid analysis and culture, and all of the pericardial fluid is aspirated. The catheter is then removed.
- Ventricular arrhythmias are common during pericardiocentesis and ECG monitoring during the procedure is recommended.
- In virtually all cases with pericardial effusion, pericardiocentesis results in rapid and marked hemodynamic improvement. Clinical signs, pulse quality, and mucous membrane perfusion improve, and heart rate decreases. However, ventricular and supraventricular arrhythmias (including atrial fibrillation) are common both during and following pericardiocentesis. These arrhythmias seldom require therapy and usually resolve spontaneously. Nevertheless, we prefer to hospitalize and monitor cases for 12 to 24 hours following pericardiocentesis and to provide supportive care as indicated.

SPECIFIC CAUSES OF PERICARDIAL EFFUSIONS, EPIDEMIOLOGY, TREATMENT, AND PROGNOSIS

Neoplastic Causes

Cardiac Hemangiosarcoma

- Hemangiosarcoma, a highly malignant neoplasm of vascular endothelium, is the most commonly diagnosed cardiac tumor in dogs. It occurs with an approximately 10-fold greater incidence than the second most common cardiac tumor, aortic body tumors. Primary and metastatic cardiac hemangiosarcoma has been reported in cats, but it is rare in this species.
- At the UMVMC, cardiac hemangiosarcoma was diagnosed either by echocardiography, or echocardiography and histopathology in 53 of 87 dogs

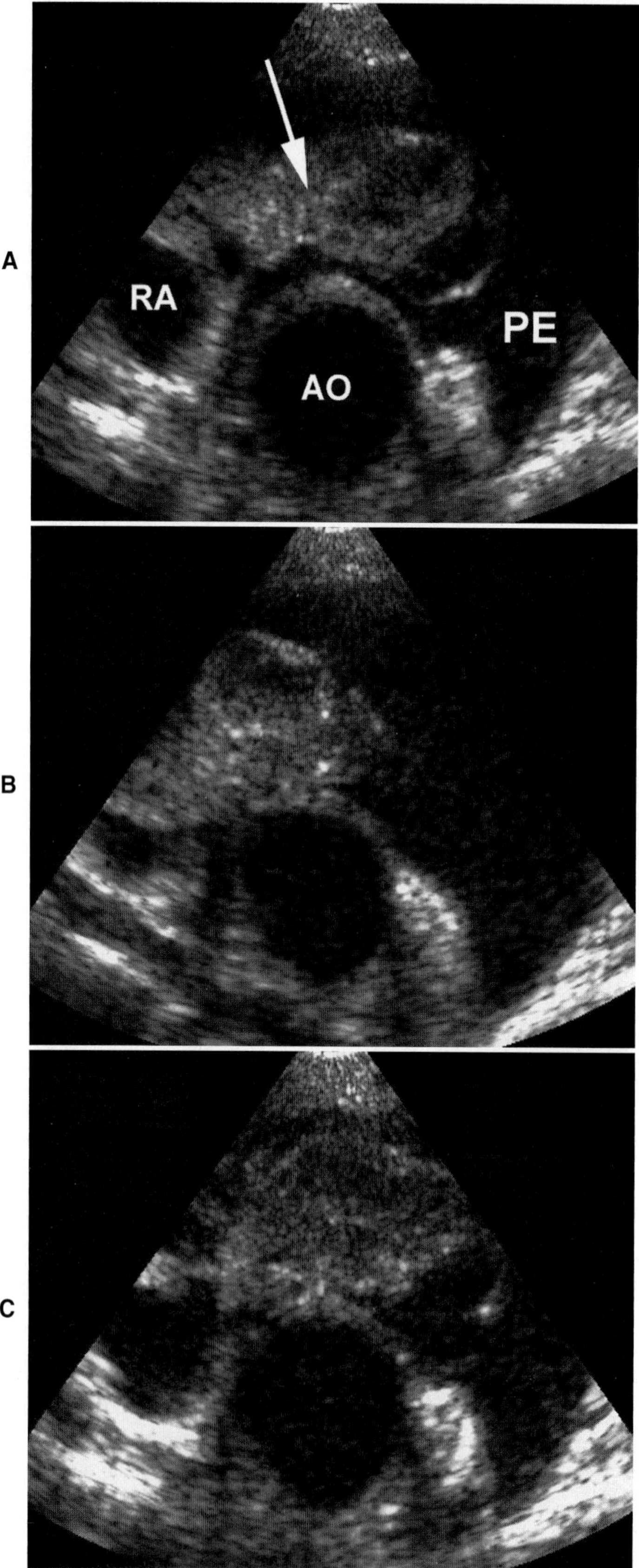

Figure 11-4. Echocardiographic images from a dog with cardiac hemangiosarcoma recorded in the short-axis view from the right parasternal location. **A,** A cavitary and cystic mass *(arrow)* is associated with the right auricle *(RA)*. **B** and **C,** The mass moves back and forth with right auricular motion during different phases of the cardiac cycle. *AO,* Aorta; *PE,* pericardial effusion.

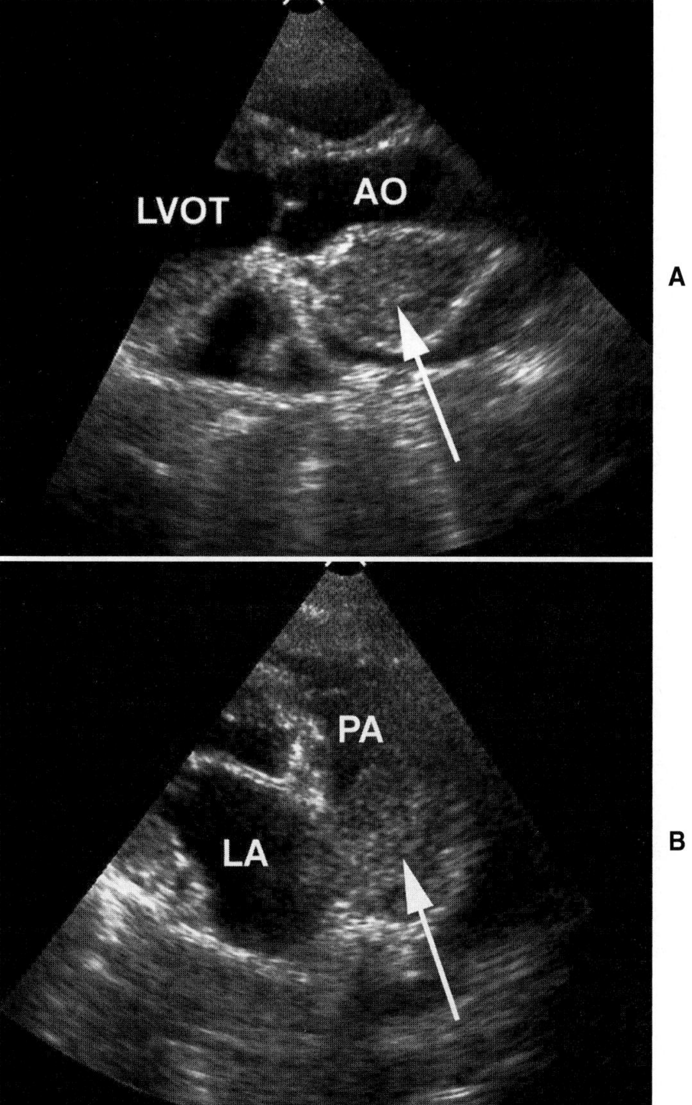

Figure 11-5. Echocardiographic images from a dog with a heart base tumor recorded from the left cranial parasternal location. **A,** A large homogeneous mass *(arrow)* is attached to the caudal aspect of the aorta *(AO).* **B,** The tumor has infiltrated the main pulmonary artery *(PA). LVOT,* Left ventricular outflow tract; *LA,* left atrium.

(61%) in the study population with pericardial effusion. Cardiac hemangiosarcoma with pericardial effusion was nearly three times more prevalent than the second most common form of pericardial effusion, idiopathic pericardial effusion.

- The average age among the affected dogs was 9.8 (±2.1) years, and their average weight was 32.0 (±12.2) kg.
- There was no sex predisposition. Although males outnumbered females (31 [58.5%] males: 22 [41.5%] females), this was not significantly different from the sex distribution among dogs in the general hospital population.
- A total of 16 of the 53 dogs (30%) were Golden Retrievers, and the breed was over-represented (odds ratio, 5.3; 95% confidence interval, 2.9 to 9.4), which is consistent with data from the Veterinary Hospital of the University of Pennsylvania.
- Treatment for all forms of hemangiosarcoma is challenging, and a diagnosis of cardiac hemangiosarcoma confers a grave prognosis. By the time of diagnosis, cardiac hemangiosarcoma usually has metastasized, and it should be considered a systemic disease.
- Many owners of dogs with cardiac hemangiosarcoma elect palliation with pericardiocentesis alone. Pericardiocentesis is predictably associated with marked clinical improvement, but clinical signs of tamponade typically recur within a few days, often resulting in death or prompting euthanasia.

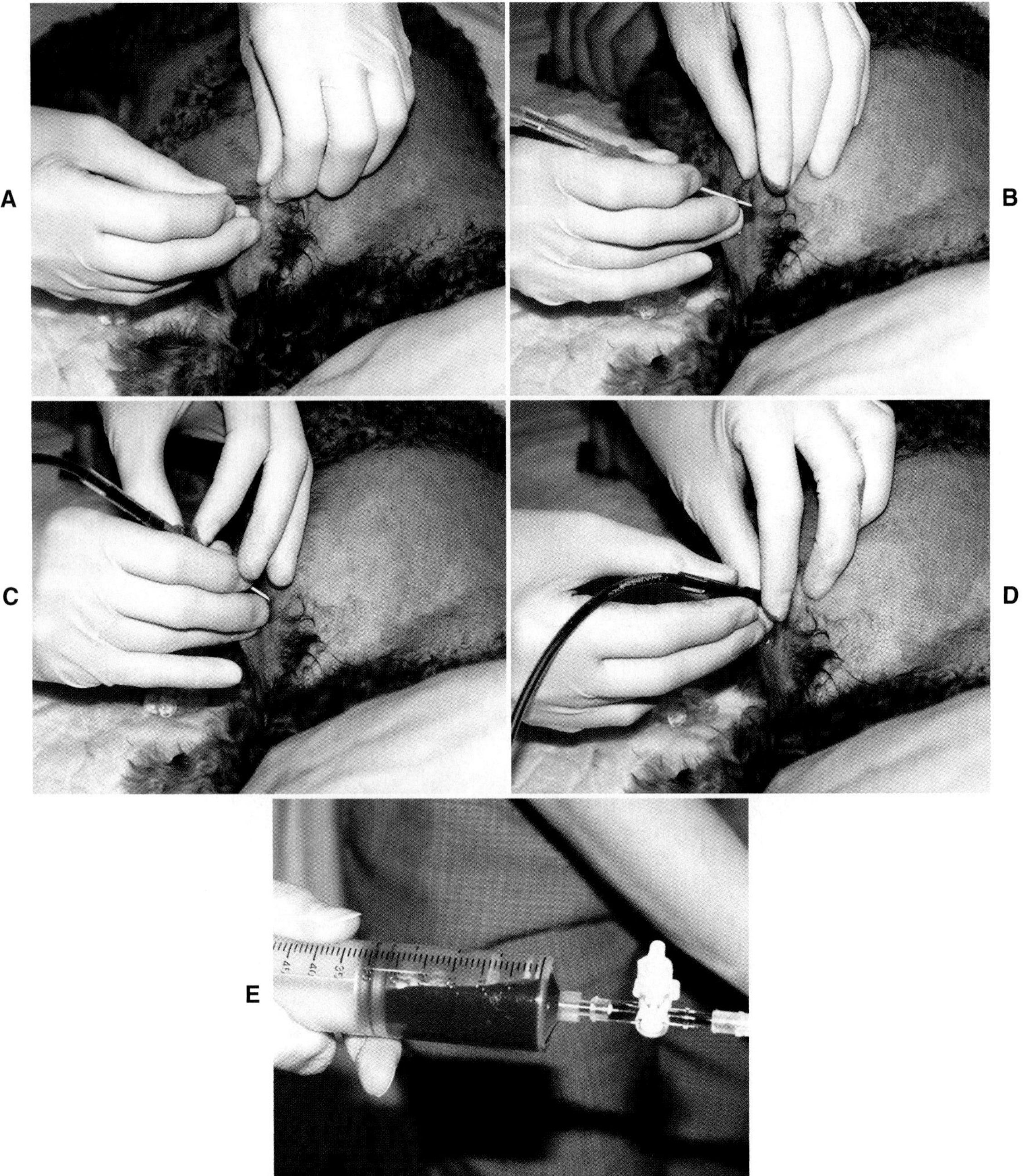

Figure 11-6. Pericardiocentesis in a dog. **A,** A small skin incision is made after local anesthetic has been administered. **B,** An over-the-needle catheter system with 2 side holes is advanced towards the pericardium. Slight negative pressure is applied via a syringe coupled to the needle by extension tubing. **C,** Pericardial fluid flows into the extension tubing, and the catheter is advanced over the needle into the pericardial space. **D,** The extension tubing is removed from the needle and coupled to the catheter. **E,** Pericardial effusion is aspirated. The gross appearance of pericardial effusion is almost invariably sanguinous, irrespective of cause.

- In the UMVMC study population, median survival time for 30 dogs with cardiac hemangiosarcoma that were treated by pericardiocentesis alone on one or more occasions was just 11 days (range, 0 to 208).
- More aggressive approaches to the treatment of cardiac hemangiosarcoma include various combinations of tumor resection, pericardectomy, chemotherapy, and splenectomy in cases with splenic metastases. A recent retrospective study from the University of Pennsylvania reported on 23 cases in which tumor resection was performed. In addition, pericardectomy was performed in 21 of the dogs, 3 had splenectomies, and 8 received adjuvant chemotherapy.

- Median survival time from time of surgery for all 23 cases was 56 days (range, 0 to 229), once again emphasizing the extremely poor prognosis associated with cardiac hemangiosarcoma. Adjuvant chemotherapy following tumor resection may prolong survival in dogs with cardiac hemangiosarcoma, especially with protocols that include doxorubicin. However, the data are not compelling and the survival advantage is small. Nevertheless, management of cardiac hemangiosarcoma should always include consultation with an oncologist to take advantage of continually emerging modalities for the treatment of this highly malignant tumor.

Heart Base Tumors

- The term *heart base tumor* is used to designate any mass located at the base of the heart in association with the ascending aorta and main pulmonary artery. Most heart base tumors in dogs are aortic body tumors, although 5% to 10% of heart base tumors in dogs are thyroid tumors (both adenomas and adenocarcinomas) that arise from ectopic thyroid tissue at the base of the heart. Aortic body tumors have occasionally been reported in cats.
- Heart base tumors were diagnosed either by echocardiography, or echocardiography and histopathology in 6 of the 87 dogs (7%) with pericardial effusion in the UMVMC study population, which is consistent with a recent review of the epidemiology of cardiac tumors in dogs. Despite being the second most common cardiac tumors in dogs, the incidence of aortic body tumors is approximately 10-fold lower than cardiac hemangiosarcoma.
- English Bulldogs, Boxers, and Boston Terriers are predisposed to aortic body tumors, although these tumors also occur in nonbrachycephalic breeds. In various studies, brachycephalic breeds have accounted for between 39% and 85% of dogs with aortic body tumors. Chronic hypoxia induces hyperplasia and neoplasia of chemoreceptors, which may explain the predisposition of brachycephalic breeds to aortic body tumors.
- Among the predisposed breeds, males may be at increased risk for developing aortic body tumors, but differences in sex predisposition are not statistically significant in all studies.
- The age range at time of diagnosis of aortic body tumors is 6 to 15 years, with an average of 10 years.
- Between 5% and 10% of tumors at the heart base are ectopic thyroid tumors.
- Aortic body tumors tend to be slow-growing and locally expansive, but local invasiveness and metastases occur in both dogs and cats. The biologic behavior of ectopic thyroid tumors at the heart base is less well described, and both ectopic thyroid adenomas and adenocarcinomas with metastases have been reported.
- Complete surgical resection of heart base tumors is seldom possible because the tumors are highly vascular, located close to major blood vessels, and usually extensive by the time of diagnosis. However, palliation with pericardectomy alone often results in prolonged survival with an excellent quality of life.
- In a recent retrospective study in dogs with aortic body tumors in which surgery was performed, only pericardectomy had a significant effect on survival, and the survival advantage was remarkable. Median survival time among dogs following pericardectomy was 730 days, whereas median survival time among those that did not have a pericardectomy was only 42 days.

Mesothelioma

- Mesothelioma, a diffuse neoplasm of the pericardium and other serosal surfaces is emerging as an increasingly important cause of pericardial effusion. Mesothelioma was confirmed in 4 of 87 dogs (5%) in the UMVMC study population of dogs with pericardial effusion.
- Average age among the affected cases at time of presentation was 9.5 (±2.2) years, average weight was 37.5 (±11.1) kg, and males and females were equally represented.
- No breed predisposition has been reported, and affected breeds in the UMVMC population were Akita, Golden Retriever, Labrador Retriever, and Springer Spaniel.
- Mesothelioma causing pericardial effusion has been described in a cat, but pericardial mesothelioma is rare in this species.
- The clinical course of pericardial effusion due to mesothelioma in the UMVMC study population followed a characteristic pattern.
  - Presenting and clinical signs were no different from other cause of pericardial effusion. In all four cases, a provisional diagnosis of idiopathic pericardial effusion was made after various diagnostic procedures, including echocardiography and pericardial fluid analysis failed to disclose a cause for the pericardial effusion.
  - Pericardiocentesis was performed, and this was repeated 31 to 133 days later, when the dogs developed recurrent effusions with clinical tamponade.

  - Pericardectomies were then performed in all cases, and histopathology of the excised pericardia was consistent with idiopathic pericarditis in three cases and mesothelioma in one.
  - Severe and unremitting pleural effusions requiring repeated thoracocentesis began 48 to 148 days following pericardectomy.
  - Intracavitary cisplatin was administered in 2 dogs, but this did not appear to significantly change the course of the disease.
  - Thoracocentesis was necessary every 2 to 3 weeks until death or euthanasia, and median survival time from the initial episode of pericardial effusion was 312 days (range, 206 to 352).
  - In all cases, mesothelioma that had spread throughout the thoracic cavity was confirmed on post-mortem examination.
- The signalment and clinical course among cases with pericardial effusion due to mesothelioma in the UMVMC study population are strikingly similar to those described by others. It is extremely difficult to distinguish between idiopathic pericardial effusion and pericardial effusion due to mesothelioma, even with pericardial histopathology and immunohistochemistry. However, accumulations of significant amounts of pleural effusion within 4 to 6 months of pericardectomy increase the index of suspicion for mesothelioma.
- In addition to being a diagnostic challenge, mesothelioma is difficult to treat. However, long-term survival has been reported in a dog in which a histopathological diagnosis of pericardial mesothelioma was made following pericardectomy for recurrent pericardial effusion. Treatment in that case was initiated 48 hours after surgery with intracavitary cisplatin and intravenous doxorubicin, and the dog was free of disease 27 months later.

KEY POINT

Pericardial mesothelioma represents both a diagnostic and therapeutic challenge. Unlike other cardiac tumors, mesothelioma does not form discrete tumor masses that are readily detectable using echocardiography. Even with pericardial biopsy with histopathology, the diagnosis may be elusive, and only after recurrent pleural or pericardial effusions result in mortality and post-mortem examination is the diagnosis confirmed.

Other Cardiac Tumors

- Cardiac lymphosarcoma, rhabdomyosarcoma, and fibrosarcoma with pericardial effusion have been reported in both dogs and cats. Cardiac lymphosarcoma is diagnosed in approximately 1% of dogs with pericardial effusion, whereas rhabdomyosarcoma and fibrosarcoma are rare. Among the various cardiac tumors, cardiac lymphosarcoma is unique because cytology of the pericardial fluid establishes the diagnosis in many cases and the tumor is amenable to combination chemotherapy.

Infections

- Bacterial, fungal, and viral infections are occasionally associated with pericardial effusions in small animals.
- Most cases of pericardial effusions due to bacterial infections are thought to arise as a consequence of intrapericardial foreign body penetration, usually by migrating foxtails (*Hordeum* spp.). In contrast to most other causes of pericardial effusion, pericardial fluid cytology and culture is crucial for the diagnosis of infectious cases. In the largest series of bacterial pericarditis reported in dogs (5 cases), treatment involved pericardectomy and removal of any foreign bodies, chest drainage, and antibiotic therapy for up to 6 months. All dogs recovered without complications, suggesting that dogs with bacterial pericarditis have a good prognosis when treated aggressively with a combination of surgical and medical therapy.
- Systemic coccidioidomycosis in dogs is occasionally associated with pericardial disease. In most cases the fungal infection results in effusive-constrictive or constrictive pericarditis. Coccidioidomycosis should be considered especially in dogs with pericardial disease that reside in or have a travel history that includes areas where the soil fungus *Coccidioides immitis* is endemic, such as the southwestern United States. Treatment involves pericardectomy, chest drainage, and anti-fungal therapy (usually beginning with Amphotericin B). Based on limited published information and experience, the prognosis for cases of coccidioidomycosis with pericardial involvement is guarded. A single case of effusive-constrictive pericarditis due to *Aspergillus niger* has been reported in a dog.
- Feline infectious peritonitis is occasionally associated with pericardial effusion in the cat. Voluminous pericardial effusion may be present in some cats suffering from this systemic and invariably fatal viral disease.

Hemorrhage

- Left atrial perforation is an uncommon cause of pericardial effusion that occurs in smaller breed dogs with chronic degenerative valve disease. At the UMVMC, left atrial perforation is diagnosed in approximately 1% of dogs with pericardial effusion. Affected cases have a history consistent with acute pericardial effusion, and a loud left apical murmur is usually apparent despite muffling of the heart sounds. Echocardiography discloses intrapericardial fluid, a mobile thrombus caudal to the left ventricle, and substantial mitral regurgitation. We have diagnosed left atrial perforation in several dogs following an episode of weakness or collapse. In many of these cases, the dog is either recovering or clinically normal by the time of their echocardiogram, and relatively little pericardial fluid and only mild echocardiographic evidence of tamponade is demonstrated. In such cases, we provide no therapy other than congestive heart failure medications if appropriate (i.e., for cases with left-sided congestive heart failure due to mitral regurgitation). Repeat echocardiograms 7 to 10 days later have demonstrated complete resolution of both the pericardial effusion and the intrapericardial thrombus. On the other hand, pericardiocentesis is required for cases with left atrial perforation that are hemodynamically compromised as a result of tamponade. Furthermore, the possibility of continued hemorrhage exists, necessitating blood transfusion and thoracotomy to remove larger clots from the pericardial space and to repair the left atrium. The prognosis in such cases is grave.
- Pericardial effusions secondary to coagulation disorders are rare causes of clinically significant tamponade. A single case of pericardial effusion and cardiac tamponade secondary to anticoagulant rodenticide toxicity has been reported in a dog. Pericardial effusions secondary to disseminated intravascular coagulation, warfarin toxicity, and other coagulopathies have been reported in cats.

Miscellaneous

- Pericardial effusion is frequently detected in both dogs and cats with congestive heart failure, but usually not in sufficient quantity to cause significant hemodynamic compromise.
- Pericardial effusion secondary to uremia has been recognized in small animals.
- A case of cholesterol-based pericardial effusion has been reported in a dog with hypothyroidism.
- Pericardial effusions associated with intrapericardial foreign bodies (e.g., pellets) are occasionally seen.

Idiopathic Causes

Idiopathic Pericardial Effusion

- Idiopathic pericardial effusion is a diagnosis of exclusion. It is made in cases with pericardial effusion where no intrapericardial masses are identified after thorough echocardiographic evaluation, and the results of ancillary tests such as pericardial fluid analysis fail to disclose an etiology. Pericardial histopathology and immunohistochemistry from dogs with idiopathic pericardial effusion demonstrate changes consistent with pericarditis of undetermined etiology.
- As with any diagnoses of exclusion, a diagnosis of idiopathic pericardial effusion should be made cautiously.
  - Small intrapericardial tumors may elude detection, especially in cases where echocardiography is performed following pericardiocentesis.
  - Mesothelioma does not result in appreciable thickening of the pericardium on echocardiography. Routine cytology of pericardial effusion does not distinguish between idiopathic pericardial effusion and mesothelioma. Consequently, mesothelioma should always be considered as an important differential diagnosis for idiopathic pericardial effusion.
  - Idiopathic pericardial effusion has not been reported in cats.
- Idiopathic pericardial effusion was diagnosed in 8 of 42 dogs (19%) with pericardial effusion in a retrospective study from the Veterinary Teaching Hospital, Colorado State University. Idiopathic pericardial effusion was provisionally diagnosed in 24 of 87 dogs with pericardial effusion in the UMVMC study population, but mesothelioma was subsequently confirmed in 4 of these cases. Thus, 20 of the 87 cases (23%) with pericardial effusion were finally diagnosed as having idiopathic pericardial effusion, which is similar to the Colorado State University data.
  - Average age among the cases with idiopathic pericardial effusion in the UMVMC study population was 9.4 (±2.2) years, average weight was 28.9 (±14.5) kg, and there was no apparent sex predisposition (11 [55%] males to 9 [45%] females).
  - Five of the 20 dogs (25%) were Golden Retrievers, and the breed was over-represented (odds ratio, 4.2; 95% confidence interval, 1.6 to 11.2).

- We have frequently treated first episodes of idiopathic pericardial effusion by pericardiocentesis alone, followed by pericardectomy in cases that develop recurrent effusions. However, the UMVMC data show that:
  - Tamponade recurs in approximately one third of dogs with idiopathic pericardial effusion within a month or two.
  - Virtually all remaining cases develop recurrent tamponade, often with effusive-constrictive pericarditis, within 3 years of pericardiocentesis.
- Consequently, the authors currently recommend surgical or minimally invasive thoracoscopic pericardectomy with the initial episode of idiopathic pericardial effusion. Although pericardectomy is by no means devoid of morbidity and mortality, it is an extremely successful procedure for idiopathic pericardial effusion. Pericardectomy avoids the risk of recurrent life-threatening cardiac tamponade and the potential for developing effusive-constrictive and constrictive pericarditis. In addition, surgical pericardectomy permits examination of thoracic and intrapericardial structures to rule out other causes of pericardial effusion, including tumors and foreign bodies.
- Colchicine, nonsteroidal anti-inflammatories, and corticosteroids are prescribed for humans with recurrent idiopathic pericarditis. Colchicine and nonsteroidal anti-inflammatories are recommended in most cases, and the use of corticosteroids is limited to very severe cases. Colchicine for the treatment of recurrent pericarditis in humans is promising, although data from large controlled prospective studies are lacking. The safety and efficacy of colchicine, nonsteroidal anti-inflammatories, corticosteroids, and any other medical therapies in the management of idiopathic pericardial effusion in small animals have yet to be established.

SUMMARY AND CONCLUSIONS

- Pericardial effusions causing clinical tamponade are common in dogs and Golden Retrievers are over-represented.
- Chief complaints, histories, and physical examination findings in dogs with pericardial effusions are diverse and often vague.
- Whereas thoracic radiography and electrocardiography may be helpful to diagnose the presence of pericardial effusion, echocardiography is the most sensitive and specific procedure to confirm its presence.
- The great majority of dogs with pericardial effusion have an associated cardiac tumor, of which hemangiosarcoma is the most common.
- Echocardiography is the method of choice to detect cardiac tumors, and the procedure should be performed before pericardiocentesis whenever the clinical condition of the patient permits.
- Pericardiocentesis provides initial patient stabilization. Pericardiocentesis alone is rarely, if ever, curative.
- Pericardial fluid analysis and cytology will only occasionally provide a definite diagnosis of the cause of pericardial effusion.
- Depending on the underlying cause, the prognoses for cases with pericardial effusions vary from grave to excellent. Pericardectomy forms part or all of the therapy in virtually all cases that have prolonged, disease-free survival.

Frequently Asked Questions

Why do dogs with pericardial effusion develop pulsus paradoxus?

Pulses paradoxus refers to the phasic change in peripheral arterial pulse quality that corresponds to the patient's phase of respiration. Dogs demonstrating pulsus paradoxus have stronger pulse quality during expiration and weaker or absent pulses during inspiration. Pulsus paradoxus is due to the limitation to cardiac filling imposed by the presence of significant pericardial effusion. When the dog inspires, intrathoracic pressure falls and increases venous return to the thorax and right side of the heart. The right heart is constrained by the presence of the pericardial effusion and right heart filling occurs at the expense of left heart volume. This phenomenon causes left heart volume and output to fall during inspiration, which produces poor systemic arterial pulse quality. The opposite effect occurs during expiration and quality of the systemic arterial pulses increases.

What are the primary clinical signs in a dog with clinically significant pericardial effusion?

Commonly, dogs with significant pericardial effusion present with three cardinal signs, historically referred to as Beck's triad. These signs include muffled heart sounds, weak femoral pulses, and jugular venous distension. Careful examination of dogs suspect for pericardial effusion usually reveals the presence of all three components of the triad. Successful inspection of the jugular veins sometimes necessitates shaving the hair from the patient's jugular groove in order to properly visualize the vein. Inspection of the jugular vein should be done with the patient standing. The finding of jugular venous distension is a quick and reliable way to help distinguish cardiac versus noncardiac causes of abdominal effusion that is often overlooked.

What are the advantages and disadvantages of surgical versus thorascopic pericardectomy?
Surgical pericardectomy using a median sternotomy allows for complete resection of the ventral two thirds of the pericardial sac. The surgical approach allows for visual inspection of the heart base and right heart in an attempt to identify small tumors that may have been undetected during cardiac ultrasound. The disadvantages of the surgical approach include increased invasiveness, morbidity, cost, and length of hospital stay as opposed to thorascopy. Thorascopy is best performed in larger dogs and enables the operator to cut a "window" into the lateral or apical pericardial surface. A lesser amount of pericardium is removed during the thorascopic technique as opposed to the subtotal pericardectomy, but resealing of the pericardium after window procedures is rare. The main disadvantage of the thorascopic procedure is the limited ability to inspect the heart base and right heart for small tumors that may have been undetected during cardiac ultrasound. Biopsy of the pericardial tissue can be accomplished using either technique.

SUGGESTED READINGS

Adler Y, Finkelstein Y, Guindo J, et al: Colchicine treatment for recurrent pericarditis: a decade of experience, Circulation 97:2183, 1998.

Alleman AR: Abdominal, thoracic, and pericardial effusions, Vet Clin Small Anim Pract 33:89, 2003.

Aronsohn MG, Carpenter JL: Surgical treatment of idiopathic pericardial effusion in the dog: 25 cases (1978-1993), J Am Anim Hosp Assoc 35:521, 1999.

Aronson AR, Gregory CR: Infectious pericardial effusion in five dogs, Vet Surg 24:402, 1995.

Balli A, Lachat M, Gerber B, et al: Cardiac tamponade due to pericardial mesothelioma in an 11-year-old dog: diagnosis, medical and interventional treatments, Schweizer Archiv fur Tierheilkunde 145:82, 2003.

Berg RJ, Wingfield W: Pericardial effusion in the dog: a review of 42 cases, J Am Anim Hosp Assoc 20:721, 1983.

Bonagura JD: Electrical alternans associated with pericardial effusion in the dog, J Am Vet Med Assoc 178:574, 1981.

Buergelt CD, Das KM: Aortic body tumor in a cat, Pathologia Veterinaria 5:84, 1968.

Capen CC: Tumors of the endocrine glands. In Moulton JE, ed: Tumors in domestic animals, ed 2, Berkeley, 1978, University of California Press.

Carpenter DH Jr, Mackin AJ, Gellasch KL: Cardiac tamponade secondary to *Aspergillus niger*–induced constrictive pericarditis, J Am Vet Med Assoc 218:1890, 2001.

Cho KO, Park NY, Park JC, et al: Metastatic intracavitary cardiac aortic body tumor in a dog, J Vet Med Sci 60:1251, 1998.

Churg A, Colby TV, Cagle P, et al: The separation of benign and malignant mesothelial proliferations, Am J Surg Path 24:1183, 2000.

Closa JM, Font A, Mascort J: Pericardial mesothelioma in a dog: long-term survival after pericardiectomy in combination with chemotherapy, J Small Anim Pract 40:383, 1999.

Cobb MA, Brownlie SE: Intrapericardial neoplasia in 14 dogs, J Small Anim Pract 33:309, 1992.

Constantino-Casas P, Rodriguez-Martinez HA, Guterrez Diaz-Ceballos ME: A case report and review: the gross, histological, and immunohistochemical characteristics of a carcinoma of ectopic thyroid in a dog, Br Vet J 152:669, 1996.

Day MJ, Martin MWS: Immunohistochemical characterization of the lesions of canine idiopathic pericarditis, J Small Anim Pract 43:383, 2002.

Dunning D, Monnet E, Orton EC, et al: Analysis of prognostic indicators for dogs with pericardial effusion: 46 cases (1985-1996), J Am Vet Med Assoc 212:1276, 1998.

Ehrhart N, Ehrhart EJ, Willis J, et al: Analysis of factors affecting survival in dogs with aortic body tumors, Vet Surg 31:44, 2002.

Fine DM, Tobias AH, Jacob KA: Use of pericardial fluid pH to distinguish between idiopathic and neoplastic effusions, J Vet Intern Med 17:525, 2003.

George C, Steinberg H: An aortic body carcinoma with multifocal thoracic metastases in a cat, J Compar Pathol 101:467, 1989.

Gliatto JM, Crawford MA, Snider TG III, et al: Multiple organ metastasis of an aortic body tumor in a boxer, J Am Vet Med Assoc 191:1110, 1987.

Gonin-Jmaa D, Paulsen DB, Taboada J: Pericardial effusion in a dog with rhabdomyosarcoma in the right ventricular wall, J Small Anim Pract 37:193, 1996.

Hayes HM, Sass B: Chemoreceptor neoplasia: a study of the epidemiological features of 357 canine cases, J Vet Med 35:401, 1988.

Heinritz CK, Gilson SD, Soderstrom MJ, et al: Subtotal pericardectomy and epicardial excision for treatment of coccidioidomycosis-induced effusive-constrictive pericarditis in dogs: 17 cases (1999-2003), J Am Vet Med Assoc 227:435, 2005.

Holt D, Van Winkle T, Schelling C, et al: Correlation between thoracic radiographs and findings in dogs with hemangiosarcoma: 77 cases (1984-1989), J Am Vet Med Assoc 200:1535, 1992.

Jackson J, Richter KP, Launer DP: Thoracoscopic partial pericardectomy in 13 dogs, J Vet Intern Med 13:529, 1999.

Johnson KH: Aortic body tumors in the dog, J Am Vet Med Assoc 152:154, 1968.

Keene BW, Rush JE, Cooley AJ, et al: Primary left ventricular hemangiosarcoma diagnosed by endomyocardial biopsy in a dog, J Am Vet Med Assoc 197:1501, 1990.

Kerstetter KK, Krahwinkel DJ Jr, Millis DL, et al: Pericardiectomy in dogs: 22 cases (1978-1994), J Am Vet Med Assoc 211:736, 1997.

MacGregor JM, Faria MLE, Moore AS, et al: Cardiac lymphoma causing pericardial effusion in 12 dogs, J Am Vet Med Assoc 227:1449, 2005.

MacGregor JM, Rozanski EA, McCarthy RJ, et al: Cholesterol-based pericardial effusion and aortic thromboembolism in a 9-year-old mixed-breed dog with hypothyroidism, J Vet Intern Med 18:354, 2004.

Maisch B, Ristic AD, Seferovic PM: New directions in the diagnosis and treatment of pericardial disease: a project of the taskforce on pericardial disease of the World Heart Federation, Herz 25:769, 2000.

Mathiesen DT, Lammerding J: Partial pericardectomy for idiopathic pericardial effusion in the dog, J Am Anim Hosp Assoc 21:41, 1985.

McDonough SP, MacLauglin NJ, Tobias AH: Canine pericardial mesothelioma, Vet Pathol 29:256, 1992.

Merlo M, Bo S, Ratto A: Primary right atrium hemangiosarcoma in a cat, J Feline Med Surg 4:61, 2002.

Owen TJ, Bruyette DS, Layton CE: Chemodectoma in dogs, Compend Cont Ed Practic Vet 18:253, 1996.

Petrus DJ, Henik RA: Pericardial effusion and cardiac tamponade secondary to brodifacoum toxicosis in a dog, J Am Vet Med Assoc 215:647, 1999.

Prosek R, Sisson DD, Oyama MA: Pericardial effusion with a clot in the pericardial space likely caused by left atrial rupture secondary to mitral regurgitation, J Am Vet Med Assoc 222:441, 2003.

Rush JE, Keene BW, Fox PR: Pericardial disease in the cat: a retrospective evaluation of 66 cases, J Am Anim Hosp Assoc 26:39, 1990.

Sadanaga KK, MacDonald MJ, Buchanan JW: Echocardiography and surgery in a dog with left atrial rupture and hemopericardium, J Vet Intern Med 4:216, 1990.

Shubitz LF, Matz ME, Noon TH, et al: Constrictive pericarditis secondary to *Coccidioides immitis* infection in a dog, J Amer Vet Med Assoc 218:537, 2001.

Sims CS, Tobias AH, Hayden DW, et al: Pericardial effusion due to primary cardiac lymphoma in a dog, J Vet Intern Med 17:923, 2003.

Sisson D, Thomas WP, Reed J, et al: Intrapericardial cysts in the dog, J Vet Intern Med 7:364, 1993.

Sisson D, Thomas WP, Ruehl WW, et al: Diagnostic value of pericardial fluid analysis in the dog, J Am Vet Med Assoc 184:51, 1984.

Speltz MC, Manivel JC, Tobias AH, et al: Primary cardiac fibrosarcoma in a Labrador retriever, Vet Pathol 44:403, 2007.

Stephens LC, Saunders WJ, Jaenke RS: Ectopic thyroid carcinoma with metastases in a Beagle dog, Vet Pathol 19:669, 1982.

Stepien RL, Whitley NT, Dubielzig RR: Idiopathic or mesothelioma-related pericardial effusion: clinical findings and survival in 17 dogs studied retrospectively, J Small Anim Pract 41:342, 2000.

Thake DC, Cheville NF, Sharp RK: Ectopic thyroid adenomas at the base of the heart of the dog, Vet Pathol 8:421, 1971.

Tilley LP, Owen JM, Wilkens RJ, et al: Pericardial mesothelioma in a cat, J Am Anim Hosp Assoc 11:60, 1975.

Tobias AH: Pericardial disorders. In Ettinger SJ, Feldman EC, eds: Textbook of veterinary internal medicine, ed 6, St Louis, 2005, WB Saunders.

Walsh KM, Diters RW: Carcinoma of ectopic thyroid in a dog, J Am Anim Hosp Assoc 20:665, 1983.

Walsh PJ, Remedios AM, Ferguson JF, et al: Thoracoscopic versus open partial pericardectomy in dogs: comparison of postoperative pain and morbidity, Vet Surg 28:472, 1999.

Ware WA, Hopper DL: Cardiac tumors in dogs: 1982-1995, J Vet Intern Med 13:95, 1999.

Weisse C, Soares N, Beal MW, et al: Survival time in dogs with right atrial hemangiosarcoma treated by means of surgical resection with or without adjuvant chemotherapy: 23 cases (1986-2000), J Am Vet Med Assoc 226:575, 2005.

Willis R, Williams AE, Schwarz T, et al: Aortic body chemodectoma causing pulmonary oedema in a cat, J Small Anim Pract 42:20, 2001.

Yates WD, Lester SJ, Mills JH: Chemoreceptor tumors diagnosed at the Western College of Veterinary Medicine: 1967-1979, Can Vet J 21:124, 1980.

CHAPTER 12

Congenital Heart Disease

Keith N. Strickland

INTRODUCTION

Incidence

- The incidence of congenital heart disease in dogs has been reported to be 6.8 to 8.0 per 1000 hospital admissions. On average, this equates to one case per 15 litters. The actual incidence is likely higher, as some defects result in neonatal death and are unreported.
- The most common congenital heart defects in dogs include patent ductus arteriosus (PDA), pulmonic stenosis (PS), aortic stenosis, ventricular septal defect (VSD), and tetralogy of Fallot (Box 12-1). Several breed predispositions have been identified (see Appendix 1: Canine Breed Predilections for Heart Disease).
- Less common defects in dogs include mitral valve dysplasia, atrial septal defects, tricuspid valve dysplasia, cor triatriatum dexter, and mitral stenosis. Rare defects include persistent truncus arteriosus, tricuspid stenosis, right ventricular hypoplasia, double outlet right ventricle, and transposition of the great vessels.
- Congenital heart disease is less common in cats than in dogs. The reported incidence is 0.2 to 1.0 per 1000 hospital admissions. No consistent breed or gender predilections have been adequately demonstrated.
- The most common congenital heart defects in cats include mitral valve dysplasia, tricuspid valve dysplasia, PDA, VSD, aortic stenosis, tetralogy of Fallot, persistent common atrioventricular canal, and endocardial fibroelastosis.
- Less common defects in cats include persistent truncus arteriosus, PS, atrial septal defect, tricuspid stenosis, and right ventricular hypoplasia.

Hereditary Aspects

- Congenital heart diseases are the most common type of heart disease in young dogs and cats, but are occasionally diagnosed in adult animals.
- Congenital heart defects are generally recognized in the young animal and usually represent a heritable trait or a defect that originated during gestation. A primary genetic mutation or environmental influences may exist, resulting in significant variation of disease severity.
- Four common forms of congenital heart disease have been shown to be inherited in dogs:
  - PDA in the Poodle
  - Subaortic stenosis in the Newfoundland
  - Tetralogy of Fallot in the Keeshond
  - PS in the Beagle

Diagnosis

- Generally, a congenital heart defect is suspected when a heart murmur is detected in a young dog or cat (Table 12-1).
- Other supporting clinical features may include:
  - Failure to thrive
  - Exercise intolerance
  - Cyanosis
  - Collapse or seizure

Box 12-1 Classification of Congenital Defects According to Pathophysiology

CANINE

Defects primarily causing volume overload

Systemic to pulmonary (left-to-right) shunting

Common
- Patent ductus arteriosus
- Ventricular septal defect

Uncommon
- Atrial septal defect
- Endocardial cushion defect
- (Pseudo) truncus arteriosus

Valvular regurgitation

Common
- Mitral dysplasia
- Tricuspid dysplasia

Uncommon
- Pulmonic insufficiency
- Aortic insufficiency

Defects primarily causing pressure overload

Common
- Pulmonic stenosis
- Subaortic stenosis

Uncommon
- Valvular aortic stenosis
- Coarctation and interruption of the aorta
- Cor triatriatum dexter

Defects primarily causing cyanosis

Common
- Tetralogy of Fallot

Uncommon
- Pulmonary to systemic shunting (ventricular septal defect [VSD])
- Pulmonary to systemic shunting (patent ductus arteriosus [PDA])
- Tricuspid atresia/right ventricular hypoplasia
- Double outlet right ventricle
- Transposition of the great vessels
- Truncus arteriosus
- Aorticopulmonary window

Miscellaneous cardiac and vascular defects

Common
- Peritoneopericardial diapharagmatic hernia
- Persistent right aortic arch
- Persistent left cranial vena cava

Uncommon
- Endocardial fibroelastosis
- Pericardial defects
- Anomalous pulmonary venous return
- Double aortic arch
- Retroesophageal left subclavian artery
- Situs inversus

FELINE

Defects primarily causing volume overload

Common
- Ventricular septal defect
- Patent ductus arteriosus
- Atrial septal defect
- Endocardial cushion defect

Uncommon
- Truncus arteriosus

Valvular regurgitation

Common
- Mitral dysplasia
- Tricuspid dysplasia

Defects primarily causing pressure overload

Common
- Dynamic subaortic stenosis

Uncommon
- Pulmonic stenosis
- Pulmonary artery branch stenosis
- Fixed subaortic stenosis
- Valvular aortic stenosis
- Cor triatriatum dexter
- Cor triatriatum sinister

Defects primarily causing cyanosis

Common
- Tetralogy of Fallot
- Endocardial cushion defect

Uncommon
- Pulmonary to systemic shunting (VSD)
- Pulmonary to systemic shunting (PDA)
- Double outlet right ventricle
- Truncus arteriosus

Miscellaneous cardiac and vascular defects

Common
- Peritoneopericardial diapharagmatic hernia
- Endocardial fibroelastosis

Uncommon
- Persistent right aortic arch

Table 12-1 Auscultatory Findings in Congenital Heart Disease

Lesion	Timing	Features	Point of Maximum Intensity	Comments
Atrial septal defect	Systolic (diastolic)	Ejection (diastolic rumble)	Left base	Systolic murmur ends prior to S_2, which is usually split; murmur (or murmurs) due to relative pulmonic (tricuspid) stenosis
(Sub) aortic stenosis	Systolic*	Ejection (crescendo-decrescendo)	Left base	Often nearly as loud at the right base; diastolic murmur of aortic regurgitation may also occur
Mitral valve dysplasia†	Systolic	Regurgitant (holosystolic)	Left apex	May radiate widely
Patent ductus arteriosus	Continuous	Machinery	Left base	Murmur peaks at S_2, often radiates to right base and thoracic inlet
Pulmonary hypertension (Eisenmenger's syndrome)	None (systolic)	Split S_2 (ejection)	Left base	Accentuated and split S2; systolic murmur of tricuspid regurgitation or blowing, decrescendo diastolic murmur of pulmonic regurgitation may also occur
Pulmonic stenosis	Systolic	Ejection (crescendo-decrescendo)	Left base	Occasional systolic ejection sound; blowing, decrescendo diastolic murmur of pulmonic regurgitation may occur
Tetralogy of Fallot	Systolic	Ejection (crescendo-decrescendo)	Left base	Murmur due to pulmonic stenosis; may be soft or absent with pulmonary artery hypoplasia
Tricuspid valve dysplasia†	Systolic	Regurgitant (holosystolic)	Right midprecordium	Often low pitched and rumbling
Ventricular septal defect	Systolic*	Regurgitant (holosystolic)	Right base	Often higher pitched and more cranially located than tricuspid regurgitation; may also be loud at left base

From Ettinger SE, Feldman EF: Texbook of veterinary internal medicine, ed 6, St Louis, 2005, WB Saunders.
*At times a diastolic murmur of aortic regurgitation may also be present.
†Mitral stenosis and tricuspid stenosis are rare but may cause diastolic murmurs over the affected valve and ventricle.
PMI, Point of maximum intensity.

    • Jugular venous distention
    • Electrocardiographic (ECG) abnormalities
    • Radiographic evidence of cardiac enlargement.
- A tentative diagnosis can be made based on results of a complete cardiovascular physical examination, routine ECG, and radiography (see Table 12-1).
- The specific diagnosis is confirmed in most cases by echocardiography, and rarely by cardiac catheterization. Information obtained echocardiographically is also helpful in determining the severity of the defect, especially if Doppler techniques are used (measurement of blood velocities within the heart).

Therapy

- Advances since the early 1990s allow for the treatment of certain stenotic lesions by balloon valvuloplasty, a technique employing a small balloon located at the end of a cardiac catheter, and

transcatheter occlusion of PDA using a Gianturco coil or similar device. Surgical correction or palliation is possible for certain defects.
- Medical treatment is primarily for the control or prevention of complications, such as congestive heart failure, arrhythmias, and endocarditis, rather than for correction of the defect. Medical therapy is discussed briefly in this chapter.

INNOCENT (FUNCTIONAL) MURMUR

Not all young dogs and cats with heart murmurs have congenital heart disease. Innocent, or functional, murmurs are created by mild turbulence within the heart and great vessels and usually diminish in intensity or resolve by 4 to 5 months of age. The following characteristics of innocent murmurs help differentiate them from pathologic murmurs.

- Innocent murmurs are systolic in timing, usually occurring early in systole and of short duration (ejection-type). They are "soft" (i.e., grade III/VI or less in intensity) and often have a low-pitched, vibrating, or musical quality.
- Innocent murmurs are usually loudest along the left sternal border and are poorly transmitted. Their intensity may vary with changes in position, with the phase of respiration, with exercise, and from day to day.
- The most important characteristic of the innocent murmur is that it is heard in the absence of any other demonstrable evidence of cardiovascular disease (e.g., lack of clinical signs or radiographic abnormalities).
- Loud systolic murmurs (grade IV/VI or greater), precordial thrills, and diastolic murmurs are indicative of cardiac disease and should prompt further diagnostics.

SPECIFIC DEFECTS

Patent Ductus Arteriosus

- In fetal circulation, the ductus arteriosus serves to shunt maternally oxygenated blood into the aorta, thereby bypassing the nonfunctional lungs. Shortly after birth, several factors contribute to effect closure of the ductus. Pulmonary vascular resistance drops dramatically, vasodilatory prostaglandin levels decrease, and oxygen tension increases, resulting in a marked increase in pulmonary blood flow and vasoconstriction of the ductus. Following closure by vasoconstriction, the ductus is permanently closed by fibrous contracture, which produces the ligamentum arteriosum. Failure of the ductus to close is termed *patent ductus arteriosus (PDA)* or *persistent ductus arteriosus*.

Pathophysiology

- The consequences of a PDA depend primarily on the diameter of the ductus and the pulmonary vascular resistance.
- When pulmonary vascular resistance is normal, blood continually shunts from the aorta (high resistance) into the pulmonary circulation (low resistance). Shunting in this fashion (systemic to pulmonary) is referred to as left-to-right and represents the most common pattern in PDA (Figure 12-1).
- When pulmonary vascular resistance increases and exceeds systemic vascular resistance, blood will shunt from the pulmonary artery into the aorta (so-called right-to-left or reversed PDA).
- Failure of ductal closure is due to an abnormal amount of elastic fibers compared to contractile smooth muscle fibers (so-called extension of the noncontractile wall structure of the aorta into the ductus arteriosus). Varying amounts of normal smooth muscle causes varying degrees of ductal closure; this creates a structure that ranges from a funnel-shaped ductus that narrows on the pulmonary artery side of the ductus (Figure 12-2) to a tubelike structure without narrowing.
- Blood flow through the ductus is also dependent upon ductal diameter. With a small ductus, the volume of blood shunted is restricted and there may be no hemodynamic effects. In cases with a large ductus and significant shunting, one of two major consequences usually occurs. In most cases, volume overloading of the left atrium and left ventricle results in eventual left-sided failure. In the largest of shunts, the excessive pulmonary blood flow induces dramatic increases in pulmonary vascular resistance, pulmonary hypertension and shunt reversal (Eisenmenger's physiology).

Diagnosis

Etiology and Breed Disposition

- PDA occurs in both the dog and cat, with higher frequency in the dog. There is also a higher frequency in the female.
- Breeds predisposed or at increased risk include Bichon Frisé, Chihuahua, Cocker Spaniel, Collie, English Springer Spaniel, German Shepherd,

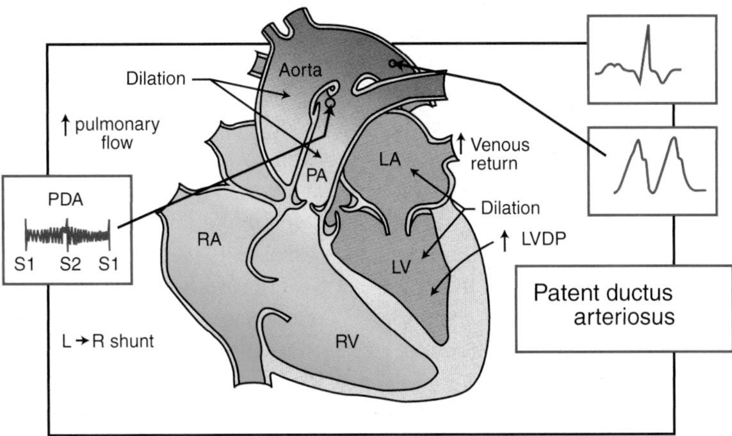

Figure 12-1. Pathophysiology and genesis of clinical findings in PDA. (Modified from Fox PR, Sisson D, Moise N, eds: Textbook of canine and feline cardiology: principles and clinical practice, ed 2, Philadelphia, 1999, WB Saunders.)

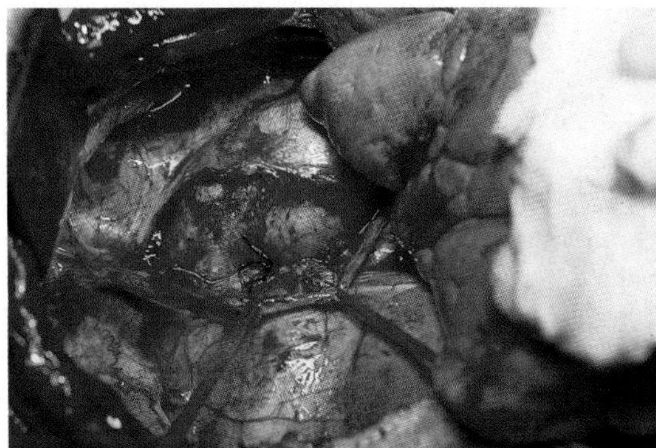

Figure 12-2. Postmortem specimen from a young German Shepherd of the transverse and proximal descending aorta on top, the pulmonary artery branches ventrally, and a left-to-right shunting patent ductus arteriosus between them. The aortic end of the PDA is wide open. The pulmonary artery end is partially constricted. This results in a funnel shape to the PDA. (From Kittleson MD, Kienle RD, eds: Small animal cardiovascular medicine, St Louis, 1998, Mosby. Courtesy Dr. Mark Rishniw.)

Keeshond, Labrador Retriever, Maltese, Newfoundland, Poodle, Pomeranian, Shetland Sheepdog, and Yorkshire Terrier.

- The defect has been shown to be inherited in the Miniature Poodle, transmitted as a polygenic trait.

History and Clinical Signs

- Clinical signs are related to the degree of shunting and may range from none to severe congestive heart failure.
- Depending on the degree of heart failure, owners may report signs such as cough, labored breathing, exercise intolerance, and collapse. Reports of seizures and cyanosis are suggestive of a right-to-left shunting PDA.
- Cats seldom display signs of cardiac failure until decompensation is advanced and life threatening.

Physical Examination

Palpation

- Water-hammer, or bounding, arterial pulses are usually present in animals with left-to-right shunting PDA. This type of pulse represents a widened pulse pressure secondary to the loss of diastolic pressure through the ductus, and elevation of systolic blood pressure from the volume-overloaded left ventricle. Usually, the larger the ductus (and therefore the shunt), the more prominent the arterial pulse.
- In the majority of cases, a precordial thrill can be palpated over the cranial left-heart base and the left apical impulse is prominent. In cases with right-to-left shunting, there is no precordial thrill, and the right apical impulse is more prominent.

General

- Caudal cyanosis is an important physical finding in animals with right-to-left shunting PDA. Owing to the location of the ductus (distal to the arteries supplying the head and forelimbs), cyanosis is limited to the caudal half of the body. This differential cyanosis is best appreciated by examining caudal mucous membranes, although occasionally cyanosis of the skin caudal to the costal arch can be seen.
- Polycythemia (packed cell volume greater than 60) is usually present in cases with right-to-left shunts.

Auscultation

- A continuous-type machinery murmur is a hallmark of left-to-right shunting PDA. The murmur is loudest in mid-to-late systole, and gradually decreases in intensity through diastole. In some cases, this characteristic murmur is restricted to the cranial left-heart base, and may be missed if auscultation is limited to the apex. The systolic component of the murmur is usually quite prominent at the cardiac apex; however, a systolic murmur secondary to mitral regurgitation because of annular dilation as the heart enlarges is also possible.
- In cases with a right-to-left shunting PDA, there is no murmur associated with the shunt (in these cases blood flows through the shunt rather than "jetting"); however, a split second heart sound is often present in these cases. Rarely, a diastolic murmur of pulmonic insufficiency is present owing to pulmonary hypertension. In cases undergoing reversal of a left-to-right shunting PDA, there is initially a loss of the diastolic component of the continuous murmur, followed by a loss of the systolic component. A murmur of tricuspid regurgitation may be present in some cases.

Diagnostic Testing

Electrocardiogram

ECG abnormalities are present in most cases of PDA. Evidence of left ventricular and left atrial enlargement includes the following:

- Tall R waves present in leads II (greater than 3.0 mV), III, and aVF
- Deep Q waves are often present in leads II, III, and aVF
- The QRS complexes are increased in duration (greater than 80 ms)
- The mean electrical axis may be shifted to the left (less than 40 degrees)
- P-mitrale (widened P wave) is often present
- Atrial fibrillation and ventricular arrhythmias may occur in association with congestive heart failure
- Animals with pulmonary hypertension may show evidence of right ventricular hypertrophy:
  - Deep S waves in leads I, II, III, and aVF; right shift of the mean electrical axis (more than 100 degrees).

Thoracic Radiographs

- The radiographic signs of PDA (Figures 12-3 and 12-4) vary considerably with the volume of blood being shunted, the age of the animal, and the degree of cardiac decompensation.
- Dorsoventral radiographs often reveal three prominences along the left cardiac silhouette.
  - The aneurysmal bulge of the aortic arch
  - The enlarged pulmonary outflow tract
  - The enlarged left atrial appendage
- Mild to moderate left ventricular and left atrial enlargement are usually present.
- Overcirculation of the lung field can often be visualized.
- Severe cardiomegaly, pulmonary congestion, and pulmonary edema will be present when there is congestive heart failure.
- Right ventricular enlargement and prominent tortuous pulmonary arteries are seen in animals with severe pulmonary hypertension (R to L PDA).

Echocardiography

- Echocardiographic changes reflect the volume-overloaded state of the left side of the heart and include left atrial dilation, left ventricular dilation, and normal to excessive wall motion (fractional shortening). In some cases the ductus can be visualized.
- Shunting of left to right blood flow through the ductus can be detected by Doppler echocardiography, and can be visualized with color-flow Doppler echocardiography.
- In cases with pulmonary hypertension and reversed-shunting, right ventricular hypertrophy is evident, along with enlargement of the main pulmonary artery; Doppler echocardiography may reveal pulmonic insufficiency.
- Contrast echocardiography can be used to confirm the presence of a right-to-left shunting PDA. In this technique, agitated saline is injected into a peripheral vein during echocardiographic examination (first injection) and abdominal aortic imaging (second injection) to detect right-to-left shunting of blood. The absence of intracardiac shunting with the presence of microbubbles within the abdominal aorta is diagnostic of reversed PDA.

Cardiac Catheterization and Angiocardiography

- Cardiac catheterization and angiocardiography should be considered when PDA is accompanied by other anomalies.
- Routinely used to characterize and measure the ductus prior to transarterial coil occlusion.

Selective Angiocardiography

- The diagnosis of a left-to-right PDA can be made by injecting contrast media into the aortic arch.

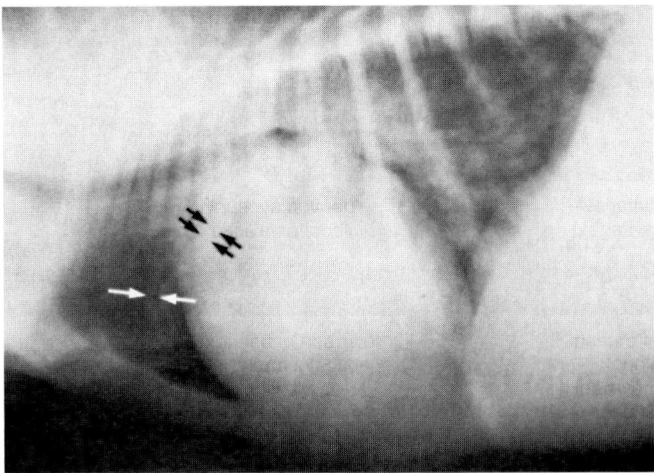

Figure 12-3. Patent ductus arteriosus (lateral projection) in a 3-month-old Poodle. There is generalized heart enlargement, engorgement of the right cranial lobar artery *(white arrows)*, and engorgement of the right cranial lobar vein *(black arrows)*. Vascular engorgement, perivascular congestion, and alveolar edema are seen in the caudal lung lobes.

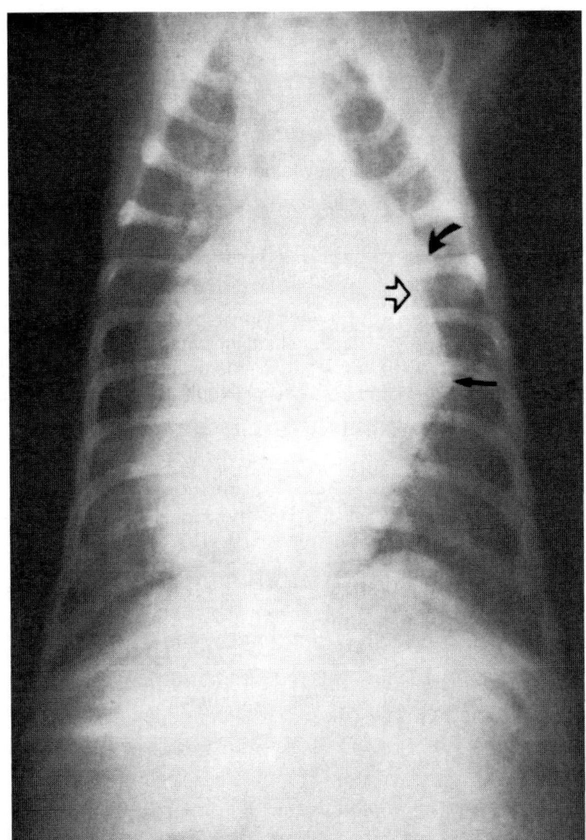

Figure 12-4. Patent ductus arteriosus (dorsoventral projection) in a 3-month-old Poodle. There is generalized heart enlargement, an aneurysm-like bulge of the descending aorta *(open arrow)*, a bulge of the main pulmonary artery *(curved arrow)*, and enlargement of the left auricle *(straight arrow)*. Alveolar infiltrate due to pulmonary edema is present in the caudal lung lobes.

The simultaneous filling of the main pulmonary artery and the aorta is diagnostic for PDA. Likewise, a main pulmonary artery contrast injection can be used to confirm the diagnosis of a right-to-left shunt (simultaneous filling of main pulmonary artery and aorta).

Nonselective Angiocardiography

- Nonselective angiocardiography is performed by injecting contrast material through a large-diameter venous catheter and taking radiographs in quick succession. Nonselective angiocardiography may be used to support the diagnosis of a right-to-left shunting PDA; however, this technique is of no value in the diagnosis of left-to-right shunts.

Differential Diagnosis

- Echocardiography or angiocardiographic studies may be used to differentiate PDA from other congenital cardiac defects. Two cardiac defects that can resemble PDA are as follows:
  - Aorticopulmonary window
    - A round or oval communication between the aorta and the main pulmonary artery close to their origin from the heart base. This rare defect usually results in severe pulmonary hypertension.
  - Concurrent aortic stenosis and insufficiency
    - The systolic murmur of aortic stenosis and the diastolic murmur of aortic insufficiency combine to mimic the machinery murmur of PDA. Echocardiography easily differentiates between these differentials.

Natural History

- Mortality is high in affected, untreated dogs; approximately 64% die before 1 year of age if left untreated.
- Constant volume overload of the left atrium and left ventricle results in chamber dilation, myocardial dysfunction, and arrhythmias.
  - Left-sided cardiac strain and pulmonary congestion leads to congestive heart failure.
  - Sudden death following exertion has been observed in young, affected dogs.
- When there is right-to-left shunting, progressive polycythemia and hypoxemia occurs. Survival to 3 to 5 years of age is not uncommon. Phlebotomy is indicated if the packed cell volume is elevated to greater than 65% and symptoms are present.

KEY POINT

- Presence of a continuous murmur should never be considered a normal physical examination finding.
- Eisenmenger's syndrome is the clinical scenario when a very large left to right shunt results in persistent pulmonary hypertension and reversal of the shunt direction.

Therapy and Prognosis

Surgery

- As discussed previously, several deleterious effects are to be expected in cases with uncorrected PDA. In addition, dogs with long-standing PDA are predisposed to the development of bacterial endocarditis; therefore, every effort should be made to correct left-to-right shunting PDA cases.
- In asymptomatic animals with left-to-right shunting PDA, surgical correction of the ductus should be performed as soon as possible. Current surgical ligation success rates are 95%. Recent studies have shown asymptomatic large dogs and older dogs (more than 2 years) have no significant added risk.
- In cases with mild to moderate left-sided heart failure, resolution of pulmonary edema must precede anesthesia and surgery.
- In cases with severe heart failure, patient stabilization should be attempted; however, these patients are poor anesthetic risks. Presence of myocardial failure and atrial fibrillation are negative prognostic indicators.

Advantages

- Best approach for patients with large PDA (frequently observed in German Shepherds)
- May be best approach for very small dogs

Disadvantages

- Requires thoracotomy and hospitalization for 48 to 72 hours with post-operative analgesia
- Success depends on the experience of the surgeon
- A thoracoscopic technique to occlude the PDA utilizing titanium ligation clips has been described and may be available as an additional option.
- Correction of PDA is contraindicated when right-to-left shunting is present. Acute right failure and death will occur, as the patent ductus functions as a relief valve for the right ventricle.

Transcatheter Occlusion

- Shunting through the ductus may be stopped by a relatively noninvasive method termed *transcatheter occlusion.* This procedure employs delivery of a Gianturco coil, resulting in embolization of the ductus.

- Coils are composed of prothrombotic poly-Dacron fibers. The size of the coil selected is based on the approximate size of the ductus (as determined by angiography or echocardiography). The device(s) are delivered from a catheter passed up the femoral artery and into the ductus (Figure 12-5). Multiple coils may be needed for full occlusion of the ductus.

Advantages

- Less invasive procedure with short hospitalization period.
- Little need for post-operative analgesia.

Disadvantages

- Difficult to catheterize femoral artery of very small dogs due to size constraints.
- Ineffective in patients with large, tubular PDA.
- Requires fluoroscopy.

Medical Management

- In cases deemed unacceptable anesthetic-surgical candidates, medical management of congestive heart failure is indicated (see Chapter 15).
- There are no drugs currently effective for closing the patent ductus in dogs and cats.

AORTIC STENOSIS

Anatomy

- Aortic stenosis is a narrowing or reduction of the left ventricular outflow tract dimension at the subvalvular (fibrous ring or muscular), valvular, or supravalvular level.
- The subvalvular form (subaortic stenosis) is the most common form in the dog. With this defect, a fibrous band or ring located just below the aortic semilunar valves impedes left ventricular emptying.
- Fixed valvular and supravalvular stenosis have been reported in the cat.
- Some patients demonstrate a dynamic subaortic stenosis associated with systolic anterior motion of the anterior mitral valve leaflet. This condition has been described in patients with fixed aortic/subaortic stenosis, hypertrophic cardiomyopathy, mitral valve dysplasia, and other conditions that cause hypertrophy of the interventricular septum.
- Some breeds (boxers, bull terriers, golden retrievers) have mildly decreased left ventricular outflow tract dimensions that result in mild elevations of transvalvular blood velocity without other structural abnormalities.

Pathophysiology

- Stenosis of the left ventricular outflow tract results in pressure overload of the left ventricle (Figure 12-6). The left ventricle responds to this chronic pressure overload by undergoing concentric hypertrophy. As blood is forced through the stenotic area, its velocity increases, resulting in turbulence, a systolic ejection murmur, and a post-stenotic dilation of the aorta. The velocity of blood through the lesion is directly proportional to the severity of stenosis. Left ventricular hypertrophy increases the myocardial oxygen demand.
- Myocardial hypertrophy, decreased capillary density, and increased wall tension all contribute to produce myocardial hypoxia/ischemia. Focal areas of myocardial infarction and fibrosis, particularly involving the papillary muscles and subendocardium, have been commonly observed in patients with severe stenosis. These cases are prone to sudden death, presumably from fatal ventricular arrhythmias induced by hypoxia.
- Infrequently, left-sided heart failure develops.
- The presence of aortic/subaortic stenosis may increase the risk of the development of infective endocarditis.

Diagnosis

Etiology and Breed Predisposition

- A polygenic inheritance pattern has been identified in the Newfoundland, which is most consistent with an autosomal dominant mode of transmission with modifying genes.
- Other commonly affected breeds include Bouvier de Flanders, Boxer, English Bulldog, German Shepherd, German Shorthair Pointer, Golden Retriever, Great Dane, Rottweiler, and Samoyed.
- Bull Terriers are predisposed to valvular aortic stenosis characterized by thickened aortic valve leaflets and a hypoplastic annulus.

History and Clinical Signs

- In mildly to moderately affected cases, there are often no clinical signs, and the suspicion of aortic stenosis occurs when a murmur is detected during routine examination.
- In severe cases, owners may report failure to thrive, exercise intolerance, collapse, and labored breathing. In some cases, the first clinical sign is sudden death.

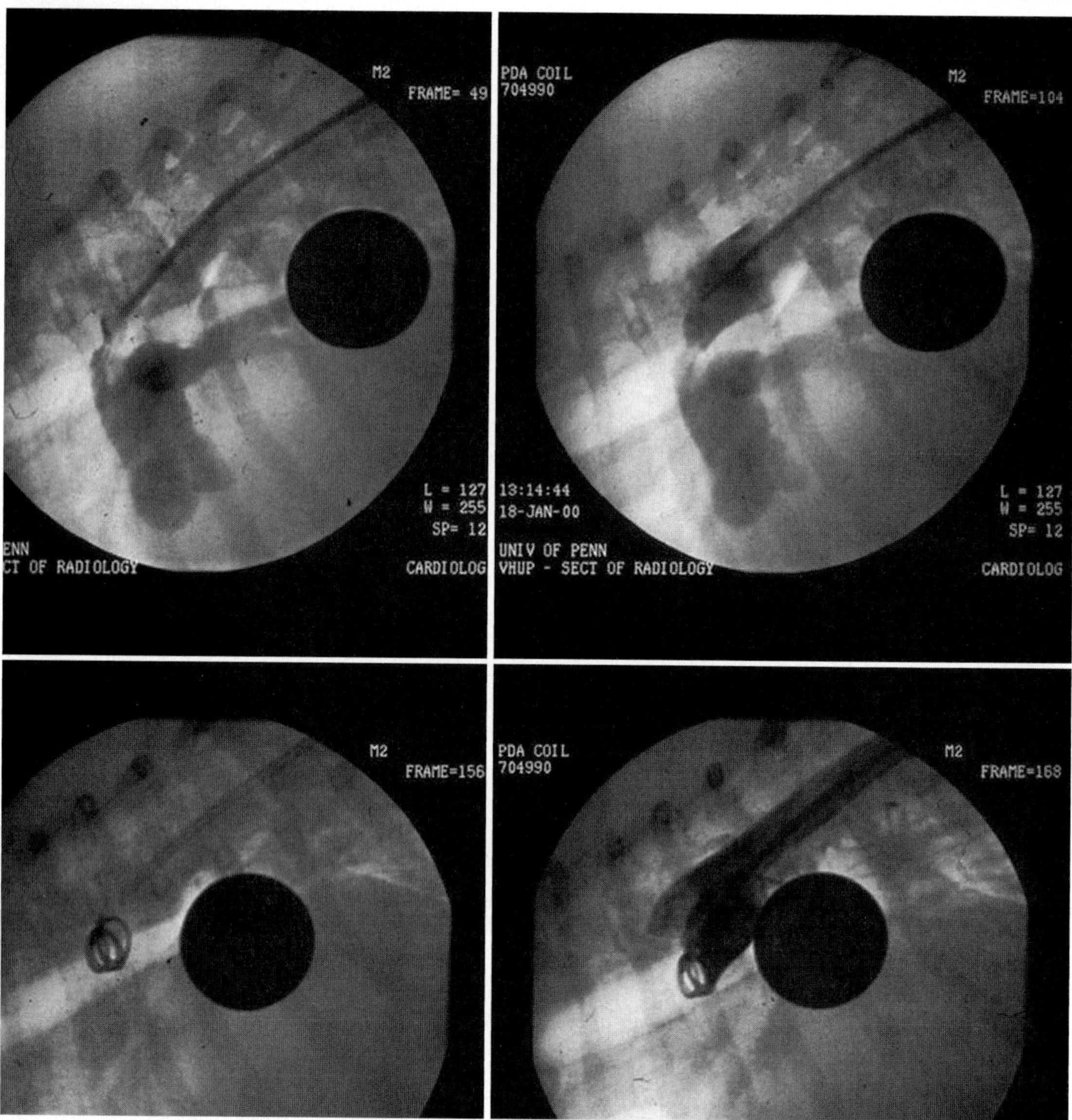

Figure 12-5. Serial angiocardiograms obtained during a PDA coil embolization procedure. Note the catheter access is via a femoral artery (right femoral artery) and the placement of one coil completely occludes contrast (and blood) flow across the ductus arteriosus.

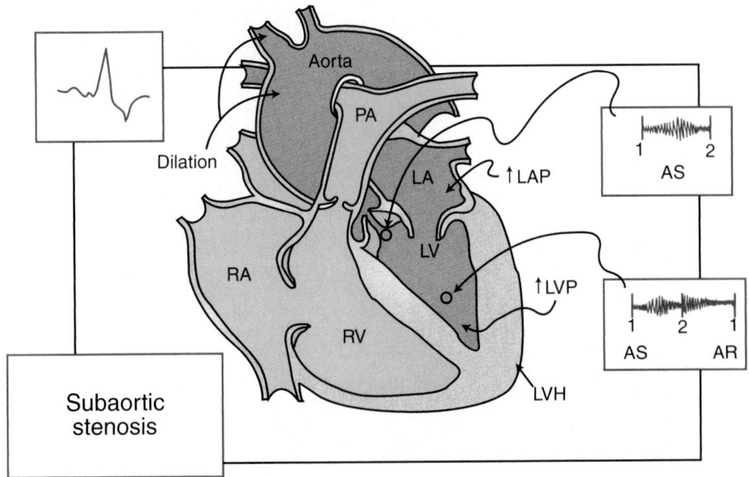

Figure 12-6. Pathophysiology and genesis of clinical signs in congenital subaortic stenosis. (From Fox PR, Sisson D, Moise NS, eds: Textbook of canine and feline cardiology: principles and clinical practice, ed 2, Philadelphia, 1999, WB Saunders.)

Physical Examination

Palpation

- Animals with aortic stenosis have easily palpable left ventricular impulses, and those with severe stenosis usually have a palpable precordial thrill over the aortic valve area. Femoral pulses are often weak and late rising (pulsus parvus et tardus).

Auscultation

- Aortic stenosis is manifested by a systolic ejection-type murmur heard best over the left fourth intercostal space at the level of the costochondral junction (aortic valve area). Frequently, the murmur radiates up the carotid artery and can be auscultated in the midcervical area. Occasionally, the murmur may be loudest in the right third or fourth intercostal space midway up the thorax. Rarely, a concurrent diastolic murmur of aortic insufficiency is present.

Diagnostic Testing

Electrocardiogram

- The ECG may be normal.
- Alternatively there may be evidence of left ventricular hypertrophy (tall R waves in leads II [greater than 3.0 mV], III, and aVF).
- Ventricular or supraventricular arrhythmias are occasionally detected.

Thoracic Radiographs

- Radiographic changes tend to parallel severity of the stenosis. Characteristic features include enlargement of the aortic arch (post-stenotic dilation) and left ventricle (Figures 12-7 and 12-8).
- Left atrial enlargement will be present in advanced cases with concurrent mitral insufficiency.

Echocardiography

- Echocardiography is the most sensitive noninvasive method to diagnose and grade subaortic stenosis.
- This technique provides visualization of the defect and secondary cardiac changes. In most cases, there is significant left ventricular hypertrophy. In severe

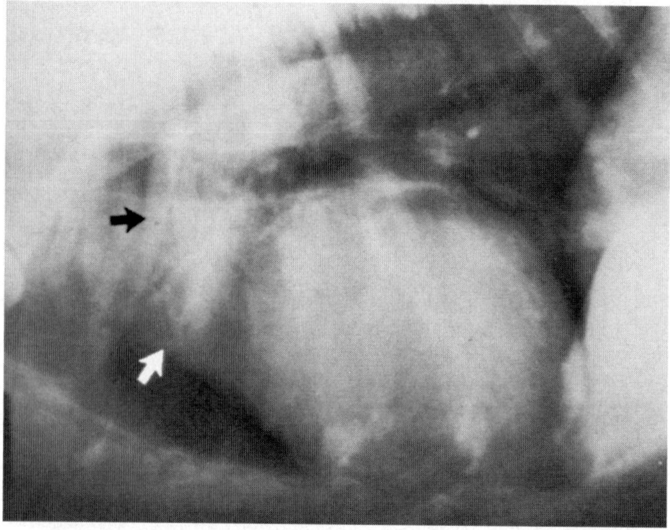

Figure 12-7. Aortic stenosis (lateral projection). There is marked enlargement of the aortic arch cranial to the heart base *(arrows)*.

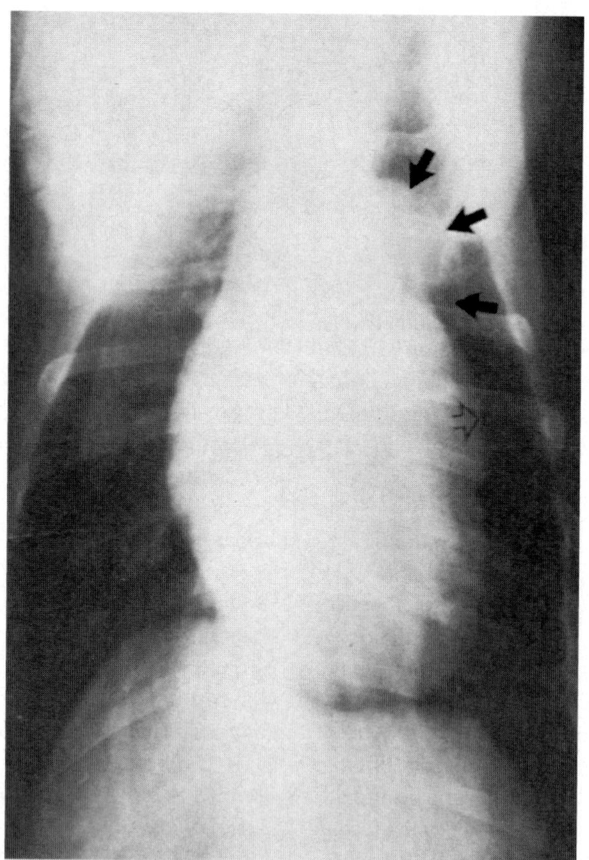

Figure 12-8. Aortic stenosis (dorsoventral projection). The enlarged aortic arch extends to the heart base *(arrows)*. The left auricle *(open arrow)* extends beyond the cardiac border, and there is slight left ventricular enlargement.

or advanced cases, the papillary muscles and myocardium become hyperechoic (bright) secondary to calcium deposition, ischemia and/or fibrosis.

- Doppler echocardiography allows measurement of blood flow velocity through the defect and provides reliable data regarding severity. The velocity of blood (m/s) through the stenosis, measured by Doppler echocardiography, provides a reliable and noninvasive measure of the pressure gradient across the stenosis. The pressure gradient

KEY POINT

The differentiation between patients with trivial to mild stenosis and normal patients with physiologic-induced accelerated transaortic velocities can be difficult, if not impossible. A diagnosis of trivial to mild subaortic/aortic stenosis based solely on elevations of transaortic velocity can be problematic; the diagnosis should include a combination of the following: accelerated transvalvular velocities, turbulent blood flow, visualization of an anatomical lesion, concurrent aortic insufficiency, and/or a distinct "step up" in velocity across a discreet region of the outflow tract.

(in mm Hg) can be readily derived with the modified Bernoulli equation:

$$\text{Pressure gradient} = 4\,(\text{maximum velocity})^2$$

- Pressure gradients between 80 to 100 mm Hg represent moderate stenosis; pressure gradients greater than 100 mm Hg are consistent with severe stenosis.

Cardiac Catheterization

- Cardiac catheterization may be used to confirm the diagnosis, but this procedure is usually unnecessary since the advent of echocardiography. Cardiac catheterization and angiography are occasionally used when multiple cardiac defects are suspected.
- Angiography will illustrate the stenosis and poststenotic dilation. Pressure measurements obtained during selective catheterization are used to determine the gradient across the stenosis. Unlike echocardiography, general anesthesia is required, which can significantly lower pressure gradients.

Natural History

- The clinical manifestations of aortic/subaortic stenosis are variable. Up to 25% of dogs with severe stenosis may die suddenly during the first 3 years of life. In others, congestive heart failure may develop. A serious, but rare complication is the development of infective endocarditis, resulting in metastatic infection and aortic insufficiency. Cardiac arrhythmias are common in affected dogs. Other affected individuals may demonstrate symptoms such as syncope or lack of exercise capacity.

Therapy and Prognosis

Surgery

- There are several surgical techniques used to relieve left ventricular obstruction. There are only a limited number of institutions currently performing these techniques owing to their complexity, special equipment requirements (cardiopulmonary bypass), and expense.
- Surgery is not indicated for cases with mild stenosis (low gradients). Surgery should only be considered for those cases with severe obstructive disease causing clinical signs such as syncope, and without evidence of irreversible myocardial damage.

Balloon Dilation

- As in PS, balloon valvuloplasty may be effective in alleviating outflow obstruction. This technique has much less morbidity than corrective surgery because it requires insertion of an arterial catheter rather than a thoracotomy.
- Studies have documented significant reductions (50%) in pressure gradients immediately following balloon dilation. However, although short-term (2 to 3 months) effects are favorable, there does not appear to be a long-term survival benefit.

Medical Management

- Beta blockers (propranolol, atenolol) are used to reduce myocardial oxygen demands. They appear to be of some benefit in reducing the frequency of arrhythmias.
- Antibiotics should be administered when bacteremia is suspected or likely (e.g., dental procedures) to reduce the chance of endocarditis developing.
- Treatment with various cardiac drugs, diuretics, low-salt diets, and rest is usually of some benefit in those severe cases that have developed congestive heart failure.

PULMONIC STENOSIS

PS is the third most commonly reported congenital defect in the dog. Obstruction to the ejection of blood from the right ventricle may occur at the following levels. The latter two types are uncommon.

- Valvular (pulmonic valve dysplasia)
- Subvalvular
- Supravalvular

Pathophysiology

- The consequences of this defect are in direct proportion to the severity of the obstruction. The major clinical manifestations are secondary to pressure overload of the right ventricle.
- Hemodynamically, valvular PS results in a pressure gradient across the stenotic valve because of resistance to right ventricular outflow (Figure 12-9). The severity of the lesion is directly related to this pressure gradient. Right ventricular hypertrophy is almost always present; the degree varies with the severity of stenosis.
- Turbulence associated with the increase in velocity of blood across the stenotic valve is the cause of the post-stenotic dilation in the main pulmonary artery segment.
- The valvular lesion may be characterized by fusion of the valve leaflets, dysplasia of the valvular apparatus, or both.
- Depending on the severity of the right ventricular hypertrophy, some patients will have a dynamic, infundibular stenosis in addition to the fixed valvular stenosis.

Diagnosis

Etiology and Breed Disposition

- PS occurs in both the dog and cat (rare).
- The defect is more common in the following breeds: Airedale Terrier, Beagle, Boykin Spaniel, Boxer, Chihuahua, Cocker Spaniel, English Bulldog, Bull Mastiff, Samoyed, Schnauzer, and West Highland White Terrier.
- A polygenic inheritance pattern has been identified in the Beagle.
- Some authors note that supravalvular stenosis occurs with increased incidence in Giant Schnauzers.

History and Clinical Signs

- Animals with mild or moderate PS are usually asymptomatic and many live apparently normal lives with mild disease.
- Symptomatic animals with PS have clinical signs of dyspnea and fatigue secondary to low cardiac output. Exercise-induced syncope may occur because of the limitation in cardiac output imposed by the stenotic valve. Approximately 35% of dogs with severe stenosis develop clinical signs.
- Decompensation and signs of right-heart failure may occur.
- Cyanosis may be present in dogs with concurrent right to left shunting patent foramen ovale or coexisting atrial septal defect or VSD.
- Similar to subaortic stenosis, severe hypertrophy can result in myocardial hypoxia and ventricular arrhythmias.

Physical Examination

Palpation

- Animals with moderate to severe PS have easily palpable right ventricular impulses. A precordial thrill is usually present at the left lower third or fourth intercostal space.
- Jugular venous distention and pulsations may be present if tricuspid regurgitation and/or congestive heart failure is present.

Auscultation

- A systolic, crescendo-decrescendo murmur is heard best at the left lower third or fourth intercostal space. If the murmur is severe, it may radiate over the cranial thorax and be audible at the thoracic inlet.
- A split second heart sound due to delayed closure of the pulmonic valve may also be present.

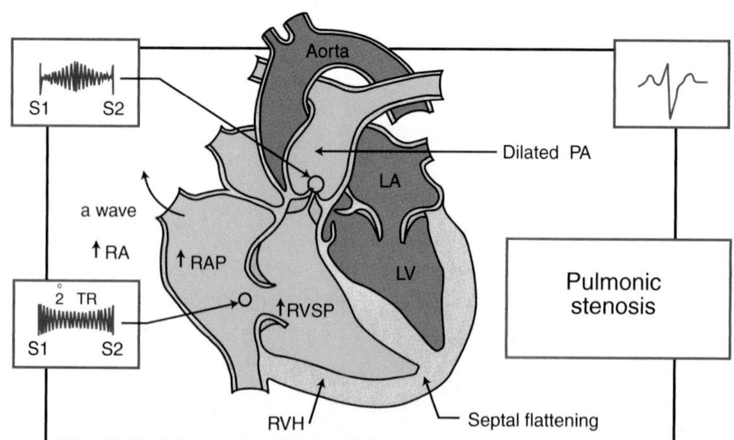

Figure 12-9. Pathophysiology and genesis of clinical signs in pulmonic stenosis. (Modified from Fox PR, Sisson D, Moise NS, eds: Textbook of canine and feline cardiology: principles and clinical practice, ed 2, Philadelphia, 1999, WB Saunders.)

- It can be difficult to differentiate between the murmurs of subaortic/aortic stenosis and PS.

Diagnostic Testing

Electrocardiogram

- Signs of right ventricular hypertrophy are present in almost all cases. There are deep S waves present in leads I, II, and III, and a right shift of the mean electrical axis in the frontal plane (more than 120 degrees).
- Ventricular arrhythmias may be present. Atrial fibrillation may be present in severe cases.

Thoracic Radiographs

- The primary radiographic features (Figures 12-10 and 12-11) include the following:
- Right ventricular enlargement and right atrial enlargement
- Enlargement of the main pulmonary segment
- Decreased pulmonary vascularity; pulmonary arteries smaller than normal

Echocardiography

- Echocardiography has proven to be highly sensitive in the diagnosis and determination of severity of PS.
- Characteristic findings include the following:
- Right ventricular dilation and hypertrophy of the right ventricular wall and interventricular septum. Owing to increased pressures within the right ventricle, the septum is typically flattened (Figure 12-12).
- The right ventricular outflow tract is often dilated, and in cases of valvular stenosis, the pulmonic valve cusps are thickened and immobile. A post-stenotic dilation of the main pulmonary artery is usually evident.
- Doppler echocardiography provides a sensitive and noninvasive method to determine the severity of stenosis by estimating the pressure gradient across the obstruction in a similar manner as with aortic stenosis: mild (less than 50 mm Hg), moderate (50 to 80 mm Hg), and severe (greater than 80 mm Hg).

Other Diagnostic Techniques

- Cardiac catheterization may be used to confirm the diagnosis of PS, but this procedure is usually unnecessary since the advent of echocardiography. Cardiac catheterization and angiography are occasionally used when multiple cardiac defects are suspected.
- Cardiac catheterization and angiography are performed routinely prior to an interventional procedure such as balloon valvuloplasty. Selective coronary angiography is required to rule out the presence of an anomalous left main coronary artery in English Bulldogs and Boxers if surgery or balloon valvuloplasty is considered.

Differential Diagnosis

- Atrial septal defect: The right ventricular volume overload associated with a left-to-right shunting atrial septal defect may result in a systolic ejection murmur over the pulmonic valve. Such murmurs are usually softer than those associated with PS.
- Innocent or physiologic murmurs: These murmurs are usually much softer than typical PS murmurs and do not typically persist beyond 6 months of age.

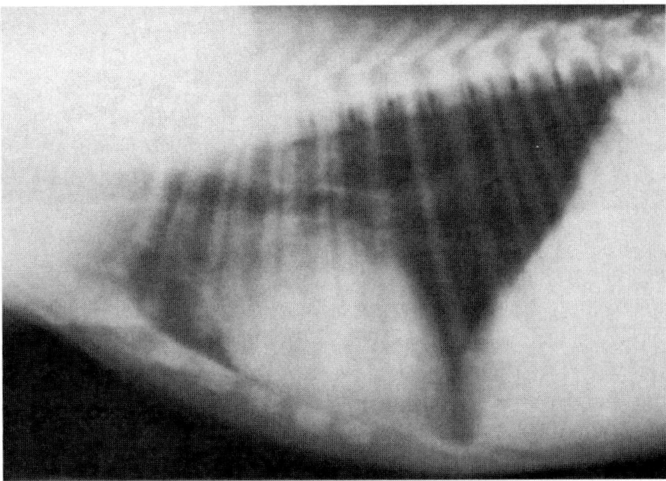

Figure 12-10. Pulmonic stenosis (lateral projection) in a 2-month-old mixed-breed dog. There is increased sternal contact of the right heart, due to right-heart enlargement, and normal to slightly diminished pulmonary vasculature.

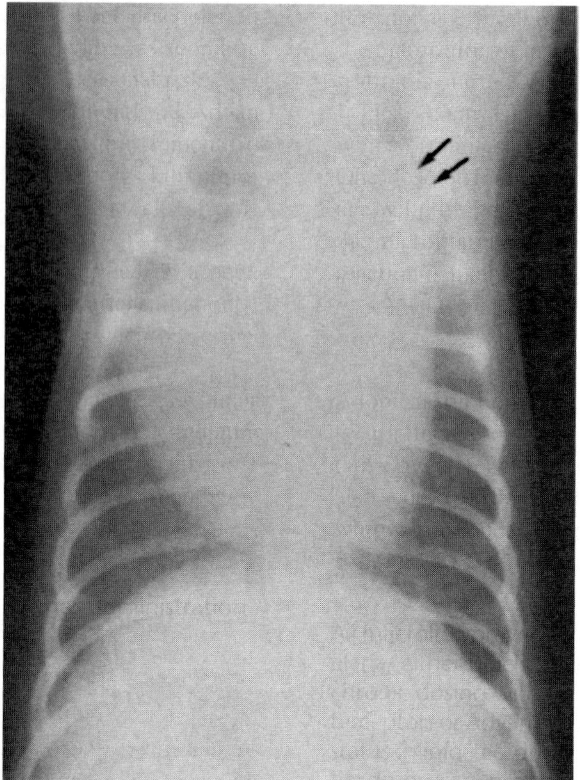

Figure 12-11. Pulmonic stenosis (dorsoventral projection) in a 2-month-old mixed-breed dog. There is marked right-heart enlargement and prominence of the main pulmonary artery *(arrows)*.

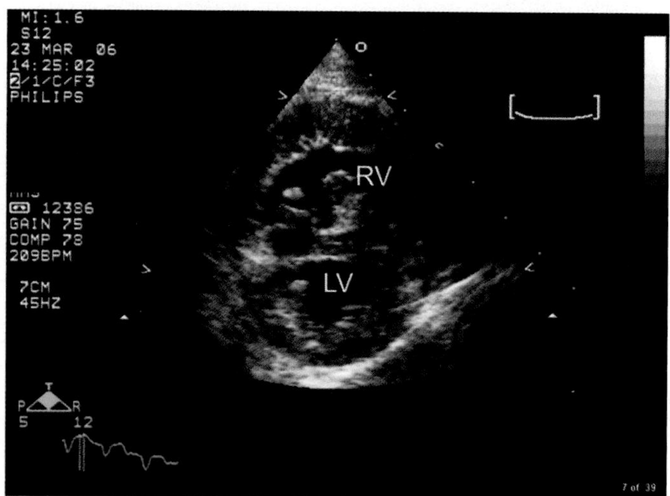

Figure 12-12. Right parasternal short-axis 2-dimensional echocardiogram obtained from a West Highland White Terrier with severe pulmonic stenosis. Note the severely thickened right ventricle. *RV,* Right ventricle; *LV,* left ventricle.

Natural History

- Uncomplicated survival to adulthood may occur in dogs with mild to moderate PS. In general, the natural history correlates well with disease severity (pressure gradient) and the degree of right ventricular hypertrophy. Dogs with moderate to severe PS may develop signs of right-sided congestive heart failure, cardiac arrhythmias, exertional syncope, and/or sudden death. Concurrent tricuspid valve dysplasia increases the risk of the development of congestive heart failure.

Therapy and Prognosis

- The need for treatment and the prognosis are dependent upon the severity of the defect as determined by Doppler echocardiography or cardiac catheterization. Cases with mild stenosis (less than 50 mm Hg; ejection velocity less than 3.5 m/s) do not require treatment and have a favorable prognosis. Those with severe stenosis (more than 80 mm Hg; ejection velocity more than 4.5 m/s) are candidates for surgery or balloon valvuloplasty, and may have a poor prognosis if uncorrected. Intermediate cases should be followed to monitor for progression of the stenosis.

Surgery

- The method of surgical correction depends on the type of stenosis present and its severity.
- Supraventricular PS may be palliated by circumventing the stenosis with a conduit.
- Repair of valvular or discrete subvalvular PS can be accomplished by pulmonary arteriotomy (using inflow occlusion). The patch graft technique is effective in young animals with valvular PS. The bistoury technique or the modified Brock procedure has also been used effectively.
- In general, surgical correction is not recommended unless the surgeon is experienced with the procedure.

Balloon Valvuloplasty

- In this procedure, a special cardiac catheter is guided through the stenotic valve, and a balloon situated at the end of the catheter is inflated, effectively enlarging the valve diameter. Balloon valvuloplasty is most effective when valves are thin and fused, and hypoplasia of the annulus is not present.
- Generally, balloon valvuloplasty results in a significant (40% to 60%) decrease in the pressure gradient and is maintained in 60% to 70% of the patients; however, the long-term effects on survival improvement have not been definitely determined.

KEY POINT

English Bulldogs and some Boxers may have an anomalous left main coronary artery arising from a single right coronary artery associated with the stenosis that precludes surgical or catheter-based intervention due to the risk of vessel rupture and subsequent death.

- This procedure is generally recommended for patients with moderate to severe stenosis, particularly those patients with symptoms such as syncope and/or decreased exercise capacity.
- Reduction in the transvalvular pressure gradient by balloon valvuloplasty may be accompanied by exacerbation of the dynamic subvalvular (infundibular) obstruction.

Medical Management

- Signs of right-sided congestive heart failure should be treated as described in Chapter 15.
- Beta blocker therapy (**atenolol** 0.25 to 1.5 mg/kg PO every 12 hours) is routinely administered to patients with moderate to severe right ventricular hypertrophy in an effort to decrease myocardial oxygen consumption and to suppress ventricular arrhythmias.

VENTRICULAR SEPTAL DEFECT

Anatomy

- The interventricular septum separates the left ventricle and the right ventricle. It is muscular at the apex and tapers to a membranous portion at the heart base near the origin of the aorta. Septal defects may occur in any area of the septum, but are most commonly located in the membranous portion.
- VSDs may occur as isolated defects, may coexist with concurrent defects (e.g., PDA and atrial septal defect), or may be a component of complex cardiac anomalies.

Pathophysiology

- There are two major factors that determine the consequences of a VSD, the size of the defect and the relative pressures (or resistances) of the ventricles. When left and right ventricular pressures are normal, blood will shunt left to right, as the left ventricular systolic pressure is roughly five times greater than right ventricular systolic pressure (Figure 12-13). In the typical VSD (left-to-right shunting membranous defect), most of the blood is shunted into the right ventricular outflow tract or the main pulmonary artery. This shunt creates a large volume overload to the pulmonary circulation, the left atrium, and the left ventricle. When pulmonary resistance remains relatively normal, the right ventricle is spared most of the effects of the shunting.
- Small defects may be of no hemodynamic significance, although they may predispose the animal

to the development of endocarditis. In some cases, small defects close spontaneously.
- Moderately sized defects may allow significant shunting and usually produce clinical signs.
- Very large defects may create a functional single ventricle with equilibration of left and right ventricular pressures.
- If right ventricular resistance increases (e.g., PS, pulmonary hypertension), right ventricular pressure will increase proportionately, thereby decreasing the shunt volume. If right ventricular pressure increases to a point where it exceeds left ventricular pressure, blood will shunt right to left, and signs of cyanosis may develop.

Diagnosis

Etiology and Breed Predisposition

- Breed studies in the keeshond have shown the defect to be polygenic.
- The English bulldog appears to have a higher incidence than other breeds, but the defect is seen in many purebred and mixed-breed dogs.
- Breed incidence in the cat has not been determined.

History and Clinical Signs

- The clinical course of animals with VSD is variable and to a large extent dependent upon the size of the defect and the ventricular pressures. Small defects may cause little or no functional disturbances and may cause no clinical signs. Moderate to large defects usually produce signs of left-sided failure subsequent to the chronic left-sided volume overload. In cases that develop pulmonary hypertension, signs of right-sided failure and cyanosis will predominate.

Physical Examination

Palpation

- In many cases, a precordial thrill is present at the right-heart base (third to fourth intercostal spaces, (just above the costochondral junctions). Volume overloading of the left ventricle often accentuates the left-sided impulse. In cases with significant pulmonary hypertension, precordial thrills are unusual, and the right apical impulse is accentuated.

Auscultation

- Typically, the murmur is harsh, holosystolic, and heard best at the right sternal border, at the second through fourth intercostal spaces.
- A murmur of functional PS may be heard over the pulmonic valve area. This is due to the extra volume of blood passing through the pulmonic valve and not related to a structural valve problem.
- A split-second heart sound occasionally is present due to slightly prolonged right ventricular ejection time.
- When the defect causes destabilization of an aortic valve cusp, a diastolic murmur of aortic insufficiency may be present in addition to the systolic murmur. This combination is referred to as a to-and-fro murmur and is not a continuous murmur.
- In cases with progressive pulmonary hypertension, elevations in right ventricular resistance result in diminished shunting. With very large defects and/or severe pulmonary hypertension, a murmur may be absent because of the lack of a pressure differential across the septum.

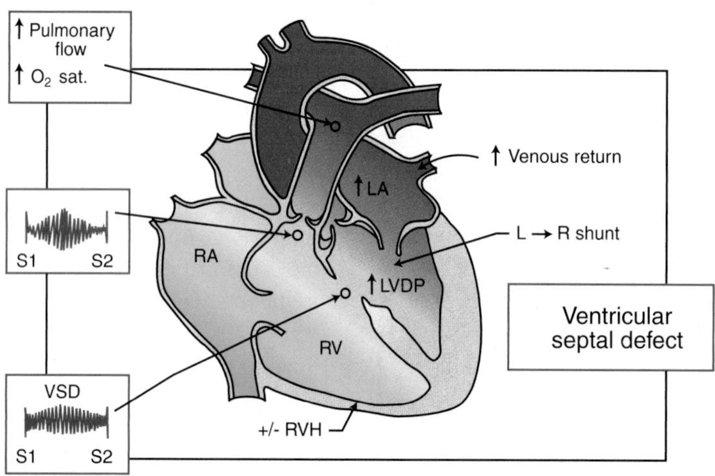

Figure 12-13. Pathophysiology and genesis of clinical findings in VSD. (Modified from Fox PR, Sisson D, Moise NS, eds: Textbook of canine and feline cardiology: principles and clinical practice, ed 2, Philadelphia, 1999, WB Saunders.)

Diagnostic Testing

Electrocardiogram

- ECG abnormalities usually parallel the degree of hemodynamic compromise.
- The ECG may be normal when a small defect is present.
- The ECG may show evidence of left, right, or biventricular enlargement, depending on hemodynamic consequences of the shunt.
- Right bundle branch block may also be observed.

Thoracic Radiographs

- Small defects usually do not cause radiographic changes.
- Left ventricular enlargement, left atrial enlargement, and increased pulmonary artery prominence are seen with larger defects resulting in significant left-to-right shunting.
- Right ventricular enlargement accompanied by prominent tortuous pulmonary arteries may be present in cases of pulmonary hypertension and right-to-left shunting (Figure 12-14).

Echocardiography

- The diagnosis of VSD can usually be confirmed by routine echocardiography. Typical findings for a moderate to large shunt include left ventricular and left atrial dilation, and a defect in the interventricular septum with 2D echocardiography. It is important to distinguish the septal dropout normally present in the membranous septum from a VSD. In most VSD cases, the interventricular septum is slightly blunted just apical to the defect, whereas the septum tapers gradually in normal animals.
- Contrast echocardiography will confirm the presence of a right-to-left shunting VSD. Agitated saline is rapidly injected into a peripheral vein, resulting in the appearance of microbubbles (contrast) within the heart. In the absence of a right-to-left shunt, all contrast remains right-sided.

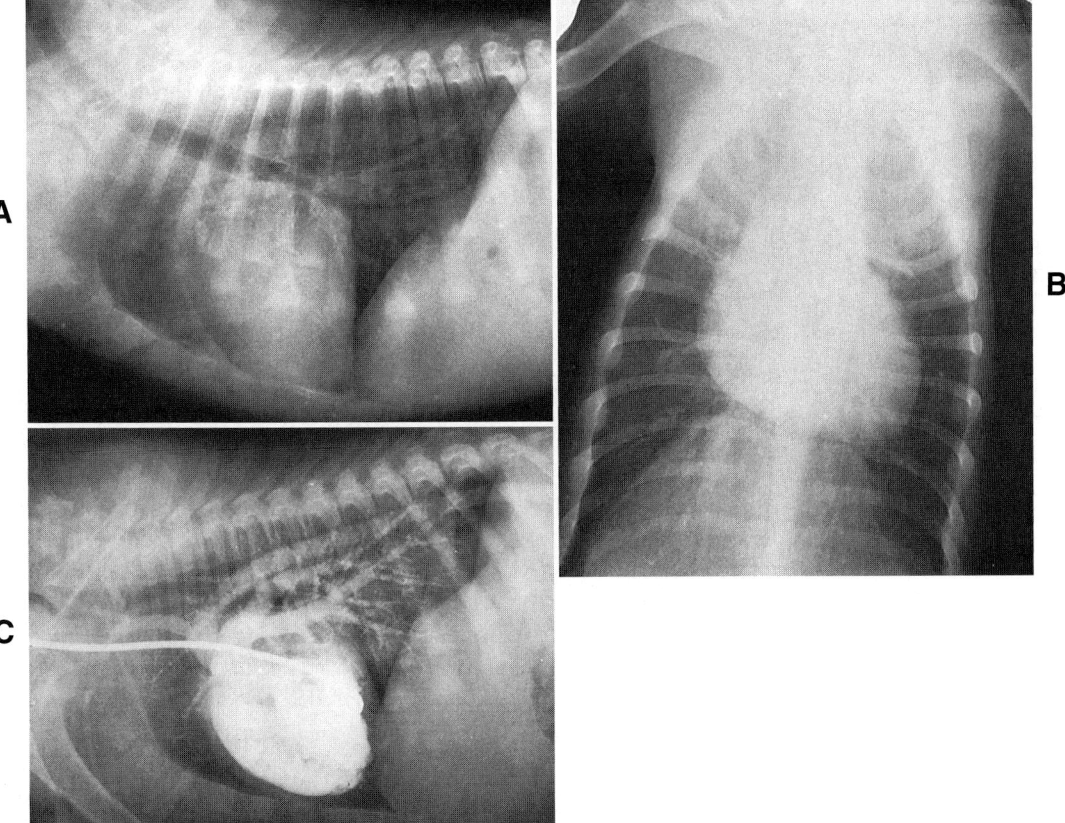

Figure 12-14. Ventricular septal defect. A routine examination of a 3-month-old Doberman revealed a grade 2 systolic murmur over the mitral and aortic valve areas. There were a weak pulse and a split R wave. **A** to **C**, The plain lateral radiograph shows fluid in an interlobar fissure and increased pulmonary vascular markings. The right heart cannot be evaluated on the lateral view because of the fluid. The lateral and dorsoventral views show left ventricular enlargement. A thymic sail is seen. Selective catheterization of the left ventricle and angiocardiography show simultaneous filling of the left and right ventricles. The aorta and the pulmonary arteries are also seen.

Continued

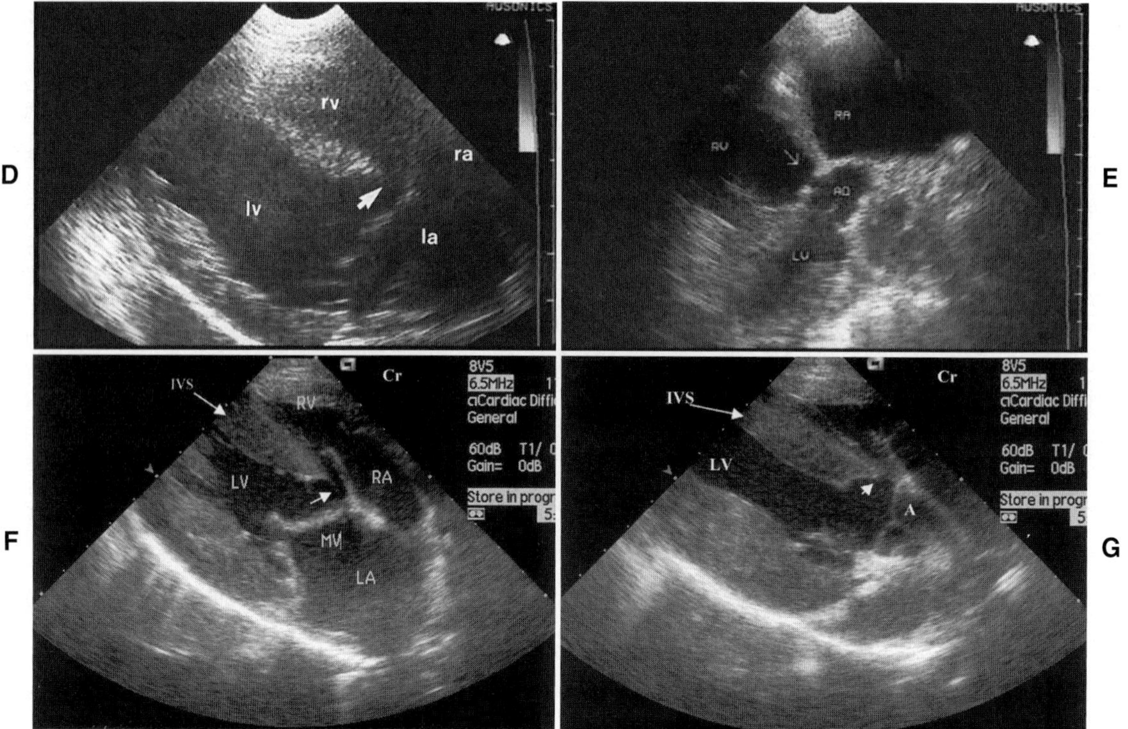

Figure 12-14, cont'd. **D,** A 4-month-old German Shepherd puppy presented for vaccination. A murmur was auscultated, and a pronounced precordial thrill was palpated. A 1-cm septal defect is seen high in the interventricular septum *(arrow).* Diagnosis: interventricular septal defect. *ra,* Right atrium; *rv,* right ventricle; *la,* left atrium; *lv,* left ventricle. **E,** A Staffordshire Bull Terrier presented for vaccination. A murmur was auscultated, and a palpable thrill was felt on the thoracic wall. A small interventricular septal defect (proved at autopsy) is seen between the left and right ventricles. The edges of the septal defect are thickened and hyperechoic. The defect was visible only when the image orientation was optimized for the left ventricular outflow tract. Diagnosis: interventricular septal defect. (From Kealey JK, McAllister H: Diagnostic radiology and ultrasonography of the dog and cat, ed 3, Philadelphia, 2000, WB Saunders.)

KEY POINT

- High-velocity flow (greater than 4.5 m/s, as defined by Doppler echocardiography) across the VSD and normal transpulmonic valvular velocities indicate that the defect is associated with a small shunting volume. These "restrictive" shunts are hemodynamically insignificant and are unlikely to be associated with clinical signs.
- Low-velocity flow (less than 4.5 m/s) across the VSD and increased transpulmonic valvular velocities indicate that the defect is associated with a large shunting volume. These "unrestrictive" shunts are hemodynamically significant and are likely to be associated with clinical signs.

In right-to-left shunting VSD, microbubbles will be seen traversing the defect.

- Doppler echocardiography will confirm the shunting of blood through the defect (Figure 12-15).

Other Diagnostic Procedures

- Cardiac catheterization and angiography may be used to confirm the diagnosis of VSD. As with other congenital defects, the use of cardiac catheterization has decreased with the availability of echocardiography. Determination of oxygen saturation of blood from each chamber may be used to confirm shunting. Left-to-right shunts produce a step-up in oxygen saturation in the right ventricle compared with the right atrium.

Therapy and Prognosis

- The prognosis and need for therapy are dependent upon the severity of the defect. With small defects, spontaneous closure may occur within the first 2 years of life. Indications for surgical intervention include a large septal defect, the presence of clinical signs, or a calculated shunt ratio of 3:1 or greater.

Surgery

- Open heart techniques have been used with reasonable success. Although curative, these techniques are available at a very limited number of

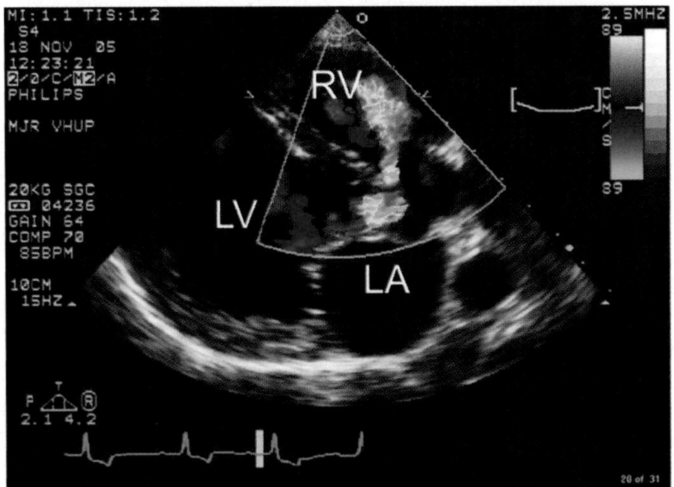

Figure 12-15. Right parasternal long-axis-2 dimensional echocardiogram obtained from a 9-week-old Golden Retriever puppy with a right sided systolic murmur. Note the aliased color flow pattern crossing the interventricular septum. This finding is consistent with a left to right shunting ventricular septal defect. *RV,* Right ventricle; *LV,* left ventricle; *LA,* left atrium.

locations and are often prohibitively expensive. Reduction of the shunt can be accomplished by pulmonary artery banding, a technique resulting in elevation of the right ventricular systolic pressure. As right ventricular pressure increases, the shunt volume decreases, and the pulmonary circulation is spared the deleterious effects of chronic volume overload.

Medical Management

- In patients where surgical correction or palliation is not an option, medical management of congestive heart failure may be required. Treatment should be tailored to the type and degree of failure (see Chapter 15). Animals with VSD should receive antibiotic prophylaxis prior to procedures likely to produce bacteremia (e.g., dental cleaning).

Prognosis

- Prognosis is excellent for animals with small defects or for those with surgically corrected defects. Cases with moderate to large defects have a variable clinical course and prognosis, depending on shunt volume.

TETRALOGY OF FALLOT

Tetralogy of Fallot is the most common cyanosis-producing defect and results from a combination of PS, high VSD, right ventricular hypertrophy, and varying degrees of dextroposition and overriding of the aorta.

- The right ventricular hypertrophy is secondary to the obstruction in right ventricular outflow. The PS may be valvular, infundibular, or both.

Pathophysiology

The hemodynamic consequences of tetralogy of Fallot depend primarily on the severity of the PS and the size of the VSD.

- The direction and magnitude of the shunt through the septal defect are dependent upon the degree of right ventricular obstruction. If the PS is mild, and right ventricular pressures are only modestly elevated, then blood will shunt primarily from left to right. Pathophysiologically, these cases are similar to VSD cases with pulmonary artery banding (i.e., the mild right ventricular obstruction protects the pulmonary vasculature from excessive shunting).
- When PS is severe, the elevated right ventricular pressures will result in right-to-left shunting. Consequences include reduced pulmonary blood flow (resulting in fatigue and shortness of breath) and generalized cyanosis (resulting in weakness).
- Owing to the shunting of venous blood into the aorta and consequent hypoxemia, the kidneys are stimulated to release erythropoietin. Chronic elevations in erythropoietin result in polycythemia. The increased blood viscosity associated with polycythemia can have significant hemodynamic effects, resulting in sludging of blood and poor capillary perfusion. Animals with severe polycythemia may seize.

Diagnosis

Etiology and Breed Predisposition

- Breeds predisposed to tetralogy of Fallot include the Keeshond, English Bulldog, Miniature Poodle, Miniature Schnauzer, and Wire-Haired Fox Terrier. This defect has also been recognized in other canine breeds, and in cats.
- Based on breeding studies and genetic analysis (primarily in the keeshond), conotruncal malformations are thought to be recessive, but not simply inherited.

History and Clinical Signs

- Typical historical features include stunted growth, exercise intolerance, cyanosis, collapse, and seizure activity.

Physical Examination

Palpation

- A precordial thrill may be felt in the third left intercostal space, near the costochondral junction.

Auscultation

- In most cases, a murmur of PS is present. The intensity of the murmur is attenuated when severe polycythemia is present.

Diagnostic Testing

Electrocardiogram

- A right ventricular enlargement pattern is usually present.
- Arrhythmias may be present.

Thoracic Radiographs

- Variable right-heart enlargement is present.
- Pulmonary vessels are undersized, and the main pulmonary artery is often diminished.

Echocardiography

- Echocardiography will confirm the diagnosis, with malposition of the aortic root, right ventricular hypertrophy, and VSD.
- Routine contrast echocardiography will demonstrate right-to-left shunting at the level of the VSD. Flow through the defect can also be determined by Doppler echocardiography.

Cardiac Catheterization

- Selective angiocardiography of the right ventricle demonstrates simultaneous filling of the aorta and pulmonary artery in cases with right-to-left shunts.
- Nonselective angiocardiography may support a diagnosis of tetralogy of Fallot, but this technique is much less sensitive than echocardiography.

Therapy and Prognosis

Surgery

- Surgical correction of tetralogy of Fallot is uncommonly performed because of the attendant mortality and expense. Palliative surgical options include the Blalock anastomosis and the Potts anastomosis. In the Blalock anastomosis, the left subclavian artery is anastomosed with the pulmonary artery in order to increase pulmonary blood flow. The Potts anastomosis consists of a side-to-side anastomosis of the aorta and pulmonary artery. These procedures are generally effective in reducing signs of pulmonary hypoperfusion and systemic hypoxia.
- In some cases, palliation can be provided by reducing PS. Surgical valvuloplasty or balloon valvuloplasty are options.

Medical Management

- Beta-adrenergic blockade has been used to reduce the dynamic component of right ventricular outflow obstruction and to attenuate beta-adrenergic–mediated decreases in systemic vascular resistance. Increases in systemic vascular resistance will lower the magnitude of right-to-left shunting.
- Polycythemia should be controlled by periodic phlebotomy. When the packed cell volume exceeds 68, intervention is indicated. Up to 20 ml/kg of blood can be removed and replaced with a crystalloid solution, such as lactated Ringer's or saline.
- If the required frequency of phlebotomy is poorly tolerated by the patient, hydroxyurea, an oral myelosuppressive agent, can be used. However, administration of this drug requires close patient monitoring with periodic complete blood and platelet counts.

ATRIOVENTRICULAR VALVE DYSPLASIA

Congenital malformation of the mitral and tricuspid valves has been reported in dogs and cats. Malformation of the valve may result in a range of hemodynamic consequences including valvular regurgitation, mitral or tricuspid stenosis, and dynamic left ventricular outflow obstruction. Congenital malformation of the mitral valve complex (mitral valve dysplasia) is a common congenital cardiac defect in the cat. In addition, several canine breeds are predisposed including Bull Terriers, German Shepherds, and Great Danes. Tricuspid valve dysplasia has been shown to have a genetic basis in Labrador Retrievers.

Anatomy

- Mitral valve dysplasia most commonly results in valvular insufficiency and systolic regurgitation of blood into the left atrium.
- Any component of the atrioventricular valve complex (valve leaflet, chordae tendineae, papillary muscles) may be malformed. Often, more than one component is defective. A wide spectrum of valvular malformations has been described: thickening of the valve leaflets; incomplete separation of the valvular structures from the ventricular wall; shortening or elongation, thickening, and fusion of the chordae tendineae; and malpositioning and/or malformation of the papillary muscles.

Pathophysiology

- Malformation of the atrioventricular valve complex can result in significant valvular insufficiency. In the case involving the mitral valve, chronic mitral regurgitation leads to volume overload to the left heart, which results in dilation of the left ventricle and atrium in the same manner as does chronic degenerative valvular disease (see Chapter 6).
- When mitral regurgitation is severe, cardiac output decreases, resulting in signs of cardiac failure.
- Dilation of the left-sided chambers predisposes affected animals to arrhythmias. Severe atrial enlargement increases the risk of tachyarrhythmias such as atrial fibrillation.
- In some cases, malformation of the mitral valve complex causes a degree of valvular stenosis as well as insufficiency.
- If the tricuspid valve is involved, then atrial and ventricular enlargement secondary to volume overload with subsequent systemic venous hypertension and right-sided congestive heart failure is a likely outcome if regurgitation is severe.

Diagnosis

History and Clinical Signs

- Clinical signs correlate with the severity of the defect. Affected animals usually display signs of left-sided heart failure, including weakness, cough, and exercise intolerance if the mitral valve is affected. Alternatively, signs of right heart failure (abdominal distention associated with ascites) may be present if the tricuspid valve is affected.

Physical Examination

Palpation

- Affected animals may have a precordial thrill over the left cardiac apex (mitral valve) or right cardiac apex (tricuspid valve).

Auscultation

- A holosystolic murmur of mitral regurgitation is most prominent at the left cardiac apex. A diastolic heart sound (gallop) is present in some cases. The murmur of tricuspid regurgitation is best heart at the right cardiac apex. Some patients with clinically significant tricuspid regurgitation may have "silent" regurgitation.

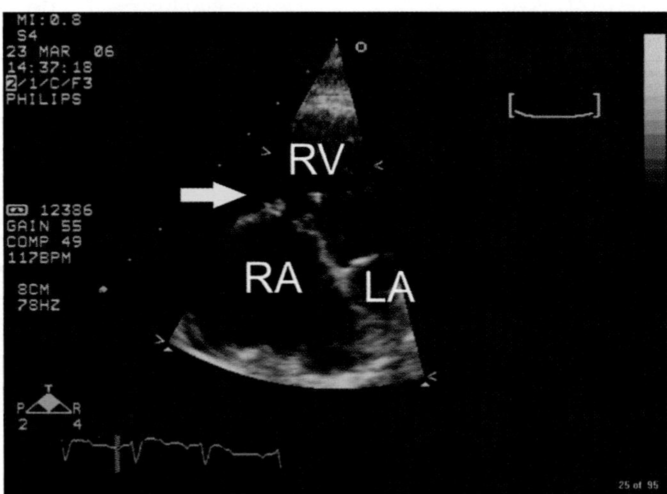

Figure 12-16. Echocardiogram from a dog with tricuspid valve dysplasia. Note the severely thickened tricuspid valve leaflets *(arrow)*. *RV*, Right ventricle; *LA*, left atrium; *RA*, right atrium.

Diagnostic Testing

Electrocardiogram

- Atrial arrhythmias (atrial premature contractions, atrial fibrillation) are common.
- Evidence of left atrial enlargement (widened P waves) and left ventricular enlargement may be present.
- Splintered QRS complexes are common ECG findings in cats and dogs with tricuspid valve dysplasia. Right heart enlargement patterns may also be present.

Thoracic Radiographs

- The most prominent abnormality with mitral valve dysplasia is severe left atrial enlargement. Left ventricular enlargement is also present. Pulmonary veins may be distended and evidence of left-sided congestive heart failure may be present.
- Right atrial and ventricular enlargement may be evident if severe tricuspid valve regurgitation is present. Distention of the caudal vena cava may be noted if right-sided congestive heart failure is present.

Echocardiography

- Echocardiography demonstrates malformation of the mitral valve complex (fused chordae tendineae and thickened, immobile valve leaflets) and left atrial and ventricular dilation.
- Doppler echocardiography demonstrates severe mitral regurgitation. If present, mitral stenosis can be identified.
- The echocardiographic findings with tricuspid valve dysplasia mirror those changes seen with mitral valve dysplasia, only involve the right heart instead (Figure 12-16).

Therapy and Prognosis

- Prognosis for the severely affected animal with clinical signs is poor. Mildly affected animals may remain free of clinical signs for several years. Therapy for progressive congestive heart failure is detailed in Chapter 15.

Frequently Asked Questions

How do I differentiate between a continuous murmur and a systolic murmur?
The differentiation between a continuous murmur and a systolic murmur is important because there is only one clinically important cause of a continuous murmur—patent ductus arteriosus.

- Continuous murmurs begin at the onset of systole, peak in intensity during mid to late systole, and continue into diastole.
- Systolic murmurs begin at the onset of systole, maintain a consistent intensity throughout the systolic period, and terminate at the end of systole. The termination of a systolic murmur may occur during or just after the second heart sound depending on the left ventricular systolic pressures and the severity of the valvular insufficiency. The duration of a systolic murmur is, for the most part, consistent regardless of the cardiac rhythm (excluding premature beats and tachyarrhythmias). In general, systole has a defined duration and, therefore, a systolic murmur has a defined duration. So even during prominent sinus arrhythmias, a systolic murmur sounds like it has a consistent duration.
- The scenario is different for continuous murmurs; the duration of the murmur changes during periods of sinus arrhythmia. In fact, the intensity of a continuous murmur during diastole may become inaudible during long pauses.

Which is the best approach for treatment of PDA: Surgical ligation or transarterial coil occlusion?
Both approaches have been demonstrated to be effective and safe when performed by experienced individuals; therefore, the best approach is the approach that is most readily available (there are geographical limitations for transarterial coil occlusion because there are a limited number of individuals trained to perform transcatheter interventional procedures).

Does the intensity of a cardiac murmur associated with congenital heart disease correlate with the severity of the disease?
In general, the intensity of the murmur roughly approximates the severity of the defect; however, there are some exceptions. Patients with small, restrictive VSDs often have very loud systolic murmurs, but are unlikely to be clinically affected. With regards to defects that cause obstruction to ventricular outflow, presence of myocardial failure can decrease the intensity of the murmur. Some patients with tricuspid valve dysplasia have "silent" regurgitation that can only be detected by echocardiography or angiocardiography. Patients with reversed PDA have severe cardiovascular derangement but often have no audible cardiac murmurs.

What is the most important diagnostic test for a patient suspected of having a congenital heart defect?
Echocardiography is the most important part of the evaluation of a patient suspected of having a congenital heart defect. Two-dimensional echocardiography provides an anatomical image of the cardiac structures that can be observed in real time for assessment of structural and functional abnormalities. M-mode echocardiography can be used to quantify cardiac dimensions and function. Doppler echocardiography is

a critical part of the echocardiographic evaluation of a patient with a cardiac murmur. Color flow Doppler allows for rapid detection of abnormal flow patterns and spectral Doppler can be utilized for quantification of blood flow characteristics such as velocity.

SUGGESTED READINGS

Bonagura JD, Lehmkuhl LB: Congenital heart disease. In Fox PR, Sisson D, Moise NS, eds: Textbook of canine and feline cardiology, Philadelphia, 1999, WB Saunders.

Kittleson MD, Kienle RD, eds: Small animal cardiovascular medicine, St Louis, 1998, Mosby.

Oyama MA, Sisson DD, Thomas WP, Bonagura JD: Congenital heart disease. p. 972. In Ettinger SJ, ed: Textbook of veterinary internal medicine, ed 6, Philadelphia, 2005, WB Saunders.

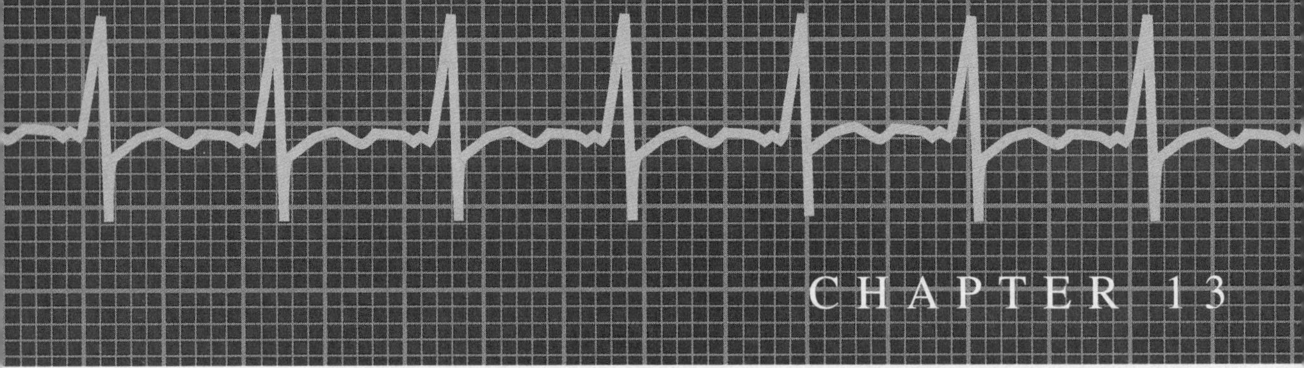

Cardiovascular Effects of Systemic Diseases

Francis W. K. Smith, Jr., Donald P. Schrope, and Carl D. Sammarco

INTRODUCTION

Many systemic diseases are capable of profoundly affecting cardiovascular structure and function (Box 13-1). The veterinarian may detect cardiovascular abnormalities as the predominant clinical sign or systemic disease manifestations may overshadow cardiac abnormalities. Although cardiovascular manifestations may sometimes be of no clinical significance, at other times they may constitute the major medical concern. Detection of cardiovascular involvement may be based on clinical signs, radiographic changes, electrocardiographic (ECG) or echocardiographic abnormalities, or laboratory findings. Emphasis in this chapter is given to diseases having the greatest cardiovascular effects or incidence in practice. The focus of discussion is the cardiovascular effects and their treatment.

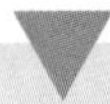

Endocrine Diseases

HYPERTHYROIDISM

- Hyperthyroidism is the most common systemic disturbance to affect cardiac function in cats and is rare in dogs. Hyperthyroid heart disease can be a severe problem, leading to heart failure in some animals.
- Hyperthyroidism is a disease of middle-aged to geriatric cats (range, 4 to 22 years; mean, 13 years) that is generally caused by a thyroid adenoma. Clinical evidence of thyrotoxic heart disease is unusual before the age of 6 years. Thyroid tumors in dogs are generally rare and nonfunctional adenocarcinomas that don't cause hyperthyroidism. Iatrogenic hyperthyroidism can result from over supplementation of thyroxin in hypothyroid dogs.

Cardiac Pathophysiology

Direct Effects

- Positive inotropic effects (i.e., increased contractility) result from an increased sodium-potassium – exchanging adenosine triphosphatase (Na^+, K^+-ATPase) activity, increased mitochondrial protein synthesis, and increased synthesis and enhanced contractile properties of myosin. Thyroid hormone favors the production of the alpha heavy chain myosin isoenzyme, which has the fastest ATPase activity, but is less efficient at converting ATP to mechanical energy. Thyroid hormones increase the number of L-type calcium channels and expression of sodium calcium ATPase, which improves the recycling of calcium by the sarcoplasmic reticulum. Systolic and diastolic performances are both altered.
- Positive chronotropic effects (i.e., increased heart rate) result from an increased rate of sinoatrial firing, decreased threshold of atrial activation, and shortened refractory period of the conduction tissue. The effect on atrial activation may increase the risk for atrial arrhythmias.

Indirect Effects

- The effect of thyroid hormones on the adrenergic system is controversial. The number of myocardial beta-adrenergic receptors and their affinity are

Box 13-1 Classification of Important Systemic Disorders That Affect the Heart

Endocrine
Thyroid gland
- Hyperthyroidism
- Hypothyroidism

Adrenal gland
- Hyperadrenocorticism
- Hypoadrenocorticism
- Pheochromocytoma

Pituitary
- Acromegaly (hypersomatotropism)

Pancreas
- Diabetes mellitus (hyperglycemia)

Metabolic
Hypercalcemia
Hypocalcemia
Hyperkalemia
Hypokalemia
Hypoglycemia
Uremia
Anemia

Neoplastic and infiltrative heart diseases
Physical and chemical agents
Hyperpyrexia (heat stroke)
Hypothermia
Carbon monoxide
Toad poisoning
Oleander toxicity
Chocolate (theobromine) toxicity
Doxorubicin cardiotoxicity

Infectious/inflammatory myocardial diseases
Bacterial (Lyme disease)
Viral (parvovirus)
Mycotic
Protozoal (trypanosomiasis)

Miscellaneous
Systemic lupus erythematosus (SLE)
Neurologic disease
Gastric dilatation-volvulus (GDV)
Pancreatitis
Traumatic myocarditis

increased in hyperthyroid animals. However, this does not always explain or result in an increased responsiveness to catecholamines. Postreceptor effects of thyroid hormone are probably mediated by changes in intracellular G protein populations that result in an enhanced response to adrenergic agonists. Circulating catecholamine levels are normal.

- Hyperthyroidism results in an increased metabolic rate, and consequently an increased tissue oxygen demand. The need for increased tissue perfusion and oxygen delivery requires greater cardiac output. Peripheral vasodilation increases tissue perfusion and decreases afterload. As blood volume increases, increased venous return to the heart and increased preload result. The combination of increased preload, increased contractility, increased heart rate, and decreased afterload results in increased cardiac output. Chronic volume overload and high metabolic rate can result in heart failure even though the cardiac output is still greater than normal. This is referred to as high-output heart failure.
- Hypertension is a frequent although usually not severe sequela of hyperthyroidism in cats, with one study showing an incidence of mild to moderate hypertension in 73% of cases. This occurs in spite of peripheral vasodilation, and probably reflects the increased stroke volume and heart rate which increases cardiac output in these animals. Blood pressure is a function of cardiac output and systemic vascular resistance.
- The combination of volume and pressure overload alters myocardial protein synthesis and degradation, which results in myocardial hypertrophy and chamber dilation. These changes are most notable in the left heart. In rare cases, hyperthyroid cats with congestive heart failure develop a cardiomyopathy of overload that resembles dilated cardiomyopathy.

KEY POINT

The net effects of hyperthyroidism on the cardiovascular system are enhanced cardiac contractility, tachycardia, cardiomegaly, left ventricular hypertrophy, high cardiac output, systemic hypertension, and occasionally high-output heart failure.

Diagnosis

History and Physical Examination

- Historical findings and clinical signs include weight loss, polyphagia, unkempt hair coat, polydipsia, diarrhea, nervousness, hyperactivity, vomiting, tremor, polyuria, lethargy, aggression, decreased appetite, weakness, episodic panting, and bulky, foul-smelling stool.
- Cardiovascular abnormalities that may be present on physical examination include tachycardia, premature heart beats, gallop rhythm, apical systolic murmur, accentuated heart sounds, forceful precordial beat, strong femoral pulses, jugular venous distention, and dyspnea when stressed.

- Noncardiac findings can include thinness, palpable thyroid gland, hyperactivity, dehydration, easily stressed, small kidneys, depression, weakness, and ventral flexion of the neck.

Electrocardiography

- ECG findings in hyperthyroid cats are sinus tachycardia (42%), right bundle branch block (7%), tall R waves in lead II (22%), left anterior fascicular block (4%), ventricular premature complexes (1%), atrial premature complexes (5%) atrial tachycardia or atrial fibrillation (2%). Ventricular tachycardia, ventricular bigeminy, ventricular pre-excitation and atrioventricular (AV) block have also been described.
- Sinus tachycardia and increased R wave voltage resolve with treatment of hyperthyroidism. Atrial and ventricular premature contractions (APCs and VPCs) may decrease in frequency or become abolished. Conduction disturbances may or may not resolve. If arrhythmias or R wave amplitude changes persist after hyperthyroidism is controlled, the patient should be evaluated for idiopathic cardiomyopathy or systemic hypertension.

Radiography

- Mild to severe cardiomegaly is seen in 50% of cases.
- Evidence of congestive heart failure (pulmonary edema or pleural effusion) is reported in fewer than 5% of cases.

Echocardiography

- Common findings in hyperthyroidism include left atrial enlargement, left ventricular wall and septal hypertrophy, increased aortic amplitude, hyperkinetic left ventricular wall and septum, left ventricular dilation (eccentric hypertrophy), and increased fractional shortening.
- A dilated form of cardiomyopathy occasionally develops and is characterized by left atrial and ventricular dilation and low fractional shortening.

Clinical Pathology

- Elevated serum values for alkaline phosphatase, aspartate aminotransaminase, and alanine aminotransaminase are common.
- Mild azotemia is present in approximately 34% of cases.
- The thyroxine (T_4) value is usually elevated and is the diagnostic screening test of choice; however, thyroid hormone levels fluctuate during the day and may dip into the normal range in mildly hyperthyroid animals.

Specialized Diagnostic Tests

- Additional diagnostic tests may occasionally be needed to confirm the diagnosis of hyperthyroidism in cats with normal resting T_4 values on repeated assessment.

Free T_4 by Equilibrium Dialysis

- Cats with mild hyperthyroidism and normal T_4 levels often have a high free T_4 level, whereas cats with nonthyroidal illness often have a normal free T_4 (specificity and sensitivity > 90%).
- Not recommended as a screening test for hyperthyroidism, as some cats with nonthyroidal illness will have a high free T_4 level.

T_3 Suppression Test

- Administer triiodothyronine (T_3) at 25 μg PO every 8 hours for seven doses for a cat. Collect blood for a T_4 determination prior to the first dose of T_3 and 2 to 4 hours after the last dose.
- A normal cat's T_4 level will suppress to less than 1.5 μg/dL. Values between 1.5 to 2 μg/dL are nondiagnostic whereas values greater than 2 μg/dL support diagnosis of hyperthyroidism. T_3 values can be measured concurrently to assess owner compliance. T_3 values should rise regardless of the cat's thyroid status.

Thyroid-Releasing Hormone Response Test

- To perform the thyroid-releasing hormone (TRH) response test, inject 0.1 mg/kg of TRH and obtain blood samples before and 4 hours after TRH injection.
- In normal cats, the post-TRH T_4 is at least 60% greater than baseline. A hyperthyroid cat's T_4 levels change less than 50% following TRH administration. Values between 50% and 60% are not diagnostic.
- The TRH response test takes less time to perform than the T_3 suppression test and does not depend on the owner's ability to medicate the cat. TRH can cause vomiting, salivation, tachypnea, and defecation following the injection. TRH is substantially more expensive than T_3.
- Results not superior to repeated assessment of total T_4 coupled with free T_4 by equilibrium dialysis, if necessary.

Thyroid Imaging

- Thyroid imaging with radioactive technetium-99m will identify the affected gland(s). This imaging study is recommended prior to surgery in any hyperthyroid cat with nonpalpable thyroid glands, because the thyroid glands can migrate into the chest, rendering them inoperable.

Therapy

Management of Hyperthyroidism

- Radioactive iodine is curative and does not require anesthesia or surgery. In most instances it is the safest and most effective treatment.
- Surgical treatment effectively cures the condition and eliminates the need for chronic medication. Medical management generally is instituted to stabilize the patient prior to surgery. The most frequent complication of surgery is transient postoperative hypocalcemia.
- Medical management generally involves administering **methimazole** (Tapazole) at 2.5 to 5 mg PO every 8 to 12 hours in cats. Start with a low dose and titrate up as needed and tolerated. A transdermal formulation in pleuronic **lecithin organo gel** can be used, but the rate of clinical improvement is slower than with oral administration. **Carbimazole** is an alternative to methimazole, available in Europe, and is dosed at 5 mg PO every 8 hours in cats. Propylthiouracil is no longer recommended because of a high incidence of side effects. These drugs inhibit the formation of thyroid hormones, but do not inhibit or block the release of already formed T_3 and T_4. Thus serum thyroid levels do not drop acutely.
- Inorganic iodine therapy is rarely used. Iodine blocks thyroid hormone synthesis and release, and thyroid levels rapidly drop. Rapid reduction of thyroid levels may benefit patients with severe congestive heart failure. Preoperative use may decrease the vascularity of the thyroid gland. Administer one dose of methimazole prior to the iodine, so that the iodine is not incorporated into new thyroid hormone. Administer one drop of saturated solution of **potassium iodide** orally once a day for 7 to 10 days.
- **Sodium** or **calcium ipodate** at 15 mg/kg PO every 12 hours blocks the conversion of T_4 to T_3. It is not effective in all cats and should be considered a treatment of last resort.

Management of Arrhythmias

- The expedient way to manage tachyarrhythmias is to start methimazole therapy. Even before euthyroidism is restored, many arrhythmias improve or are abolished. In this fashion, ancillary therapy is usually unnecessary.
- Severe tachyarrhythmias (i.e., atrial tachycardia, multiform VPCs, ventricular tachycardia) in patients without heart failure are best managed with beta blockers such as **atenolol** (3.125 to 6.25 mg PO every 12 hours) or **propranolol** (2.5 to 7.5 mg PO every 8 hours). Higher than normal doses of beta blockers may be needed because of an increased rate of metabolism and elimination. Supraventricular arrhythmias in asthmatic cats should be managed with **diltiazem** (7.5 mg PO every 8 hours).
- Supraventricular arrhythmias in patients with congestive heart failure can be managed with digoxin, beta blockers, or diltiazem. Exercise caution when using beta blockers in the presence of congestive heart failure, because these agents depress cardiac contractility and may exacerbate heart failure. Cats with hyperthyroidism almost always have increased contractility, so worsening of congestive heart failure with beta blockade is rare. Ideally, congestion should be treated and controlled with diuretics before prescribing a beta blocker. Diltiazem also depresses contractility, but less so than beta blockers. The vasodilating effects of diltiazem usually offset its negative inotropic effects.

Management of Hypertension

- Usually accomplished with control of the hyperthyroid state. The use of beta blockers, vasodilators (e.g., angiotensin-converting enzyme [ACE] inhibitors, **amlodipine**), and other agents is occasionally indicated.

Management of Congestive Heart Failure

- Diuretics are used to control pulmonary edema and pleural effusion.
- **Nitroglycerin** ointment can be used in patients with critical congestion or in those refractory to diuretics alone. **Enalapril** or **benazepril** also may be helpful in refractory cases.
- Treat arrhythmias as discussed previously.
- **Digoxin** may be useful in cases where chronic hyperthyroidism results in dilated cardiomyopathy.

Prognosis

- The prognosis for remission of sinus tachycardia, voltage changes, arrhythmias, and congestive heart failure is generally favorable when the hypermetabolic state is controlled through the medical or surgical techniques discussed.
- The prognosis is poor if dilated cardiomyopathy has developed secondary to chronic overload of the heart.

HYPOTHYROIDISM

- Hypothyroidism is a common endocrinopathy in dogs and is rarely encountered as a naturally occurring condition in cats. It is most commonly diagnosed in middle-aged dogs (22% are 2 to 3 years old; 32% are 4 to 6 years old; 22% are 7 to 9 years old). Many breeds are affected, and there appears to be a breed predilection in the Golden Retriever, Doberman Pinscher, Dachshund, Irish Setter, Miniature Schnauzer, Great Dane, Poodle, and Boxer. There is no gender predilection. Hypothyroidism is rare in cats and generally limited to postoperative cases following surgical removal of unilateral or bilateral functional thyroid tumors.

- The cardiac effects of hypothyroidism are generally the opposite of those found in hyperthyroidism. The cardiac effects of hypothyroidism rarely have severe consequences. However, hypothyroidism can aggravate heart failure and complicate the management of cardiac patients.

Cardiac Pathophysiology

- Cardiac contractility is decreased as a result of decreased Na^+,K^+-ATPase activity, decreased mitochondrial protein synthesis, and decreased synthesis of contractile properties of myosin.
- Cardiac conduction is decreased as a result of a decreased rate of sinoatrial firing, increased threshold of atrial activation, and prolonged refractory period of the conducting tissue. Enhanced vagal tone in hypothyroidism also slows the heart rate and accentuates sinus arrhythmias.

KEY POINT

Evaluate the thyroid status in any dog in congestive heart failure with an inappropriately slow heart rate.

- Thyroid hormone plays an important role in lipid and cholesterol metabolism. Hypothyroidism predisposes animals to increased levels of cholesterol and, to a lesser extent, triglycerides. Although rare in dogs, hypercholesterolemia can result in atherosclerosis and myocardial infarction. Lipid abnormalities resolve with thyroid hormone supplementation.
- Hypothyroidism decreases the metabolic rate, thus lessening the required cardiac output. Correcting hypothyroidism increases the workload on the heart. This is important to remember when treating animals in congestive heart failure.
- Hypothyroidism decreases digoxin clearance, predisposing patients to digoxin toxicity.

Diagnosis

History and Physical Examination

- Historical findings in hypothyroid animals include alopecia and other dermatologic problems, lethargy, weakness, depression, infertility, and diarrhea.
- Cardiovascular abnormalities noted on physical examination can include muffled heart sounds, weak apex heart beat, weak pulses, and bradycardia.
- Noncardiac physical findings can include symmetric alopecia, seborrhea, myxedema, pyoderma, hypothermia, depression, and lameness.

Electrocardiography

- ECG changes in hypothyroidism reflect decreased automaticity of pacemaker tissue and depressed conduction. Changes that reflect decreased automaticity may include sinus bradycardia, pronounced sinus arrhythmia, and atrial and ventricular arrhythmias. Changes that reflect depressed conduction may include AV block, widened QRS complexes, and inverted T waves. The most common findings reported in dogs are sinus bradycardia and inverted T waves.
- Low-voltage QRS complexes are frequently seen in hypothyroid animals.
- Atrial fibrillation in giant-breed dogs occasionally accompanies hypothyroidism, usually in association with dilated cardiomyopathy. Supplementation with thyroid hormone rarely causes conversion to sinus rhythm.
- Radiographs are generally normal.

Echocardiography

- May reveal mild to marked decreases in indices of cardiac contractility and mild chamber enlargement. Decreased contractility is documented by increase in left ventricular interval diameter in systole, prolongation of the preejection period, decrease in left posterior wall thickness in systole and decrease in septal wall thickness in systole and diastole. There is a decrease in aortic root diameter, decrease in velocity of circumferential shortening and decrease fractional shortening.
- Always check thyroid status when depressed contractility is noted in an animal of a breed not predisposed to dilated cardiomyopathy.

Clinical Pathology

- The hemogram may reveal a low-grade nonregenerative anemia.
- The most common abnormality on the serum chemistry profile is hypercholesterolemia and, occasionally, hypertriglyceridemia.

- A normal serum T_4 value generally is sufficient to rule out hypothyroidism. Unfortunately, a low serum T_4 does not confirm the diagnosis. Concurrent systemic ailments and numerous drugs can cause depressed serum T_4 values in animals with normal thyroid function (euthyroid sick syndrome) (Box 13-2). To make a diagnosis in these cases requires integration of the history, physical findings, and other blood test results, or confirmation by specialized diagnostic tests.
- Serum T_3 values are less reliable than T_4 values at diagnosing hypothyroidism.

Specialized Diagnostic Tests

- The thyroid-stimulating hormone (TSH) response test has been the "gold standard" in veterinary medicine for diagnosing hypothyroidism. Animals with hypothyroidism have low baseline T_4 values and fail to increase their T_4 values above a predetermined level following administration of TSH. Animals with euthyroid sick syndrome will also have low baseline T_4 levels, but following TSH administration, their T_4 values will increase above an absolute cutoff value. Unfortunately, TSH is often difficult to obtain and expensive.
- Free T_4 by equilibrium dialysis as a diagnostic test of canine hypothyroidism has a sensitivity of 98% and specificity of 92%, versus a total T_4 sensitivity of 90% and specificity of 90%. The free T_4 by ED should be low in a hypothyroid animal.
- Canine TSH levels as a diagnostic test for canine hypothyroidism has a sensitivity of 75% and specificity of 90%. The TSH level should be high in a hypothyroid animal.
- When the endogenous TSH is high and the free T_4 by equilibrium dialysis is low, the diagnostic accuracy approaches 100%.

Box 13-2 Some Drugs and Diagnostic Agents that Can Alter Basal Serum Thyroid Hormone Concentrations in Humans and Possibly Dogs

Decrease T_4 and/or T_3	Increase T_4 and/or T_3
Amiodarone (T_3)	Amiodarone (T_4)
Androgens	Estrogens
Cholecystographic agents	5-Fluorouracil
Diazepam	Halothane
Dopamine	Insulin
Flunixin	Narcotic analgesics
Furosemide	Radiopaque dyes (ipodate)
Glucocorticoids	Thiazides
Heparin	
Imidazole	
Iodide	
Methimazole	
Mitotane	
Nitroprusside	
Penicillin	
Phenobarbital	
Phenothiazines	
Phenylbutazone	
Phenytoin	
Primidone	
Propranolol	
Propylthiouracil	
Radiopaque dyes (ipodate) (T_3)	
Salicylates	
Sulfonamides (sulfamethoxazole)	
Sulfonylureas	

From Feldman EC, Nelson RW: Canine and feline endocrinology and reproduction, 3rd ed. St Louis: WB Saunders, 2004.

Therapy

- Treatment of hypothyroidism is simple and inexpensive. **L-Thyroxin** is administered at 20 μg/kg PO every 12 hours, or 0.5 mg/m^2 every 12 hours with a maximum dose of 0.8 mg/dose for a dog. After 6 to 8 weeks, evaluate a serum T_4 value 4 to 6 hours after a dose of L-thyroxin. If the post-pill T_4 value is normal and clinical signs have resolved, you can try decreasing the frequency to once a day. Ideally, a post-pill T_4 value should then be obtained in another month at 4 to 6 and 24 hours after a dose of thyroxin. This is important to make sure that there is an adequate duration of effect with once daily dosing.
- Treatment in patients with congestive heart failure is more complicated. Supplementation will increase the metabolic rate and demand on the heart. If the failing heart is unable to meet these demands, heart failure will worsen. Therefore, implement thyroid hormone supplementation gradually in patients with cardiac disease, especially if they are already in failure. Start with one fourth of the standard dose and increase it by one-fourth dose weekly. It should be emphasized that hypothyroidism rarely causes heart failure, but may significantly exacerbate cardiac function in an animal with underlying heart disease.
- The risk of digoxin toxicity is increased in hypothyroid states. Monitor hypothyroid animals closely for signs of digoxin toxicity, and consider

assessing thyroid status in any animal with normal renal function that develops digoxin toxicity on reasonable doses of digoxin. Ideally the digoxin level on a sample obtained 8 hours postdose should be between 0.5 to 1 ng/dL.

Prognosis

- There are few complications in the treatment of hypothyroidism.

HYPOADRENOCORTICISM (ADDISON'S DISEASE)

- Hypoadrenocorticism is a potentially life-threatening endocrinopathy that is uncommon in dogs and rare in cats. The disease is more common in female dogs and usually occurs in young to middle-aged animals. Approximately 76% of cases occur before 7 years of age, with an age range of 5 weeks to 16 years.
- Primary hypoadrenocorticism (Addison's disease) results from destruction of the zona glomerulosa and zona fasciculata of the adrenal gland. These areas of the adrenal gland produce aldosterone and cortisol, respectively. Destruction is generally immune mediated, but also can occur secondary to infection, neoplasia, infarction, and drugs such as o,p′-dichlorodiphenyldichloroethane (o,p′-DDD) (Lysodren, [mitotane]).
- Secondary hypoadrenocorticism results from decreased production or release of adrenocorticotropic hormone (ACTH) from the pituitary gland. Secondary adrenal insufficiency may occur following acute withdrawal of long-term, high-dose glucocorticoid therapy that has suppressed the hypothalamic-pituitary-adrenal axis. These patients have normal mineralocorticoid activity, so electrolyte values are normal. Cortisol values are depressed.
- Adrenal destruction occurs gradually, so basal hormone levels remain normal. It is only when the animal is stressed and the adrenal reserve is inadequate that signs develop. Eventually, the destruction proceeds to the point that basal hormone levels are depressed and clinical signs are present without stress.

Cardiac Pathophysiology

Cardiovascular Effects of Cortisol

- Cortisol is important in maintaining vascular integrity and responsiveness to catecholamines. Cortisol deficiency predisposes animals to hypotension.
- Cortisol has a positive inotropic effect on the heart.
- Cortisol affects the distribution and elimination of body water.
- Cortisol is important in helping the body deal with stress. This is why so many addisonian crises follow stress, and why glucocorticoid supplementation must be increased during periods of stress.

Cardiovascular Effects of Aldosterone

- Aldosterone acts on the distal renal convoluted tubule and collecting duct to enhance sodium retention and potassium elimination. Aldosterone deficiency results in hyponatremia and hyperkalemia.
- Hyponatremia decreases plasma osmotic pressure, causing fluid shifts out of the vascular compartment. This contributes to hypovolemia and hypotension.
- Hyperkalemia alters cardiac conduction, resulting in numerous arrhythmias. The cardiac effects of hyperkalemia are aggravated by low sodium, low calcium, and acidosis.

> **KEY POINT**
>
> Net cardiovascular effects of hypoadrenocorticism are hypovolemia, systemic hypotension, altered cardiac conduction, and depressed myocardial function. These changes can be fatal if not rapidly diagnosed and aggressively treated.

Diagnosis

History and Physical Examination

- A history of waxing and waning of clinical signs, with more severe signs during periods of stress, generally is present.
- Patients often present with history of anorexia, vomiting, diarrhea, depression, weakness, and cardiovascular collapse. Other signs include weight loss, polyuria, polydipsia, melena, and shivering.
- Transient improvement after intravenous fluid therapy or corticosteroid administration followed by subsequent relapse days or weeks later can occur.
- Findings on physical examination include depression, weakness, dehydration, hypothermia, slow capillary refill time, shaking, bradycardia, and weak femoral pulses.

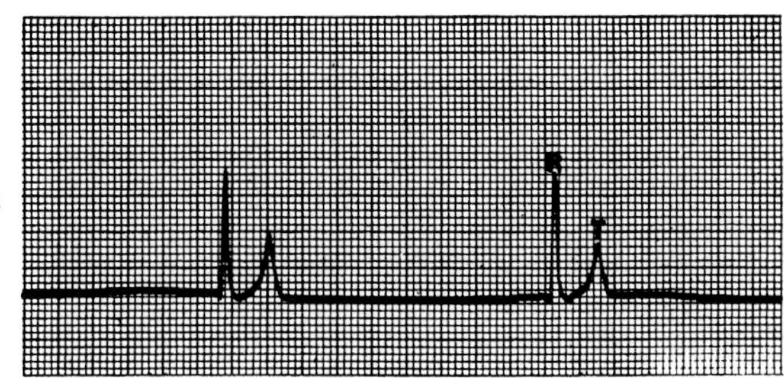

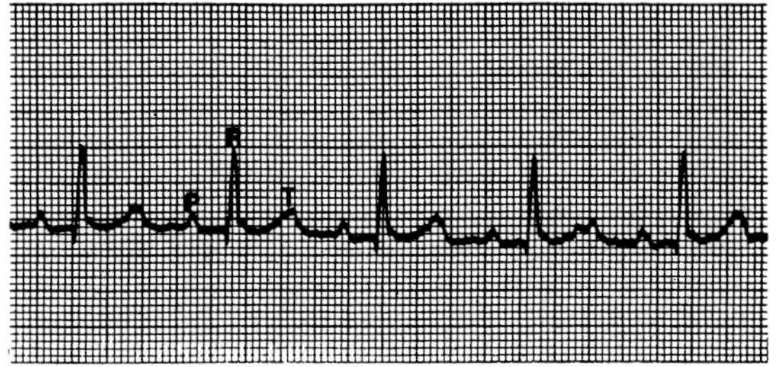

Figure 13-1. **A,** Hyperkalemia in a dog in cardiovascular collapse, consistent with an Addisonian crisis. P waves are absent (atrial standstill), and T waves are tall and peaked. Serum potassium was 8.4 mEq/L. **B,** After institution of therapy, P waves are present, and the T wave is of smaller amplitude. Serum potassium is now 4.8 mEq/L. (From Tilley LP: Essentials of canine and feline electrocardiography: interpretation and treatment, ed 3, Malvern, Penn, 1992, Lea & Febiger.)

Electrocardiography

- ECG changes vary with the magnitude of the hyperkalemia and are aggravated by hyponatremia, hypocalcemia, and acidosis. The following ECG findings are seen with experimentally induced hyperkalemia (Figure 13-1):
  - Peaking of the T wave with a narrow base is the earliest ECG abnormality and may be observed when serum K^+ exceeds 5.7 to 6.0 mEq/L.
  - P wave morphology is altered, its amplitude reduced, intra-atrial conduction delayed, and PR interval prolonged when serum K^+ exceeds 7.0 mEq/L.
  - P waves become unrecognizable (atrial standstill) at plasma K^+ levels greater than 8.5 mEq/L.
  - The QRS widens uniformly at plasma K^+ levels greater than 9 mEq/L.
  - Sinoatrial exit block or junctional rhythms with and without escape complexes may be present.
  - Ventricular fibrillation and ventricular asystole may occur at plasma K^+ levels greater than 10 mEq/L.
  - In clinical cases, ECG changes do not correlate as closely with potassium concentrations as they do in published experimental studies.
  - The rhythm with atrial standstill secondary to hyperkalemia is generally slow and may be regular or irregular. It is a sinoventricular rhythm. The sinus node continues to fire, and impulses are transmitted to the AV node and ventricles by internodal pathways. P waves are absent because atrial myocytes are not activated.

KEY POINT

Hyperkalemia is the most common cause of atrial standstill. Atrial standstill also occurs with fibrous replacement of atrial muscle cells secondary to severe atrial distention (valve disease, cardiomyopathy) in dogs and cats, with cardiac arrest, and secondary to an atrial myopathy in dogs, a condition most commonly seen in English springer spaniels.

Radiographs

- Approximately 80% of untreated dogs have one or more radiographic abnormalities. Abnormalities in order of reported frequency include narrow caudal vena cava, microcardia, narrow cranial lobar pulmonary artery and microhepatica. These changes are the result of hypovolemia and rapidly resolve with steroid and volume replacement.

Clinical Pathology

- A low-grade normocytic, normochromic nonregenerative anemia is present in 25% of cases, but may be masked by the effects of hemoconcentration. Eosinophilia and lymphocytosis may also be present.
- A serum chemistry profile frequently reveals azotemia, hyponatremia, and hyperkalemia. A sodium: potassium ratio of less than 27 supports hypoadrenocorticism, but is not pathognomonic for the disease. Hypercalcemia and hypoglycemia are not uncommon.
- Mild-to-moderate metabolic acidosis is common during a crisis.
- It is unusual for a dog with untreated Addison's disease to have a urine specific gravity greater than 1.030, and it is often less than 1.020.
- In patients with secondary hypoadrenocorticism, sodium and potassium levels are normal. The other abnormalities described above may be present.

Specialized Diagnostic Tests

- A tentative diagnosis is frequently obtained from the history and results of the complete blood count and serum chemistry profile. However, there are numerous causes of hyperkalemia, and acid-base and electrolyte changes associated with severe gastrointestinal disease and renal failure can cause an abnormal sodium: potassium ratio that would erroneously suggest Addison's disease.

- An ACTH response test is helpful in confirming Addison's disease and essential for documenting secondary hypoadrenocorticism.

Therapy

Addisonian Crisis Therapy

- Patients that present with cardiovascular collapse and atrial standstill require aggressive therapy. Therapy is directed at rapidly correcting hypovolemia, correcting rhythm disturbances, correcting electrolyte imbalances, and replacing mineralocorticoids and glucocorticoids.
- Volume replacement and correction of hyponatremia and hypochloremia is initially achieved with rapid infusion of **0.9% saline** at 60 to 80 ml/kg/hr for 1 to 2 hours and then modified according to patient needs. The ACTH response test can be performed while saline is being administered.
- Glucocorticoid deficiency is corrected with either **methylprednisolone sodium succinate** (1 to 2 mg/kg IV) or **dexamethasone sodium phosphate** (0.5 to 2 mg/kg IV) and then repeated every 2 to 6 hours. After the initial high dose of a rapidly acting water-soluble glucocorticoid has been administered, glucocorticoid therapy can be continued with **dexamethasone** at a dosage of 0.05 to 0.1 mg/kg PO every 12 hours added to the IV fluids. Once the patient is stable, switch to oral prednisone. It should be noted that prednisolone interferes with cortisol assays, so ideally it should be started after the ACTH response test is performed. Dexamethasone has no mineralocorticoid effects and does not interfere with the cortisol assay.
- Mineralocorticoid deficiency is initially corrected (after the ACTH response test is performed) with **desoxycorticosterone pivalate (DOCP)** at 2.2 mg/kg IM or **fludrocortisone acetate (Florinef)** at 0.02 mg/kg/day PO if the dog is not vomiting
- Hyperkalemia is corrected in several different ways.
- Saline infusion results in rapid dilution of potassium and is often the only treatment needed.
- Severe hyperkalemia associated with significant cardiac conduction abnormalities often requires more aggressive therapy. Treatment options include **sodium bicarbonate** (1 to 2 mEq/kg) given slowly IV over 5 minutes *or* a combination of **regular insulin** (0.5 U/kg IV) and **50% dextrose** (1 g/kg IV). Dextrose can also be administered alone, as it will stimulate endogenous insulin secretion.
- If life-threatening cardiac arrhythmias are noted, administer **calcium gluconate** (10%) at 0.5 to 1 ml/kg slowly IV over 10 to 15 minutes. Monitor the ECG while administering calcium. Calcium will temporarily correct rhythm disturbances by countering the effect of potassium on the conduction tissue. Calcium has no effect on serum potassium levels. Calcium overdose can also cause severe cardiac disturbances, so careful monitoring is required.

Maintenance Therapy

- Mineralocorticoid replacement is initiated with either **fludrocorticosterone acetate** at 0.02 mg/kg/day given orally or **DOCP** at 2.2 mg/kg every 25 days given IM. These doses—and dose interval for DOCP—are adjusted as needed to maintain normal electrolyte balance. Therapy must be individualized to the patient. A large trial with DOCP showed a dose and interval range of 1.5 to 2.2 mg/kg every 25 to 30 days.
- Glucocorticoid replacement is achieved with either **prednisone** at 0.2 mg/kg PO every 24 hours or **cortisone** at 1.0 mg/kg PO every 24 hours. Some patients receiving fludrocorticosterone acetate or DOCP do not need glucocorticoid supplementation except during periods of stress.

Prognosis

- Excellent prognosis with therapy
- Many dogs appear to do better with a small daily maintenance dose of prednisone or cortisone. During illness or other stressful periods, however, larger doses of glucocorticoids are necessary to avoid relapse into acute adrenal crisis.

HYPERADRENOCORTICISM (CUSHING'S DISEASE)

- Hyperadrenocorticism is a common endocrinopathy in older dogs and is rarely reported in cats. The syndrome is associated with excessive levels of cortisol that result from excess pituitary ACTH or excess ACTH from ectopic nonendocrine tumors, functional adrenocortical adenoma, or carcinoma. Iatrogenic Cushing's syndrome occurs with excessive glucocorticoid administration.
- Pituitary-dependent hyperadrenocorticism accounts for 80% to 85% of cases of hyperadrenocorticism. It is a disease of middle-aged and older dogs (usually older than 6 years), although a few cases have been diagnosed under 1 year of age. There is no sex predilection. Poodles, Dachshunds, and Beagles may be at increased risk.

- Dogs with functional adrenocortical tumors tend to be older, ranging from 6 to 16 years of age with a mean age of 11 years. Females are affected more frequently. German Shepherds, Toy Poodles, Dachshunds, and Terriers are most commonly affected.
- Hyperadrenocorticism rarely produces significant cardiac disease; however, signs and side effects of hyperadrenocorticism can mimic cardiac disease. Systemic effects of hyperadrenocorticism can also exacerbate underlying cardiac disease.

Pathophysiology

Systemic Hypertension

- Hypercortisolism increases vascular resistance by increasing smooth muscle sensitivity to catecholamines and increasing production of angiotensinogen. Mineralocorticoid properties of cortisol enhance the renal resorption of sodium and secondary fluid retention, resulting in an increased vascular volume. Hypertension is present in 57% to 82% of cushingoid dogs.
- Systemic hypertension may cause myocardial hypertrophy.
- Many affected dogs have coexisting AV valvular insufficiency and its associated cardiac changes. Hypertension might exacerbate underlying cardiac problems.

Pulmonary Thromboembolism

- Patients with hyperadrenocorticism are predisposed to pulmonary thromboembolism, with most cases diagnosed while the animal is being treated for Cushing's disease. Factors causing thromboembolism with Cushing's disease include obesity, high hematocrit, hypertension, and increased levels of clotting factors.
- Pulmonary thromboembolism should be suspected in any cushingoid patient with a history of acute onset of dyspnea or cyanosis.

Panting and Dyspnea

- Altered ventilation mechanics are often present owing to weakness in the muscles of respiration, increased thoracic fat deposition (decreasing chest wall compliance), and increased diaphragmatic abdominal pressure resulting from adipose tissue and hepatomegaly. Mild respiratory distress or rapid respiratory rate at rest often results.
- Many cushingoid dogs have variable degrees of lower airway disease or parenchymal disease.
- The triad of mitral/tricuspid insufficiency, respiratory disease, and Cushing's syndrome may create intractable dyspnea due to cardiopulmonary failure.

Diagnosis

History and Physical Examination

- The major historical features are systemic manifestations of hypercortisolism; they include polydipsia, polyuria, polyphagia, panting, alopecia, anestrus, exercise intolerance, and lethargy.
- Findings on physical examination may include abdominal enlargement, hepatomegaly, muscle weakness, testicular atrophy, symmetric alopecia, skin atrophy, hyperpigmentation, calcinosis cutis, bruising, and obesity.
- ECGs show no characteristic changes. ECG evidence of left ventricular enlargement is often present in cushingoid dogs with mitral valvular insufficiency.

Radiography

- Hypercortisolism causes changes on thoracic radiographs that include calcification of the tracheal and bronchial rings and osteoporosis of the thoracic vertebrae. Metastatic pulmonary lesions are seen infrequently with adrenal tumors.
- Radiographic changes associated with pulmonary thromboembolism include hypoperfusion of the infarcted lung lobes, overcirculation within the normal lung lobes, pleural effusion, and blunting and thickening of the pulmonary arteries. Thoracic radiographs may be normal.
- Echocardiography is rarely part of the workup of Cushing's disease.

Clinical Pathology

- The excessive production of cortisol may result in neutrophilia, lymphopenia, eosinopenia, and erythrocytosis (females).
- Chemistry abnormalities include fasting hyperglycemia, high serum alkaline phosphatase (sometimes extremely elevated), high alanine aminotransferase, high cholesterol, lipemia, and low blood urea nitrogen.
- Urinalysis shows specific gravity less than 1.015 and often less than 1.008. Proteinuria, glycosuria, and bacterial cystitis are sometimes noted.

Specialized Diagnostic Tests

- A urine cortisol:creatinine ratio is a quick screening test for Cushing's disease. This test has a high sensitivity, but low specificity for Cushing's disease. The ACTH response test and low-dose dexamethasone suppression tests are the standard tests used to confirm the diagnosis.

- A high-dose dexamethasone suppression test or serum ACTH level is used to try to differentiate between adrenal tumors and pituitary-dependent Cushing's disease.
- Ultrasound or computed tomography scan can be used to try to differentiate pituitary-dependent Cushing's disease from adrenal tumors in patients that do not suppress with the high-dose dexamethasone suppression test.

Therapy

Pituitary-Dependent Hyperadrenocorticism

- Chemotherapy using **mitotane** (Lysodren) is the standard treatment. Lysodren selectively, and usually reversibly, destroys the zona fasciculata (cortisol) and zona reticularis (sex hormones) of the adrenal gland. The zona glomerulosa (aldosterone) is occasionally affected.
- **Ketoconazole** (Nizoral) can be substituted in animals that do not tolerate Lysodren. Ketoconazole blocks an enzymatic step that is necessary for the production of cortisol.
- **Trilostane** (Vetoryl) inhibits adrenal steroidogenesis through enzyme inhibition and can also be substituted for Lysodren. This drug is not currently approved by the FDA but is licensed for use in dogs in Europe.
- Hypophysectomy and bilateral adrenalectomy with replacement hormone therapy are rarely used alternatives to medical management.

Adrenocortical Tumor

- Surgical removal of the affected adrenal gland(s) is recommended if possible.

KEY POINT

There is a high morbidity associated with surgery. Ideally, the patient is stabilized first by decreasing cortisol synthesis with ketoconazole.

- If the tumor is inoperable or metastasis is identified, manage the patient with either **mitotane** or **ketoconazole**. Very high doses of mitotane are usually required in patients with adrenal tumors. Many dogs with adrenal tumors respond poorly to medical management.
- Replacement steroid therapy is necessary both during and after surgery.
- Management of pulmonary embolism and systemic hypertension, if present, is undertaken through standard therapeutic protocols (see Chapters 9 and 15).

Prognosis

- Excellent prognosis is confirmed with resectable, benign adrenal tumors.
- Nonresectable or metastatic adrenal adenocarcinomas have a poor prognosis.
- Chemotherapy with o,p′-DDD (Lysodren) or ketoconazole for pituitary-dependent hyperadrenocorticism has potential side effects, but most treated dogs respond well to therapy. Average survival in one study was 2 years, with a range of 18 days to 7 years. Clinical experience with trilostane is not as extensive as with o,p′-DDD, but side effects with trilostane are negligible and therapy appears to be efficacious in most dogs.
- Systemic hypertension generally resolves with control of hypercortisolism.

HYPERSOMATOTROPISM (ACROMEGALY) IN CATS

- Acromegaly is a syndrome associated with high levels of growth hormone (hypersomatotropism).
- In cats, acromegaly occurs secondary to a pituitary tumor. It is a rare endocrinopathy that is seen in middle-aged to old cats (mean age: 10 years; median age: 9 years; range: 4 to 17 years). It is most common in males and rarely seen in females.
- In dogs, hypersomatotropism is associated with progestogen treatment or endogenous progestogens that are produced during diestrus. It does ot cause clinically significant cardiac problems in dogs. The syndrome is seen in females and is reversible with discontinuation of progestogen therapy or resolves spontaneously with the end of diestrus.

Cardiovascular Pathophysiology

- The trophic effect of growth hormone results in generalized organomegaly, including the heart. Cardiac changes are those of myocardial hypertrophy, interstitial fibrosis, myocytolysis and intramural arteriosclerosis. Heart failure is a common sequela of acromegaly in cats.
- Systemic hypertension is seen frequently in humans with acromegaly. Systemic hypertension is sometimes present in cats with acromegaly

and is usually accompanied by evidence of renal insufficiency.

Diagnosis

History and Physical Examination

- Most cats present with a history of polyuria, polydipsia, and weight gain.
- Cardiac abnormalities noted on physical examination may include a systolic murmur, gallop rhythm, and signs of congestive heart failure (dyspnea, cyanosis, muffled heart sounds, or crackles).
- Other abnormalities include hepatomegaly, nephromegaly, large head, arthritis, prognathism, pot belly, large tongue, and circling.
- ECG abnormalities have not been observed in these patients.
- Radiographs of the thorax usually demonstrate cardiomegaly and, less commonly, pulmonary edema or pleural effusion.
- Echocardiograms generally reveal hypertrophy of the intraventricular septum and left ventricular free wall.

Clinical Pathology

- The hemogram is generally unremarkable, but some cats have erythrocytosis.
- All cases are hyperglycemic and glucosuric. Most cats are also hyperproteinemic, azotemic, and hyperphosphatemic. Hypercholesterolemia, high alanine aminotransferase, high serum alkaline phosphatase, and ketonuria are seen less frequently.

Specialized Diagnostic Tests

- A commercially available validated growth hormone assay is not currently available for cats.
- Insulin-like growth factor I level was high in two cats with acromegaly that were tested. This test is commercially available.
- Computed tomography can be used to identify the pituitary tumor.
- Evaluate blood pressure in any suspected or confirmed cases.

Therapy

- Treatment options include hypophysectomy, radiation therapy, and medical management with **bromocriptine** or **octreotide** (a somatostatin analogue). Hypophysectomy has not been reported in cats. Radiation therapy is difficult to obtain and has only resulted in transient improvement to date. Medical management is generally unsuccessful.
- Supportive medical care includes high doses of insulin for insulin-resistant diabetes mellitus and diuretics for congestive heart failure.

Prognosis

- Survival in cats with acromegaly ranges from 4 to 60 months (generally 1.5 to 3 years) from time of diagnosis.
- Most cats die or are euthanized owing to severe congestive heart failure, renal failure, or expanding pituitary tumor.

Note: Hypersomatotropism without acromegaly has been associated with hypertrophic cardiomyopathy in some cats. A total of 31 cats with hypertrophic cardiomyopathy were shown to have growth hormone levels that were four times the control levels. None of the cats that were examined postmortem had pituitary tumors, and none demonstrated hyperinsulinism or diabetes mellitus.

PHEOCHROMOCYTOMA

- These tumors of adrenal medullary origin are uncommonly detected in dogs. They are typically seen in old dogs (mean age, 11 years, with range of 1 to 16 years) and extremely rare in cats.
- Pheochromocytomas are catecholamine-producing tumors derived from chromaffin cells.
- In addition to important effects on the cardiovascular system, catecholamines have significant metabolic effects, stimulating glycogenolysis and gluconeogenesis.

Cardiac Pathophysiology

- The cardiovascular effects of pheochromocytomas result from the alpha-1, beta-1, and beta-2 effects of norepinephrine and epinephrine. Stimulation of alpha and beta-adrenergic receptors generally causes opposite effects. The dominant effect varies with relative receptor density and activation thresholds. For example, in vascular smooth muscle, alpha adrenergic effects predominate. Thus, hypertension results when both alpha- and beta-adrenergic receptors are stimulated.
- Beta-1 adrenergic effects include sinus tachycardia, increased cardiac conduction velocity, and increased contractility.
- Beta-2 adrenergic effects on the cardiovascular system include venous and arteriole vasodilation.
- Alpha-1 adrenergic effects on the cardiovascular system include venous and arteriole

vasoconstriction. Approximately 50% of dogs with pheochromocytomas are hypertensive at the time of testing.

- Myocardial injury may result from catecholamine excess (i.e., myonecrosis with subsequent fibrosis and interstitial inflammation is reported in some humans with pheochromocytomas) and coronary vasoconstriction.

Diagnosis

History and Physical Examination

- Historical observations include weakness, collapse, anorexia, vomiting, weight loss, panting, dyspnea, lethargy, diarrhea, whining, pacing, polyuria, polydipsia, shivering, and epistaxis.
- Abnormalities noted on physical examination include lethargy, tachypnea and dyspnea, arrhythmias, systolic murmur, pulmonary crackles, tachycardia, weak pulses, pale mucous membranes, and muscle wasting.
- Other physical findings are emaciation, peripheral edema, ascites, and abdominal mass.
- Many signs and physical findings are reported to be episodic because of the episodic release of catecholamines by the tumor.

Electrocardiography

- Nonspecific ST segment and T wave changes may be noted.
- Arrhythmias can occur, especially ventricular premature complexes and paroxysmal ventricular tachycardia.

Radiography

- Generalized cardiomegaly and pulmonary edema can develop, probably owing to sustained chronic hypertension.
- Adrenal tumors can be identified in one third of the cases.

Clinical Pathology

- No consistent abnormalities are present on the hemogram or chemistry profile.
- Demonstration of elevated 24-hour urinary excretion of vanillylmandelic acid, total metanephrines, fractionated catecholamines, and plasma catecholamines is diagnostic in humans.

Special Diagnostic Tests

- Abdominal ultrasound may be helpful as a localizing procedure. The presence of an adrenal mass on ultrasound with no evidence of Cushing's disease is highly suggestive.
- Angiography can be used in some situations to evaluate adrenal masses invading the caudal vena cava.
- Computed tomography, nuclear imaging, and provocative testing to induce hypertension (with histamine, tyramine, and glucagon) or hypotension (with phentolamine) may be useful, but rarely are practical or available in general practice.

Therapy

- Alpha- and beta-adrenergic blocking drugs may help control hypertension and arrhythmias, respectively. Always start with an alpha-adrenergic blocker such as **phenoxybenzamine** (0.2 to 1.5 mg/kg PO every 12 hours). If a hypertensive crisis is identified, administer **phentolamine** at 0.02 to 0.1 mg/kg IV, followed by an intravenous infusion. If tachyarrhythmias remain a problem, then add a beta blocker such as **propranolol**. Using a beta blocker without alpha blockade can result in severe hypertension.
- Surgical tumor removal is the only definitive treatment. This should be attempted after medical stabilization in patients without metastasis.

Prognosis

- Dogs with inoperable lesions have a poor prognosis. Long-term alpha- and beta- adrenergic blockers may be used in these instances.

DIABETES MELLITUS

- Diabetes mellitus causes devastating cardiovascular problems in humans. The cardiovascular systems of dogs and cats are relatively immune to the effects of hyperglycemia. Recent studies reported hypertension (defined as a pressure higher than 160 mm Hg systolic, 100 mm Hg diastolic, and 120 mm Hg mean) in 46% of 50 dogs with diabetes. Subclinical reduction of myocardial contractility has also been reported

Cardiac Pathophysiology

- Systemic hypertension in diabetic dogs is associated with the duration of disease and an increased urine albumin to creatinine ratio. Severity of mean and diastolic hypertension correlated with duration of disease. In humans, severity of hypertension correlates with degree of glycemic control. This association has not been reported in dogs. Hypertension is rarely reported in cats with diabetes.

- The cause of hypertension is not known, but may relate to changes in vascular compliance secondary to changes in lipid profile, generalized glomerular hyperfiltration, and immune mediated microangiopathy affecting the basement membrane.
- Diabetic cardiomyopathy occurs in humans and is associated with myocardial hypertrophy, fibrosis, microvascular disease and glycoprotein accumulation. Myocardial changes result in diastolic and systolic dysfunction. In the absence of coronary microvascular disease and systemic hypertension, diabetic cardiomyopathy in humans is a mild condition. In alloxan-induced diabetes in dogs, mild reductions in fractional shortening and left ventricular ejection fraction have been reported along with increased aortic stiffness and increased collagen type I and type III protein content. Diastolic changes have been mild and inconsistent. Functional coronary artery hyperemia is attenuated and the balance between coronary blood flow and myocardial metabolism is impaired in alloxan-induced diabetic dogs.
- Dysfunction of the autonomic nervous system is common complication of diabetes mellitus with parasympathetic dysfunction typically preceding sympathetic dysfunction. Cardiac manifestations of autonomic dysfunction in human diabetics include sinus tachycardia, arrhythmias, blunted response to vagal maneuvers and pharmacologic autonomic interventions, postural hypotension and increased incidence of cardiac arrest under anesthesia. ECG studies in alloxan induced diabetes in dogs have not demonstrated any evidence of impaired parasympathetic autonomic function.

KEY POINT

Decreased cardiac performance in dogs with diabetes mellitus is mild and unlikely to cause clinical problems unless accompanied by other forms of heart disease such as dilated cardiomyopathy.

Diagnosis

History and Physical Examination

- No cardiovascular signs associated with diabetes
- *Polyuria, polydipsia, polyphagia with weight loss, cataracts (dogs)*

Electrocardiography

- No changes related to diabetes

Radiography

- No changes related to diabetes

Clinical Pathology

- Fasting hyperglycemia, hypercholesterolemia, hypertriglyceridemia, increased alanine aminotransferase activity, increased alkaline phosphatase activity
- Glucosuria, variable ketonuria; sometimes proteinuria, microalbuminuria, and bacteriuria
- High fructosamine and glycosylated hemoglobin

Special Diagnostic Tests

- Evaluation is systemic blood pressure may reveal hypertension.
- Echocardiography may demonstrate mild reduction in fractional shortening, increase in pre-ejection period (PEP), decrease in left ventricular ejection time (LVET) and increase in PEP/LVET.

Therapy

- Treat hypertension with an ACE inhibitor (e.g., **enalapril** or **benazepril**), **amlodipine**, or a beta blocker (see Chapter 12).
- Manage diabetes with insulin. Optimizing glycemic control should reduce the risk of secondary cardiovascular complications.

Prognosis

- Cardiac complications with diabetes mellitus in dogs and cats are generally mild and easy to control.

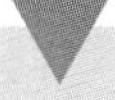

Metabolic Disturbances

DISORDERS ASSOCIATED WITH HYPERKALEMIA

- Over 95% of body potassium is intracellular, with only 2% to 5% extracellular. Therefore, serum potassium values are not always reliable indicators of total body potassium stores.
- Clinical causes of hyperkalemia include the following:
  - Excessive administration of oral potassium supplements or potassium supplemented fluids
  - Decreased renal elimination associated with oliguric or anuric renal failure
  - Hypoadrenocorticism (Addison's disease)
  - Drugs (potassium-sparing diuretics and ACE inhibitors)

- Ruptured urinary tract and urethral obstruction
- Translocation from intracellular to extracellular space (metabolic acidosis, rapid release from tissue during severe injury such as aortic thromboembolism)

Diagnosis, Therapy, and Prognosis

- ECG changes caused by hyperkalemia are dependent on magnitude and also rate of development of hyperkalemia (see p. 247).

KEY POINT

Majority of patients with clinically significant hyperkalemia will have bradycardia but uncommonly tachycardia can also develop (Figure 13-2).

- Identification and treatment of the underlying cause of hyperkalemia are essential. See Hypoadrenocorticism (Addison's Disease).

DISORDERS ASSOCIATED WITH HYPOKALEMIA

- When severe potassium loss has occurred, severe muscle weakness or paralysis may develop.
- Clinical causes of hypokalemia include the following:
  - Decreased intake (anorexia, especially when combined with potassium-deficient fluid administration)
  - Excessive gastrointestinal loss
    - Chronic vomiting
    - Severe diarrhea
  - Overuse of enemas, laxatives, or exchange resins
  - Excessive urinary loss
    - Renal (renal tubular acidosis, postobstructive diuresis, chronic pyelonephritis)
    - Drugs (diuretics, amphotericin B)
  - Secondary hyperaldosteronism (liver failure, congestive heart failure, nephrotic syndrome)
  - Extracellular to intracellular transfer
    - Metabolic alkalosis
    - Insulin and glucose administration
    - Hyperinsulinism (insulinoma)
    - Ketoacidotic diabetes mellitus

Cardiac Pathophysiology

- Severe hypokalemia causes hyperpolarization of nerve and muscle fiber membranes.
- ECG changes are manifested in delayed and abnormal repolarization, increased automaticity, and increased duration of the action potential.

Diagnosis

History and Physical Examination

- Muscle weakness may be mild or present as profound weakness and depression.
- Ventroflexion of the head is frequently seen in symptomatic cats.
- Polyuria and polydipsia may occur.

Electrocardiography

- QT interval prolongation and U waves may occur.
- ST segment may become depressed (Figure 13-3), with a gradual blending of T waves and what appears to be a tall U wave.
- Ventricular and supraventricular arrhythmias may occur.
- Clinical pathology may be reflective of the underlying disease process contributing to hypokalemia. Urine concentrating ability may be impaired.

Therapy

- Treat the primary disease process.
- Parenteral replacement with potassium chloride is recommended when potassium loss is severe and the animal is symptomatic for hypokalemia (Table 13-1).

KEY POINT

When administering potassium chloride, do not exceed 0.5 mEq/kg/hr.

- Parenteral administration may initially decrease the serum K^+ level. This effect is minimized by avoiding dextrose-containing fluids, administering K^+ at correct rate and concentration, and starting oral potassium gluconate supplementation early.
- Return to alimentation and treatment of the primary disease responsible for hypokalemia will replace potassium deficits. Therefore, prolonged oral maintenance therapy is rarely indicated except when ongoing excessive loss of potassium owing to diuretic administration or polyuric renal disease is present.
- Hypokalemia markedly increases the likelihood of toxicity when digitalis is being administered. Serum potassium should be promptly checked and corrected when digitalis toxicity is suspected.

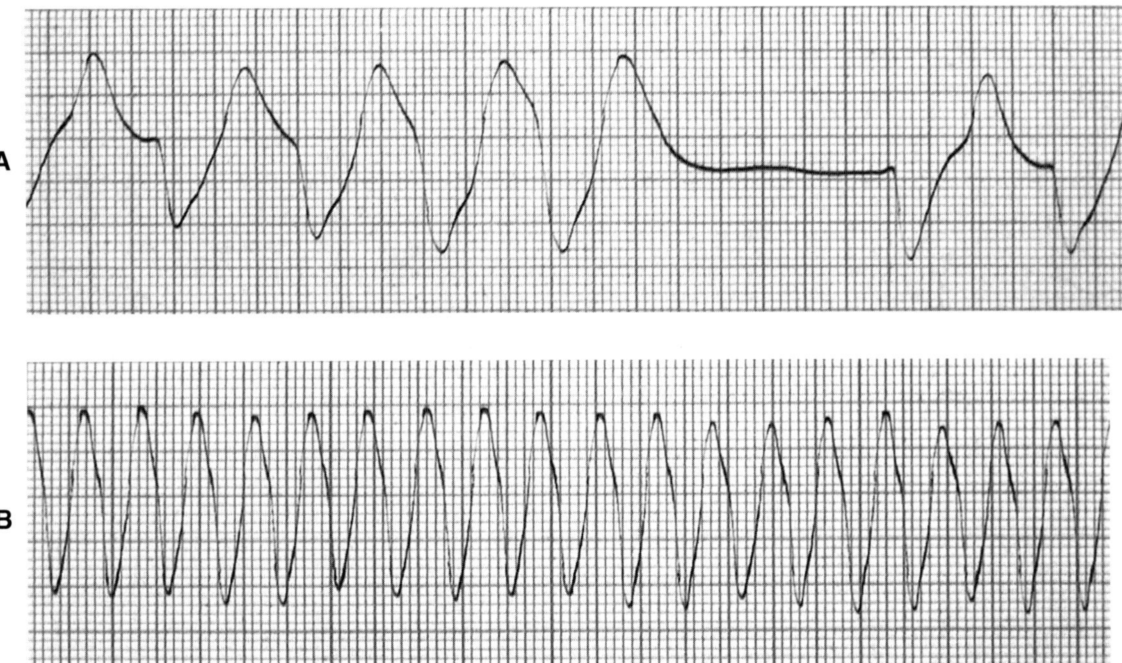

Figure 13-2. **A,** Hyperkalemia in cat with urinary obstruction resulting in a wide-complex bradycardia. **B,** Same cat developed wide complex tachycardia as treatment with insulin and dextrose was initiated. Normal sinus rhythm developed as treatment was continued.

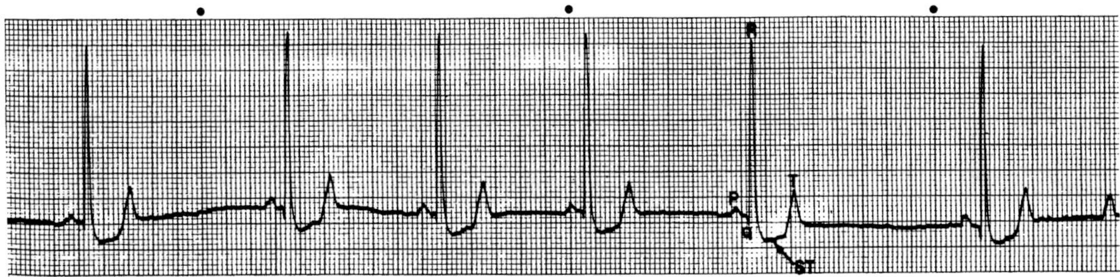

Figure 13-3. ST segment depression in a dog with hypokalemia (serum potassium 3.3 mEq/L) secondary to respiratory alkalosis. (From Tilley LP: Essentials of canine and feline electrocardiography: interpretation and treatment, ed 3, Malvern, Penn: 1992, Lea & Febiger.)

Table 13-1 Guidelines for Potassium Supplementation

Serum Potassium (mEq/L)	mEq KCl to Add to 250 mL Fluid	Maximum Fluid Rate (mL/kg/hr)
< 2.0	20	6
2.1-2.5	15	8
2.6-3.0	10	12
3.1-3.5	7	18
3.6-5.0	5	25

From Greene RW, Scott RC: Lower urinary tract disease. In Ettinger SJ ed: Textbook of Veterinary Internal Medicine. Philadelphia, 1975, WB Saunders.

- Hypokalemia increases the risk of ventricular arrhythmias and decreases the responsiveness to class I antiarrhythmic agents (lidocaine, mexiletine, procainamide, quinidine). Serum potassium should be promptly checked and corrected when refractory ventricular arrhythmias are identified.

Prognosis

- The prognosis is good if the underlying condition can be corrected or managed.

DISORDERS ASSOCIATED WITH HYPERCALCEMIA

- Hypercalcemia occurs when serum calcium concentration consistently exceeds 12 mg/dL in mature dogs and 11 mg/dL in cats. Young, actively growing dogs may normally have calcium values of greater than 12.0 mg/dL.
- Many different conditions can cause hypercalcemia. Hypercalcemia results from calcium bone resorption, increased gastrointestinal calcium absorption, increased serum protein binding of calcium, increased calcium binding to anions, and decreased renal and intestinal calcium removal from serum.
- The following conditions are associated with hypercalcemia:
  - Young growing puppy (normal)
  - Paraneoplastic syndromes (lymphoma, anal sac apocrine gland adenocarcinoma, occasionally other soft tissue tumors, primary and metastatic bony tumors)
  - Hypoadrenocorticism
  - Renal failure
  - Skeletal lesions (septic osteomyelitis, disuse osteoporosis, hypertrophic osteodystrophy)
  - Nutritional (hypervitaminosis D, hypervitaminosis A, calcium administration)
  - Primary hyperparathyroidism
  - Other (hemoconcentration, hyperproteinemia, severe hypothermia, laboratory error)

Cardiac Pathophysiology

- Cardiovascular effects of experimentally induced acute hypercalcemia include elevated systolic and diastolic blood pressure, especially with renal failure.
- Clinically, elevated calcium levels have little if any direct adverse effect on cardiac function. In hypercalcemic crisis (more than 16 mg/dL serum calcium), cardiac arrhythmias or arrest may occur.
- Animals with hypercalcemia may be more predisposed to complications of digitalis intoxication.
- Long-standing hypercalcemia may predispose to calcification of myocardium, blood vessels, and other soft tissues.

Diagnosis

History and Physical Examination

- Regardless of its cause, hypercalcemia affects the kidney (renal dysfunction, polyuria, polydipsia, nocturia, nephrocalcinosis, renal failure, uremia), gastrointestinal system (anorexia, constipation, and vomiting from decreased gastrointestinal smooth muscle excitability), and nervous system (generalized skeletal muscle weakness from decreased neuromuscular activity).

Radiography

- Thoracic radiographs may indicate mediastinal mass(es), metastasis, abnormal bony densities, or osteolysis.
- Abdominal radiographs may show organomegaly, abnormal bone density, sublumbar masses, or sublumbar lymphadenopathy.

- Skeletal survey radiographs may exhibit isolated bony lesions that could account for hypercalcemia. Osteopenia, metastatic calcification, or focal bony lesions may be present.

Electrocardiography

- The characteristic ECG finding is a short QT interval. In extreme cases, the ST segment may fuse with the upstroke of the T wave.

KEY POINT

ECG changes do not correlate closely with serum calcium concentration.

- With severe hypercalcemia, bradycardia may occur.
- Hypercalcemia may predispose to arrhythmias of digitalis intoxication.
- ECG changes resolve after normalization of serum calcium.

Clinical Pathology

- Hypercalcemia often causes diminished urinary concentrating ability. The urine is usually hyposthenuric or isosthenuric.
- Renal failure with azotemia may develop from progressive structural and functional alterations in the kidney.
- Hypophosphatemia or hyperphosphatemia may be recorded, depending on the presence or absence of renal failure and the underlying etiology of hypercalcemia.
- Serum alkaline phosphatase may be elevated if severe bone disease or concomitant hepatic disease is present.
- A hemogram may be normal, display hemoconcentration or anemia, or occasionally show evidence of leukemia (when this disease is associated with the underlying etiology).
- Bone marrow evaluation may be unremarkable or disclose evidence of lymphoma, leukemia, or multiple myeloma.

Therapy

- Initial treatment is directed at reducing the systemic effects of hypercalcemia.
  - Preexisting dehydration should be corrected and hydration maintained.
  - Administration of **0.9% saline** should be used to enhance the renal excretion of calcium.
  - **Furosemide** (5 mg/kg IV bolus initially then 2 to 4 mg/kg PO every 8 to 12 hours thereafter) and/or **sodium bicarbonate** (1 mEq/kg IV every 10 to 15 minutes, up to 4 mEq/L maximum dose) may also help in cases of moderate-to-severe hypercalcemia.
  - Glucocorticosteroids may limit bone resorption, decrease intestinal calcium absorption, increase renal calcium excretion, and be cytolytic in certain neoplasms. Administration may interfere with diagnosis of neoplasia.
- Definitive treatment is directed at the underlying etiology.

Prognosis

- The prognosis depends on early detection, ability to establish a definitive diagnosis, and success of treatment. The prognosis of many causes of hypercalcemia is guarded to poor.

DISORDERS ASSOCIATED WITH HYPOCALCEMIA

- Hypocalcemia, although infrequently encountered, can cause profound clinical signs. It occurs when serum calcium concentration is less than 8 mg/dL in the dog and less than 7 mg/dL in the cat (ionized calcium less than 5 in dogs and less than 4.5 in cats).
- The following conditions may be associated with hypocalcemia:
  - Renal failure
  - Eclampsia (puerperal tetany)
  - Canine acute pancreatitis
  - Hypoparathyroidism
  - Idiopathic
  - Postoperative (during bilateral thyroid surgery)
  - Ethylene glycol toxicity
  - Hyperphosphatemia
  - Hypocalcemia due to hypoalbuminemia, where calcium values are not adjusted for serum protein concentration

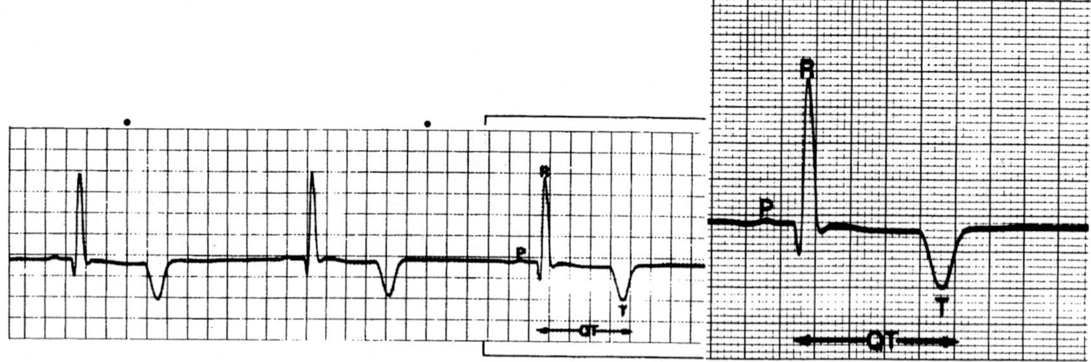

Figure 13-4. Prolonged QT interval in a dog with severe hypocalcemia (2.2 mg/dL) secondary to ethylene glycol toxicity. (From Tilley LP: Essentials of canine and feline electrocardiography: interpretation and treatment, ed 3, Malvern, Penn: 1992, Lea & Febiger.)

Cardiac Pathophysiology

- Hypocalcemia causes an excitatory effect on nerve and muscle cells. Neuromuscular irritability, tetany, and seizures may result.
- Animals with coexisting congestive heart failure may experience decreased cardiac function that improves with restoration of calcium levels (owing to the augmenting effect of calcium on myocardial contractility).
- Acutely induced hypocalcemia (i.e., treatment with chelating agents) can potentially cause sharp reductions in blood pressure resulting in cardiovascular shock.

Diagnosis

History and Physical Examination

- Tetany, seizures, anorexia, vomiting, and abdominal discomfort are the predominant signs in affected animals.
- Aggressive rubbing of the ears, nose, face, and eyes can also be seen.
- Handling or stress may precipitate tetany.

Electrocardiography

- The typical ECG manifestation of hypocalcemia consists of QT prolongation, but is heart rate dependent. (Figure 13-4)

Clinical Pathology

- Clinical pathology will reflect abnormalities associated with the underlying disease process. Hypocalcemia is usually diagnosed when low serum calcium levels are detected during clinical investigation of tetany, seizures, renal failure, pancreatitis, or other disorders through analysis of a serum biochemical profile.

Therapy

- Severe hypocalcemia (less than 6 mg/dL) is a life-threatening emergency.
  - **Ten percent calcium gluconate** is administered intravenously (0.5 to 1.5 ml/kg) slowly over a 15- to 30-minute interval.
    - **Calcium** should be administered slowly as ECG changes do not closely conform to serum calcium levels, especially when other electrolyte and acid/base disturbances are present.
    - ECG monitoring should accompany administration.
    - Calcium infusion should be temporarily interrupted if ST segment elevation or bradycardia occurs, to be reinstated at a slower rate when these changes have abated.
    - Gradual QT interval shortening from its prolonged state may accompany calcium infusion.

KEY POINT

Calcium is cardiotoxic if replaced too quickly; even a normal concentration of serum calcium may be toxic if replenished to that level too rapidly.

- Subsequent intravenous calcium administration may be repeated every 6 to 12 hours, or as needed.
- Clinical signs of hypocalcemia may abate slowly, despite calcium infusion. Resolution of clinical signs may not provide a reliable guide as an end point of adequate calcium administration. Some hypocalcemic signs may persist (i.e., weakness, anorexia) if cardiotoxic doses of calcium are infused.
- **Vitamin D** therapy may be required in some disorders to maintain control of hypocalcemia.

In treatment of postoperative parathyroid insufficiency, care must be taken to detect recovery of parathyroid function in order to avoid vitamin D–associated hypercalcemia.

Prognosis

- For most causes of hypocalcemia that are carefully managed, the prognosis is good to excellent.

DISORDERS ASSOCIATED WITH HYPOMAGNESEMIA AND HYPERMAGNESEMIA

- Abnormalities in magnesium levels rarely affect cardiac function directly, but they may potentiate problems caused by other electrolyte derangements.
- Causes of hypomagnesemia are very similar to causes of hypokalemia.

Cardiac Pathophysiology

- Abnormalities of magnesium have minimal effects on the ECG with normal calcium and potassium levels.
- Hypomagnesemia will exacerbate problems due to hypocalcemia.
- Hypomagnesemia predisposes to digitalis-induced arrhythmias.
- Hypomagnesemia prevents correction of hypokalemia.

Diagnosis

- Consider hypomagnesemia with conditions that lead to hypokalemia.
- Consider hypomagnesemia when there is difficulty correcting hypokalemia.

Therapy

- Treat the underlying disease process.
- Parenteral replacement if there is evidence of cardiac complications or if there is difficulty correcting hypokalemia. **Magnesium sulfate** at 0.75 to 1.0 mEq/kg/day in 5% dextrose in water (D_5W) as a constant rate infusion could be considered.

HYPOGLYCEMIA

- Hypoglycemia may be caused by:
  - Hyperinsulinism due to a functional islet cell pancreatic carcinoma.
  - Insulin overdose for the treatment of diabetes mellitus.
  - Nonpancreatic tumors
  - Glycogen storage diseases
  - Neonatal/juvenile hypoglycemia
  - Septic shock
  - Addison's disease
  - Hepatic disease

Cardiac Pathophysiology

- Irrespective of the etiology, hypoglycemia triggers catecholamine release, which causes tachycardia, increases in myocardial oxygen demand, and, potentially, arrhythmias.

Diagnosis

History and Physical Examination

- Clinical manifestations of hypoglycemia range from lethargy to episodic weakness and seizures.

Electrocardiography

- ECG findings can include:
  - ST depression
  - T wave flattening
  - QT prolongation
  - Supraventricular and/or ventricular arrhythmias
  - ECG changes usually resolve with correction of hypoglycemia

Laboratory Findings

- A low blood glucose level (less than 60 mg/dL) is usually present. A fasting blood glucose level may be needed to confirm hypoglycemia.
- Elevated insulin levels or amended insulin: glucose ratio may be demonstrated with insulinomas.

Therapy

- Hypoglycemic crisis, regardless of cause, is managed by slow, intravenous administration of **50% dextrose** to effect. A slow IV bolus of 0.5 to 1.0 mg/kg could be considered.
- Treat underlying disease or improve diabetic regulation.

Prognosis

- Resolution of neurologic signs due to hypoglycemia is usually abrupt and virtually complete.
- Prolonged, untreated hypoglycemia may result in cerebrocortical hypoxic damage. Lack of

symptom amelioration after therapy may indicate cerebral hypoxia and edema.

UREMIA

- Uremia is generally associated with renal failure.
- Uremia is common in geriatric populations.
- Renal failure can affect cardiac function and reduce elimination of many cardiac drugs (digoxin, most ACE inhibitors, many beta blockers).

Cardiac Pathophysiology

- Hypertensive cardiovascular disease, electrolyte imbalance, fluid overload, and anemia can contribute to the production of cardiac disturbances.
- Renal failure can cause elevations or reductions of potassium and calcium; associated changes may register on the ECG.
- Systemic hypertension is a common sequela of chronic renal failure in dogs and cats and is reported in 50% to 93% of dogs and 65% of cats.
- Pericardial effusion is reported as an uncommon sequela of uremia in cats and dogs. The effusion may occur secondary to uremic serositis.
- Pulmonary thromboembolism may occur associated with protein-losing glomerulopathy. (Figure 13-5)
- Uremic pneumonitis can uncommonly cause noncardiogenic pulmonary edema.

KEY POINT

Uremic toxins have a cardiodepressant effect.

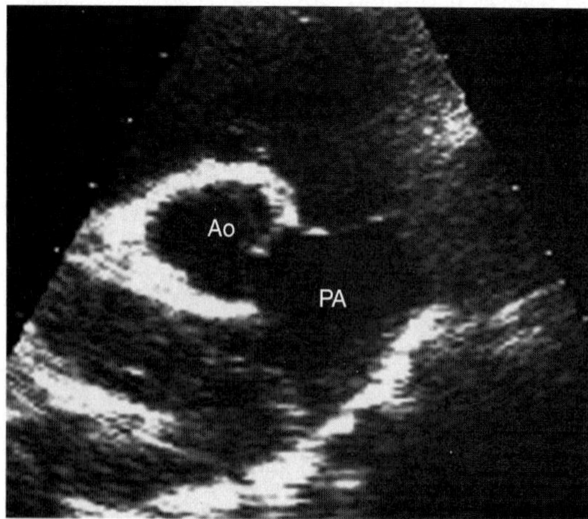

Figure 13-5. Right parasternal short-axis view at the base of the heart in a dog with protein-losing nephropathy. A well circumscribed thrombus can be seen at the bifurcation of the pulmonary artery. *Ao,* Aorta; *PA,* pulmonary artery.

Diagnosis

History and Physical Examination

- Signs that may accompany uremia include polyuria, polydipsia, depression, anorexia, lethargy, vomiting, diarrhea, and weight loss.
- Uremic pneumonitis and metabolic acidosis cause dyspnea and/or tachypnea that may be confused with signs of congestive heart failure.

Electrocardiography

- Nonspecific ECG abnormalities may be attributed to hypertension, anemia, electrolyte abnormalities, and pericarditis.
- Conduction defects or arrhythmias may occur.

Echocardiography

- Echocardiography may show changes consistent with hypertension and chronic anemia.

Clinical Pathology

- Clinical pathology may reveal abnormalities in the hemogram, urinalysis, and biochemistry profile consistent with uremia (increased blood urea nitrogen, creatinine, and phosphorus, nonregenerative anemia, and isosthenuria).

Therapy

- Treatment is directed at managing uremia and its underlying causes. Therapy generally includes parenteral fluids, protein and phosphorus restriction, phosphate binders, and sometimes calcitriol and erythropoietin.
- Management of severe azotemia in patients with concurrent heart disease is extremely challenging and often frustrating.
  - Azotemia identified while treating congestive heart failure may be prerenal and/or renal in origin.
  - Rehydrate cautiously.
    - Consider low-sodium fluids (half-strength saline)
    - Consider reduced administration rates (start at maintenance rate)
    - May take 48 hours to see improvement in azotemia.
  - Monitor clinically and radiographically for development of congestive heart failure.
  - Reduce doses or avoid cardiac drugs eliminated by the kidneys. If using ACE inhibitors or digoxin, monitor kidney function and electrolytes frequently. Monitor digoxin levels periodically. **Pimobendan**, or **hydralazine**

and **nitroglycerin** can be substituted for ACE inhibitors.
- Monitor and control hypertension, electrolyte, and acid-base disturbances.

Prognosis

- Resolution of the uremic state may improve ECG abnormalities but arrhythmias may persist.
- The development of congestive heart failure in the face of severe azotemia carries a poor prognosis.

ANEMIA

- Anemia is a sign of a disease, not a disease entity.
- Evaluation should emphasize history (drug or toxin exposure), clinical signs related to other disorders complicated by anemia (fever, lethargy, bleeding, weight loss), physical examination (petechiae, lymphadenopathy), and clinical pathology.
- Symptoms of reduced cardiac reserve associated with anemia depend on the severity of anemia, rate of anemia development, and on the presence and extent of underlying cardiac disease.

Cardiac Pathophysiology

- The combination of tissue hypoxia and reduced blood viscosity leads to decreased systemic vascular resistance. The body responds to decreased systemic vascular resistance by increasing sodium and water retention resulting in an increased stroke volume and cardiac output.
- Tissue hypoxia may also result in sinus tachycardia.
- When anemia is associated with increased viscosity (multiple myeloma or macroglobulinemia), cardiac output may fail to rise.
- Physiologic consequences depend on the developmental rate of anemia.
  - With acute blood loss (i.e., hemorrhage), hypovolemic shock may predominate.
    - Acute blood loss leads to volume depletion and a resultant decrease in cardiac output. Additionally, acute anemia can lead to myocardial hypoxia and resultant depressed cardiac function.
  - With chronic anemia blood volume is maintained but cardiac output may rise as described previously.
    - The augmented stroke volume associated with the increased cardiac output may result in cardiac dilation and hypertrophy. Chronic anemia is usually well tolerated because of compensatory mechanisms that include increased cardiac output, redistribution of blood flow, and decreased oxygen affinity of red blood cells.
  - Uncommonly the volume overload can result in congestive heart failure. In many of these cases, pre-existing subclinical heart disease may be a factor.
  - Pulmonary thromboembolism may occur with autoimmune hemolytic anemia.

Diagnosis

History and Physical Examination

- Chronic anemia produces variable symptoms that may include fatigue and mild exertional dyspnea. In rare situations chronic anemia can lead to syncope.
- Acute anemia may present with collapse, weakness, lethargy, stupor, and dyspnea.
- Physical exam may reveal precordium that is hyperkinetic, bounding or pistol shot arterial pulses, pale or icteric mucous membrane color, and prolonged capillary refill time.
- A soft, systolic murmur at the left apex, generally grade I to III/VI, is common with severe anemia.
- Heart sounds may be accentuated.

Radiology

- Thoracic radiographs may display cardiac enlargement, but this will vary depending on the presence and extent of previously existing heart disease.
- Uncommonly cardiac changes can result in evidence of pulmonary venous congestion, pulmonary edema, and/or pleural effusion.

Electrocardiography

- Sinus tachycardia is often present. The heart rate varies with the rate of onset and degree of anemia.
- Ventricular premature complexes may be seen.
- Evidence of left ventricular enlargement (wide QRS complex and/or tall R waves) may be present.

Echocardiography

- May show evidence of left ventricular, left atrial, right ventricular, and/or right atrial dilation.
- Hyperdynamic cardiac function (increased fractional shortening, decreased end-systolic left ventricular diameter) is usually seen in the presence of volume overload.

- Evidence of pre-existing cardiac disease may be present.

Clinical Pathology

- The laboratory database varies considerably depending on the cause of anemia.

Therapy

- Treatment of anemia depends on the underlying cause.
- Animals with congestive heart failure secondary to anemia should be given furosemide as needed. Once the anemia is controlled, chronic cardiac therapy may not be necessary.
- Animals with concurrent congestive heart failure and life-threatening anemia should be given furosemide and transfused simultaneously. Packed red blood cells may be more appropriate than whole blood owing to the smaller volume that can be administered to correct the anemia.
- Caution with fluid administration should always be exercised when cardiomegaly is present in the face of significant anemia.
- A decision as to when to transfuse a patient is based on the clinical assessment, which includes the rate of anemia development, the patient's state of compensation, and progression of continued red blood cell loss.

Prognosis

- Successful management of anemia and underlying causes confers a good short-term prognosis. Long-term prognosis depends on the cause of the anemia.

Neoplastic and Infiltrative Heart Diseases

HEMANGIOSARCOMA

- Tumor originates from endothelial cells.
- Can be seen in any portion of the heart, but appears to be more common in the wall of the right atrium (Figure 13-6).
- Rare in cats
- Average age of affected dogs is 10 years; no gender predilection; incidence increased in German Shepherds.
- Metastasis is common.
- Other common sites of hemangiosarcoma include the spleen, liver, and lungs.

CHEMODECTOMA

- Tumor originates from neuroepithelial cells most commonly found in the aortic bodies.
- Masses are typically seen at the heart base. Because of the complexity of the heart base, small masses can be difficult to identify (Figure 13-7).
- Rare in cats.

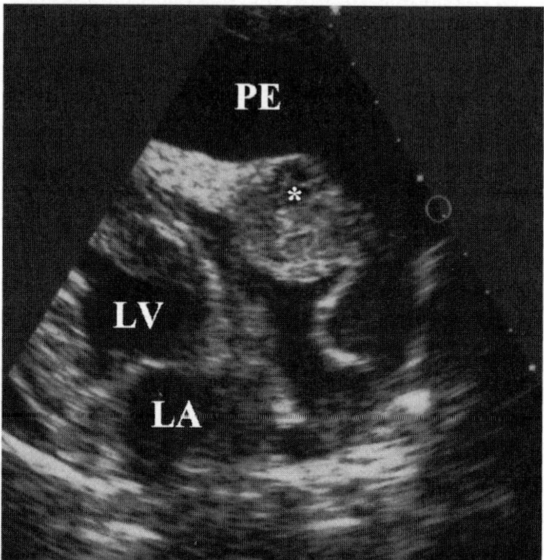

Figure 13-6. Slightly oblique right parasternal long-axis view. A large soft tissue mass effect *(*)* can be seen in the wall of the right atrium. Moderate pericardial effusion *(PE)* is present resulting in diastolic collapse of the right atrium. *LV,* Left ventricle; *LA,* left atrium.

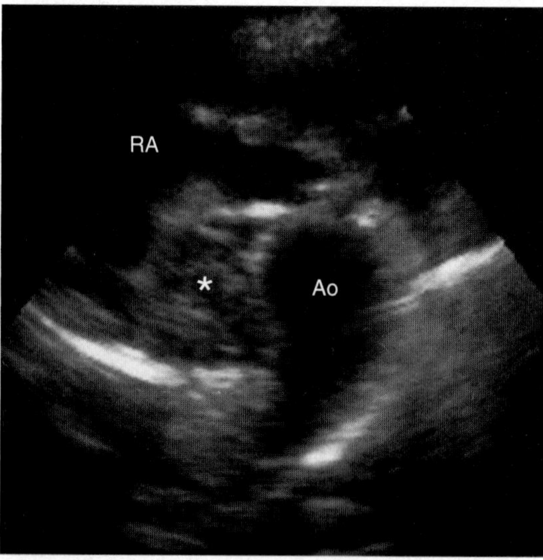

Figure 13-7. Slightly oblique right parasternal short-axis view high on the base above the left atrium. A small soft tissue mass effect *(*)* can be seen associated with the aorta and above the left atrium. Mild to moderate pericardial effusion is also present. *Ao,* Aorta; *RA,* right atrium.

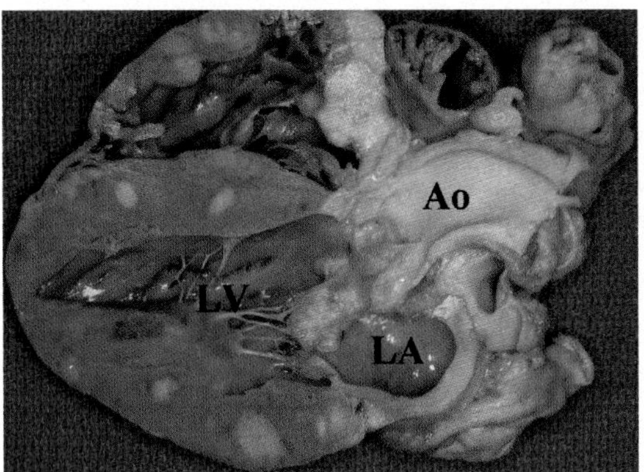

Figure 13-8. Transverse section through the heart of a dog diagnosed with cardiac lymphoma. Multiple pale nodules can be seen in the left and right ventricular myocardium. *Ao,* Aorta; *LV,* left ventricle; *LA,* left atrium.

- More common in dogs over 6 years old; no gender predilection; increased incidence in boxers and Boston Terriers.
- Metastasis is uncommon, but can appear in lungs, liver, lymph nodes, and bone.

OTHER ETIOLOGIES

- Lymphoma is the most common tumor that metastasizes to the heart in cats but also can be seen in dogs. (Figures 13-8 and 13-9)
- Ectopic thyroid carcinomas occur at the heart base and, rarely, in the right ventricular outflow tract.
- Cardiac myxomas are rare but are more common in the right heart (right atrial lumen). (Figure 13-10)
- Rarely, cardiac fibroma, fibrosarcoma, and rhabdomyosarcoma are diagnosed in young dogs.
- Infiltrative myocardial disease (e.g., amyloidosis, hypereosinophilic syndrome) involving non-neoplastic cells is rare in dogs and uncommon in cats.

Cardiac Pathophysiology

- Tumors from other tissues gain access to the heart by invasive growth from adjacent structures or spread by hematogenous or lymphatic vessels.
- The relative infrequency of cardiac metastasis has been attributed to metabolic peculiarities of striated muscle, rapid coronary blood flow, efferent lymphatic drainage from the heart, and the vigorous kneading action of the myocardium.
- Myocardial neoplasia may cause congestive heart failure owing to diastolic dysfunction, obstruction to ventricular inflow or outflow, pericardial tamponade, or arrhythmias.

Diagnosis

History and Physical Examination

- Cardiac involvement may not always lead to clinical signs. Signs depend on the site and extent of metastasis. Resultant cardiac dysfunction may cause signs of congestive heart failure, weakness, and/or syncope.
- Pericardial effusion and tamponade may lead to similar clinical signs.
- Possible physical findings include muffled heart sounds on auscultation, jugular venous distention, ascites, weakness (often acute), hypokinetic pulses, tachypnea, weight loss, and pale mucous membranes.

Radiography

- Radiographic evidence of a cardiac mass is uncommonly seen (Figure 13-11).
- Cardiac enlargement and rounding of the cardiac silhouette may be observed if pericardial effusion is present.
- Dilation of the caudal vena cava may present secondary to cardiac tamponade or obstruction to blood flow within the lumen of the right heart. In general, the diameter of the caudal vena cava should be less than the length of the vertebra above the carina.
- Pneumopericardiography or angiocardiography may assess the thickness and any irregularities of the pericardium, epicardium, and endocardium.
- The use of magnetic resonance imaging may allow visualization of a cardiac mass.

Electrocardiography

- Reduced QRS voltage on the ECG and electrical alternans occur in many, but not all, cases with pericardial effusion.
- Atrial or ventricular arrhythmias, conduction disturbances, and complete heart block can occur.

Echocardiography

- Echocardiographic evidence of pericardial effusion may be demonstrated. Diastolic right atrial or right ventricular collapse signifies pericardial tamponade. Dilation of the abdominal vena cava and/or hepatic veins is also typically seen with tamponade.
- Two-dimensional echocardiography may facilitate identification of cardiac neoplasia. Unfortunately due to the elusive nature of some cardiac masses, the lack of a mass on echocardiogram does not rule out neoplasia.

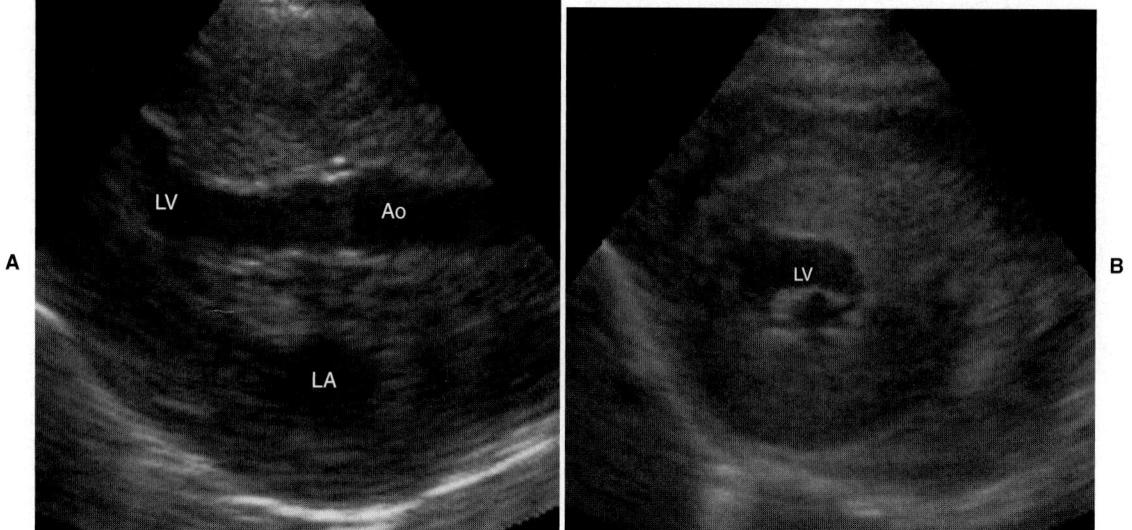

Figure 13-9. Right parasternal long-axis **(A)** and short-axis **(B)** views in a cat with cardiac lymphoma confirmed on histopathology. Note the marked thickening of the left ventricular and left atrial myocardium. *Ao,* Aorta; *LV,* left ventricle; *LA,* left atrium.

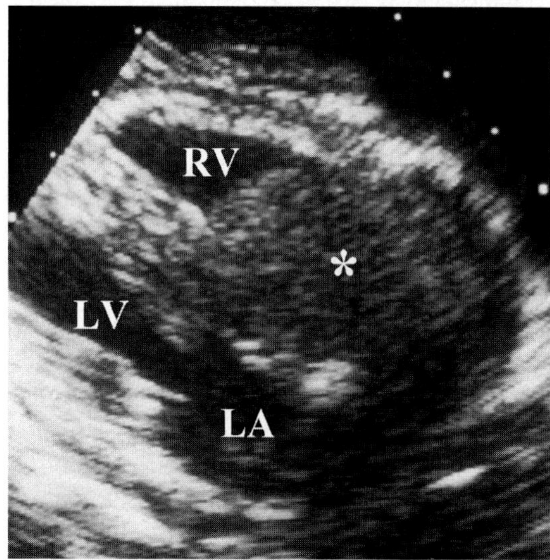

Figure 13-10. Right parasternal long-axis view in a dog. A large, well-circumscribed mass effect *(*)* is seen filling the majority of the right atrial lumen. The mass was confirmed as a myxoma on histopathology.

- Whenever safely possible, an echocardiogram should be performed while pericardial fluid is present. The fluid can be helpful in identifying a mass.
- Pericardiocentesis may detect cytologic evidence of neoplasia. The majority of the time, though, fluid analysis will come back as nonspecific hemorrhagic effusion.
- Uncommonly, biopsy of the tumor is possible without thoracotomy using techniques such as myocardial biopsy or thoracoscopy.

Therapy

- Pericardiocentesis may offer temporary relief from cardiac tamponade.
- If recurrent pericardiocentesis is necessary, then partial pericardectomy via thoracotomy, or a pericardial window via thoracoscopy could be considered.
- Surgery would likely improve the patient's quality of life but may not prolong life.
- Other than standard thoracotomy concerns and risks, the main complication with surgery is ongoing hemorrhage from the tumor. This can result in hemothorax.
- Animals with myocardial infiltration of tumors sensitive to chemotherapy or radiotherapy may respond favorably, but this is uncommon.
- Congestive heart failure and arrhythmias resulting from cardiac neoplasia can be difficult to treat.
- Surgical resection or debulking of cardiac masses is uncommonly possible.
- Masses confined to the right atrial appendage can periodically be removed with resection of the appendage.
- Some intraluminal cardiac masses can be removed using cardiac bypass or inflow occlusion. Studies with long-term follow-up with such patients are not available.

Prognosis

Hemangiosarcoma

- Surgical resection may be possible, but distant microscopic metastasis is almost always present.

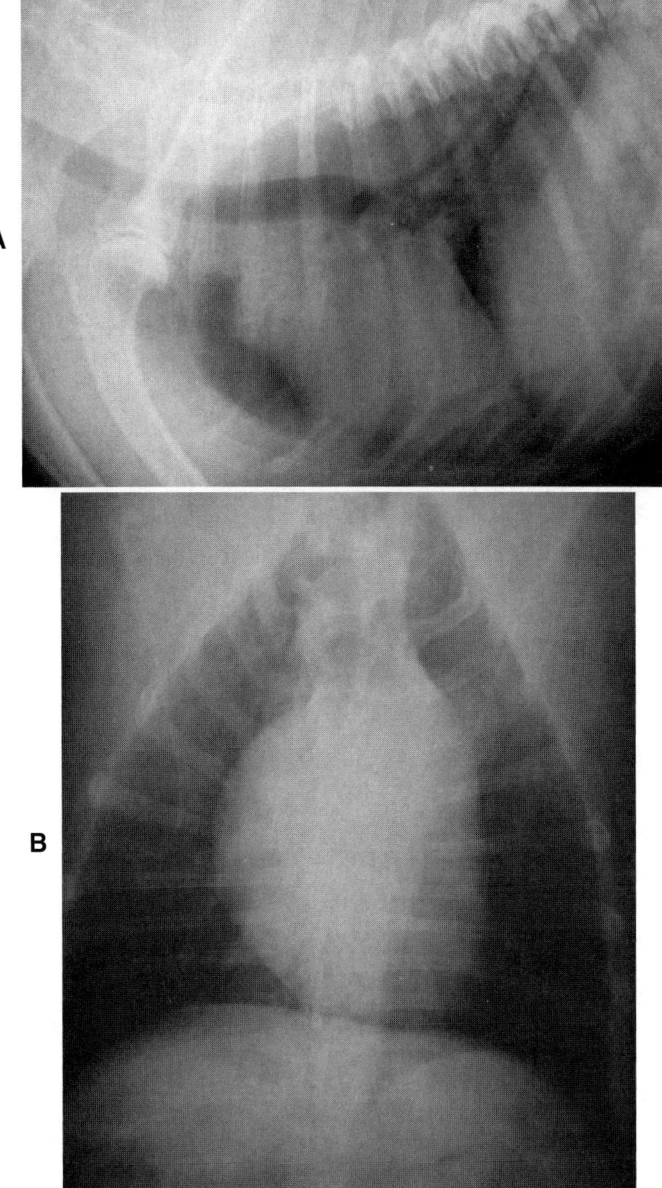

Figure 13-11. Lateral **(A)** and ventrodorsal **(B)** radiographs in a Boxer with a large heart base mass. A bulge in the area of the cranial waist of the cardiac silhouette can be seen on the lateral. A similar bulge can be seen on the ventrodorsal projection at the 2 o'clock position on the cardiac silhouette.

- Poor response to chemotherapy in general although a combination of surgical resection and chemotherapy may improve the prognosis to some degree.
- Pericardectomy may improve quality of life.

Chemodectoma

- Debulking surgery is an option, but complete resection of the tumor is rarely possible.
- Pericardectomy may improve quality of life.
- Radiation therapy may be beneficial in some cases, but general response to chemotherapy is poor.

KEY POINT

In general, long-term prognosis with cardiac cancer is poor owing to difficulty in surgical resection, minimal response to chemotherapy and radiation therapy, and detrimental side effects of chemotherapy and radiation therapy on the heart.

Physical and Chemical Agents that Affect the Cardiovascular System

- Many noninfectious stimuli can cause myocardial injury. Damage can be acute and transient or chronic and lead to permanent myocardial change. Effects are usually related to the severity, dose, and rate of exposure.

HYPERPYREXIA (HEAT STROKE)

- Hyperpyrexia is usually associated with heat stroke when the rectal temperature rises to 41° to 44° C (106° to 111° F). Experimentally, signs of heat stroke develop consistently at temperatures above 43° C (109° F) in dogs.
- Heat stroke develops in animals exposed to high environmental temperatures, or during heavy activity in warm environmental temperatures. It commonly occurs in animals left in unventilated automobiles during the summer months.
- High humidity reduces evaporation of water from the oral and nasal cavities, and reduces the ability of small animals to regulate their temperatures.
- Animals that are obese, brachycephalic, very young or old, or have cardiopulmonary disease are predisposed to heat stroke.
- Malignant hyperthermia is a rare but potentially fatal abnormal response to anesthetic agents. It is characterized by an acute, rapid rise in body temperature and severe biochemical changes accompanied by muscle rigidity.

Cardiac Pathophysiology

- Heat-induced vasodilation results in hypotension and decreased organ perfusion.
- Respiratory alkalosis may result from panting.
- Dehydration with hemoconcentration may occur, as well as mild hyperkalemia and hypophosphatemia.
- Tachyarrhythmias and cardiogenic shock can occur owing to myocardial hemorrhage, ischemia, and necrosis.
- Disseminated intravascular coagulopathy (DIC) may develop owing to destruction of clotting factors.
- Right-heart dilation may occur.
- Mechanisms suggested for myocardial injury include direct thermal effects, circulatory collapse with secondary myocardial hypoxia, decreased coronary blood flow, and secondary metabolic injury.
- Animals that recover from heat stroke may be prone to subsequent occurrences owing to heat-induced damage to the thermoregulatory zone of the hypothalamus.

Diagnosis

History and Physical Examination

- The diagnosis is usually made on the reported history of an animal being exposed to high environmental temperatures. However, some cases have more subtle history.
- Depending on the duration and severity of the heat stroke, clinical signs may include panting, sinus tachycardia, bright red oral mucous membranes, and hyperthermia. Extremities become hot to the touch.
- Red mucous membranes may turn pale because of diminished circulation or vasoconstriction.
- Watery diarrhea may occur, which can progress to bloody diarrhea.
- Stupor and coma with respiratory arrest can follow.
- With malignant hyperthermia, an acute, profound temperature elevation may be the first noticeable sign to the surgeon.
- If the heart rate is monitored, tachycardia may be the earliest indication.
- Skeletal muscle hypertonus may occur.
- ECG may show tachycardia, extrasystoles (especially if DIC develops), and ST segment and T wave abnormalities.
- Clinical pathologic alterations relate to the stage and severity of the hyperpyrexia.

Therapy

- Therapy should begin with lowering body temperature. Submergence in cool water and wetting the extremities with rubbing alcohol are useful techniques. Rectal temperature should be recorded every 5 to 10 minutes. Discontinue cooling when the body temperature drops below 39.5° C (103° F), to avoid hypothermia.
- If laryngeal paralysis, laryngeal edema, and tracheal stenosis are present, they may impede heat loss through the respiratory system. If these conditions are present, then a temporary tracheotomy or endotracheal intubation may have to be performed.
- Supportive care should include isotonic fluid therapy (0.45% saline or half-strength lactated Ringer's solution, with 2.5% dextrose), correction of acid-base and electrolyte abnormalities, and treatment for DIC.

- Nonsteroidal anti-inflammatory drugs or antipyretics (e.g., aspirin, flunixin meglumine) are contraindicated. The use of glucocorticoids remains controversial, but they are often used when cerebral edema is suspected.
- When malignant hyperthermia is anesthetic related, all inhalation agents and relaxants should be discontinued. Hyperventilation with 100% oxygen should be started.
- For malignant hyperthermia, dantrolene, 2 mg/kg IV up to 10 mg/kg IV has been used in the dog. No proven efficacy is known. Its use is based on experience from humans, horses, and pigs. Dantrolene exhibits muscle relaxation activity by direct action on muscle.
- Administer **mannitol** (0.25 to 2 gm/kg of a 20% solution over 15 to 20 minutes) if cerebral edema is suspected or if stupor or coma develops.
- The patient should be monitored for several days for the development of complications, such as renal failure and DIC.

Prognosis

- The prognosis for heat stroke is guarded to good if detected and treated early.
- Malignant hyperthermia is rare, but seems to offer a worse prognosis.
- Coagulopathy and renal failure confer a worse prognosis.

HYPOTHERMIA

- Lowering of body temperature can occur accidentally, owing to deep cooling from external cold, drugs, or interference with thermoregulatory centers during anesthesia. Physiologic consequences of hypothermia depend on the extent and duration of exposure.

Cardiac Pathophysiology

- Cardiac dilation with epicardial and subendocardial hemorrhage can result from severe hypothermia. Microinfarcts can occur in myocardial tissue.
- Lesions may result from circulatory collapse, hemoconcentration, sludging of blood in capillaries, or decreased cellular metabolism.

Diagnosis

History and Physical Examination

- Signs vary with the degree of hypothermia (reduction in core temperature), mild (32° to 35° C or 89.6° to 95° F), moderate (28° to 32° C or 82.4° to 89.6° F) and severe (lower than 28° C or 82.4° F).
- Signs include lethargy, ataxia, stupor, shivering and bradycardia. Cardiopulmonary arrest may occur with severe hypothermia.

Electrocardiography

- Mild hypothermia results in prolongation of the PR interval, QRS duration, and QT interval; atrial premature complexes; and inverted T waves.
- Moderate hypothermia produces atropine-resistant bradycardia and ventricular arrhythmias.
- Severe hypothermia may cause cardiac arrest secondary to ventricular fibrillation or asystole.

Therapy

- Treatment initially involves warming the patient.
- Active external warming with warm-water blankets is recommended for mild to moderate hypothermia. External warming causes vasodilation of skin vessels, which may initially transfer cooled blood to the body core, further lowering internal temperature. This is rarely a significant clinical complication with mild to moderate hypothermia.
  - Internal (core) warming is recommended if the rectal temperature is less than 30° C (86° F) or the cardiovascular status is unstable. This is accomplished by peritoneal dialysis with dialysate fluids warmed to 45° C (113° F).
  - Appropriate supportive care (e.g., intravenous fluids, ventilation) must be administered. Severe hypothermia can cause cardiopulmonary collapse. Keep these patients well oxygenated, and administer warmed intravenous fluids.
  - Cardiac output and ECG abnormalities improve after warming.
- Evaluation of the patient for underlying systemic disorders that could have predisposed it to hypothermia should be made once normothermia has been achieved.

CARBON MONOXIDE TOXICITY

- Carbon monoxide is a colorless, odorless, tasteless, toxic gas that has the molecular formula CO. CO is produced by the incomplete combustion of the fossil fuels—gas, oil, coal and wood used in boilers, engines, oil burners, gas fires, water heaters, solid fuel appliances and open fires. CO is a commercially important chemical. It is also formed in many chemical reactions and in the thermal or incomplete decomposition of many organic materials.

- Dangerous amounts of CO can accumulate when as a result of poor installation, poor maintenance or failure or damage to an appliance in service, the fuel is not burned properly, or when rooms are poorly ventilated and the CO is unable to escape.

Cardiac Pathophysiology

- CO competes with oxygen for binding sights on hemoglobin, diminishing oxygen transport capacity. This results in myocardial hypoxia. Myocardial hemorrhage and necrosis may occur.

Diagnosis

History and Physical Examination

- The history often supports exposure to fumes from a gasoline-burning engine.
- Clinical signs are often associated with cardiac hypoxia (sudden death) or hypoxia to the brain (convulsions, disorientation, coma).
- The physical examination is often unremarkable.
- A blood sample will be cherry red.

Electrocardiography

- ECG abnormalities can include ST segment changes, conduction abnormalities, or arrhythmias.

Specialized Diagnostic Test

- Carboxyhemoglobin blood levels can be measured.

Treatment

- One hundred percent oxygen should be administered.
- Any arrhythmias should be treated as needed.
- Supportive care should include correction of electrolyte and acid-base imbalances.

Prognosis

- Clinical recovery usually occurs if the situation is detected and treated early.

TOAD POISONING

- The Colorado river toad (*Bufo alvaritus*) and the marine toad (*Bufo marinas*) secrete toxins from the parotid glands that can cause profound cardiotoxicity. The parotid gland secretions contain epinephrine, norepinephrine, dopamine, serotonin, bufotenine, bufagenins, and bufotoxins. The animal does not have to ingest the toad to become poisoned. Toxic parotid secretions can be absorbed through the oral mucous membranes just holding the toad in its mouth.

Cardiac Pathophysiology

- Bufagenins and bufotoxins can have digitalis-like effects on the heart.

Diagnosis

History and Physical Examination

- The pet is often observed playing with the toad.
- Clinical signs occur within minutes and may include hypersalivation, vomiting, diarrhea, weakness, pulmonary edema, and seizures. Coma and death can occur within 30 minutes.

Electrocardiography

- In experimental studies, the digitalis-like effect of the toxin may result in any type of arrhythmia. In natural exposure, arrhythmias are rare. The most common rhythms noted are sinus arrhythmia and sinus tachycardia.
- Severely intoxicated dogs with bradycardia, tachycardia, neurologic disability or signs of shock should get an initial ECG. Monitoring the ECG is recommended if significant arrhythmias are noted.

Therapy

- The patient's mouth should be rinsed immediately. Atropine may help decrease salivation, but is reserved for patients with heart rates less then 50 bpm. Using atropine to treat excess salivation in dogs with normal heart rates or tachycardia can lead to more severe arrhythmias.
- Vomiting should be induced if ingestion was recent. The venom may enter enterohepatic circulation. Therefore, multiple doses of activated charcoal should be administered. Sorbitol cathartic is advised.
- Provide supportive care, including anticonvulsive and antiarrhythmic medication as needed.
- Pentobarbital anesthesia will control seizures.
- **Propranolol** is quite effective for tachyarrhythmias. In patients without asthma or pre-existing heart disease, doses of 0.5 to 2 mg/kg can be given slowly IV, to effect.

OLEANDER TOXICITY

- Oleander (*Nerium oleander*) is an ornamental shrub found mostly in the southeast United States.

Cardiac Pathophysiology

- The toxin of oleander is a digitalis-like glycoside.

Diagnosis

History and Physical Examination

- Signs of vomiting and diarrhea occur within 2 to 3 hours.
- ECG may reveal any type of arrhythmia due to the digitalis-like compounds.

Therapy

- Supportive care that includes fluid therapy, electrolyte replacement, and control of vomiting and diarrhea is recommended.
- Arrhythmias should be treated as needed.

CHOCOLATE TOXICITY

- Toxic effects of chocolate are due to methylxanthines, in particular theobromine and caffeine
- The median lethal dose of theobromine and caffeine is 100 to 200 mg/kg (0.2 to 0.5 oz baking chocolate/kg). Mild signs can occur with 20 mg/kg, severe signs at 40 to 50 mg/kg and seizures at 60 mg/kg.

Cardiac Pathophysiology

- Theobromine increases cyclic adenosine mono phosphate, causes release of catecholamines, blocks adenosine receptors, and increases calcium uptake by the sarcoplasmic reticulum.
- The net effect is to increase heart rate and the force of contractions.

Diagnosis

History and Physical Examination

- Clinical signs associated with chocolate toxicity include vomiting and diarrhea, hyperactivity, ataxia, hyperthermia, muscle tremors, coma, and death.
- Tachycardia is frequently noted, as well as bradycardia.
- ECG findings may include sinus tachycardia, sinus bradycardia, and ventricular arrhythmias.

Therapy

- Symptomatic therapy should include prevention of absorption, increasing elimination, maintenance of life support, and control of cardiac arrhythmias and seizures.
- Vomiting should be induced if ingestion was recent. **Activated charcoal** (1 to 4 g/kg orally) should be administered. Because methylxanthines undergo enterohepatic recirculation, giving repeated doses of activated charcoal is usually beneficial in symptomatic animals.
- Arrhythmia management
  - Lidocaine is used for control of ventricular arrhythmias, if needed. Beta blockers can be added if additional control and maintenance therapy is required. Because propranolol hydrochloride reportedly delays renal excretion of methylxanthines, metoprolol succinate or metoprolol tartrate is the beta blocker of choice, if available.
  - Treat supraventricular tachycardia with beta blockers (i.e., propranolol, metoprolol, atenolol).
  - Seizure control can be done with diazepam or barbiturate.

DOXORUBICIN CARDIOTOXICITY

- Doxorubicin is an anthracycline antibiotic used for its antineoplastic properties. Its mechanism of action as a chemotherapeutic agent is inhibition of nucleic acid synthesis. Cardiotoxicity manifested as arrhythmias or dilated cardiomyopathy usually develops after cumulative doses of 240 mg/m^2 in dogs, but toxicity can occur at dosages as low as 130 mg/m^2 (dog range, 135 to 265 mg/m^2; cat range, 130 to 320 mg/m^2). Clinical studies in humans have shown a reduced incidence of cardiomyopathy when people are treated with prolonged infusions (24 hours) of doxorubicin. Prolonged infusion therapy in dogs is still under investigation.
- Acute cardiotoxicity is manifested by arrhythmias during or shortly after administration. Dilated cardiomyopathy may develop with chronic treatment. Although histologic lesions and echocardiographic changes may develop, clinical signs of congestive heart failure are uncommon in cats treated with doxorubicin.

Cardiac Pathophysiology

- The mechanism by which doxorubicin causes cardiotoxicity is unknown, but free radical generation and lipid membrane peroxidation may be

involved in the pathogenesis. The heart rate at the time of drug administration may also determine the degree of cardiac toxicity, with slower heart rates associated with less toxicity.
- Histologic lesions consist of myocyte vacuolization, myocytolysis, and, occasionally, interstitial fibrosis.

Diagnosis

History and Physical Examination
- Clinical signs and physical findings are associated with dilated cardiomyopathy and include exercise intolerance, dyspnea and coughing, hepatomegaly, and ascites. Congestive heart failure usually develops acutely.

Electrocardiography
- In dogs, ECG abnormalities include ST segment and T wave changes, decreased QRS voltages, intraventricular conduction abnormalities, and atrial and ventricular arrhythmias. ECG changes are rare in cats treated with doxorubicin.
- ECG changes can occur acutely during drug administration. In this situation, stopping the drip and then reinstituting it at a slower rate may resolve the problem.

Radiography
- With dilated cardiomyopathy, radiography may show cardiomegaly, pulmonary edema, pleural effusion, hepatomegaly, and ascites.

Echocardiography
- The most consistent abnormalities with doxorubicin cardiotoxicity are increased left ventricular end-systolic internal dimensions and decreased fractional shortening. As cardiac function deteriorates, progressive left atrial enlargement can be seen.

Therapy

- If congestive heart failure develops, the patient should be treated accordingly. Unfortunately, the therapeutic response is poor. An ECG is recommended prior to each doxorubicin treatment, especially in dogs. If arrhythmias develop, doxorubicin treatment should be discontinued. An echocardiogram is recommended after the third cycle in dogs or fifth cycle in cats, and every one to three cycles thereafter. Doxorubicin treatment should be discontinued if contractility is impaired.
- Protection from cardiomyopathy has been demonstrated with dexrazoxane (Zinecard).
- The mechanism for cardioprotection is not understood. One suggested mechanism is dexrazoxane prevents the formation of the free radicals and subsequent lipid peroxidation that occurs from free iron and iron associated with the doxorubicin-iron complex.
- It is FDA approved for use in women with doxorubicin administration against metastatic breast cancer.
- It has been shown in studies to protect mice, rats, hamsters, pigs and dogs.
- It appears to prevent cardiotoxicity, but does not protect against other toxic effects by anthracyclines.
- Dexrazoxane ameliorates anthracycline extravasation lesions.
- The recommended dose ratio of **dexrazoxane to doxorubicin** is 10:1. It is given as an infusion over 15 minutes, 30 minutes prior to using doxorubicin.
- Expense of the drug limits its routine use.

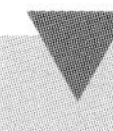

Infectious/Inflammatory Diseases

- The heart can be involved in an inflammatory process owing to many infectious agents. Myocardial cells, interstitium, or vessels may be affected.

Cardiac Pathophysiology

- Myocardial injury can occur from direct myocardial invasion of an infectious agent, from a myocardial toxin produced by the agent, or from a secondary immune-mediated reaction.
  - Important causes of myocardial injury in small animals include the following:
    - Bacterial myocarditis
      - Pyogenic bacteria originate in septicemic states or from other septic foci.
      - Clinical signs range from subclinical and nonspecific (weight loss, lethargy) to apparent and specific (arrhythmias, congestive heart failure).
    - Viral myocarditis has been associated with canine parvovirus and distemper virus in dogs, and with suspected but not yet identified viral pathogens in cats. Clinical abnormalities include cardiomegaly, arrhythmias, and nonspecific ECG abnormalities. The severity of the cardiac changes ranges from congestive heart failure with canine parvovirus to subclinical myocarditis with canine distemper virus.

- Fungi and algae can infect the heart secondary to a disseminated disease process, often in conjunction with reduced host defense.
- Protozoal myocarditis can occur in dogs with canine trypanosomiasis (*Trypanosoma cruzi*) or in dogs and cats with toxoplasmosis (*Toxoplasma gondii*).
  - Trypanosomiasis is discussed later.
  - Toxoplasmosis can produce signs dominated by the extent and severity of multiorgan system involvement.

Therapy

- Treatment is often supportive and usually focused on the most prominent systemic manifestation of the disease process.

BORRELIOSIS (LYME DISEASE)

- Borreliosis is caused by the spirochete *Borrelia burgdorferi.* Transmission is by ticks of the *Ixodes* species. The incidence of cardiac involvement is unknown in animals. In humans, 10% of patients with borreliosis have cardiac involvement. Borreliosis in animals is usually acute and cured by antibiotics. However, the prognosis may be poor if second-stage disease involving the heart, kidneys, or central nervous system (CNS) develops.

Cardiac Pathophysiology

- Spirochetes have been isolated from myocardial biopsies in humans.
- DCM has been reported in a few humans with Lyme disease. Cardiac damage may involve an immune-mediated mechanism.

Diagnosis

History and Physical Examination

- Ticks may be found on dogs, or owners may report recent exposure to ticks in endemic areas.
- Although nonspecific, clinical signs include anorexia, depression, and lameness.
- Physical examination reveals fever, joint pain, and lymphadenopathy.

Electrocardiography

- The most common ECG finding in humans is AV block.
- Ectopic beats and ST segment abnormalities have also been reported in humans.
- AV block secondary to *B. burgdorferi* in the dog has been reported in one case.

Specialized Diagnostic Tests

- Commercial test kits are available, but titers should be interpreted in view of the history, physical examination, and clinical signs. False-positive and false-negative titers are not uncommon.

Therapy

- Antibiotics are the treatment of choice for borreliosis. **Tetracycline, doxycycline, ampicillin,** or **amoxicillin** appear to be the most effective first-line agents.
- Humans with cardiac involvement are often treated with IV ceftriaxone or cefotaxime.
- A 5- to 7-day course of anti-inflammatory doses of corticosteroids may be helpful for heart block that does not rapidly resolve with appropriate antibiotic therapy.

TRYPANOSOMIASIS (CHAGAS DISEASE)

- Trypanosomiasis is a rare disease caused by the protozoan *T. cruzi.* It usually occurs in young dogs in the southeastern United States. Transmission is via the bite of a reduviid bug.

Cardiac Pathophysiology

- During the acute stage (2 to 4 weeks after infection), cardiac damage occurs when trypomastigotes rupture from myocardial cells. This causes myocardial failure, conduction disturbances, and arrhythmias.
- If animals survive the acute stage, they may remain asymptomatic for months. During this time, myocardial degeneration occurs, and DCM develops. Myocardial damage during this stage may be related to immune mechanisms or to the release of toxic parasitic products.

Diagnosis

History and Physical Examination

- Clinical signs during the acute stage are related to left- and (mainly) right-heart failure. Collapse and sudden death may be noted in a previously healthy dog. Gastrointestinal signs of anorexia and diarrhea are also common. The lymph nodes will be enlarged during the acute stage.
- Clinical manifestations during the chronic stage are associated with dilated cardiomyopathy, with signs of right-sided heart failure often predominating. Various cardiac arrhythmias also occur. The cardiomyopathy is not curable and responds poorly to treatment.

- Physical findings associated with heart failure—pale mucous membranes, weak femoral pulses, and ascites—can be seen during acute and chronic stages.

Electrocardiography

- Conduction disturbances, ectopic beats, and sustained arrhythmias can be seen during the acute and chronic stages.

Radiography

- Radiography may show cardiomegaly, pulmonary edema, pleural effusion, hepatomegaly, and ascites.

Echocardiography

- Echocardiography is normal during the acute phase. As the disease becomes chronic, ventricular contractility and wall thickness decrease, and cardiac chambers dilate.

Specialized Diagnostic Tests

- Trypomastigotes may be seen on a blood smear during the acute stage. The patient becomes aparasitemic 2 to 4 weeks after infection.
- Indirect fluorescent antibody, direct hemagglutination, and complement fixation tests confirm antibodies to *T. cruzi*.
- Blood cultures can be performed, but they are time consuming.

Therapy

- Treatment of this disease is very unrewarding. By the time the diagnosis is made, the disease is often no longer responsive to antiprotozoal medication.
- Various therapeutic recommendations include oral **benzimidazole** (5 mg/kg PO once daily for 2 months), **allopurinol** (30 mg/kg PO every 12 hours for 100 days), or **nifurtimox** (2 to 7 mg/kg PO every 6 hours for 3 to 5 months).
- Alert owners and veterinary staff to potential zoonotic risk.

PARVOVIRUS

- Parvovirus has caused cardiac disease when it infected puppies less than 2 weeks of age. Current cases of parvoviral myocarditis are very rare.

Cardiac Pathophysiology

- Viral multiplication occurs in rapidly dividing myocardial cells, resulting in cell death and scarring.

Diagnosis

History and Physical Examination

- The cardiac form of parvovirus often results in sudden death.
- Some puppies that survived the acute phase developed heart failure weeks to months later, and died from cardiac arrhythmias or dilated cardiomyopathy 6 to 12 months later.
- ECG reveals atrial or ventricular arrhythmias.

Echocardiography

- In some infected dogs, echocardiography revealed abnormalities consistent with dilated cardiomyopathy, including decreased fractional shortening, left atrial and ventricular enlargement, and increased E-point septal separation.

Therapy

- Heart failure is managed with diuretics, digoxin, and ACE inhibitors.
- Arrhythmias should be treated accordingly.

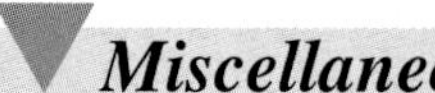

Miscellaneous Diseases

SYSTEMIC LUPUS ERYTHEMATOSUS

- Cardiac disease due to systemic lupus erythematosus (SLE) is a common finding in humans, rare in dogs, and not reported in cats. Pericarditis is the most common cardiac abnormality associated with SLE in humans. Other abnormalities in humans include myocarditis, congestive heart failure, and valvular heart disease. Ventricular arrhythmias were reported in two dogs and heart failure in one dog diagnosed with SLE.

Cardiac Pathophysiology

- Pericarditis occurs secondary to vasculitis.
- Myocarditis and endocarditis can also occur.

Diagnosis

History and Physical Examination

- Clinical signs associated with heart disease are usually overshadowed by systemic signs of SLE.
- Clinical findings associated with arrhythmias or heart failure may be present.
- ECG may reveal ventricular arrhythmias.

- Echocardiographic abnormalities have not been reported in dogs or cats with SLE.

Specialized Diagnostic Tests

- A diagnosis of SLE can be made with a positive ANA titer in conjunction with clinical signs.

Therapy

- Immunosuppressive doses of **prednisone** (2 mg/kg PO every 12 hours) is advised. If there is no improvement after 7 days, more aggressive immunosuppressive therapy should be considered.
- Pericardiocentesis is recommended if pericardial effusion is present.

NEUROGENIC CARDIOMYOPATHY

- CNS disease has been associated with myocardial lesions in clinical cases in all domestic species except the cat. Experimentally, stimulation of specific areas of cat's brains can cause myocardial necrosis. Most cases involve trauma to the brain or spinal cord. CNS neoplasia, infection, encephalomalacia, and ruptured intervertebral discs can also result in myocardial damage.

Cardiac Pathophysiology

- Histologic lesions include degeneration or disintegration of myocardial cells, with necrosis and mineralization. Scar formation may develop. The endocardium is most frequently involved, with occasional involvement of the subepicardium.
- Myocardial necrosis may be evident as early as 3 days after the CNS damage, and generally is present within 5 to 10 days in affected animals. Cardiac arrhythmias are the most frequent clinical sequela.
- The myocardial lesions probably occur owing to increased sympathetic tone and release of catecholamines.

Diagnosis

History and Physical Examination

- Clinical signs are usually referable to the CNS disease and sometimes arrhythmias.

Electrocardiography

- Atrial and ventricular arrhythmias, ST segment depression, prolonged QT interval, and T wave abnormalities have been reported.
- The diagnosis is often made on necropsy.

Therapy

- Appropriate therapy for the CNS disease is advised. Treat arrhythmias as necessary.

GASTRIC DILATION-VOLVULUS COMPLEX

- Gastric dilation-volvulus complex (GDV) is a life-threatening emergency in the dog. It is most common in large, deep-chested dogs. No specific etiology has been determined, but GDV is often associated with exercise following a large meal. Cardiac arrhythmias occur in up to 40% of patients with GDV. Most arrhythmias are ventricular in origin. Atrial arrhythmias have also been reported. Arrhythmias usually occur within 36 hours of admission. The presence of arrhythmias does not worsen the prognosis.

Cardiac Pathophysiology

- The exact mechanism for the arrhythmias is unknown. Theories include acid-base imbalances, autonomic imbalances, myocardial hypoxia, electrolyte imbalances, or a myocardial depressant factor.

Diagnosis

History and Physical Examination

- Clinical signs are restlessness, pacing, lethargy, weakness, attempts to vomit, and abdominal distention.
- The physical examination findings often include pale mucous membranes, rapid heart rate, weak femoral pulses, pain upon abdominal palpation, distended, tympanic stomach, and signs associated with shock.

Electrocardiography

- The ECG may reveal ventricular and occasionally atrial arrhythmias. The most common appears to be an accelerated idioventricular rhythm (AIR). The terminology for this arrhythmia is still in dispute. Other terms for this ventricular rhythm are slow ventricular tachycardia, fast idioventricular rhythm, or idioventricular tachycardia.
- The features of AIR are a wide, bizarre complex rhythm, typically with a rate similar to the underlying sinus rate. As the sinus rate slows, the ventricular rate may "capture" the heart rhythm. Commonly, fusion beats are seen as the rhythm waxes between the sinus and the ventricular

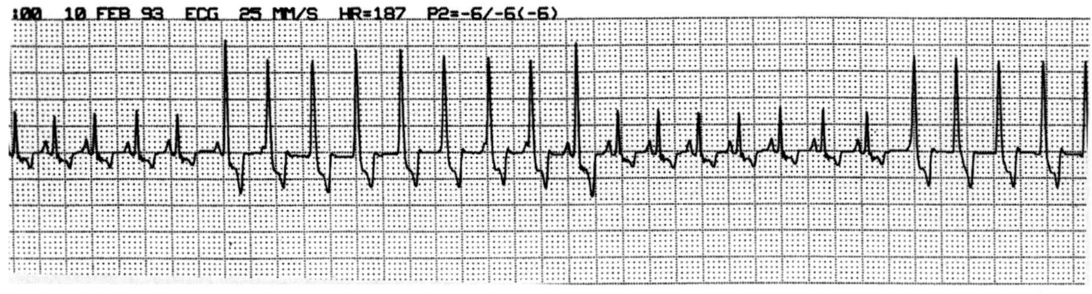

Figure 13-12. Accelerated idioventricular rhythm. Beats 7 through 13 and the last four beats on the right are ventricular in origin. These beats represent an accelerated ventricular rhythm. Beats 6 and 14 are fusion beats, a hybrid of the sinus beat and the ventricular focus.

rhythm. As the underlying sinus rate slows, the ventricular rate may slow also (Figure 13-12)
- ST segment and T wave changes may be evident.

Radiography
- The stomach is gas-filled, distended, and often rotated.
- The cardiac silhouette may be small owing to decreased venous return.

Treatment

- Treatment should be directed toward gastric decompression and shock therapy.
- Any arrhythmias should be treated as needed.

PANCREATITIS

- Pancreatitis is a disease most frequently diagnosed in middle-aged, obese dogs and cats. Although many factors have been associated with pancreatitis, the etiology is often unknown.

Cardiac Pathophysiology

- A myocardial depressant factor is released from the pancreas, which can result in decreased myocardial contractility and arrhythmias.
- Activated pancreatic enzymes may also damage the myocardium directly or play a role in thrombus formation, resulting in myocardial ischemia.
- Acid-base and electrolyte imbalances may also contribute to arrhythmias.

Diagnosis

History and Physical Examination
- Clinical signs are nonspecific and include vomiting, diarrhea, anorexia, and depression.
- Physical examination may reveal abdominal pain, fever, dehydration, and shock.
- Sudden death associated with cardiac complications can occur.

Electrocardiography
- Atrial and ventricular arrhythmias and ST segment changes have been reported.

Radiography
- Abdominal radiographs may reveal an increased density, calcification, or gas in the area of the pancreas.

Clinical Pathology
- Leukocytosis, hyperglycemia, high liver enzymes, and high amylase and lipase in serum and peritoneal fluid are common findings in animals with pancreatitis.

Therapy

- It is important to decrease pancreatic secretions by withholding food and water.
- Supportive care should include fluid and electrolyte replacement along with antibiotics.
- Cardiac arrhythmias should be treated as needed, although most arrhythmias will resolve spontaneously with resolution of the underlying disease.

TRAUMATIC MYOCARDITIS

- The term traumatic myocarditis is a catchall phrase for arrhythmias that may occur following blunt trauma. The arrhythmias seen following blunt trauma include supraventricular tachycardia, ventricular arrhythmias, or bradyarrhythmias. The trauma does not have to occur directly to the chest.

Cardiac Pathophysiology

- Blunt trauma mechanisms include the following: (1) unidirectional force, (2) bidirectional force (compressive), (3) indirect force, (4) decelerative force, and (5) concussive force.

- The actual mechanism for the cause of the arrhythmias is not known. Direct damage to the heart from the trauma does not have to occur to result in the arrhythmias. Autonomic imbalance or reperfusion of ischemic tissue may have a role.

Diagnosis

- Various arrhythmias, both atrial and ventricular, may be seen following trauma. The most common appears to be an AIR. The terminology for this arrhythmia is still in dispute. Other terms for this ventricular rhythm are slow ventricular tachycardia, fast idioventricular rhythm, or idioventricular tachycardia.
- The features of AIR are a wide, bizarre complex rhythm, typically with a rate similar to the underlying sinus rate. As the sinus rate slows, the ventricular rate may "capture" the heart rhythm. Commonly, fusion beats are seen as the rhythm waxes between the sinus and the ventricular rhythm. As the underlying sinus rate slows, the ventricular rate may slow also (see Figure 13-12).

Therapy

- The main goal of therapy is supportive care for the underlying disease: fluid therapy, control of hemorrhage, oxygen therapy, analgesia, and correction of electrolyte imbalance.
- Therapy for the ventricular arrhythmias may be necessary only if the tachycardia is persistent and the clinician feels it has a role in the patient's hypotension. If therapy is felt to be necessary, then **lidocaine** by intravenous route is recommended at 2 to 4 mg/kg as a bolus. The maximum dose to be given over a 10-minute period is 10 mg/kg. Lidocaine can cause nausea, vomiting, hypotension, and seizures. If this suppresses the arrhythmias, then a constant-rate infusion of lidocaine can be given at 40 to 100 μg/kg/min. A repeat 4- to 8-mg bolus of lidocaine may be needed once, after starting the lidocaine infusion, if more than 10 minutes elapses after injection of the original test bolus. It is not unusual for the constant-rate infusion of lidocaine to lose its effect after several hours.
- If lidocaine is not effective, then **procainamide** may be tried. The intravenous dose of procainamide is 2 to 3 mg/kg over 2 to 3 minutes. The total dose given over a 20-minute period should not exceed 20 mg/kg. The constant-rate infusion for procainamide is 20 to 50 μg/kg/min. Alternatively, oral or intramuscular dosing could be initiated following the IV dose if the dog is receiving nothing by mouth.
- Other therapies such as beta blockers or magnesium (IV) have been suggested.

Prognosis

- Fortunately, the arrhythmias are generally not lethal. They have a tendency to resolve over the next 3 to 5 days, as the patient improves clinically. Generally, progression of the underlying disorders, and not the arrhythmia, causes the patient's demise.
- If the patient requires antiarrhythmic therapy, this is usually discontinued prior to discharge, or within several days of discharge.

Frequently Asked Questions

How useful is the ECG in diagnosing electrolyte disturbances and what changes would you expect to see?

The ECG can be helpful in raising suspicion regarding the presence of some electrolyte abnormalities, most notably hyperkalemia, but it is not a very sensitive test for detecting electrolyte abnormalities. One of the reasons that the ECG is not very sensitive is that the morphology of the ECG complexes is influenced by several electrolytes (e.g., sodium, potassium, calcium) and further influenced by the patient's acid base status. As potassium levels rise above normal, T waves become peaked with a narrow base, P wave amplitude decreases, and the P-R interval prolongs. If potassium is very high, QRS complexes widen and P waves disappear (atrial standstill) and with further elevation in potassium, conduction delays lead to ventricular fibrillation and ventricular asystole. Hypokalemia produces prolonged QT intervals, U waves, and ST segment depression, with possible ventricular and supraventricular arrhythmias. Hypocalcemia may cause QT interval prolongation, whereas hypercalcemia may shorten the QT segment and with severe hypercalcemia, bradycardia may develop.

A patient presents with a ventricular arrhythmia. What systemic disturbances should be considered?

VPCs may be seen with a variety of noncardiac conditions including pancreatitis, GDV, traumatic myocarditis, splenic disease and neoplasia, cardiac masses, hypokalemia, trypanosomiasis, shock, heat stroke and pyrexia. Drugs and plant toxins such as doxorubicin, methylxanthines (chocolate, theophylline), digoxin, sympathomimetics, oleander can all cause VPCs.

Continued

A dog presents with echocardiographic evidence of myocardial failure based on depressed indices of systolic function (stroke volume, fractional shortening). What needs to be considered in addition to idiopathic dilated cardiomyopathy?

Systolic function can be depressed secondary to several systemic diseases, nutritional deficiencies and toxic insults. Systemic abnormalities associated with depressed myocardial function include hypothyroidism, pancreatitis, sepsis and shock and trypanosomiasis. Taurine and L-carnitine deficiencies can lead to dilated cardiomyopathy. Adriamycin toxicity leads to myocardial failure. Note that in some animals, especially large breed dogs, fractional shortening may be slightly below normal values established for smaller breeds and represent a normal variant.

A cat presents with left ventricular hypertrophy on the echocardiogram. What systemic disturbances need to be considered along with idiopathic hypertrophic cardiomyopathy?

Consider the possibility of systemic hypertension, acromegaly, hyperthyroidism or infiltrative processes such as lymphoma. Dehydration causes a reduction in the size of the left ventricular lumen and as a result can give the impression of left ventricular hypertrophy.

SUGGESTED READINGS

Appel MJ: Lyme disease in dogs and cats, Compend Cont Ed 12:617, 1990.

Atkins C: The role of non-cardiac disease in the development and precipitation of heart failure, Vet Clin North Am Small Anim Pract 21:5, 1991.

Atkins CE: Cardiac manifestations of systemic and metabolic disease. In Fox PR, Sisson D, Moise NS, eds: Textbook of canine and feline cardiology, Philadelphia, 1999, WB Saunders.

Barr SC: American trypanosomiasis in dogs, Compend Cont Ed 13:745, 1991.

Carson TL: Toxic gases. In Kirk RW, ed: Current veterinary therapy IX, Philadelphia, 1986, WB Saunders.

Chew DJ, Nagode LA, Carothers M: Disorders of calcium: hypercalcemia and hypocalcemia. In DiBartola SP, ed: Fluid therapy in small animal practice, Philadelphia, 1992, WB Saunders.

DiBartola SP, deMorais HSA: Disorders of potassium: hypokalemia and hyperkalemia. In DiBartola SP ed: Fluid therapy in small animal practice, Philadelphia, 1992, WB Saunders.

Feldman EC, Nelson RW: Canine and feline endocrinology and reproduction, ed 3, St Louis, 2004, WB Saunders.

Fisch C: Electrolytes and the heart. In Hurst JW, ed: The heart, ed 5, New York, 1982, McGraw-Hill.

Hooser SB, Beasley VR: Methylxanthine poisoning (chocolate and caffeine toxicosis). In Kirk RW, ed: Current veterinary therapy IX, Philadelphia, 1986, WB Saunders.

Kienle RD, Bruyette D, Pron PO: Effects of thyroid hormone and thyroid dysfunction on the cardiovascular system, Vet Clin North Am 24:495, 1994.

King JM, Roth L, Haschek WM: Myocardial necrosis secondary to neural lesions in domestic animals, J Am Vet Med Assoc 180:144, 1982.

Kintzer PP, Peterson ME: Primary and secondary canine hypoadrenocorticism, Vet Clin North Am 27:349, 1997.

Loar AS, Susaneck SJ: Doxorubicin-induced cardiotoxicity in five dogs, Semin Vet Med Surg 1:68, 1986.

Melian C, Stefanacci J, Peterson ME, Kintzer PP: Radiographic findings in dogs with naturally-occurring primary hypoadrenocorticism, J Am Anim Hosp Assoc 35(3):208-212, 1999.

Mount ME: Toxicology. In Ettinger SJ, ed: Textbook of veterinary internal medicine, ed 3, Philadelphia, 1989, WB Saunders.

Muir WM: Gastric dilatation-volvulus in the dog, with emphasis on cardiac arrhythmias, J Am Vet Med Assoc 180:739, 1982.

Nichols R: Complications and concurrent disease associated with canine hyperadrenocorticism, Vet Clin North Am 27:309, 1997.

O'Keefe DA, Sisson DD, Gelberg HB, et al: Systemic toxicity associated with doxorubicin administration in cats, J Vet Intern Med 7:309, 1993.

Palumbo ME, Perri SF: Toad poisoning. In Kirk RW, ed: Current veterinary therapy VIII, Philadelphia, 1983, WB Saunders.

Peterson ME, Taylor RS, Greco DS, et al: Acromegaly in 14 cats, J Vet Intern Med 4:192, 1990.

Rosenthal DS, Braunwald E: Hematologic-oncologic disorders and heart disease. In Braunwald E, ed: Heart disease, ed 4, Philadelphia, 1992, WB Saunders.

Ruslander D: Heat stroke. In Kirk RW, ed: Current veterinary therapy XI, Philadelphia, 1992, WB Saunders.

Sennello KA, Schulman RL, Prosek R, Siegel AM: Systolic blood pressure in cats with diabetes mellitus, J Am Vet Med Assoc 223(2):198-201, 2003.

Sisson D, O'Grady MR, Calvert CA: Myocardial diseases of dogs. In Fox PR, Sisson D, Moise NS, eds: Textbook of canine and feline cardiology, Philadelphia, 1999, WB Saunders.

Struble AL, Feldman EC, Nelson RW, Kass PH: Systemic hypertension and proteinuria in dogs with diabetes mellitus, J Am Vet Med Assoc 213(6):822-825, 1998.

Tilley LP, Bond BR, Patnaik AK, Liu S-K: Cardiovascular tumors in the cat, J Am Anim Hosp Assoc 17:1009, 1981.

Williams GH, Lilly LS, Seely EW: The heart in endocrine and nutritional disorders. In Braunwald E, ed: Heart disease, ed 5, Philadelphia, 1997, WB Saunders.

Yates RW, Weller RE: Have you seen the cardiopulmonary form of parvovirus infection? Vet Med April 1988, p 380.

CHAPTER 14

Systemic Hypertension

Rosemary A. Henik and Scott A. Brown

INTRODUCTION

Hypertension may exist transiently due to fear or excitement, or be sustained and pathologic. Small animal patients most commonly have secondary hypertension, with an underlying disease triggering increased blood pressure (BP). A diagnosis of systemic hypertension is established when reliable BP measurements demonstrate a sustained elevation of systolic (= 160 mm Hg) or diastolic (= 120 mm Hg) BP. The prevalence of idiopathic, hypertension in dogs and cats is unknown.

POPULATION AT RISK

Cats

- Chronic kidney disease, with or without proteinuria, and hyperthyroidism are the two most common causes of hypertension in cats. Although effective resolution of hyperthyroidism may reduce BP, some cats will become hypertensive only after therapy for this endocrinopathy.
- Occasionally, diseases such as hyperaldosteronism, pheochromocytoma, or other endocrine diseases may also be associated with hypertension.
- Many cats that are not hypertensive initially will become hypertensive when fluid therapy, steroids, erythropoietin, or vasoconstricting drugs are given.
- Some clinicians are incorporating the routine measurement of BP into geriatric wellness exams. This practice may occasionally identify a hypertensive cat with subclinical kidney disease; however, it should be realized that the risk of a false positive result (i.e., high BP measurement) increases when the prevalence of a disease is low (as in a healthy population).
- BP measurement is advised in all cats with:
  - Kidney disease
  - Endocrinopathy
  - Compatible ocular signs (e.g., hemorrhage, detachment, retinal vessel tortuosity)
  - Neurologic signs (e.g., nystagmus, head tilt, other cranial nerve signs, or seizures)
  - A cardiac murmur or gallop
  - Radiographic cardiomegaly
  - Echocardiographically determined cardiac wall hypertrophy (although this is not a consistent change in hypertension)

Dogs

- Chronic glomerular disease or tubulointerstitial disease associated with proteinuria are most commonly associated with hypertension in dogs.
- Endocrine diseases including hyperadrenocorticism, diabetes mellitus, pheochromocytoma, and hyperaldosteronism may be associated with hypertension.
- Metabolic abnormalities including obesity or hypercholesterolemia may result in hypertension.

- Resolution of the endocrinopathy may not restore normal BP in dogs.
- BP measurement is advised in any dog with:
  - Kidney disease
  - Endocrinopathy
  - Ocular signs or neurologic signs as described previously
  - Cardiac hypertrophy (although rare in the dog as an acquired change), which should also prompt the clinician to perform BP measurement

KEY POINT

Chronic kidney disease and endocrinopathies are most commonly associated with systemic hypertension in cats and dogs.

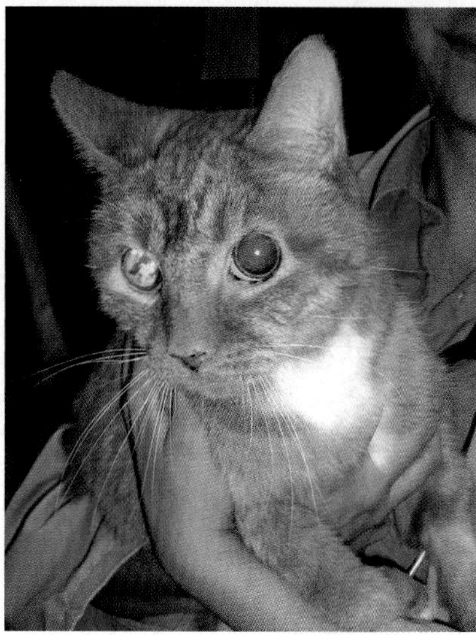

Figure 14-1. A cat with acute blindness due to systemic hypertension secondary to an aldosterone-secreting adrenal tumor. This cat presented with a systolic blood pressure > 300 mm Hg. There are severe ocular hemorrhages bilaterally.

CONSEQUENCES AND CLINICAL SIGNS OF HIGH BLOOD PRESSURE

Ocular Signs

- Severe systemic hypertension can lead to ocular injury. Findings associated with hypertensive injury include hemorrhage within the retina, vitreous, or anterior chamber; retinal detachment and atrophy; retinal edema; perivasculitis; retinal vessel tortuosity; and glaucoma.
- A sudden onset of blindness due to retinal hemorrhage and detachment is a common presenting complaint (Figure 14-1).

Neurologic Signs

- Signs consistent with cerebrovascular hemorrhage (head tilt, depression, seizures) have been seen clinically in cats and dogs with uncontrolled hypertension, and are often associated with a poor prognosis.
- Rarely, cats suffering from severe systemic hypertension (systolic BP > 300 mm Hg) develop a syndrome of progressive stupor, head pressing, or seizures that rapidly resolves with effective antihypertensive therapy. This syndrome is probably due to cerebral edema caused by high intracapillary hydrostatic pressure that develops once the systemic arterial pressure exceeds the autoregulatory range.

Renal Signs

- Persistent elevation of systolic BP to values > 160 mm Hg is associated with progressive renal injury in dogs and the severity of renal injury has been correlated to the degree of elevation. Potential renal pathologic changes induced by systemic hypertension include both glomerular and tubulointerstitial changes and can result in ischemia, necrosis, atrophy and exacerbation of proteinuria. These gradual and additive changes may be difficult to quantify in living animals with preexisting kidney disease, but systolic hypertension at the time of presentation (> 160 mm Hg) increases the odds of uremic crisis and of death in dogs with chronic kidney disease. Hypertension with systolic BP > 160 mm Hg is also likely to be a risk factor for progressive renal damage in cats.
- Proteinuria is perhaps the best marker that high BP is injurious to the kidney. The presence of microalbuminuria or an elevated urine protein-to-creatinine ratio (>0.5 in dogs, > 0.4 in cats) in a hypertensive animal (systolic BP > 160 mm Hg) should be considered an indication of ongoing renal damage.

Cardiac Signs

- Because the heart is working against an increased arterial pressure (i.e., afterload), diastolic dysfunction, left ventricular hypertrophy and secondary valvular insufficiency may develop. Changes may regress with antihypertensive treatment.
- Cardiac murmurs or gallops commonly occur.

- Congestive heart failure secondary to systemic hypertension is rare.

MEASUREMENT OF BLOOD PRESSURE

Patient Selection

- Currently there is no evidence to suggest that BP should be measured in all animals.
- BP should be measured in those animals that present with clinical signs attributable to high systemic arterial BP, such as blindness, hyphema, seizures, ataxia, or sudden collapse (signs compatible with cerebral vascular hemorrhage, edema, or stroke).
- Animals with azotemic kidney disease, hyperadrenocorticism, hyperthyroidism, pheochromocytoma, mineralocorticoid-secreting tumor, marked obesity, or cardiac hypertrophy should also be evaluated for hypertension.

Methods

- BP may be measured by either direct or indirect methods. Direct BP measurement is the "gold standard," but is technically difficult in unsedated dogs and cats, may be painful to the patient, and may be associated with hematoma formation and other complications.
- The indirect techniques are more applicable to a clinical setting, as they require less restraint and are technically easier to perform. Indirect techniques of BP measurement include the auscultatory, ultrasonic Doppler, oscillometric, and photoplethysmographic methods.
- All of the indirect techniques employ an inflatable cuff wrapped around an extremity. The pressure in the cuff is measured with a manometer or pressure transducer. A squeeze bulb is used to inflate the cuff to a pressure in excess of systolic BP, thereby occluding the underlying artery. As the cuff is gradually deflated, changes in arterial flow are detected by one of several means; the value for cuff pressure at various levels of deflation is then correlated with systolic, diastolic, or mean BP. This detection method varies among different indirect methods.
- For the auscultatory method, a stethoscope is placed over the artery distal to the cuff, and the listener hears a tapping sound when the inflation pressure falls below systolic pressure. In animals, the arterial (Korotkoff) sounds are low in both amplitude and frequency, and the auscultatory technique is difficult in dogs and cats.
- Doppler flow meters detect blood flow as a change in the frequency of reflected sound (Doppler shift) due to the motion of underlying red blood cells. BP is read by the operator from an aneroid manometer connected to the occluding cuff placed proximal to the Doppler transducer.
- Devices utilizing the oscillometric technique detect pressure fluctuations produced in the occluding cuff resulting from the pressure pulse. Machines using the oscillometric technique generally determine systolic, diastolic, and mean arterial pressures as well as pulse rate.
- Another device for measuring BP indirectly is the photoplethysmograph, which measures arterial volume by attenuation of infrared radiation, and is designed for use on the human finger. It can be employed in cats and small dogs weighing less than 10 kg.
- We have evaluated the ultrasonic Doppler and oscillometric methods in conscious dogs and cats. In both species, the oscillometric devices tend to underestimate BP by increasing amounts as pressure increases. Another problem with the oscillometric devices is the excessive time required to obtain readings in cats. The major limitation of the Doppler technique is the imprecise discrimination of the sounds designating the diastolic, and therefore mean, pressures. Owing to this fact, the Doppler method of BP measurement may be unreliable for the routine diagnosis and surveillance of patients with diastolic hypertension.
- On the basis of our studies in conscious animals, devices using the Doppler principle are recommended for use in cats; either the oscillometric or the Doppler devices are recommended in dogs. For comparative purposes, the same device should be used each time in an individual animal.

KEY POINT

Doppler is the preferred method of measurement in unsedated cats; the oscillometric technique may be used in dogs.

Cuff Size and Placement

- A complete range of pediatric cuff sizes should be available for an optimal patient limb circumference to cuff width ratio.

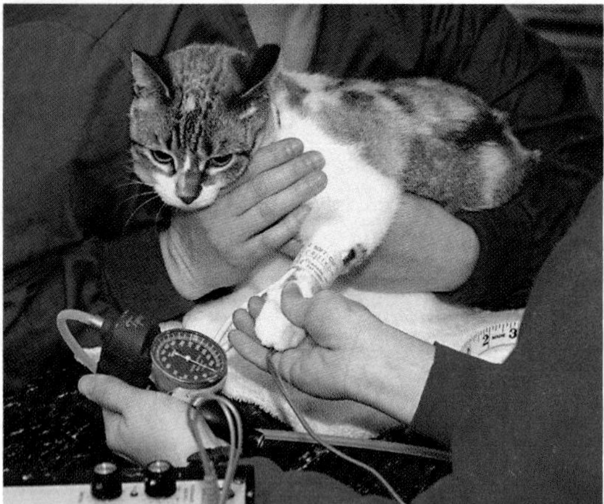

Figure 14-2. Demonstration of the technique to obtain systemic blood pressure measurements using a Doppler transducer in a cat.

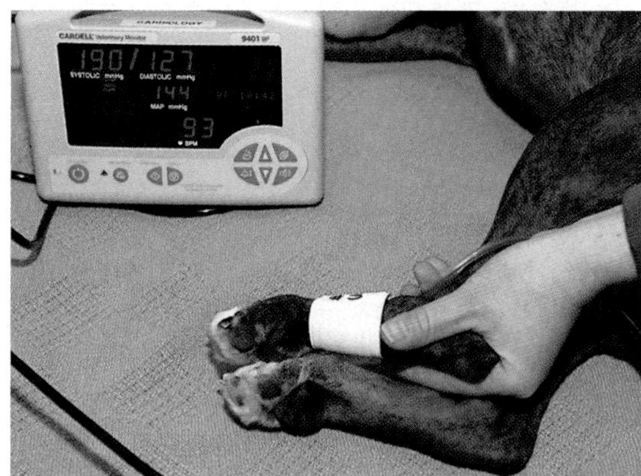

Figure 14-3. Demonstration of cuff placement over the cranial tibial artery in a dog. The oscillometric unit is most reliable in medium- and large-breed dogs.

- For dogs, a cuff width that measures 40% of the circumference of the limb should be used; for cats, a width of 30% to 40% of the limb circumference should be used. The cuff width should be noted in the medical record for future reference.
- An oversized cuff may give erroneously low recordings; an undersized cuff may give erroneously high recordings. If the ideal cuff width is midway between two available sizes, the larger cuff should be used, because it will theoretically produce the least error.
- The cuff may be placed around the brachial, median, or cranial tibial artery, or around the medial coccygeal artery.
- Generally, for the Doppler technique, the cuff is placed over the median artery, and the transducer is placed between the carpal and the metacarpal pads (Figure 14-2). Clipping the hair and applying acoustic gel at the site of transducer placement may enhance the signal, but clipping the hair may increase stress-artifact.
- For the oscillometric technique, our studies demonstrated that the coccygeal or cranial tibial artery in dogs may provide more reliable values than other sites (Figure 14-3).
- For comparative purposes, the same site for cuff placement should be used each time in an individual animal and recorded in the medical record.
- The cuff should be placed at the level of the aortic valve. If not, a compensation can be made for gravitational effect, with a 1.0 mm Hg rise in BP expected for each 1.3 cm of vertical distance between the level of the cuff and the level of the aortic valve.

Environment and Personnel

- Provide an environment that is quiet and away from other animals.
- The owner may be present to help calm the animal.
- Allow for a quiet equilibration time for the animal of 5 to 15 minutes.
- The same individual (preferably a technician) should perform all BP measurements following a standard protocol.
- Measurements should be obtained only in a patient that is calm, minimally restrained, and motionless. A blanket on the floor or table will allow the patient to be more comfortable.

Record Keeping

- A standard form for recording results of the BP measurement should be developed for the medical record. The following data should always be noted, along with each measurement obtained:
  - Cuff size (30% to 40% of limb circumference in cats; 40% in dogs)
  - Limb used (including left vs. right)
  - Time of day
  - Time of medication
  - Technique used (i.e., Doppler or oscillometric)
  - Degree of agitation, restlessness, or limb movement
  - Technician performing measurement
- If a different room or unusual environmental conditions exist (i.e., long wait prior to BP measurement with noisy dogs present), then this should be also noted if higher than normal values are obtained.

Techniques

Doppler

- In cats, a Doppler flow meter is used exclusively, whereas dogs can be evaluated with either the Doppler or oscillometric unit. Cuff size is determined after measuring the foreleg above the carpus, and the cuff is snugly wrapped around the foreleg and secured with a piece of tape.
- The position of the patient and cuff should be one that is well tolerated with the cuff at, or close to, the level of the right atrium. An excellent blood flow signal can usually be obtained from the median artery between the carpal and metacarpal pads by wetting down the hair with alcohol, followed by the application of coupling gel and the 10 MHz (i.e., pediatric) Doppler transducer.
- The transducer should be aligned parallel to blood flow, so the wire from the transducer is parallel with the limb (i.e., it emerges from under the paw). Unlike in the operative setting, the transducer is held in place, not taped.
- The cuff is inflated to a pressure 30 to 40 mm Hg higher than that required to obliterate the pulse, and then slowly deflated (about 2 to 5 mm Hg/second). A slower heart rate requires a slower deflation time in order to accurately determine systolic pressure. Too slow of a deflation time, however, will result in discomfort to the animal.
- The first sound heard as blood begins to flow through the artery is the systolic pressure. The cuff should be completely deflated prior to reinflation for the next measurement.
- Four to six measurements are advised over a 5- to 10-minute period because BP often falls with repeated measurements as the patient adjusts to the feel of the cuff inflating and deflating. The first measurement should be discarded and the average of three to five consecutive, consistent indirect measurements should be obtained. Any measurement obtained during limb movement should be discarded.
- If BP measurements are thought to be borderline or falsely high, the animal may be hospitalized for several hours in a quiet room to acclimate to the environment and BP measurement repeated.

Oscillometric Techniques

- In dogs, the oscillometric method gives reliable systolic results, with the addition of diastolic and mean arterial pressures. The rear limb is preferred for the oscillometric technique in dogs in our hospital, and the circumference of the metatarsus (i.e., below the hock) is measured for cuff width determination.
- Medium- and large-breed dogs are positioned on a blanket on the floor with the technician, who snugly wraps the cuff as described previously.
- The oscillometric unit is activated, and the same number of readings is obtained as described above for cats. If for any reason the oscillometric technique yields spurious results (as in very small dogs), the Doppler method is used.
- The average of all values obtained, or the average of all values obtained after the highest and lowest pressure readings are discarded, should be taken as the final value. Each measurement, in addition to the information mentioned previously in "Record Keeping," should be recorded.
- If results are borderline or inconsistent, repeat the measurement session on another day.

Anxiety-Induced Artifact: The "White Coat Effect"

The visit to the veterinary clinic, hospitalization, a strange environment, restraint in the examination room, clipper noise and vibration, cuff placement, cuff inflation, and other unusual stimuli in the setting of a veterinary hospital may induce anxiety in an animal during BP measurement. As a consequence, a falsely elevated value for BP may be obtained secondary to catecholamine release associated with this anxiety. The magnitude of this effect may be minimized by doing the following:

- Obtain BP measurements prior to a physical examination or other manipulations to which the animal may object.
- Perform all measurements in a quiet room utilizing a calm and reassuring manner.
- Allow the animal to acclimate to its surroundings for at least 5 minutes before obtaining BP measurements.

CHOICE OF ANIMALS TO TREAT

There is a clear association between ocular injury and marked systemic hypertension in dogs and cats. However, most other adverse effects of systemic hypertension are theorized on the basis of extrapolation from clinical studies in humans, or from experimental studies in laboratory rodents.

Treatment Guidelines

- In light of the uncertainty and the difficulties associated with BP measurement in dogs and cats, only those animals with severe elevations

of indirectly measured BP, or with clinical abnormalities directly attributable to hypertensive injury, should be considered candidates for treatment.
- The authors consider antihypertensive treatment to be indicated in any dog or cat with a sustained systolic BP > 200 mm Hg or a diastolic BP > 120 mm Hg, regardless of other clinical findings.
- In both species, an animal with a systolic/diastolic BP that consistently exceeds 160/100 mm Hg should be considered for treatment if clinical evaluation has identified abnormalities (e.g., retinal lesions or chronic kidney disease) that could be caused or exacerbated by systemic hypertension.
- In animals in which the BP is moderately elevated (systolic/diastolic BP that consistently exceeds 160/100 mm Hg), but no clinical abnormalities related to systemic hypertension are identified, the rationale for therapy is less clear. Currently, some clinicians recommend treatment for animals in this range, whereas others do not.
- Animals with no clinical signs and mildly elevated BP (systolic BP 120 to 160 mm Hg and diastolic BP 80 to 100 mm Hg) should not be treated.

KEY POINT

Animals with normal BP *or in which BP has not been measured* should not be treated with antihypertensive agents.

ANTIHYPERTENSIVE THERAPY

General

- Systemic arterial BP is the product of the cardiac output and the total peripheral resistance, so antihypertensive therapy is generally aimed at reducing cardiac output, total peripheral resistance, or both.
- Therapy may be loosely classified as dietary and pharmacologic.
- Treatment is generally conducted by sequential trials. Generally, dosage adjustments or changes in treatment should be instituted no more frequently than every 2 weeks, unless extreme hypertension necessitating emergency treatment is present.
- When using pharmacologic agents, a wide range of dosages should be considered, with initial dosages at the low end of the range.
- If an agent or combination of agents is incompletely effective, the dosage(s) may be increased, or additional agents may be added. Often, especially in dogs, multiple agents are used concurrently.
- It is usually not possible to restore BP to normal values when treating a hypertensive animal. It should be the veterinarian's goal to lower the BP to < 160/100 mm Hg, with emphasis given to the systolic value.

Duration of Treatment

- The diagnosis of hypertension associated with chronic kidney disease necessitates lifelong antihypertensive treatment, with periodic dosage adjustments based upon BP measurements.
- Hypertension associated with hyperthyroidism or hyperadrenocorticism can be expected to resolve within 1 to 3 months following effective treatment of the underlying condition, unless chronic kidney disease is also present. Occasionally, dogs with well-controlled hyperadrenocorticism remain hypertensive.
- In other patients, the duration of treatment cannot be predicted, but it may be required lifelong. Periodic dosage adjustments based upon BP measurements are indicated.

Dietary Therapy

- Though poorly studied, a low-sodium diet that provides less than 0.25% sodium on a dry-weight basis may be introduced. Dietary sodium restriction may be employed as a first step if hypertension is mild (i.e., < 170 mm Hg) and there is no target organ damage present.
- In animals with chronic kidney disease and hypertension, it may be more important to maintain adequate caloric intake rather than to insist that a low-sodium diet be fed. Therefore, drug therapy is instituted first, and when BP is stabilized, the animal may be switched to a lower sodium diet.
- Obesity can elevate systemic arterial pressure in human beings and dogs and, perhaps, in cats. Consequently, weight loss is desirable in obese, hypertensive animals.

Pharmacologic Agents: General

- Medical treatment of hypertension in dogs and cats has, until recently, been extrapolated from human protocols. Recommendations for medical therapy have included:

- Vasodilators (e.g., angiotensin-converting enzyme inhibitors [ACEI])
- Dihydropyridine calcium channel blockers
- Hydralazine
- Phenoxybenzamine
- Prazosin
- Diuretics
- Beta blockers
- These agents are generally given in concert with dietary sodium restriction.
- In animals with systemic hypertension and kidney disease, ACEI are the preferred initial choice in dogs, and ACEI and amlodipine are the preferred initial choice in cats, because of the renoprotective effects of the ACEI.

Vasodilators

- Vasodilators are considered first line drugs for hypertension in veterinary patients
- **ACE inhibitors** (e.g., **enalapril** 0.5 mg/kg PO twice a day or **benazepril** 0.5 mg/kg once or twice a day) will lower BP in many hypertensive dogs. In cats, the role of the renin-angiotensin-aldosterone system in the maintenance of systemic hypertension is less clear, but ACEI are administered for renoprotection. Benazepril may be every 24 hours given to those animals with kidney disease due to its predominantly biliary excretion, especially in cats.
- **Amlodipine besylate** (0.625 mg every 24 hours in cats or 0.1 to 0.5 mg/kg every 24 hours in dogs), a long-acting dihydropyridine calcium antagonist, reduces total peripheral resistance and has been used successfully as a single agent in hypertensive cats. Larger cats (more than 4 kg) may require 1.25 mg orally once daily. BP decreases significantly during amlodipine treatment, and significant adverse effects (i.e., azotemia, hypokalemia, and weight loss) are not frequently identified. Because amlodipine has a slow onset of action, adverse effects such as hypotension and loss of appetite are usually avoided. In dogs with chronic kidney disease, a dosage of 0.05 mg/kg given orally once daily lowered BP in initial pharmacokinetic trials, but in many spontaneously hypertensive dogs, amlodipine appears to be less effective.
- Recently, concern has been raised about the potential for deleterious effects of calcium channel antagonists. These concerns arise from studies in humans and diabetic dogs in which renal injury or proteinuria is exacerbated during therapy with calcium channel antagonists. In addition, there are theoretical rationales for preferring the use of an ACEI over other antihypertensive agents in animals with pre-existing kidney disease. However, the co-administration of a calcium channel antagonist and an ACEI may block adverse effects of calcium channel antagonism alone. In addition, because calcium channel antagonists are usually very effective in cats with systemic hypertension, they should be considered appropriate agents for use in affected cats until further information regarding long-term effects on renal function in cats becomes available.
- Direct-acting arterial vasodilators, such as **hydralazine** (0.5 to 2.0 mg/kg twice a day), are added to ACEI and amlodipine for refractory hypertension. Hydralazine acts quickly, resulting in a rapid decrease in pressure, and therefore may result in clinical signs of hypotension (e.g., tachycardia, ataxia, syncope, lethargy). Hydralazine should always be started at the low end of the dose and starting at half the recommended dose is useful in animals already receiving ACEI. Because the renin-angiotensin-aldosterone system is activated by hydralazine, ACEI, and possibly spironolactone to counteract aldosterone, should be given with hydralazine.
- **Phenoxybenzamine** (0.25 mg twice a day in dogs or 2.5 mg twice a day in cats), an alpha-receptor antagonist, lowers systemic arterial BP by lowering peripheral vascular resistance. It is indicated for those animals diagnosed with pheochromocytoma and is given with a beta blocker to block the effects of catecholamines on the cardiovascular system.

KEY POINT

ACEI are first line drugs for hypertensive dogs, and amlodipine is the antihypertensive of choice in cats (with the addition of benazepril to amlodipine if kidney disease is present).

Beta Blockers

- Beta blockers exert an antihypertensive effect by reducing cardiac output and decreasing renin release, but their efficacy in hypertensive veterinary patients is poor. In hyperthyroid, hypertensive cats, a cardioselective beta-1 antagonist, such as **atenolol**, may be given at a dosage of 6.25 mg twice a day (or approximately 1.0 mg/kg twice a day) for cats to block the cardiotoxic effects of thyroid hormone. The addition of amlodipine, however, may be needed to lower BP effectively. Beta blockers are not used routinely in hypertensive dogs unless pheochromocytoma is present.

Diuretics

- **Spironolactone**, an aldosterone-antagonist, is both a diuretic at higher doses (1 to 2 mg/kg PO twice a day), and neurohormone blocker at lower doses. It is a potassium-sparing diuretic, and limits the effects of excess aldosterone (hypokalemia, hypertension) associated with hyperaldosteronism. Aldosterone rebounds in the face of ACEI treatment; therefore, spironolactone may limit fibrosis and fluid retention associated with elevated aldosterone levels.
- Loop diuretics (**furosemide**, 2 to 4 mg/kg PO twice a day in dogs, and 1 to 2 mg/kg PO twice a day in cats) are rarely used in hypertensive animals. These agents lower extracellular fluid volume and cardiac output. The thiazide diuretics, which are commonly used as first line drugs in hypertensive people, may cause a profound decrease in serum potassium concentration.
- Adverse effects include dehydration, volume depletion, and worsening azotemia. Hypokalemia may occur with loop diuretics as well as with the thiazides, so plasma potassium and creatinine concentrations should be carefully monitored in all animals with chronic kidney disease that are receiving a diuretic.

EMERGENCY MANAGEMENT OF HYPERTENSION

Patient Selection

- Animals with neurologic signs or severe ocular manifestations of hypertension, such as retinal detachment, warrant aggressive treatment. **Sodium nitroprusside** (1.0 to 10.0 μg/kg/min constant-rate infusion), an arterial (predominantly) and venous vasodilator acting as a donor of nitric oxide inside vascular smooth muscle cells, can be used for the initial treatment of animals in hypertensive crisis. This drug must be given by constant-rate infusion, can be titrated very precisely according to the BP response, and usually does not cause reflex tachycardia. Amiodipine is an excellent choice, especially in cats.
- If a constant rate of infusion and intensive monitoring are not available in a veterinary hospital, then **hydralazine** and **furosemide** can be used in combination. The hydralazine dose can be repeated after 2 hours to titrate the effect.
- Regardless of initial therapy chosen for the management of an acute hypertensive crisis, a drug of choice for long-term management of systemic hypertension should be instituted soon after presentation to facilitate the eventual transition to long-term maintenance therapy.

FOLLOW-UP CARE AND ADDITIONAL MEDICATIONS

- In all animals treated for systemic hypertension, the routine examination should include a fundic examination, evaluation of any underlying diseases, and measurement of body weight, BP, and serum concentrations of creatinine and electrolytes. The owner should be questioned for evidence of drug toxicity, which may include lethargy, increased time spent sleeping, ataxia, or anorexia. Animals on multiple drug regimes are more likely to exhibit adverse effects than are those on a single antihypertensive agent.
- Once BP is controlled, the animal should be evaluated at 3-month intervals. A complete blood count, biochemical panel, and urinalysis should be evaluated at least once every 6 months.
- Many hypertensive animals have kidney disease. Other treatments for chronic kidney disease should accompany antihypertensive therapy, as appropriate. Potassium supplementation is often needed in cats with chronic kidney disease. Because animals with renal dysfunction generally have impaired ability to adapt to sudden changes in sodium input, the administration of electrolyte solutions can lead to volume overload, worsened systemic hypertension, and pleural effusion (or peripheral edema) in animals with renal azotemia. Similarly, a sudden reduction in dietary sodium intake in an animal with renal azotemia can lead to extracellular fluid volume depletion. Some treatments, such as the administration of recombinant erythropoietin to elevate hematocrit, may exacerbate systemic hypertension and should not be used until systemic hypertension is controlled.

Frequently Asked Questions

Because dogs are often more refractory to the effects of antihypertensive treatment than cats, what is a reasonable stepwise approach to antihypertensive therapy in dogs?

Hypertensive dogs (i.e., those with a sustained systolic BP > 160 mm Hg) are likely to be proteinuric given the underlying diseases associated with systemic hypertension in that species.

- ACE inhibitors (e.g., enalapril, benazepril, etc) have been shown to decrease proteinuria and cause balanced vasodilation, therefore they are usually the

Continued

starting drug in the treatment of canine hypertension. Enalapril (0.5 mg/kg) is given twice daily, and BP is measured after 2 weeks of treatment.

- If hypertension is still present, then amlodipine (0.1 mg/kg PO every 24 hours) can be administered with the enalapril. This combination of an ACE inhibitor and a calcium channel blocker may be effective; however, sustained hypertension warrants the addition of drugs that act by different mechanisms of action.
- Hydralazine, a direct-acting arterial vasodilator, can be given at a starting dose of 0.5 mg/kg PO twice a day, and slowly titrated up in 0.5 mg/kg increments to a maximum dose of 2.0 mg/kg. BP and serum creatinine should be monitored with each incremental increase in dose.
- Because hydralazine activates the renin-angiotensin-aldosterone axis, and aldosterone concentrations increase in spite of ACEI therapy, the addition of spironolactone (1 to 2 mg/kg PO twice a day) is advised to block the effects of aldosterone.
- If BP remains above 160 mm Hg, then amlodipine may be increased to 0.1 mg/kg twice a day (or 0.2 mg/kg once daily), or a beta blocker may be added in order to decrease heart rate and renin release.

Cats and dogs with chronic kidney disease often exhibit systemic hypertension. What is the causative factor in this relationship and how should these animals be managed? How can you tell if hypertension is damaging to the kidney?

This has often been referred to as a chicken-and-egg question but it is more properly seen as an example of a complex positive feedback loop that complicates therapy in animals affected with both problems. High systemic arterial BP produces baro trauma within the microvasculature of the kidney, effectively destroying renal tissue over time (weeks to months). On the other hand, chronic kidney disease produces abnormalities in body fluid volumes and can alter neurohumoral control of BP. These factors combine to make high BP relatively common in dogs and cats with chronic kidney disease. Furthermore, it is still generally accepted that something has to be wrong with the kidney for sustained systemic hypertension to be present.

- Interestingly, in the short-term, high BP tends to improve glomerular filtration rate. This is why the level of azotemia should always be assessed shortly (5 to 14 days) after any changes in antihypertensive therapy.
- Furthermore, vasodilators with intrarenal effects are often preferred for antihypertensive therapy in animals with kidney disease, largely because the vasodilatory effect may help to preserve renal function.
- Typical agents to select for initial therapy when both hypertension and renal azotemia are present in dogs would be an ACEI such as enalapril or benazepril (0.5 mg/kg once to twice daily) and in cats a calcium channel blocker such as amlodipine (0.1 mg/kg PO every 24 hours).
- Perhaps the best index of hypertensive damage of the kidney is proteinuria. The presence of microalbuminuria or an elevated urine protein-to-creatinine ratio (>0.5 in dogs, >0.4 in cats) is generally an indication for the use of an ACEI (e.g., enalapril or benazepril 0.5 mg/kg once daily in cats or once to twice daily in dogs).

SUGGESTED READINGS

Binns SH, Sisson DD, Buoscio DA, et al.: Doppler ultrasonographic, oscillometric sphygmomanometric, and photoplethysmographic techniques for noninvasive blood pressure measurement in anesthetized cats, J Vet Intern Med 9:405, 1995.

Bodey AR, Michell AR, Bovee KC, et al.: Comparison of direct and indirect (oscillometric) measurements of arterial blood pressure in conscious dogs, Res Vet Sci 61:17, 1996.

Brown CAJ, Munday J, Mathur S, et al: Hypertensive encephalopathy in cats with reduced renal function, Vet Pathol 42:642-649, 2005.

Brown S, Finco D, Navar L: Impaired renal autoregulatory ability in dogs with reduced renal mass, J Am Soc Nephrol 5:1768, 1995.

Brown S, Atkins C, Bagley R, et al.: Guidelines for the identification, evaluation, and management of systemic hypertension in dogs and cats: ACVIM Consensus Statement, J Vet Intern Med 21:542-558, 2007.

Brown SA, Brown CA: Single-nephron adaptations to partial renal ablation in cats, Am J Physiol 269:R1002, 1996.

Brown SA, Finco DR, Crowell WA, et al.: Single-nephron adaptations to partial renal ablation in the dog, Am J Physiol 258:F495, 1990.

Brown SA, Walton CL, Crawford P, et al.: Long-term effects of antihypertensive regimens on renal hemodynamics and proteinuria, Kidney Int 43:1210, 1993.

Cowgill LD: Systemic hypertension. In Kirk RW, ed: Current veterinary therapy IX, Philadelphia, 1986, WB Saunders.

Cowgill LD, Kallet AJ: Recognition and management of hypertension in the dog. In Kirk RW ed: Current veterinary therapy VIII, Philadelphia, 1983, WB Saunders.

Finco DR: Association of systemic hypertension with renal injury in dogs with induced renal failure, J Vet Intern Med 18:289, 2004.

Henik R, Snyder P, Volk L: Treatment of systemic hypertension in cats with amlodipine besylate, J Am Anim Hosp Assoc 33:226, 1997.

Jacob F, Polzin DJ, Osborne CA, et al.: Association between initial systolic blood pressure and risk of developing a uremic crisis or of dying in dogs with chronic renal failure, J Am Vet Med Assoc 222:322, 2003.

Jensen J, Henik RA, Brownfield M, et al: Plasma renin activity, angiotensin I and aldosterone in feline hypertension associated with chronic renal disease, Am J Vet Res 58:535, 1997.

Kallet A, Cowgill L, Kass P: Comparison of blood pressure measurements in dogs by use of indirect oscillometry in a veterinary clinic versus at home, J Am Vet Med Assoc 210:651, 1997.

Labato MA, Ross LA: Diagnosis and management of hypertension. In August JR, ed: Consultations in feline internal medicine, Philadelphia, 1991, WB Saunders.

Littman MP: Spontaneous systemic hypertension in 24 cats, J Vet Intern Med, 8:79, 1994.

Littman MP, Robertson JL, Bovee KC: Spontaneous systemic hypertension in dogs: five cases (1981-1983), J Am Vet Med Assoc 193:486, 1988.

Ortega TM, Feldman EC, Nelson RW, et al.: Systemic arterial blood pressure and urine protein/creatinine ratio in dogs with hyperadrenocorticism, J Am Vet Med Assoc 209:1724, 1996.

Remillard RL, Ross JN, Eddy JB: Variance of indirect blood pressure measurements and prevalence of hypertension in clinically normal dogs, Am J Vet Res 52:561, 1991.

Ross LA: Hypertension and chronic renal failure, Semin Vet Med Surg Small Anim 7:221, 1992.

Snyder PS, Henik RA: Feline systemic hypertension. Proc Twelfth Annual Vet Med Forum. San Francisco, 1994, p. 126.

Stiles J, Polzin DJ, Bistner SI: The prevalence of retinopathy in cats with systemic hypertension and chronic renal failure or hyperthyroidism, J Am Anim Hosp Assoc 30:564, 1994.

SECTION III

Treatment of Cardiovascular Disease

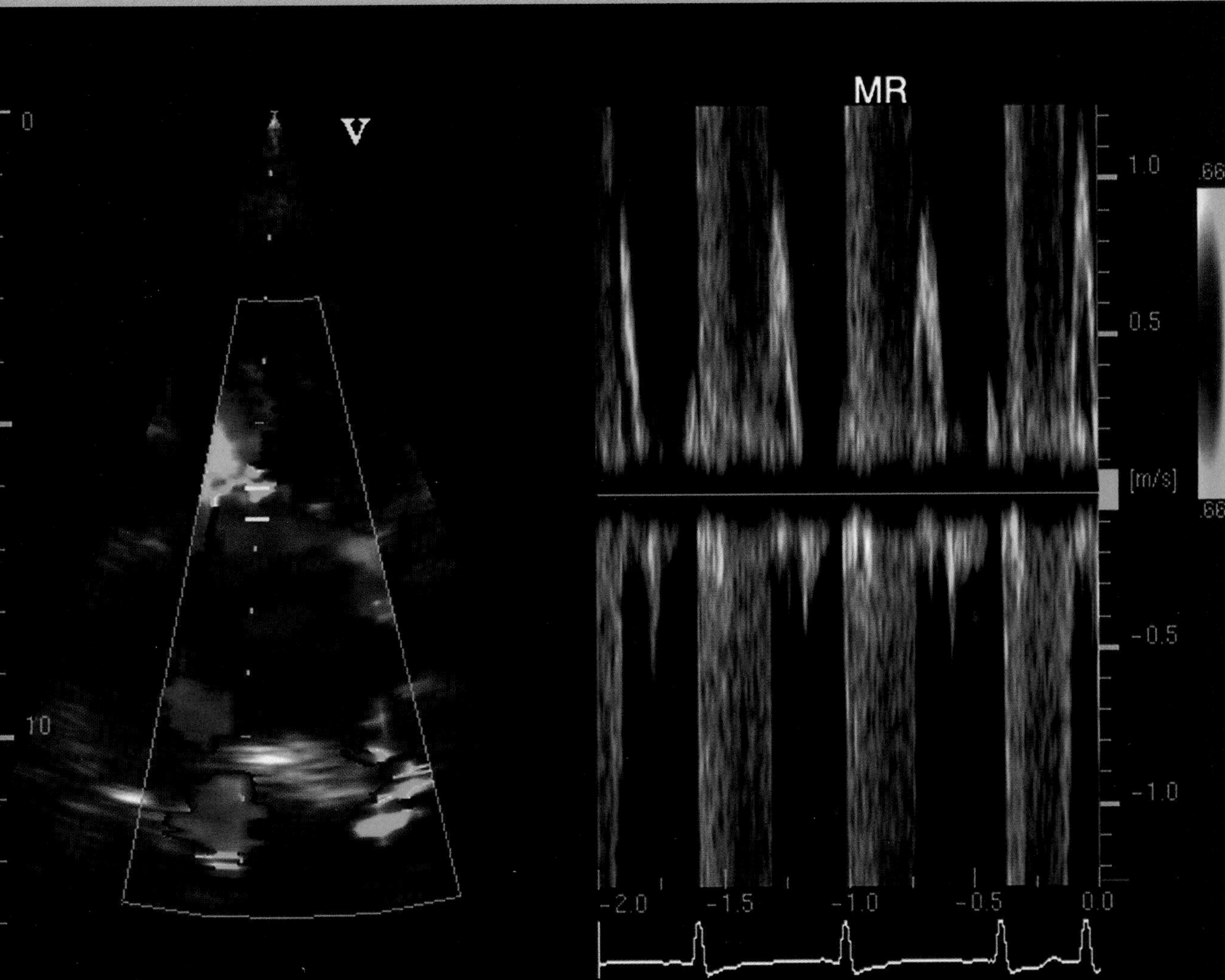

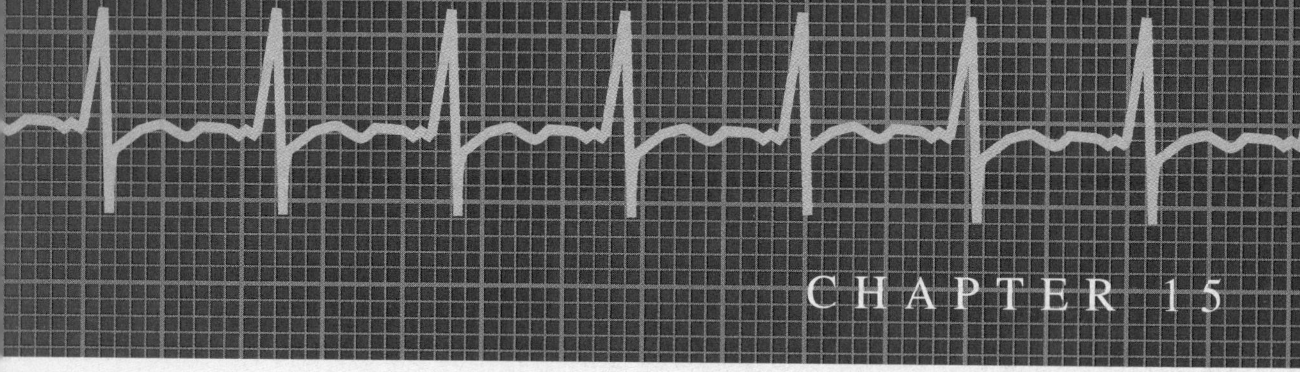

Pathophysiology and Therapy of Heart Failure

Keith N. Strickland

INTRODUCTION

Definitions

- Heart disease is any structural (microscopic or macroscopic) abnormality of the heart that may or may not result in heart failure.
- Heart failure is the pathophysiologic state that occurs when the heart is unable to function at a level commensurate with the requirements of the metabolizing tissues or can only do so at elevated filling pressures.
- Preload is the degree of muscle fiber stretch just prior to contraction. This correlates to the volume of blood within the ventricle just prior to contraction (cardiac preload, venous return)
- Afterload is the load against which a muscle exerts its contractile force. Cardiac afterload refers to the blood pressure the ventricle must overcome in order to eject blood.

Overview

- The function of the cardiovascular system is to maintain normal arterial blood pressure and flow (cardiac output) while maintaining normal venous and capillary pressures during rest and exercise. This function is necessary to provide adequate blood flow for oxygen and nutrient delivery to vital tissues (such as the brain, the heart, and the kidneys) as well as for the removal of metabolic waste products from these tissues.
- Heart failure results in a reduction in the previously described functions of the cardiovascular system. If blood pressure and cardiac output are not maintained, or if venous and capillary pressures are markedly increased, then death can occur within hours to weeks (depending on the severity of the abnormality). Heart failure can be associated with systolic or diastolic dysfunction.

HEART FAILURE

Pathophysiology

Our understanding of the progression from asymptomatic heart disease to symptomatic heart failure has changed from the traditional concept of biomechanical dysfunction to a concept emphasizing neuroendocrine dysfunction secondary to chronic biomechanical dysfunction.

- The current model embodies the idea that some cardiac damage or dysfunction results in chronically altered hemodynamics that lead to activation of neurohumoral mechanisms designed to promote cardiac function and tissue perfusion. Chronic activation of these compensatory mechanisms leads to progressive cardiovascular dysfunction culminating in life-threatening congestive heart failure (CHF) low-output failure or sudden death.
- Cardiac dysfunction that leads to the clinical syndrome of heart failure can be subdivided into systolic and diastolic dysfunction. Systolic

dysfunction occurs when the ability of the heart to pump blood in a forward direction is impaired. Components of systolic function include myocardial contractility, valvular competence, preload, afterload, and heart rate.

Phases of Heart Failure

- Phase 1: Cardiac Injury
- Phase 2: Compensatory mechanisms
- Phase 3: Cardiac failure with clinical signs of cardiac dysfunction

KEY POINTS

- CHF occurs when cardiac diastolic filling pressures result in elevated venous and capillary hydrostatic pressures with subsequent edema formation. Therapy for CHF is directed toward reducing cardiac diastolic filling pressures so that edema fluid can be mobilized.
- Low-output failure occurs when cardiac function does not produce adequate cardiac output to maintain blood pressure and tissue perfusion.

Myocardial Failure

- Impaired contractility may occur with primary heart disease (idiopathic dilated cardiomyopathy [DCM]) or secondary heart disease.
  - Chronic heart disease of varying causes may mimic primary cardiomyopathy. Systolic failure following chronic overload may be secondary to chronic valvular insufficiency and left-to-right shunting lesions, such as patent ductus arteriosus or ventricular septal defect.
  - Nutritional deficiencies, such as taurine deficiency, have been recognized as a cause of myocardial failure in the cat, and have been associated with DCM in certain breeds of dogs (American Cocker Spaniels, Golden Retrievers, Dalmatians, Boxers, Welsh Corgis, Newfoundlands). Myocardial deficiency of L-carnitine has been reported in Boxers and Doberman Pinschers.
  - Metabolic cardiomyopathies include feline hyperthyroidism, canine hypothyroidism, and chronic uremia.
  - Toxic cardiomyopathy: doxorubicin-induced DCM
  - Infiltrative cardiomyopathy: neoplastic (e.g., lymphosarcoma), amyloidosis

Valvular Insufficiency

- Valvular insufficiency is one of the most common causes of systolic dysfunction encountered in veterinary medicine. Incompetency of an atrioventricular valve (endocardiosis, endocarditis, congenital malformation) allows retrograde ejection (regurgitation) of blood into the corresponding atrium during systole, reducing forward flow and decreasing cardiac output. Severe regurgitation also increases atrial and ventricular filling pressures, with the risk of CHF.
- Valvular insufficiency can be primary (myxomatous degeneration) or secondary (associated with other conditions that alter valvular function such as ventricular hypertrophy, ischemia, etc.).

Excessive Afterload

- Normally, an abrupt increase in afterload causes a positive inotropic effect (Anrep effect). However, when the hemodynamic overload is severe or chronic, myocardial contractility may be depressed. Chronically increased afterload leads to a reduction in the rate of ejection and the amount of blood ejected at any given preload, and increased myocardial oxygen consumption with the risk of ischemic damage.
- Pulmonary/systemic hypertension or ventricular outflow obstructions (aortic or pulmonic stenosis) are examples of clinically significant causes of increased afterload.

Inadequate Preload

- In cases in which inadequate preload is the primary hemodynamic abnormality (such as cardiac tamponade), the reduction in preload decreases stroke volume and cardiac output. Normally, the reduced preload may be compensated for by systemic mechanisms that result in increased venous return and ventricular end-diastolic volume; however, significant pericardial effusion obstructs venous inflow and limits the end-diastolic volume, precluding the circulatory system from fully compensating for the reduced cardiac output.

Diastolic Dysfunction

- Diastolic dysfunction may result in heart failure. Indeed, most cases of overt heart failure have some degree of diastolic dysfunction. Adequate

ventricular filling is dependent on several factors:
- Ventricular relaxation
- Ventricular elasticity (change in muscle length for a change in force)
- Ventricular compliance (change in ventricular volume for a given change in pressure).

- Ventricular relaxation may be decreased in several diseases or disorders (e.g., idiopathic hypertrophic cardiomyopathy, ischemia).
- Ventricular compliance may be reduced when elevated filling pressure are required. This change can be associated with:
  - Volume overloading
  - An increase in muscle mass or wall thickness, as with myocardial concentric hypertrophy
  - A decrease in ventricular distensibility (usually associated with extrinsic compression of the heart)
  - Diseases that result in myocardial fibrosis (e.g., restrictive cardiomyopathy, ischemic heart disease) also cause a decrease in ventricular compliance.
- Diastolic dysfunction may increase ventricular end-diastolic pressure, which is then transmitted to the corresponding atrium and the venous system. Elevation in venous and capillary pressures may result in interstitial and alveolar pulmonary edema or ascites through hydrostatic factors.

COMPENSATORY MECHANISMS IN CHRONIC HEART FAILURE

Frank-Starling Mechanism

- The Frank-Starling mechanism is an adaptive mechanism by which an increase in preload enhances cardiac performance. Venous return determines the preload of the ventricle. Physiologic increases in ventricular end-diastolic volume are associated with increases in myocardial fiber length. This allows the sarcomere to function near the upper limit of its maximal length (optimal length), where it is able to generate the maximal amount of force during contraction.
- To better understand the role of the Frank-Starling mechanism, consider the hemodynamic changes associated with exercise. Cardiac output is increased during exercise through the following mechanisms: (1) increased heart rate and contractility through increased sympathetic nervous system (SNS) activity, (2) increased venous return (preload) with a more vigorous contraction (Frank-Starling mechanism), and (3) reduced afterload associated with reduced peripheral vascular resistance. In this way cardiac performance is enhanced during exercise in the absence of heart failure. In the presence of heart failure, cardiac output and ventricular performance may be maintained within normal limits at rest only because the ventricular end-diastolic fiber length and the preload are elevated (ventricular performance is maintained through the Frank-Starling mechanism).
- In the failing heart, these factors that normally help increase cardiac output during exercise are chronically active and cause increased preload and ventricular end-diastolic pressures (especially in a noncompliant, dilated ventricle), with the threat of edema formation. Exercise drives the ventricle along the flat portion of the ventricular performance curve, where increases in ventricular volume and diastolic pressure do not increase ventricular performance.

Renin-Angiotension-Aldosterone System

- The renin-angiotensin-aldosterone system (RAAS) is a complex neurohormonal compensatory system that functions to maintain relatively normal blood pressure and tissue perfusion when cardiac output is reduced. Reduced renal perfusion detected by renal baroreceptors results in release of renin (Figure 15-1). Other factors causing release of renin include decreased sodium delivery to the macula densa, and SNS stimulation of beta-1 adrenoceptors in the juxtaglomerular apparatus of the kidney. Renin initiates a cascade resulting in the formation of angiotensin II, a potent vasoconstrictor. Angiotensin II also causes activation of the SNS, increases synthesis and release of aldosterone from the zona glomerulosa of the adrenal cortex and release of antidiuretic hormone.
- Aldosterone causes sodium retention in the distal renal tubules to promote fluid retention. Aldosterone also promotes fibrosis of the myocardium and vascular smooth muscle.
- The RAAS can be subdivided into:
  - Systemic or renal RAAS
  - Tissue RAAS
- The tissue RAAS (brain, vascular, and myocardial tissues) can generate angiotensin II independently of the circulating RAAS.
- Angiotensin II stimulates the release of growth factors that promote remodeling of the vessels

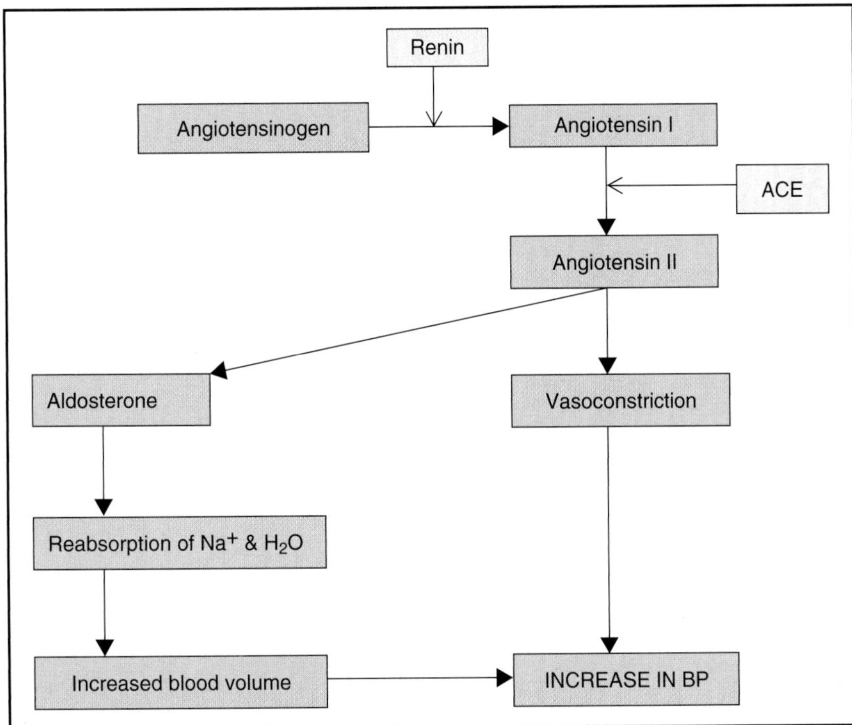

Figure 15-1. RAA cascade. Reduced renal perfusion is the primary stimulus for renin release, which leads to activation of the angiotensin-aldosterone system. RAAS activation results in sodium and water retention and peripheral vasoconstriction.

and myocardium. Vascular remodeling (smooth muscle cell growth and hyperplasia, hypertrophy, and apoptosis; cytokine activation; myocyte and vascular wall fibrosis) results in decreased vascular responsiveness to alterations in blood flow, decreased vascular compliance, and increased afterload. Angiotensin II also causes pathologic ventricular hypertrophy, exerts cytotoxic effects resulting in myocardial necrosis and loss of myocardial contractile mass with resultant cardiac dysfunction.

Sympathetic Nervous System Activation

Sympathetic Nervous System Activation

- The autonomic nervous system plays a crucial role in the compensation of heart failure. The activity of the SNS is increased in part by baroreflex-mediated parasympathetic withdrawal, as well as by activation by the RAAS. Early activation of the SNS helps to maintain cardiac output, blood pressure, and tissue perfusion by increasing venous return to the heart (vasoconstriction of the splanchnic vessels), vasoconstriction of other various vascular beds, and positive inotropic and chronotropic cardiac effects. Activation of the SNS early in heart failure is beneficial, but becomes maladaptive when chronically activated (Figure 15-2).

Sympathetic Desensitization:

- Chronic activation of the SNS is associated with elevated levels of plasma norepinephrine (NE), cardiac NE depletion, down-regulation and desensitization of beta-1 adrenergic receptors, and abnormal baroreflex function. Plasma NE levels appear to be increased because of a combination of increased release of NE from adrenergic nerve endings and reduced uptake of NE by adrenergic nerve endings. The depletion of myocardial NE (serum NE levels increase and myocardial levels decrease) probably represents the depletion of the neurotransmitter in adrenergic nerve endings.
    - The down-regulation of beta-1 adrenergic receptors occurs relatively soon (24 to 72 hours) after the initial SNS activation, making it progressively more difficult for the SNS to counter impaired contractility.
- **Chronic activation of the SNS** also overloads the heart by increasing venous return (to a heart that is already volume-overloaded), by increasing myocardial oxygen consumption (by increasing heart rate and volume overloading of the heart)

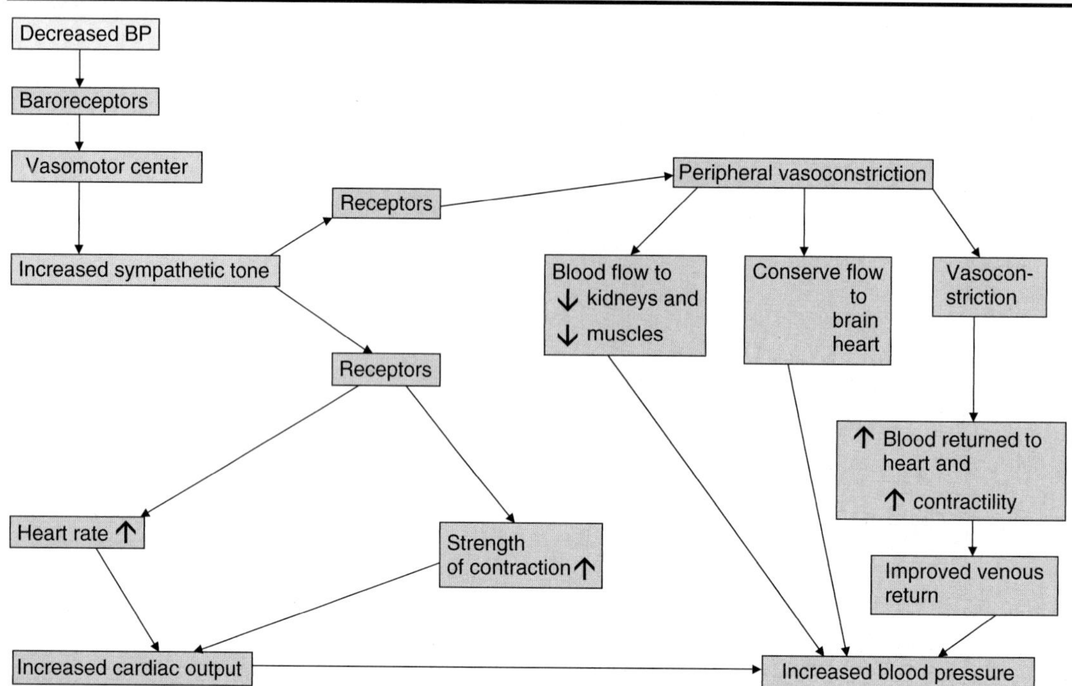

Figure 15-2. Effect of compensatory sympathetic system in response to a reduction in blood pressure. Decreased systemic blood pressure results in activation of the sympathetic nervous system and a cascade of consequences which are deleterious in the long term.

and by damaging the myocardium, creating a substrate for arrhythmogenesis.

Myocardial Hypertrophy

Myocardial hypertrophy occurs as a compensatory mechanism directed toward normalizing cardiac output, wall tension, and filling pressures. The hemodynamic load imposed on the heart (either volume or pressure overloading) determines the type of hypertrophy (eccentric vs. concentric). Chronic activation of the RAAS and the SNS produces pathologic changes (remodeling) within the ventricular myocardium, which contribute to cardiac dysfunction. The result can be myocardial failure with low-output signs or elevated filling pressures with the risk of CHF.

- Eccentric myocardial hypertrophy (or volume-overload hypertrophy) occurs with heart disease as a compensatory mechanism to allow the ventricle to pump a relatively normal amount of blood in spite of abnormal systolic function. Eccentric hypertrophy is characterized by chamber dilation, a response to the increase in blood volume and venous return associated with activation of the RAAS and SNS. More specifically, the increased venous return is secondary to sodium (aldosterone effect) and water (antidiuretic hormone/vasopressin effect) retention as well as to venoconstriction of the splanchnic vascular bed (RAAS and SNS effect). Chronic heart failure represents a nonosmotic (mediated by SNS and RAAS, instead of osmotic hypertonic) stimulus for antidiuretic hormone release from the hypothalamus. Antidiuretic hormone probably plays a limited role in the pathogenesis of CHF. However, chronic volume overload causes an increase in diastolic wall stress, and this leads to replication of sarcomeres in series, elongation of myocytes, and ventricular dilation.
- Concentric myocardial hypertrophy (or pressure-overload hypertrophy) is characterized by thickening of the ventricular walls in response to increased systolic wall stress, and occurs as a compensatory mechanism to normalize systolic wall tension. Increased systolic wall stress stimulates the replication of sarcomeres in parallel, increasing myocardium thickness and thereby normalizing systolic wall stress (via the La Place relationship, wall tension = pressure × radius/wall thickness). The increase in thickness of the ventricular wall compensates for the increased systolic wall stress in a pressure-overloaded ventricle. If the compensatory concentric hypertrophy is inadequate and the systolic wall stress is increased, then afterload-mismatch

and decompensation occur. Interestingly, when significant eccentric hypertrophy occurs in a volume-overloaded ventricle, systolic wall tension is increased secondary to the increase in ventricular diameter. Therefore, both eccentric and some degree of concentric hypertrophy are present in severely volume-overloaded ventricles.

KEY POINTS

In the syndrome of heart failure, changes in ventricular mass and geometry are a culmination of compensatory hypertrophy (in response to pressure or volume overload) and pathologic hypertrophy (in response to activation of the RAAS and SNS).

- These compensatory mechanisms require days to weeks to become fully activated. If the cardiac dysfunction is acute and severe, then the compensatory mechanisms do not have sufficient time to become fully activated (with the exception of the SNS, which is immediately activated).
  - For example, most dogs with idiopathic DCM have insidious, progressive cardiac dysfunction that worsens over a period of years, therefore allowing the compensatory mechanisms to become fully activated. Although these dogs have compensated heart failure chronically, at some point they may acutely decompensate, mimicking an acute disease process.
  - Conversely, a dog with a peracute disease syndrome (such as a very rapid supraventricular tachyarrhythmia like atrial fibrillation) may develop heart failure without activating compensatory mechanisms other than the SNS.

Additional Compensatory Mechanisms/ Neuroendocrine Mechanisms

- Endothelins, a vasoactive family of peptides that are released from endothelial cells, play an important role in the regulation of vascular tone and blood pressure. Endothelin-1 is a strong, vasoconstrictive agent with inotropic and mitogenic actions; it is a strong stimulus for activation of the RAAS and SNS. Additionally, Endothelin-1 may play an important role in the pathogenesis of pulmonary hypertension.
- Natriuretic peptides are regulators of salt and water homeostasis and blood pressure control with potential value as diagnostic and prognostic markers in patients with CHF. Natriuretic peptide levels are elevated in many disease conditions resulting in expanded fluid volume (such as DCM and chronic valvular insufficiency in dogs, and cardiomyopathy in cats).
- Atrial, brain, and C-type natriuretic peptides have been identified (ANP, BNP, and CNP, respectively)
- BNP is primarily produced in the atria and is released in response to atrial stretch resulting in natriuresis, diuresis, and balanced vasodilation.
- Natriuretic peptides antagonize the RAAS and SNS, inhibit release of antidiuretic hormone, prevent myocardial fibrosis, and modulate cell growth and myocardial hypertrophy.
- Circulating natriuretic peptide levels may be used to differentiate between symptoms associated with cardiac disease and from symptoms associated with primary pulmonary disease. Lack of elevated BNP levels does not support a diagnosis of symptomatic heart failure.
- Inflammatory and immune mediators such as tumor necrosis factor alpha, interleukins (IL-1, IL-2, and IL-6), nuclear factor-kappa-B, and reactive oxygen species are thought to play a role in the progression of heart failure. The "cytokine hypothesis" suggests that heart failure progresses because cytokine pathways are activated in response to cardiac dysfunction and exert negative effects on the cardiovascular system.

Course of Events: Compensatory Mechanisms

- Reduced cardiac output leads to decreased tissue perfusion
- Activation of baroreceptors in kidney, carotid arteries, aorta, and heart results in SNS activation and parasympathetic nervous system withdrawal
- SNS activation (positive inotropic and chronotropic activity, vasoconstriction to increase venous return and maintain blood pressure, stimulation of antidiuretic hormone and renin)
- RAAS activation associated with the reduced renal perfusion, decreased sodium delivery to the macula densa, and SNS activation
- Renal sodium and water retention to increase blood volume and, therefore, venous return to the heart
- Myocardial hypertrophy (dilation of the affected atrium and ventricle) to maintain relatively normal cardiac output and systolic wall tension while preventing diastolic filling pressures from rising
- Stretch-induced release of atrial natriuretic factor serves to facilitate sodium excretion. The effects of this factor are quickly negated owing to

degradation by neutral endopeptidases and the effects of overstimulation of the RAAS and SNS.
- Initially, these mechanisms allow the body to compensate for the decreased cardiac output by increasing blood volume and blood pressure. However, with chronicity, the compensatory mechanisms are maladaptive and facilitate progression of heart failure.
- Overstimulation of inflammatory/immune mediators (tumor necrosis factor–alpha, IL-1, IL-2, IL-6, reactive oxygen species) exert deleterious effects on the heart and circulation.
- The sustained effects of the SNS and RAAS continue to increase the workload of the heart by increasing blood volume and venous return to a heart that has maximized its ability to compensate by eccentric hypertrophy. Ventricular filling pressures begin to increase, with the threat of edema formation. The onset of edema formation is variable, depending on the severity and onset of ventricular dysfunction. Dogs with cardiomyopathy may have mild edema for days to weeks and only show minimal clinical signs, such as tachypnea and exercise intolerance.

TYPES OF HEART FAILURE

Myocardial Failure

- Myocardial failure is associated with decreases in contractility. It can be associated with:
  - Primary myocardial disease (idiopathic DCM)
  - Secondary myocardial diseases (chronic congenital and valvular heart disease, thyrotoxicosis, taurine deficiency, infectious/inflammatory and infiltrative diseases)
  - Myocardial failure causes systolic dysfunction and activation of compensatory mechanisms which increase sodium and water retention to increase venous return to the heart. The ventricles must obtain a larger end-diastolic dimension to maintain a relatively normal total stroke volume (TSV). As the myocardial function deteriorates (as noted by a decrease in fractional shortening and a decrease in ejection fraction), the ventricles progressively enlarge so that the TSV is maintained, even though the percentage of blood being ejected is decreasing. Severe left ventricular dilation causes distortion and dilation of the mitral valve annulus, resulting in mitral regurgitation (MR) and further volume overloading of the left ventricle.
  - Once the compensatory limits are reached, further increases in blood volume (associated with sodium and water retention) and venous return cause an increase in cardiac filling pressures, with threat of CHF development.

Volume Overload

- Volume overload is associated with two common causes of heart failure:
  - Valvular insufficiency
  - Shunts

Atrioventricular Valvular Insufficiency

- Atrioventricular valvular insufficiency can result from:
  - Degenerative valvular disease
  - Valvular endocarditis
  - Congenital valvular dysplasia
  - Chamber dilation
  - Valvular insufficiency may result in systolic dysfunction and activation of compensatory mechanisms which maintain cardiac output and tissue perfusion by vasoconstriction and fluid retention. As with impaired contractility, valvular insufficiency forces the ventricle to achieve larger end-diastolic dimensions to compensate for the decrease in forward stroke volume. The difference between volume overloading secondary to impaired contractility (DCM) and valvular insufficiency (MR) is associated with the changes in TSV (end-diastolic volume minus end-systolic volume). In MR without myocardial failure, TSV is increased to compensate for the amount of blood leaking through the incompetent valve. The end-diastolic volume increases, but the end-systolic volume remains normal (evidence of normal contractility), thereby resulting in an increased TSV. With impaired contractility, TSV is normal or decreased (depending on the stage of the disease) because both end-diastolic and end-systolic volumes have increased. End-diastolic volumes increase to compensate for the increased end-systolic volumes, reflecting impaired contractility.
- Shunts such as patent ductus arteriosus, ventricular septal defect, and arteriovenous fistula are similar to valvular leaks in that the heart increases TSV to compensate for the reduction in forward flow.

Pressure Overload

- Lesions that cause increased intraventricular systolic pressures usually do not cause CHF because the heart is usually able to compensate for the increased intraventricular systolic pressures with concentric hypertrophy (La Place principle), and the ventricular systolic function remains relatively normal. Only when the obstruction to flow is severe (critical stenosis) or acute does pressure overload result in myocardial failure and heart failure. More commonly, CHF occurs when there is a concurrent valvular insufficiency (e.g., pulmonic stenosis with tricuspid regurgitation, subvalvular aortic stenosis with MR or aortic regurgitation, pulmonary hypertension with tricuspid regurgitation).
- Alternatively, sudden death may occur in dogs with severe (noncritical) congenital subvalvular aortic stenosis or possibly valvular pulmonic stenosis. When the ventricle is severely hypertrophied, coronary perfusion is impaired, and regions of the myocardium (especially the papillary muscles and subendocardial regions) are at risk of hypoxia. Myocardial hypoxia can result in impaired contractility as well as ventricular tachyarrhythmias which may degenerate into ventricular fibrillation, leading to sudden cardiac death.

Decreased Ventricular Compliance or Abnormal Ventricular Relaxation

- In idiopathic hypertrophic cardiomyopathy, the increase in ventricular or septal wall thickness is associated with decreased ventricular compliance (increased ventricular stiffness). Myocardial or endocardial fibrosis (restrictive cardiomyopathy) can also increase ventricular stiffness.
- Decreased ventricular compliance and abnormal ventricular relaxation may result in elevated diastolic intraventricular pressures (filling pressures), even though the ventricular diastolic volume is not increased. During the course of diastole, for any increase in preload, there is an abnormal increase in intraventricular pressure. Over time, the corresponding atrium dilates to compensate for the elevated filling pressure. Once compensatory dilation of the atrium has reached its limit, further elevation of the ventricular filling pressure results in the development of edema (or pleural effusion in cats).
- Pericardial disease with cardiac tamponade is the clinical syndrome in which there is compression of the heart by fluid within the pericardial space (pericardial effusion), resulting in signs of right-heart failure and low-output failure. Elevation of intracardiac pressure, progressive limitation of ventricular diastolic filling, and reduction of stroke volume and cardiac output characterize cardiac tamponade. The clinical course depends on the size and rate of accumulation of the effusion, and the compliance of the pericardial sac.
  - **Acute tamponade** is usually associated with an acute hemorrhage from a neoplastic lesion, such as hemangiosarcoma, but may also be associated with rupture of the left atrium secondary to chronic severe MR. As the effusion accumulates, intrapericardial pressures increase and eventually exceed the diastolic pressures in the right atrium and ventricle, thereby restricting the venous inflow to the right heart. The restriction of venous return causes a reduction in right ventricular cardiac output, pulmonary blood flow, and left-sided venous return that is associated with a reduction in left ventricular stroke volume and cardiac output, and signs of low-output heart failure.
  - **Chronic tamponade** associated with the slow accumulation of pericardial effusion differs from acute tamponade in that the body has time to compensate for the impediment of cardiac inflow, secondary reduction in stroke volume, and cardiac output. Although compensation may somewhat normalize cardiac output, signs of right-sided CHF are often present (jugular distention and ascites).

CLINICAL DESCRIPTIONS OF HEART FAILURE

- CHF is the accumulation of fluid in tissues associated with increased capillary hydrostatic pressures and elevated diastolic intra-atrial and intraventricular pressures. Diseases that cause diastolic or systolic dysfunction are capable of increasing cardiac filling pressures, leading to CHF.
- Low-output failure can be defined as poor cardiac output, resulting in reduced tissue perfusion and inadequate tissue oxygenation. Generally, the term low-output failure is used to describe clinical scenarios in which cardiac output is dramatically reduced by end-stage, primary, systolic dysfunction.
- Right-sided heart failure may result when the right atrium or right ventricle develops elevated filling pressures associated with valvular insufficiency, pericardial disease, outflow tract

obstruction, or pulmonary hypertension. Volume and pressure overloading of the right ventricle can cause hepatic congestion accompanied by ascites, pleural effusion, and, rarely, peripheral subcutaneous edema. These diseases may also reduce the forward flow of blood into the pulmonary circulation and the left heart, resulting in reduced stroke volume, cardiac output and, possibly, signs of low-output heart failure.

- Left-sided heart failure may result when the left side of the heart develops elevated filling pressures associated most commonly with valvular insufficiency, impaired contractility, or diastolic dysfunction. Elevated left ventricular filling pressures are transmitted to the left atrium and pulmonary venous and capillary beds, with the threat of fluid accumulation in the interstitial and alveolar spaces (pulmonary edema). In dogs, pleural effusion may develop when biventricular or right ventricular failure is present. Cats may develop pleural effusion with pure left-sided heart failure apparently because the visceral pleural lymphatics drain into the pulmonary venous circulation. Pulmonary venous hypertension creates a functional obstruction, thereby restricting the ability of the lymphatics to maintain a normal amount of fluid in the pleural space.

DIAGNOSIS OF HEART FAILURE

KEY POINTS

- The diagnosis of CHF is considered to be a multimodal diagnosis, based on a careful history, physical examination, and ancillary diagnostics including electrocardiography, thoracic radiography, and echocardiography.
- Good quality thoracic radiographs should always be obtained.
- Exclude diseases that mimic CHF (e.g., chronic broncho-interstitial disease is often present in patients with cardiac disease).

History

- A complete medical history is important to establish the clinical course of the presenting complaint, as well as the presence of concurrent diseases that may complicate heart disease.
- Coughing, tachypnea, dyspnea (respiratory distress), exercise intolerance, lethargy, and weakness are common complaints of clients with pets with symptomatic heart disease or heart failure. Additionally, pets with heart failure may have a history of inappetence, weight loss, and syncope.
- Coughing is a very common historical finding in dogs with heart failure, especially those with chronic MR. In this scenario, a cough reflex is associated with left atrial compression of the left mainstem bronchus. Alternatively, dogs with severe alveolar pulmonary edema may also cough. It is important to be cognizant that other, noncardiac diseases may also cause coughing, and that coughing is not specific for heart failure. Diseases such as tracheal collapse and chronic pulmonary disease also cause coughing and may occur concurrently with heart disease.
- Tachypnea (increased respiratory rate) is a common sign of heart failure. Tachypnea can be caused by many nonpathologic mechanisms and is often overlooked by the client and the clinician. Left-sided CHF with interstitial pulmonary edema causes stimulation of receptors within the pulmonary interstitium that reflexively increase the respiratory rate. The increase in respiratory rate can occur with or without the presence of hypoxia. Because of this concept, the resting respiratory rate may be used effectively to monitor the status of patients with left-sided CHF. The normal resting respiratory rate for most small animals is usually below 30 to 35 breaths per minute. Typically, trends of increasing resting respiratory rate indicate progressive decompensation of left-sided heart failure and the need for cardiac medication adjustments (i.e., an increase in furosemide dosage or frequency of administration).
- Dyspnea (perception of difficult breathing) usually accompanies severe heart failure that has resulted in pulmonary edema or pleural effusion. Dyspnea is exacerbated by exercise in patients capable of exercising.
- Orthopnea (difficult breathing during recumbency) may occur before dyspnea. Often, the client may recognize orthopnea because the patient is reluctant to lie down or because the patient has difficulty breathing when it is lying down.
- Nocturnal coughing or dyspnea typically occurs after the patient has been recumbent for some time. It is not specific for left-sided CHF.

- Exercise intolerance may be a very early sign of heart failure in animals that are active; however, it may be difficult to identify in animals that are inactive. Reduced tolerance for exercise results because cardiac function is abnormal, and the metabolic demands of tissues (especially the working muscles) are not met, leading to hypoxia, lactic acidemia, muscle weakness, and fatigue.
- Abdominal distention secondary to ascites may be associated with right-sided or biventricular failure and must be differentiated from effusions associated with other conditions, such as hypoproteinemia, liver disease, and abdominal neoplasia. Evaluation of the jugular and abdominal subcutaneous veins may aid in determining that ascites is associated with right-sided CHF. With right-sided heart failure, these vessels are often distended and engorged.

Cardiovascular Physical Examination Findings

Murmur

- A cardiovascular murmur is a series of auditory vibrations associated with turbulent (nonlaminar) blood flow and, occasionally, with vibrating valve leaflets. When blood flow velocities are supraphysiologic (i.e., higher than normal physiologic velocities), or when blood viscosity is reduced (e.g., with anemia), blood flow tends to be nonlaminar and turbulent. Nonlaminar blood flow generates acoustic energy that vibrates the structures within the heart or the associated vessel(s). The intensity (loudness), timing in the cardiac cycle, frequency (pitch), configuration (shape), quality, duration, location, and direction of radiation of the sound created by the blood flow are important characteristics of cardiac murmurs.
  - The intensity of the murmur refers to the loudness of the murmur and is graded on a scale from 1 to 6 (1 being the least audible murmur, and 6 being the loudest).
  - The timing is defined as being systolic, diastolic, or continuous.
  - The configuration of the murmur refers to the shape of the sound created by the abnormal blood flow, and is described as being either a plateau (regurgitant murmur) or a crescendo-decrescendo (ejection murmur) sound.
  - A cardiac murmur is present in many dogs with heart failure, but the presence of a cardiac murmur is not specific for heart failure.

Cardiac Rhythm Disturbances

- Arrhythmias are relatively common in animals with heart failure.
  - Atrial fibrillation is a common supraventricular arrhythmia present in some dogs with DCM and chronic MR secondary to primary valve disease, as well as in cats with cardiomyopathy.
  - Ventricular tachyarrhythmias may be present in dogs with heart failure or with extracardiac disease, such as thoracic trauma, splenic disease, and gastric dilatation-volvulus. Ventricular arrhythmias are especially common in Boxers and Doberman Pinschers with cardiomyopathy.
  - Bradyarrhythmias such as third-degree (complete) atrioventricular block may cause signs of reduced cardiac output (lethargy, weakness, and exercise intolerance) and, occasionally, CHF.
  - Gallop sounds are abnormal heart sounds in dogs and cats that are often associated with heart failure. A third heart sound (S_3) gallop occurs just after the second heart sound (S_2) during the rapid diastolic phase of ventricular filling. An S_3 gallop occurs commonly in dogs with heart failure associated with volume overload, particularly dogs with DCM. During early diastolic filling, blood rushes out of the atrium into a noncompliant ventricle, which then vibrates, resulting in a low-frequency sound just after S_2. A fourth heart sound (S_4) gallop occurs just before the first heart sound (S_1) and is associated with atrial contraction. Ventricular filling in late diastole associated with atrial contraction vibrates the noncompliant ventricle, creating a low-frequency sound just before S_1 and the onset of systole. S_4 gallop are commonly auscultated in cats with hypertrophic or restrictive cardiomyopathy. Summation gallops (S_3 and S_4) may occur during periods of tachycardia.

Diagnostics

Electrocardiography

- Electrocardiography is used to detect cardiac rhythm disturbances, chamber enlargement, or conduction abnormalities that may be associated with cardiac disease. Electrocardiographic abnormalities are not specific for heart failure and therefore should not be used to determine the presence of heart failure. Furthermore, a normal electrocardiogram does not rule out the possibility of severe heart disease with secondary chamber enlargement.

Thoracic Radiography

- Thoracic radiography is important in the evaluation of patients with suspected heart disease or CHF. In general, with respect to heart disease and heart failure, three questions should be answered when evaluating a thoracic radiograph:
  - Is cardiomegaly present? If so, which side of the heart is affected?
  - What is the pulmonary vascular pattern (e.g., normal, undercirculated, overcirculated, venous distention, or arterial distention)?
  - Is there evidence of heart failure (pulmonary edema, pleural effusion, or ascites)?
  - With compensated left-heart failure, the earliest evidence of pulmonary edema formation is pulmonary venous congestion (stage I of pulmonary edema formation). That is, the pulmonary veins are distended and larger than their respective arteries. At this time pulmonary capillary pressures are approximately 15 to 20 mm Hg.
- As pulmonary venous and capillary pressures progressively increase with left-sided heart failure, decompensation occurs, and fluid leaks into the interstitium (interstitial edema, stage II).
- As pulmonary venous and capillary pressures continue to rise (e.g., 30 to 40 mm Hg), the alveoli are flooded with edema fluid, and stage III (alveolar edema) is present.
- Pulmonary edema may be primarily perihilar (centrally located) in distribution, or it may be diffuse and generalized. In cats, pulmonary edema may appear as a patchy mixed interstitial-alveolar pattern that is not primarily located in the perihilar region.
- Pleural effusion may be evident in cases with biventricular or severe right-sided heart failure in dogs, and may be present with left-sided or biventricular heart failure in cats.

Echocardiography

- The three principal modalities of echocardiography are two-dimensional, M-mode, and Doppler evaluation of the heart. Because of the noninvasive nature of echocardiography, it has essentially replaced cardiac catheterization in the diagnosis of heart disease in small animals. Echocardiography enables the trained specialist to identify diseases that may cause or be associated with heart failure, such as:
  - Valvular leaks
  - Myocardial failure
  - Intracardiac or extracardiac shunts
  - Decreased ventricular compliance
  - Pericardial disease
- The combination of thoracic radiographs and echocardiography allows the clinician to define structural heart disease and identify CHF in most cases. Typically, heart failure is not present without atrial enlargement (with the exception of pericardial diseases and some other uncommon diseases). The atria are usually compliant and enlarge as filling pressures increase.

Differential Diagnoses

- Primary pulmonary disease may mimic cardiac disease or failure because both may cause coughing, abnormal bronchovesicular sounds, and respiratory distress. The presence of pulmonary crackles, a respiratory sinus arrhythmia, and respiratory distress in a dog without a cardiac murmur is almost always associated with pulmonary disease rather than with heart failure.
- Ascites and pleural effusion may occur secondary to diseases other than heart failure. Evaluation of the jugular veins may aid in differentiating ascites associated with heart failure from ascites associated with hypoproteinemia secondary to liver or renal disease.

Therapy of Heart Failure

- The medical management of heart failure is aimed at relieving symptoms and cardiac dysfunction because, in most cases, heart disease and heart failure are not curable entities. In addition to relieving heart failure symptoms, heart failure therapy is also directed toward increasing the survival time of the patient.
- Signs of congestion can be treated with agents that reduce cardiac filling pressures (preload reducers such as diuretics and venodilators) and agents that facilitate cardiac performance (positive inotropes and arterial dilators). Modulation of the compensatory mechanisms that exacerbate chronic heart failure has become increasingly important in the therapy of heart failure as understanding of the genesis of heart failure (especially chronic heart failure) has evolved.
- Monotherapy with diuretics and simply restricting dietary sodium intake are no longer accepted therapies for treating chronic heart failure. In fact, these therapies may actually promote the activation of the compensatory mechanisms that are responsible for overloading the failing heart.
- It is important to note that the appropriate therapy for a given patient is determined by the clinical

signs present, the severity of the clinical signs, and the underlying disease entity.

- In general, combinations of angiotensin-converting enzyme (ACE) inhibitors, diuretics, ± a positive inotrope represent the conventional therapy for chronic heart failure. Adjunctive therapy in selected patients may include additional agents for heart rate control, nutritional supplementation (e.g., taurine), or additional medications for refractory symptomatic heart failure.
  - *Occult heart disease* refers to heart disease that has resulted in the first detectable changes associated with heart disease (myocardial dysfunction, chamber dilation, arrhythmias). This description is usually used to describe cardiomyopathic patients (e.g., Doberman Pinschers with idiopathic DCM). Therapy with ACE inhibitors and, potentially, beta-adrenergic receptor blocking agents is advocated in these cases in hopes of slowing the progression of heart dysfunction and increasing the time before clinical signs associated with heart failure appear. However, there is no peer-reviewed evidence supporting their effectiveness in altering the disease course in canine chronic valve disease or DCM. In any case, these patients typically have a good to guarded prognosis for long-term survival (i.e., years).
  - Mild heart failure is associated with clinical signs such as exercise intolerance. These clinical symptoms are usually apparent only when the patient is pushed beyond its heart's capacity to maintain an appropriate cardiac output during exercise. These patients show minimal signs of heart failure and, in general, are compensating. Radiographically, cardiomegaly and pulmonary venous congestion are present. In cases such as these, ACE inhibitors and possibly a positive intrope/negative chronotrope such as digoxin and/or a positive inotrope/vasodilator such as pimobendan are indicated. These patients typically have a guarded prognosis for long-term survival (i.e., months to years).
  - Moderate heart failure is associated with more persistent clinical signs such as coughing, exercise intolerance, and tachypnea at rest. These patients have pulmonary edema (or ascites depending on which side of the heart is affected) and require more aggressive therapy with ACE inhibitors, a diuretic such as furosemide, and possibly digoxin and/or pimobendan. These patients typically have a guarded prognosis for long-term survival (i.e., months).
  - Severe heart failure is characterized by the presence of overt clinical signs associated with heart failure at rest. These patients are critically ill and may require intensive monitoring and aggressive therapy, including combinations of ACE inhibitors, furosemide, pimobendan, digoxin, nitrates, and sympathomimetic agents such as dopamine or dobutamine. The prognosis for severe heart failure is guarded to poor, and these patients generally have short survival times (i.e., days to weeks).

THERAPEUTIC STRATEGIES FOR THE MANAGEMENT OF HEART FAILURE

Dietary Modifications

- A reduction in dietary sodium intake can blunt the tendency to conserve sodium and to develop edema. Theoretically, the use of low-sodium diets in combination with vasodilators and ACE inhibitors may allow for less reliance on diuretics to control edema and signs of congestion. Early in the course of heart failure, dietary sodium restriction should be in the form of elimination of high-salt–containing snacks. We tend to rely on diuretics in combination with vasodilators and ACE inhibitors early in the course of heart failure, and to institute salt restriction when excessively high diuretic dosages are required to control signs. Chronic administration of salt-restricted diet may cause sodium conservation through the RAAS, causing further progression of heart failure. Reduced dietary sodium intake stimulates the synthesis and secretion of aldosterone. Another disadvantage to salt-restricted diets is the unpalatable nature of such diets. Salt makes food taste good, so without it, the patient may be reluctant to eat the food, and this may lead to client noncompliance.

KEY POINTS

The general theme regarding sodium restriction in patients with heart failure is to avoid treats or foods with excessive sodium content.

- **L-Carnitine** supplementation may be indicated in patients that have myocardial failure associated with definitive myocardial L-carnitine deficiency. Some Boxers with cardiomyopathy may respond to L-carnitine supplementation. In most cases, however, it is likely that myocardial L-carnitine deficiency is a result of the underlying disease

and myocardial failure rather than the etiology of the myocardial failure. The dosage for L-carnitine supplementation in dogs is 50 to 100 mg/kg PO three times a day.
- Taurine supplementation (sometimes in combination with L-carnitine) has been effective in reversing some secondary DCMs associated with taurine deficiency in cats, American Cocker Spaniels, and other Spaniel breeds. The addition of taurine to feline diets after 1987 dramatically reduced the incidence of taurine deficiency–induced DCM in cats. Although DCM secondary to taurine deficiency in cats is uncommonly encountered today, it is prudent to evaluate plasma taurine levels or to supplement taurine on a trial basis in all cats with DCM. In patients suffering from taurine deficiency–induced DCM, supplementation with taurine results in clinical and echocardiographic improvement typically within 2 to 3 months. Dosage for taurine supplementation:
  - Dogs: 500 to 1000 mg PO once or twice a day
  - Cats: 250 to 500 mg PO once or twice a day
- n-3 polyunsaturated fatty acids levels are reduced in dogs with CHF and fish oil supplementation can normalize these plasma fatty acid abnormalities. The author currently recommends a fish oil dosage to provide 40 mg/kg/day **EPA (eicosapentaenoic acid)** and 25 mg/kg/day **DHA (docosahexaenoic acid)** for patients with anorexia and/or cardiac cachexia.

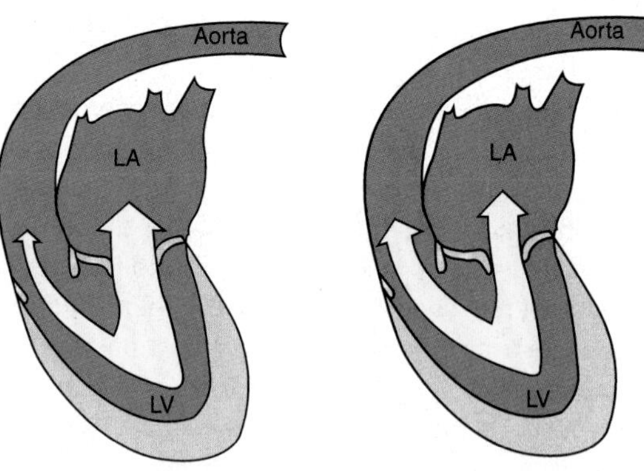

Figure 15-3. Drawings of the left heart from a dog with severe mitral regurgitation before and after administration of an afterload reducing agent. Note that forward flow (out the aorta) increases with afterload reduction because of the reduction in systemic vascular resistance. *LV,* Left ventricle; *LA,* left atrium.

Vasodilator Therapy

- Indications: Arterial vasodilators are used to reduce systemic vascular resistance in patients with CHF. In doing so, cardiac function is improved. Myocardial systolic wall tension is an important determinant of myocardial oxygen consumption. By decreasing systemic vascular resistance (and, therefore, afterload and systolic wall tension), arterial vasodilators reduce myocardial oxygen consumption. Additionally, the reduction in afterload results in an increase in cardiac output. Arterial vasodilators decrease the volume of regurgitation across an insufficient valve, and, therefore, increase forward flow in patients with mitral or aortic regurgitation (Figure 15-3). Arterial vasodilators may lessen the magnitude of left-to-right shunting in patients with ventricular septal defects. However, arterial vasodilators may exacerbate right-to-left shunting in patients with tetralogy of Fallot or with nonrestrictive ventricular septal defects.
- Indications: Venous vasodilators are used to reduce congestive symptoms by redistributing blood volume within the circulatory system (the capacitance vessels and the splanchnic veins) and reducing venous return, which results in lower filling pressures (preload).
  - Classification of vasodilators based on vessels affected:
    - Arterial (e.g., hydralazine)
    - Venous (e.g., nitroglycerin, isosorbide dinitrate)
    - Mixed (e.g., nitroprusside, prazosin, ACE inhibitors, pimobendan)
  - Classification of vasodilators based on mechanism of action:
    - Direct acting (e.g., nitroprusside, nitroglycerin, isosorbide dinitrate, hydralazine)
    - Alpha-adrenergic blocking agents (e.g., prazosin)
    - Calcium channel blocking agents (e.g., amlodipine, verapamil, diltiazem)
    - ACE inhibitors (e.g., captopril, enalapril, lisinopril, benazepril)
    - Phosphodiesterase inhibitors (e.g. pimobendan)

Angiotensin-Converting Enzyme Inhibitors

- ACE inhibitors cause mixed vasodilation by preventing the conversion of angiotensin I to angiotensin II. Angiotensin II is a potent vasoconstrictor. The decrease in angiotensin II levels results in a reduction in the level of vasoconstriction, as well as decreased SNS activity. Furthermore, ACE inhibition also results in decreased aldosterone synthesis and secretion, so that there is less sodium and water retention, among many other benefits beyond the scope of this discussion.

- Large, multicenter clinical trials have demonstrated the safety and efficacy of ACE inhibitors in the therapy of CHF secondary to DCM and primary valve disease. ACE inhibitors appear to significantly decrease the clinical signs of heart failure when used in combination with conventional therapy (diuretics with or without digoxin). Enalapril has been extensively studied in veterinary medicine and is approved for the use in dogs in the United States:
  - The Invasive Multicenter Prospective Veterinary Enalapril (IMPROVE) study showed a decrease in pulmonary capillary wedge pressure and improvement of heart failure status with enalapril.
  - The Cooperative Veterinary Enalapril (COVE) study showed that enalapril with digoxin and/or furosemide significantly decreased clinical signs of heart failure in DCM or MR.
  - The Enalapril Long-Term Efficacy Study showed increased survival times for dogs treated with enalapril.
  - Enalapril studies in cats in the late 1990s appear to suggest that ACE inhibitors improve control of CHF associated with hypertrophic and other forms of cardiomyopathy.
  - Benazepril therapy has been demonstrated to be effective in the treatment of systemic hypertension secondary to chronic renal disease or hypertrophic cardiomyopathy, as well as in the control of CHF.
- The earliest time at which ACE inhibition is indicated has not been accurately determined, but it may be reasonable for ACE inhibitor therapy to be initiated in dogs and cats with signs of advanced, compensated heart failure (e.g., cardiomegaly and pulmonary venous congestion), regardless of their symptoms. ACE inhibitor therapy in asymptomatic Doberman Pinschers with occult DCM may delay the onset of symptomatic CHF.
- However, there is no indication for therapy with ACE inhibitors in patients with asymptomatic, chronic valve disease. A large multicenter placebo controlled double blind study in Europe was unable to demonstrate a delay in symptomatic heart failure in patients with chronic valve disease when given enalapril.
- ACE inhibitors should not be used as a primary agent (monotherapy) in emergency treatment for acute CHF. Significant clinical improvement attributable to ACE inhibition may not be evident until 2 to 3 weeks after initiation of therapy.
- Side effects associated with ACE inhibitor therapy occur infrequently.
- Anorexia or inappetence, vomiting, hypotension, and azotemia are the most common side effects of ACE inhibitor therapy. Azotemia secondary to decreased renal perfusion represents the most important clinical consideration. Azotemia and renal dysfunction secondary to a decrease in renal perfusion result from loss of protective mechanisms to maintain filtration pressures. Angiotensin II causes vasoconstriction of the renal efferent arterioles in an effort to maintain glomerular filtration pressures in the face of decreased renal perfusion. The relative decrease in angiotensin II can significantly decrease glomerular perfusion and filtration, resulting in azotemia. Furthermore, renal dysfunction is more likely to occur in patients with pre-existing renal disease. As a result, renal function should be evaluated before and 5 to 7 days after instituting ACE inhibitor therapy, especially during concurrent diuretic therapy.
- Most complications are likely to occur shortly after beginning therapy, in association with acute cardiac decompensation, or in conjunction with systemic disease that may alter the patient's hydration status (e.g., vomiting or diarrhea). Side effects are much more likely to occur with captopril than with the other commonly used ACE inhibitors.

KEY POINTS

ACE inhibitors are recommended for patients with asymptomatic myocardial dysfunction; in patients with symptomatic CHF secondary to chronic valvular disease, DCM, and other causes of CHF; and in patients with systemic hypertension.

- Agents and dosages
  - **Captopril** (Capoten)
    - Dogs: 0.5 to 2.0 mg/kg PO three times a day
  - **Enalapril** (Enacard, Vasotec)
    - Dogs: 0.5 mg/kg PO once or twice a day
    - Cats: 0.25 to 0.5 mg/kg PO twice a day to every other day
  - **Lisinopril** (Zestril)
    - Dogs: 0.5 mg/kg PO once daily
  - **Benazepril** (Lotensin)
    - Dogs: 0.25 to 0.5 mg/kg PO once or twice a day
    - Cats: 0.25 to 0.5 mg/kg PO once or twice a day

Calcium Channel Blocking Agents

- Verapamil, diltiazem, nifedipine, and amlodipine are calcium channel blocking agents. In general, they differ with regard to their antiarrhythmic effects, their vasodilating effects, and their negative inotropic effects.

- Verapamil is used primarily (intravenously) for the short-term control of supraventricular arrhythmias (negative chronotropic effect). It possesses minimal vasodilating properties, but exerts a significant and sometimes detrimental negative inotropic effect in patients with heart failure.
- Nifedipine is a more potent vasodilator with more limited direct effects on the heart when compared with verapamil. Nifedipine is not commonly used in veterinary medicine.
- Diltiazem's (Cardizem, Dilacor) vasodilating action is weaker than that of nifedipine and more pronounced than that of verapamil. Diltiazem exerts a negligible negative inotropic effect in normal, conscious dogs, but when given rapidly intravenously, it may cause a pronounced negative inotropic effect in animals with heart failure. The antiarrhythmic and negative chronotropic effects of diltiazem are similar to those of verapamil. A positive lusitropic (enhanced relaxation) effect may also be associated the administration of diltiazem to cats with hypertrophic cardiomyopathy.
  - Agents and dosages
    - **Diltiazem** (Cardizem, Cardizem CD, Dilacor)
      - Dogs: 0.5 to 2.0 mg/kg PO two or three times a day
      - Cats: 7.5 mg PO two or three times a day or 45 to 60 mg PO every day of sustained-release formulations
  - **Amlodipine** (Norvasc)
    - Primarily used as therapy for systemic hypertension in cats and dogs.
      - Dogs: 0.05 to 0.2 mg/kg PO once or twice a day
      - Cats: 0.625 to 1.25 mg PO once or twice a day
- In general, we use calcium channel blockers (1) to control heart rate and to facilitate ventricular filling and relaxation in cats with hypertrophic cardiomyopathy; (2) as supplemental therapy for control of the ventricular response rate in some supraventricular tachycardias such as atrial fibrillation in dogs and cats; and (3) in the treatment of systemic (amlodipine) and pulmonary (diltiazem) hypertension.

KEY POINTS

Amlodipine can be added to the protocol for patients with chronic valve disease for additional afterload reduction in selected cases. A systemic systolic blood pressure (as determined noninvasively) around 100 mm Hg is the target blood pressure range.

Direct-Acting Arterial Vasodilators

Hydralazine

- Hydralazine has been evaluated in dogs with spontaneous CHF secondary to MR.
- Hydralazine has been shown to decrease MR, increase forward flow, reduce left atrial pressures, and improve exercise capacity. Whereas these studies provide a reasonable basis for the short-term use of hydralazine in dogs with decompensated left-heart failure caused by MR, poor patient tolerance and lack of owner compliance limit the usefulness of hydralazine for long-term therapy.
- We currently use hydralazine only in cases with refractory heart failure associated with MR that no longer are responding well to ACE inhibitor–diuretic–digoxin (or pimobendan) combination therapy.
- Onset of action for orally administered hydralazine is approximately 1 hour, the peak effect is achieved within 3 hours, and the effect remains stable for several hours, with a total duration of effect of about 12 hours.

Agents and Dosages

- **Hydralazine** (Apresoline):
  - Dogs: Initial dose at 0.5 mg/kg PO; the dose is gradually increased until a clinical response is elicited or up to a maximum dose of 3.0 mg/kg BID. The endpoints of drug titration can be determined by monitoring blood pressure, by the patient's clinical response, and by obtaining radiographic evidence that pulmonary edema has resolved.
  - Cats: 2.5 mg PO once or twice a day
- Hydralazine may play a role in emergency therapy for severe MR secondary to ruptured chordae tendineae.
- The author rarely uses hydralazine in cats with heart failure.
- Many side effects are associated with administration of hydralazine and limit its usefulness:
  - Hypotension
  - Gastrointestinal disturbances
  - Reflex tachycardia
  - Furthermore, there is evidence of enhanced neurohormonal activity (increased aldosterone levels) in dogs receiving hydralazine.

Sodium Nitroprusside

- Nitroprusside is the only direct-acting mixed vasodilator available (not approved) for use in dogs with CHF. It is an extremely potent vasodilator that is primarily used to rescue dogs with severe, decompensated CHF associated with MR or DCM.

- The indications for nitroprusside therapy are short-term treatment of refractory, life-threatening CHF in dogs with MR or DCM or critical systemic hypertension. Combination therapy with dobutamine, digoxin and/or pimobendan, and diuretics provides the best effect.
  - Agents and dosages
    - **Nitroprusside** (Nipride):
      - Dogs: intravenous (IV) constant rate infusion at an initial rate of 1.0 μg/kg/min (following dilution in 5% dextrose), titrated to effect, by monitoring blood pressure and pulmonary capillary wedge pressure, to a maximum dose of 10 μg/kg/min.
  - Hypotension, tachycardia, nausea, and vomiting are the most significant adverse effects of nitroprusside administration.
  - Cyanide poisoning may also occur with chronic administration.
  - Hypotension is easily managed by slowing the rate or by discontinuing the infusion (nitroprusside has a very short half-life).

Venous Vasodilators (Nitroglycerin, Isosorbide Dinitrate)

- These nitrate vasodilators are excellent preload reducers. The development of nitrate tolerance limits the continuous use (i.e., more than 36 hours) of these agents. Tolerance may be avoided by intermittent use (24 hours on and 24 hours off) and possibly concurrent use of ACE inhibitors.
  - Agents and dosages
    - **2% nitroglycerin** paste (Nitrol, Nitro-BID)
      - Dogs: ¼ to 2 inches cutaneously three or four times a day; ½ inch per 2.27 kg of body weight
      - Cats: ⅛ to ¼ inch three or four times a day
      - Nitroglycerin paste should be applied to hairless areas such as the pinna or the axillary region. If perfusion to the ears is poor (e.g., ears are cold), the axilla or groin will provide better absorption. Because nitroglycerin is absorbed transcutaneously, gloves should be worn during administration.
  - **Isosorbide dinitrate** (Isordil)
    - Dogs: 0.2 to 1.0 mg/kg PO three times a day

Alpha-Adrenergic Receptor Antagonists (Prazosin)

- The use of prazosin has been reported in dogs with CHF, but neither its short-term hemodynamic nor long-term clinical effects have been documented. Current indications for its use appear to be limited to the short-term treatment of acute heart failure when other agents are ineffective or contraindicated. Rarely used in veterinary medicine.
  - Agents and Dosages: **Prazosin** (Minipress), titrated to effect
  - Small dogs and cats: 0.25 to 1 mg PO three times a day
  - Medium dogs (<40 lb): 1 to 3 mg PO three times a day
  - Large dogs (>40 lb): 3 to 10 mg PO three times a day

Diuretic Therapy

Loop Diuretics
Furosemide (Lasix)

- The mechanism of action of loop diuretics is the reversible inhibition of the sodium/potassium/chloride co-transporter in the thick ascending limb of the loop of Henle.
- Furosemide is the most commonly used agent in this class of diuretics because it is the most potent and has a fast onset of action. The result is the obligatory loss of sodium and water into the urine. Intravenous and intramuscular furosemide acutely increases venous capacitance secondary to release of vasodilatory prostaglandins. This vasodilatory effect occurs within the first 20 minutes after IV or intramuscular (IM) administration, and the peak diuretic effect occurs after 30 to 45 minutes.
- Of interest to the clinician, there is a bioavailability difference between Lasix and generic oral formulations; we therefore do not recommend switching back and forth from one formulation to the other.
- The peak effect after oral administration of Lasix is 30 minutes to 2 hours.
- Agents and dosages: **Furosemide** (Lasix, Salix)
  - Chronic oral administration
    - Dogs: 1 to 2 mg/kg PO two to four times a day
    - Cats: 1 to 2 mg/kg PO twice a day
  - Parenteral administration (IM or IV)
    - Dogs: 2 to 8 mg/kg as needed to control edema
    - Cats: 1 to 2 mg/kg as needed to control edema
    - Continuous-rate infusion: 0.66 mg/kg IV bolus followed by 0.66 mg/kg/hour
- Adverse side effects of furosemide (Lasix) include electrolyte abnormalities, such as hypokalemia, hyponatremia, and hypochloremia (hypochloremic metabolic alkalosis).
- Typically, withdrawal of the drug or a reduction in the dose usually results in resolution of the alkalosis. Severe metabolic alkalosis can be treated with judicious use of half-strength saline with

or without 2.5% dextrose. Overzealous diuretic therapy may cause dehydration, low cardiac output, and, possibly, circulatory collapse. Furthermore, diuretics activate systemic compensatory mechanisms, such as the RAAS and SNS.
- In the therapy of heart failure, furosemide should always be used in combination with an ACE inhibitor; chronic monotherapy with furosemide is not recommended.

KEY POINT

The lowest dose of furosemide effective in controlling the clinical signs of congestion should be used. Monitoring of the patient's resting respiratory rate can facilitate achieving the appropriate maintenance dose. Once clinical signs of congestion have resolved, the dose is tapered to the lowest effective dose based on the patient's resting respiratory rate. There is no recommended goal number for resting respiratory rate in dogs or cats; however, trends of increasing rate suggest the development of interstitial pulmonary edema (stimulation of J-type receptors in the pulmonary interstitium that stimulate tachypnea). A trend of increasing resting respiratory rate may suggest that the maintenance dose of furosemide is inadequate, and that dosage adjustment is indicated.

Thiazide Diuretics (Chlorothiazide, Hydrochlorothiazide)

- Thiazide diuretics act by inhibiting distal tubule electrolyte reabsorption. These diuretics are less potent natriuretic agents and are usually not successful in controlling signs of congestion when used as a monotherapy. In general, thiazide diuretics are administered when heart failure is refractory and conventional therapy (digoxin and/or pimobendan, ACE inhibitor, and furosemide) fails to control the clinical signs of congestion.
  - Agents and Dosages
    - **Chlorothiazide** (Diuril): 20 to 40 mg/kg PO once or twice a day
    - **Hydrochlorothiazide** (Hydrodiuril): 2 to 4 mg/kg PO once or twice a day

Potassium-Sparing Diuretics

Spironolactone

- Generally, the potassium-sparing diuretics are weak diuretics that are rarely used as single-agent therapy to control edema in heart failure patients. They are most commonly used together with a more potent diuretic to control refractory edema.
- Because of their potassium-sparing effects, they should be used with caution with concurrent ACE inhibitor therapy.
- Spironolactone (Aldactone), an aldosterone antagonist, is usually used in conjunction with Lasix or Diuril.
- Aldosterone antagonism may serve a cardioprotective effect by reversing and inhibiting myocardial and vascular fibrosis. The anti-aldosterone effect may prove to be an important part in the management of chronic heart failure, particularly in patients with "aldosterone escape" (a non-RAAS associated increase in aldosterone).
- Agents and Dosages: **Spironolactone** (Aldactone):
  - 1 to 2 mg/kg PO twice a day

KEY POINT

- The appropriate timing for the initiation of spironolactone or other aldosterone antagonist therapy is not clear at this time. The author routinely administers spironolactone to patients with refractory heart failure.
- Administration of spironolactone may also be appropriate in patients with evidence of myocardial remodeling.
- Spironolactone may reduce the risk of hypokalemia in patients treated with chronic furosemide therapy.

Digitalis Glycoside Therapy

Digoxin

- Digoxin acts by inhibiting sarcolemmal Na^+, K^+-ATPase, which causes an accumulation of sodium which is then available for exchange with extracellular calcium through the Na^+-Ca^{++} exchanger. The exchange results in increased intracellular calcium. Calcium is then available for interaction with the sarcoplasmic reticulum (calcium-induced release of sarcoplasmic reticular calcium), and therefore the release of more calcium for interaction with the contractile elements (positive inotropic effect). Digitalis glycosides shift the Frank-Starling curve upward by increasing the velocity and force of contraction of the myocardium at any given level of preload. Additionally, digitalis glycosides slow conduction through the atrioventricular node by both direct and vagal effects. Digoxin may also partially restore baroreceptor reflexes that are desensitized by the chronically elevated sympathetic tone associated with CHF.

- Indications for digoxin therapy:
  - Theoretically, digoxin is indicated in virtually every patient with CHF and a supraventricular tachycardia (e.g., atrial tachycardia, flutter, or fibrillation). Digoxin is also indicated for echocardiographically documented myocardial failure and systolic dysfunction (i.e., reduced fractional shortening); however digoxin has only modest positive inotropic effects. Digoxin is not indicated in patients with pericardial disease, hypertrophic cardiomyopathy with outflow tract obstruction, or restrictive myocardial disease, unless these conditions are accompanied by myocardial failure or supraventricular tachycardias.
- Method of administration:
  - Oral and intravenous routes of administration are available for digoxin. The urgency of digitalization determines the route of administration. The intravenous route is reserved for patients with severe acute heart failure and a fast, sustained supraventricular tachyarrhythmia (i.e., atrial fibrillation at a rate of more than 240 bpm). In most cases, digoxin can be administered orally at maintenance levels, with the desired effect occurring 3 to 5 days after initiation of the drug (depending on the patient).
- Agents and Dosages: **Digoxin** (Cardoxin, Lanoxin)
  - Rapid IV digoxin:
    - Dogs: 0.0025 mg/kg IV bolus, repeat hourly 3 to 4 times (total up to 0.01 mg/kg).
    - Arrhythmias ("any arrhythmia in the book") may be the first sign of toxicity with IV digoxin.
  - Rapid oral digoxin:
    - Dogs: Rapid oral digitalization can be employed in animals that require therapeutic blood levels prior to the 72 to 92 hours required with maintenance dosage schedules; however, rapid oral digitalization (similar to IV digitalization) is usually not necessary. A variety of methods that involve giving five times the daily maintenance dose over 48 hours, or giving the maintenance dose three times instead of twice a day for the first 1 or 2 days (not to exceed 1.5 mg/day), have been employed. We typically administer digoxin at the maintenance dose instead of rapid digitalization.
  - Maintenance oral digoxin dose
    - Dogs: 0.22 mg/m^2 PO twice a day, or 0.005 to 0.01 mg/kg PO twice a day
    - Cats: One fourth of a 0.125 mg tablet PO every day or every other day (approximately 0.008 mg/kg every day or every other day). Serum digoxin levels should be determined 5 to 7 days after initiation of therapy (therapeutic serum levels = 1.0 to 2.0 ng/ml in most laboratories [8 to 12 hours post dosing]). The oral dose is then adjusted based on this trough serum level.

KEY POINT

The author initiates digoxin at a chronic oral maintenance dosage of 0.005 mg/kg every 12 hours and never uses the other methods (intravenous or rapid oral) to initiate therapy with digoxin. The most common indications for digoxin therapy include heart rate control in patients with supraventricular tachyarrhythmias, myocardial failure, or chronic heart failure.

- There are several special tips regarding the use of digoxin. A 20-lb dog usually gets 1 ml of the 0.05 mg/ml elixir; a 10-lb dog gets 0.5 ml, and so forth. *Do not use the elixir in cats, as it makes them froth at the mouth.* The elixir has a small amount of alcohol in it, which may cause gastrointestinal disturbance without drug toxicity. Signs of digitalization include the following: slowing of the heart rate, relief of clinical signs of heart failure, increased PR interval (unreliable), and demonstration of therapeutic blood levels (a therapeutic trough level of digoxin is 1 to 2 ng/ml, animals with serum levels greater than 3 ng/ml usually demonstrate signs of toxicity).
- *Determinants of digoxin dosages:*
  - Many factors (such as dosage form, electrolyte status, renal status, thyroid status, and concurrent medications) affect the serum levels attained in a particular patient receiving digoxin.
  - Digoxin elixir is more completely absorbed than the tablet form, resulting in higher blood levels at a given dosage. Do not switch patients back and forth from one to the other.
  - Hypokalemia and hypercalcemia are associated with the development of digitalis toxicity at lower digoxin doses. Electrolyte status should be monitored periodically (every 2 to 3 months), or after changes in therapy (i.e., increases in furosemide or ACE inhibitor), or changes in the patient's clinical status.
  - Concurrent medications such as quinidine, verapamil, and drugs that inhibit hepatic microsomal enzymes (tetracycline, chloramphenicol) may result in increased digoxin serum levels,

requiring a reduction in digoxin dosage. Use an alternative medication in place of quinidine whenever possible (e.g., procainamide).

- Hypothyroid animals often require less digoxin than euthyroid animals. Hyperthyroid animals may also require a decreased dose. Digoxin is excreted primarily by the kidneys. The presence of renal dysfunction often necessitates a reduction in digoxin dosage or frequency of administration.
- Dosage should be based on lean body weight. Obesity, pregnancy, or the presence of ascites should be noted, and the dose should be adjusted accordingly.

Adverse and toxic effects of digitalis glycosides:

- Caution must be used when administering digitalis glycosides intravenously. When given rapidly intravenously, they have direct vasoconstrictive effects.
- The main determinants of myocardial oxygen consumption are ventricular wall tension, heart rate, and the state of contractility. Increased contractility associated with digoxin therapy results in increased myocardial oxygen consumption that is usually offset by the decrease in heart rate and ventricular size (and thus wall tension) and increased coronary perfusion.
- The signs of toxicity are variable, but in general fall into one or more of three categories:
  - Neurologic (lethargy and depression)
  - Gastrointestinal (inappetence, anorexia, diarrhea, nausea, vomiting)
  - Cardiac (arrhythmia)
- With oral administration, gastrointestinal signs almost always occur before arrhythmias. Some of the more common arrhythmias associated with digitalis toxicity are first and second-degree atrioventricular block, accelerated junctional rhythms, ventricular premature complexes, ventricular tachycardias, and atrioventricular dissociation. A nonrespiratory sinus arrhythmia in a patient receiving digoxin may indicate high serum levels.
- The treatment of digoxin toxicosis is based on the elimination half-life of the drug and the goal is to return digoxin serum levels to within therapeutic range (1 to 2 ng/ml). In healthy dogs, the serum half-life of digoxin is approximately 24 to 36 hours. Therefore, it takes about 1½ days to decrease the serum level to half the original level.
- **CASE EXAMPLE:** if the starting serum level is 6 ng/ml, then if the drug is discontinued for 1½ days, the serum level should be around 3 ng/ml (still in the toxic range). If the drug is discontinued for yet another 1½ days, the serum level should drop from 3 ng/ml to 1.5 ng/ml. Therefore, in this example, the digoxin should be discontinued for approximately 3 to 4 days and then continued at approximately one third of the original dose to achieve serum levels in the therapeutic range. Check electrolyte status and correct hypokalemia if present. Life-threatening arrhythmias may be treated with atropine, lidocaine, or a beta blocker (depending on the arrhythmia present). Additionally, a specific antidote (Fab-antibody fragments that scavenge the free drug from the body) is available, but its use may be cost prohibitive.

Pimobendan (The "Inodilator")

- Pimobendan is a phosphodiesterase (PDE) III inhibitor that has positive inotropic activity (via increasing the sensitivity of the contractile apparatus to calcium) and vasodilatory (via phosphodiesterase inhibition) effects. Current studies have demonstrated it to increase survival time and quality of life in CHF patients with DCM or with chronic valve disease.
- There are several clinical trials (some only in abstract form) assessing the use of pimobendan in patients with chronic valve disease, include the PITCH Trial, the Edinburgh Study, the Guelph Study, the PERMIT Study, and the VetSCOPE Study. The general consensus at this time is that pimobendan has beneficial effects, with regards to survival and quality of life, when administered to patients with symptomatic chronic valve disease or DCM.
  - Dosage:
    - Dogs: 0.1 to 0.25 mg/kg PO every 12 hours; give 1 hour prior to food ingestion
    - Cats: no current recommended dosage

Miscellaneous Agents/Adjunctive Therapy for Heart Failure

- Bronchodilators, antitussives, sympathomimetics, positive inotropes, and sedatives/tranquilizers are all agents used as adjunctive therapy in the management of CHF. None of these agents when used as monotherapy is capable of effectively ameliorating the signs of CHF. However, these agents may be useful in decreasing some of the signs associated with heart failure (coughing, cardiac asthma, and signs of low-output failure).

Bronchodilators

- Theophylline (Theo-Dur) is a bronchodilating agent by inhibition of phosphodiesterase. Phosphodiesterase is the enzyme responsible for reducing intracellular levels of cyclic adenosine monophosphate (cAMP). Inhibition of this enzyme results in the accumulation of AMP, which causes increased calcium influx. An increase in calcium influx in the smooth muscles of the airways results in smooth muscle relaxation and bronchodilation. Additionally, the change in calcium ion movement in other tissues, such as nodal and myocardial tissue, results in a positive chronotropic and inotropic effect. This agent may be helpful in dyspneic patients with fatigue of the muscles of respiration. Dogs and cats may experience transient gastrointestinal disturbance (usually self-limiting and resolving within the first 2 weeks of drug administration), tachycardia, and hyperexcitability and/or restlessness. Occasionally, we use theophylline in patients with complete atrioventricular block that are not candidates for permanent pacemaker implantation.
- Agents and dosages:
  - **Theophylline** (Theo-Dur)
    - Dogs: 9 to 20 mg/kg PO two to four times a day
    - Cats: 4 mg/kg PO three times a day
  - **Aminophylline** (Aminophyllin)
    - Dogs: 11 mg/kg PO two to four times a day
    - Cats: 5 mg/kg PO three times a day

Cough Suppressants

- Cough suppressants may be effective in reducing the frequency of coughing in dogs with left mainstem bronchial compression secondary to left atrial enlargement. If chronic airway disease is also present, the long-term results of antitussive therapy are often disappointing.
  - **Hydrocodone** (Hycodan)
    - Dogs: 0.22 mg/kg PO every day to four times a day
    - Cats: Do not use.
  - **Butorphanol** (Torbutrol)
    - Dogs: 0.05 to 1 mg/kg PO two to four times a day
    - Cats: No established antitussive dose

Sedatives and Tranquilizers

- May be useful in selected cases. Respiratory distress may cause anxiety and stress in a patient with CHF. Agents with minimal cardiovascular effects should be chosen to prevent exacerbation of the CHF by causing hypotension or reduced contractility.
  - **Morphine sulfate** (reduces anxiety, decreases sympathetic tone):
    - Dogs: 0.1 to 1.0 mg/kg SQ, IM
  - **Acepromazine** (reduces anxiety, vasodilator):
    - Dogs: 0.1 to 0.2 mg/kg SQ, IM
  - **Butorphanol:**
    - Dogs, cats: 0.1 to 0.3 mg/kg IV or IM

Potassium Supplements

- Usually not necessary in most patients with CHF as long as they are eating and drinking. Dogs and, especially, cats may become hypokalemic as a result of inappetence/anorexia and aggressive concurrent diuretic therapy. Potassium supplement dose; cats: 2 to 6 mEq PO per day.

Oxygen Therapy

- As needed in cases with acute pulmonary edema

Positive Inotropic Therapy

- The bipyridines, amrinone and milrinone, are agents that are referred to as inotropic vasodilators because they have mild arteriolar dilating properties in addition to their inotropic effects. The mechanism of action is an increase in cardiac levels of cAMP by inhibition of phosphodiesterase. Increased cAMP levels mediate increased calcium delivery to the contractile elements of the myocyte, as well as possibly increasing calcium availability by augmenting the storage and release of calcium by the sarcoplasmic reticulum. Increases in cAMP in vascular smooth muscle result in muscular relaxation and a direct-acting arterial vasodilator effect.
- The indications for bipyridine therapy are similar to those for digoxin. Amrinone and milrinone are more potent inotropic agents than digoxin, but lack the antiarrhythmic properties. Both agents tend to increase heart rate and may potentiate arrhythmias in some patients.
- Their use at the present time is limited to the treatment of severe refractory myocardial failure. The route of administration for amrinone and milrinone is intravenous. Amrinone is approved only for short-term IV administration in humans.
  - **Amrinone** (Inocor):
    - Dogs: 1.0 to 3.0 mg/kg IV bolus or 10 to 80 μg/kg/min as a continuous rate infusion
- Adverse and toxic effects associated with amrinone and milrinone have been described. Thrombocytopenia, a dose-related increased heart rate, gastrointestinal signs (diarrhea, anorexia), and hypotension (at high doses) have been reported. Additionally, these agents appear to be arrhythmogenic (i.e., potentiate the development of arrhythmias) in some humans and dogs with heart failure.

- The presence of serious ventricular arrhythmias represents a contraindication for the use of these agents. Because the half-life of the parental formulations is quite short, discontinuing the medication is the treatment for toxicosis. We rarely use these agents in the therapy of heart failure in dogs and cats.

Sympathomimetics (Dobutamine, Dopamine, and Isoproterenol)

- Sympathomimetics are agents that mimic the actions of the SNS (i.e., alpha- and beta-adrenergic receptor agonists).
- Dobutamine and dopamine are used only in the therapy of acute severe heart failure. Both dobutamine and dopamine exert a positive inotropic effect by stimulating myocardial beta-1 adrenergic receptors, which results in increased cAMP levels through adenylate cyclase stimulation. The increased levels of cAMP cause an increase in the slow inward calcium currents as well as an increase in calcium storage by the sarcoplasmic reticulum, making more calcium available to the contractile elements. Dobutamine stimulates both beta-1 and beta-2 adrenergic receptors in the peripheral vasculature, and this combination results in no major changes in blood pressure.
- The positive chronotropic effect that is seen with dobutamine at higher doses should be avoided in most cases. The effects of dopamine are similar to dobutamine with the exception of the following:
  - Dobutamine favors blood flow to myocardial and skeletal muscle, whereas dopamine favors flow to the renal and mesenteric systems.
  - Dopamine infusion rates above 10 µg/kg/min may be associated with vasoconstriction.
  - Dopamine may increase diastolic intraventricular pressures.
- All sympathomimetic agents are best suited to short-term IV use. Isoproterenol stimulates beta-1 and beta-2 receptors, resulting in increased myocardial contractility, increased heart rate, and peripheral vasodilation. Isoproterenol is used mainly for the temporary control of heart rate in animals with symptomatic bradycardia. The chronotropic and arrhythmogenic effects make it unsuitable for the treatment of animals with CHF.
- Agents and dosages:
  - **Isoproterenol hydrochloride** (Isuprel):
    - Dogs: 0.04 to 0.1 µg/kg/min IV infusion following dilution in dextrose
  - **Dobutamine** hydrochloride (Dobutrex):
    - Dogs: 5 to 20 µg/kg/min IV continuous infusion diluted in 5% dextrose (monitor closely for arrhythmia)
  - **Dopamine hydrochloride** (Intropin):
    - Dogs: 2 to 8 µg/kg/min IV continuous infusion diluted in 5% dextrose

KEY POINT

"Quick Dobutamine Drip Tip:" Dilute 1 ml dobutamine (Dobutrex, 250 mg in a 20 ml vial or 12.5 mg/ml) for each 20 lb of body weight in 250 ml of 5% dextrose. Deliver by continuous rate infusion at a rate of 1 ml/min (1 drop every 4 seconds) to obtain a dose of 5 µg/kg/min if using a venoset delivery system.

- The adverse and toxic effects associated with sympathomimetic administration are usually dose related and may include:
  - Tachycardia
  - Arrhythmias
  - Gastrointestinal disturbances (anorexia, nausea)
  - Hypertension (dopamine)
  - Hypotension (isoproterenol)
  - Phlebitis may occur if the agent goes extravascular.
- Dobutamine should not be initiated prior to digitalization for heart rate control in patients with severe heart failure and rapid atrial fibrillation. Prior digitalization is necessary for ventricular rate control because administration of dobutamine may speed atrioventricular nodal conduction and increase the ventricular response rate to atrial fibrillation.
- The treatment for catecholamine toxicity involves stopping or slowing the administration of the drug.

KEY POINT

Therapy with positive inotropic agents in veterinary medicine is, for the most part, limited to the use of dobutamine or dopamine in emergency scenarios, digoxin for chronic heart failure, and, more recently, pimobendan for chronic heart failure.

Beta-Adrenergic Receptor Blockers

- **Beta**-adrenergic receptor blockers (selective beta-1 agents such as atenolol and nonselective agents such as propranolol or carvedilol) are agents that in the past have primarily been used as antiarrhythmic agents in the control of the ventricular response rate to atrial fibrillation. Recent evidence has suggested that beta blockade may be effective in the therapy of mild to moderate CHF. Chronic SNS stimulation results in down-regulation and desensitization of cardiac beta receptors. Beta blockers have been demonstrated to up-regulate myocardial beta receptors and to improve myocardial function in dogs, using certain models of heart failure.

- However, if severe heart failure is present, beta blockade must be used very cautiously.
- Patients with pathologic concentric hypertrophy (e.g., hypertrophic cardiomyopathy, aortic or pulmonic stenosis, and tetralogy of Fallot) benefit from administration of beta blockers. These patients may become symptomatic during exercise because of myocardial ischemia or dynamic outflow tract obstruction. Marked concentric hypertrophy predisposes the myocardium to hypoxia, and tachycardia exacerbates this scenario. Beta blockers reduce myocardial oxygen consumption by reducing the heart rate. Additionally, the negative inotropic effects of beta blockers may reduce the dynamic outflow tract obstruction seen in some of these patients.
  - **Carvedilol** (CoReg), a third-generation, nonselective beta blocker with alpha-1 blocking activity as well as antioxidative effects, can be administered to stable patients with heart failure for cardioprotective effects at a dosage of 1.56 mg PO every 24 hours for 1 to 2 weeks, then 1.56 mg PO every 12 hours, and then upward titration to the maximal tolerated dosage (0.4 mg/kg PO every 12 hours).

KEY POINT

In general, beta blockers in patients with advanced cardiac disease should be used only under the guidance of a specialist.

Novel Vasodilators (Sildenafil)

- Sildenafil is a phosphodiesterase V inhibitor that has been shown to improve both exercise tolerance and quality of life in humans with pulmonary hypertension.
- Initial clinical observations indicate that sildenafil may also have a positive effect in dogs with acquired pulmonary hypertension secondary to chronic valve disease, congenital heart disease, chronic pulmonary disease, and heartworm disease.
- Can be used in combination with pimobendan (Vetmedin) for additional inodilator effect.
- Dosage: **Sildenafil** (Viagra): 0.5 to 1.0 mg/kg PO two or three times a day

TREATMENT PROTOCOLS

- When considering heart failure therapy for dogs with chronic valve disease or DCM, it is helpful to think of patients with heart disease and/or heart failure as being on a continuum of stages ranging from:
  - Stage A (risk for heart disease)
  - Stage B (heart disease is present; no symptoms)
  - Stage C
    - C1: stabilized CHF
    - C2: mild to moderate CHF
    - C3: severe and/or life threatening CHF
  - Stage D (refractory CHF)

Stage A

- This refers to those patients with a risk of developing heart disease such as those with certain genetics, a family history of heart disease, a breed predisposition, or concurrent systemic disease with cardiovascular implications. Examples include the following: cavalier King Charles Spaniels are at risk for developing chronic valve disease; Doberman Pinschers are at risk for developing DCM; Boxers are at risk for developing arrhythmogenic right ventricular cardiomyopathy, and so on.
  - No therapy is indicated for dogs in stage A
  - Manage predisposing conditions
  - Manage systemic hypertension, if present
  - No dietary sodium modifications necessary

Stage B

- Heart disease is present, but there are no clinical signs of CHF.
  - Same as in stage A
  - Increase the awareness of signs of CHF (tachypnea, dyspnea, coughing)
  - Periodic reevaluation for signs of disease progression and complications
  - For patients with chronic valve disease, there is no evidence indicating that there is any beneficial effect of using an ACE inhibitor or pimobendan at this stage
  - For patients with DCM, there are no drugs recommended for routine use; however, ACE inhibitors, pimobendan, digoxin (if atrial fibrillation is present), or beta blockers may be initiated in selected patients.

Stage C1

- Stabilized CHF; historical signs of CHF, but no symptoms are currently present
  - Goals are to keep clinical signs stabilized, use the minimum effective dosage of furosemide, ACE inhibitor at not less than minimum recommended dosage, modulate neurohormones (optional aldosterone antagonist and/or beta blocker), and to preserve renal and myocardial function. Additional drugs may be added at this stage for their cardioprotective effects.
  - Drugs for routine use: furosemide (mandatory), ACE inhibitor, pimobendan
  - Drugs for selected patients: spironolactone, digoxin, thiazide, amlodipine/hydralazine or other vasodilator
  - Avoid, if possible, excessive sodium intake, beta blockers, corticosteroids, IV fluids (unless required for concurrent disease; requires careful monitoring of the respiratory rate trend)

> **KEY POINT**
>
> The dose of furosemide should be adjusted (within a range specified by clinician) based on the resting respiratory rate trend and other clinical signs as monitored by the owners.

Stage C2

- Mild to moderate CHF is present
  - Goals are to attain stage C1 (eliminate pulmonary edema and/or effusions), improve hemodynamics, and to modulate neurohormonal activation.
  - In patients with chronic valve disease, the use of furosemide is mandatory and the addition of ACE inhibitor with or without pimobendan is recommended. There is currently no consensus on which to use first in combination with furosemide, although initiation of both agents is reasonable (at this time there are no studies that have evaluated the efficacy of the combination of an ACE inhibitor and pimobendan with furosemide). Digoxin (with or without diltiazem) is recommended to control the ventricular response rate if atrial fibrillation is present. Beta blockers should not be used.
  - In patients with symptomatic DCM, furosemide, ACE inhibitor, and pimobendan are recommended. Digoxin (with or without diltiazem) is recommended to control the ventricular response rate if atrial fibrillation is present. Beta blockers should not be introduced at this time, but may be continued if the patient is already receiving them.
  - Avoid, if possible, excessive sodium intake, beta blockers, corticosteroids, IV fluids (unless required for concurrent disease; requires careful monitoring of the respiratory rate trend).

Stage C3

- Severe or life threatening CHF
  - Treat hypoxemia, increase cardiac output, continue previous cardiac drugs (see Stage C2), and stabilize the patient in hospital with intravenous drugs.
  - Drugs for routine use: as for stage C2 plus oxygen, IV furosemide, nitroglycerin
  - Drugs for selected patients: dobutamine, nitroprusside

> **KEY POINT**
>
> Aggressive diuresis (repeated IV boluses or continuous rate infusion of furosemide) is indicated when life threatening CHF is present.

Stage D

- Refractory, chronic CHF.
  - Drugs for routine use: continue current cardiac medications as in stage C plus spironolactone, thiazides, digoxin, subcutaneous furosemide, repeated centesis for effusions, and very low sodium intake.
  - Drugs for selected patients: As per stage C3
    - For chronic valve disease, consider additional vasodilation with amlodipine or hydralazine.
    - For DCM, dobutamine (continuous rate infusion for 48 hours every 3 weeks) may be helpful.

Specific Disease Treatment

Chronic Valve Disease: Mitral Regurgitation without Congestive Heart Failure (Stage B)

- ACE inhibitor therapy is initiated when there is clinical evidence that the heart disease present has led to heart failure and activation of compensatory mechanisms (RAAS). Compensated heart failure can usually be identified with thoracic radiography. For example, the presence of pulmonary venous congestion with left atrial and ventricular enlargement in a 10-year-old Miniature Poodle with a loud left apical holosystolic Murmur secondary to MR Probably represents compensated heart failure.

- In this scenario, enalapril (0.5 mg/kg) or some other ACE inhibitor may be initiated (with pretreatment and 1-week post-treatment renal evaluations) once daily, although there is no evidence that this therapy will delay the onset of clinical signs. Some dogs with primary valve disease develop significant left atrial enlargement secondary to MR. These dogs become symptomatic (coughing) because there is compression of the left mainstem bronchus by the enlarged left atrium.
- These cases require the therapeutic efforts to be aimed at reducing the MR (vasodilation with ACE inhibitors, preload reduction with diuretics, and heart rate control with digoxin) and suppressing the cough reflex (butorphanol or hydrocodone). Coughing in these patients often becomes refractory to medical therapy.

Chronic Valve Disease with Symptomatic Congestive Heart Failure (Stage C)

- Decompensated heart failure usually leads to the clinical signs of moderate CHF. The earliest signs of decompensation are usually not noticed by the pet's owner. Elevated respiratory rates during rest (tachypnea) may be mistaken for panting, and are often overlooked. Tachypnea is associated with the onset of interstitial (stage II) pulmonary edema.
- In addition to tachypnea, dogs with moderate CHF may also exhibit exercise intolerance or coughing. Again, thoracic radiography can reveal the presence of interstitial pulmonary edema (increased interstitial pattern, enlarged pulmonary veins with fuzzy, indistinct borders, and concurrent left atrial and ventricular enlargement) as well as bronchial compression, if present.
- The appropriate therapy for this patient includes ACE inhibitor therapy (**enalapril** 0.5 mg/kg PO twice a day), **furosemide** (2 to 4 mg/kg PO two or three times a day), with or without **pimobendan** (0.25 mg/kg PO every 12 hours on an empty stomach). Digoxin is usually initiated if:
  - Myocardial failure is present
  - Atrial fibrillation or other supraventricular tachycardia is present
  - Therapy with ACE inhibitors, pimobendan and diuretics has not produced an adequate response.
- The resting respiratory rate can be used to monitor the response to therapy. A trend of decreasing resting respiratory rate indicates adequate preload reduction. Once the respiratory rate has stabilized in the normal range (usually less than 30 breaths per minute), the diuretic dose is tapered down to the lowest dose capable of controlling the signs of CHF.
- A trend of increasing resting respiratory rate suggests worsening of the pulmonary edema and the need for higher dosages of diuretics or the addition of other medications such as intermittent nitrate therapy (nitroglycerin ¼ to 1 inch cutaneously every 8 to 12 hours). Beware of nitroglycerine tolerance as described previously.

Chronic Valve Disease with Symptomatic Congestive Heart Failure (Stage C3)

- Dogs with severe CHF secondary to primary valve disease are symptomatic at rest and may require aggressive therapy to control pulmonary edema. These patients typically require relatively high doses of furosemide as well as optimized doses of ACE inhibitor and pimobendan.
- If the patient is dyspneic, hospitalization is indicated to provide oxygen therapy in addition to close monitoring and parenteral administration of furosemide. Adjunctive therapy with nitroglycerin is also indicated.
- Thoracocentesis may be necessary if pleural effusion is present. Furosemide (2 to 4 mg/kg IV) is administered, and the respiratory rate is monitored for a trend of decreasing respiratory rate. If no decline in respiratory rate is observed within 1 to 2 hours, furosemide is again administered at the same or a slightly higher dose. The respiratory rate is again monitored, and the preceding is repeated if there is no improvement. As the respiratory rate decreases, the dosage and frequency of administration are reduced to the lowest dose effective in controlling the pulmonary edema. Pretreatment evaluation of renal function and hydration status aids in selecting the appropriate furosemide dose.
- In the presence of refractory, severe, chronic CHF, the addition of spironolactone with or without a thiazide to conventional therapy may help control edema formation. Furthermore, intermittent therapy with nitrates, such as nitroglycerin or isosorbide dinitrate, may also aid in reducing ventricular filling pressures and the formation of edema.

Mild Heart Failure Secondary to Dilated Cardiomyopathy (Stage B)

- The presence of ventricular ectopy, chamber dilation, or evidence of myocardial failure (reduced fractional shortening percentage and increased mitral valve E-point septal separation), particularly in dogs that are predisposed to idiopathic DCM (e.g., Doberman Pinschers and others), suggests a diagnosis of occult DCM.

- Although these dogs are usually asymptomatic, they often have progressive heart failure. ACE inhibitor therapy (enalapril 0.5 mg PO once or twice a day or benazepril 0.25 mg PO once a day) can be initiated in these dogs in an attempt to prolong the asymptomatic phase of the disease course.
- Beta-adrenergic blocking agents may also be indicated in these patients.
- Digoxin and/or pimobendan therapy is also indicated in patients with myocardial failure, however therapy is usually not initiated unless CHF is present. Some Spaniel breeds (American Cocker Spaniels) may develop DCM secondary to taurine deficiency. Therefore, plasma taurine levels should be evaluated and taurine supplementation instituted (500 mg PO twice a day) if indicated.

Moderate Heart Failure Secondary to Dilated Cardiomyopathy with Symptomatic Congestive Heart Failure (Stage C)

- As heart failure progresses, filling pressures eventually become elevated and pulmonary edema may develop.
- The therapeutic protocol in this patient is essentially the same as that for a patient with moderate heart failure secondary to MR. The only difference is that pimobendan and/or digoxin is initiated earlier in the disease course of cardiomyopathy.
- Conventional therapy for this patient with symptomatic heart failure consists of an ACE inhibitor, furosemide, and pimobendan. These patients frequently have cardiac rhythm disturbances that may be associated with symptoms or may be aggravating the CHF. In this scenario, antiarrhythmic therapy is indicated (e. g., digoxin with or without diltiazem to control the ventricular response to atrial fibrillation). Antiarrhythmic therapy is typically not indicated in patients with arrhythmias that are not associated with clinical signs of reduced cardiac output and poor tissue perfusion.

Severe Heart Failure Secondary to Dilated Cardiomyopathy (Stage C3)

- Aggressive therapy is indicated in patients with severe symptomatic heart failure. Oxygen therapy, ACE inhibitors, pimobendan, furosemide, and, possibly, dobutamine and nitroprusside may be necessary to control pulmonary edema in life-threatening heart failure.
- Furosemide (up to 6 to 8 mg/kg IV) may be given every 1 to 2 hours until the resting respiratory rate is decreasing. Then administer furosemide (2 to 4 mg/kg IV) every 4 to 8 hours, depending on the status of the patient. The goal is to taper the dose to the lowest effective dose and the frequency of administration to two to three times a day as quickly as possible.
- If intravenous dobutamine/nitroprusside therapy is necessary to control the symptoms of heart failure, the nitroprusside dose should be adjusted to decrease mean or systolic arterial blood pressure by 15 to 30 mm Hg. The long-term survival of dogs with severe, life-threatening heart failure is poor.

Feline Cardiomyopathy (Dilated Cardiomyopathy, Restrictive Cardiomyopathy, and Hypertrophic Cardiomyopathy)

- The medical approach for the feline with cardiomyopathy is based on the type of cardiomyopathy present and the presence of symptoms (i.e., symptomatic CHF). Evaluation of the patient with electrocardiography, thoracic radiography, and echocardiography usually enables the clinician to characterize the cardiomyopathy as being associated with myocardial systolic failure (DCM and, sometimes, restrictive cardiomyopathy [RCM]) or diastolic dysfunction (hypertrophic cardiomypathy [HCM] and RCM).
- In general, cats with primary systolic dysfunction are symptomatic at diagnosis. These cats receive combinations of digoxin (a fourth of a 0.125 mg tablet PO once a day or every other day, with dose adjustment based on trough serum levels about 2 weeks after initiation of therapy), enalapril (1 to 2 mg PO every other day to twice a day for cats depending on renal status), and furosemide (6.25 to 12.5 mg PO once or twice a day).
- There seems to be an increased risk of intracardiac thrombus formation if marked left atrial enlargement is present. In this scenario, aspirin (25 mg/kg PO every 3 days) or warfarin sodium (Coumadin) can be initiated. The initial dose for warfarin is 0.5 mg every 24 hours for a 3- to 5-kg cat, monitored with either prothrombin time (PT), activated partial thromboplastin time, or proteins induced by vitamin K antagonists. Anticoagulants (warfarin-based products) may be more effective at preventing thromboembolic episodes when compared with antiplatelet agents such as aspirin. However, serious side effects (hemorrhage) and the need for close monitoring of bleeding times may limit their use. Furthermore, the recurrence rate for thromboembolism in cardiomyopathic

cats is high, regardless of the agent used. There is some evidence that Plavix (clopidogrel; 18.75 mg PO every 24 hours) may prevent thrombus formation in cats at risk of intracardiac thrombus formation. Low-molecular-weight heparins such as dalteparin (Fragmin; 100 U/kg subcutaneously every 24 hours) or enoxaparin (Lovonox; 1 to 1.5 mg/kg subcutaneously every 12 to 24 hours) may also have beneficial effects in cats at risk. However, these dosages have largely been borrowed from the human literature and specific dosages have not been established in cats.

- Cats with HCM may be completely asymptomatic or may present with tachypnea and dyspnea associated with decompensated diastolic heart failure.
- There is some controversy as to which agent is the drug of choice in cats with diastolic dysfunction. Calcium channel blockers (diltiazem) and beta blockers (atenolol) facilitate diastolic function, but in different ways. Beta blockers probably facilitate diastolic function only by decreasing the heart rate and myocardial oxygen consumption. Calcium channel blockers facilitate diastolic function by improving myocardial relaxation through normalization of abnormal myocardial calcium currents as well as by coronary vasodilation to improve myocardial perfusion.
- In asymptomatic cats with HCM, the therapy is based on the presence of tachycardia, dynamic left ventricular outflow obstruction, and the severity of concentric hypertrophy and left atrial enlargement. If tachycardia (heart rate more than 200 beats per minute), dynamic left ventricular outflow obstruction, and marked hypertrophy are present, therapy with a beta blocker is initiated (atenolol 6.25 to 12.5 mg PO once or twice a day). Beta blockers appear to be more effective than calcium channel blockers in controlling the heart rate in tachycardic cats. Additionally, beta blockers are probably more effective in reducing the dynamic outflow tract obstruction seen in some cats with HCM. Beta blockers should be avoided if decompensated CHF is present.
- Tachycardia, CHF, and thromboembolism are considered to be negative prognostic indicators in cardiomyopathic cats.
- The number one priority when presented with a cat with CHF is to avoid stressing the patient with diagnostic tests such as radiographs or electrocardiograms. Cats with symptomatic heart failure typically have pulmonary edema or pleural effusion. If the cat is dyspneic, suffering from life-threatening heart failure, a thoracocentesis is performed to rule out the presence of pleural effusion. Preload reducers such as furosemide (1 to 4 mg/kg IM or IV every 3 to 4 hours) and topical 2 % nitroglycerin (¼ to ½ inch every 8 hours) are usually effective in reducing filling pressures, therefore facilitating the resolution of the pulmonary edema. The dosing frequency and dosage of furosemide are reduced once clinical improvement is noted, as evidenced by a reduction in resing respiratory rate.
- In addition to preload reducers, an agent to improve diastolic function (beta blocker or calcium channel blocker) may be used. Caution should be exercised when administering beta blockers to patients with severe CHF and possible myocardial failure. Oxygen therapy is also indicated.
- The medical management of feline RCM is similar to the therapy for DCM because systolic dysfunction is usually present in both. Combinations of enalapril, digoxin, and furosemide are currently recommended.

Pericardial Disease

- The management of chronic pericardial effusion and cardiac tamponade is quite straightforward. An echocardiogram is performed to confirm the diagnosis of pericardial effusion and to attempt to ascertain if the underlying cause is neoplasia. If the prognosis is favorable, pericardiocentesis is performed to relieve the compression on the heart by the elevated intrapericardial pressure. If the effusion returns more than once, a pericardectomy is recommended (see Chapter 11).

Congestive Heart Failure Associated with Chronic Heartworm Disease:

- The approach to dogs with CHF associated with chronic heartworm disease involves cage rest, diuretic therapy, and heartworm adulticide therapy. These patients are cage rested a minimum of 1 week before adulticide therapy (staged melarsomine adulticide protocol). Heart failure medications (ACE inhibitors, furosemide, spironolactone, pimobendan, sildenafil) may be discontinued in some patients 4 to 8 weeks after adulticide therapy (see Chapter 10).

Frequently Asked Questions

When is activation of the SNS maladaptive to the cardiac health of the animal? Select one.

A. in a normal animal that is in a flight or fight stress response
B. in an animal with RAAS activation
C. in an animal with early heart failure
D. in an animal with chronic heart failure

D Is the correct answer.

Rationales:
A. The activation of the SNS is essential for the animal under stress. By increasing heart rate, cardiac output, and selective vasoconstriction (e.g., to gut) and vasodilation (e.g., to muscles) the animal may engage the cardiovascular system effectively to deal with an acute threat.
B. The acute activation of the SNS results in stimulation of beta-1 adrenergic receptors in the juxtaglomerular apparatus of the kidney. Angiotensin II also causes activation of the SNS so these two systems are closely intertwined, not maladaptive.
C. Early activation of the SNS in early stages of heart failure helps to maintain:

- Blood pressure
- Tissue perfusion
- Cardiac output

(How? By increasing venous return to the heart via vasoconstriction of the splanchnic vessels, vasoconstriction of other various vascular beds, and positive inotropic and chronotropic cardiac effects)
D. This is a maladaptive situation because chronic SNS overactivity produces:

- Down-regulation and desensitization of beta-1 adrenergic receptors
- Abnormal baroreflex function.
- Overloads the heart by increasing venous return
- Increases myocardial oxygen consumption (by increasing heart rate)
- Cardiac NE depletion and elevated plasma NE
- Damage to the myocardium, resulting in potential arrhythmogenesis

How are natriuretic peptide levels useful in assessment of heart disease?
Though not yet widely used, these assays may be an important addition to the diagnostic toolkit for selected heart diseases. Circulating natriuretic peptide levels may be used to differentiate between symptoms associated with cardiac disease versus primary pulmonary disease.

Natriuretic peptides are salt and water homeostasis regulators, and are involved in blood pressure control so changes in these parameters may help us to understand the stage of the cardiovascular condition. Their potential value is as diagnostic and prognostic markers in patients with CHF particularly.

Natriuretic peptide levels are elevated in many disease conditions resulting in expanded fluid volume (e.g., DCM, chronic valvular insufficiency in dogs, and cardiomyopathy in cats).

SUGGESTED READINGS

Bulmer BJ and Sisson DD: Therapy of heart failure. In Ettinger SJ ed: Textbook of veterinary internal medicine, ed 6, Philadelphia, 2005, WB Saunders.

Colucci WS, Braunwald E: Pathophysiology of heart failure. In Braunwald E, ed: Heart disease: a textbook of cardiovascular medicine, ed 5, Philadelphia, 1997, WB Saunders.

Fox PR, Sisson DD: Angiotensin-converting enzyme inhibitors. In Bonagura JD, ed: Kirk's current veterinary therapy XII, Philadelphia, 1995, WB Saunders.

Goodwin JK, Strickland KN: The emergency management of dogs and cats with congestive heart failure, Vet Med 93:818-823, 1998.

Goodwin JK, Strickland KN: The role of dietary modification and nondrug therapy in dogs and cats with congestive heart failure, Vet Med 93:919-926, 1998.

Goodwin JK, Strickland KN: Managing arrhythmias in dogs and cats with congestive heart failure, Vet Med 93:818-823, 1998.

Hamlin RL: Physiology of the failing heart. In Fox PR, Sisson D, Moise NS eds: Textbook of canine and feline cardiology: principles and clinical practice, ed 2, Philadelphia, 1999, WB Saunders.

Kelly RA, Smith TW: Drugs used in the treatment of heart failure. In Braunwald E, ed: Heart disease: a textbook of cardiovascular medicine, ed 5, Philadelphia 1997, WB Saunders.

Kittleson MD: Management of heart failure. In Kittleson MD, Kienle RD, eds: Small animal cardiovascular medicine, St Louis, 1998, Mosby.

Kittleson MD: Pathophysiology of heart failure. In Kittleson MD, Kienle RD, eds: Small animal cardiovascular medicine, St Louis, 1998, Mosby.

Sisson D, Kittleson MD: Management of heart failure: principles of treatment, therapeutic strategies, and pharmacology. In Fox PR, Sisson D, Moise NS, eds: Textbook of canine and feline cardiology: principles and clinical practice, ed 2, Philadelphia, 1999, WB Saunders.

Smith TW, Kelly RA, Stevenson LW, Braunwald E: Management of heart failure. In Braunwald E, ed: Heart disease: a textbook of cardiovascular medicine, ed 5, Philadelphia, 1997, WB Saunders.

Strickland KN: Advances in antiarrhythmic therapy. In Goodwin JK, ed: Advances in cardiovascular diagnostics and therapy, Vet Clin North Am Small Anim Pract, 28:1515-1546, 1998.

Strickland KN: Canine and feline caval syndrome, Clin Tech Small Anim Pract 13:88-95, 1998.

Strickland KN: Management of chronic congestive heart failure, Vet Med 93:913-919, 1998.

CHAPTER 16

Treatment of Cardiac Arrhythmias and Conduction Disturbances

Marc S. Kraus, Anna R. M. Gelzer, and Sydney Moise

INTRODUCTION TO TREATMENT OF CARDIAC ARRHYTHMIAS

Cardiac arrhythmias are defined as variations of the cardiac rhythm from normal sinus rhythm. Some cardiac arrhythmias are benign and clinically insignificant and require no specific therapy whereas other arrhythmias may cause severe clinical signs such as syncope or degenerate into malignant arrhythmias (i.e., ventricular fibrillation [VF]) leading to cardiac arrest and sudden death. The goal of this section is to discuss treatment strategies for management of arrhythmias.

General Remarks

Antiarrhythmic drugs commonly target two general areas of the heart due to their specific electrophysiologic properties:

- Sinoatrial and Atrioventricular (AV) nodal tissue: Depolarization is calcium channel driven. To treat arrhythmias that originate from the sinoatrial and AV nodal tissue calcium channel blockers (CCB) and beta blockers (BBs) are primarily used. The most commonly prescribed CCB for treatment of arrhythmias is diltiazem (available PO and IV). The beta-1 selective BB atenolol and esmolol (IV only) are the most frequently used antiarrhythmic BB. Digoxin has a vagomimetic effect and can therefore indirectly prolong AV node conduction time. Its antiarrhythmic application is limited to the treatment of atrial fibrillation (AF). For drug dosages consult Table 16-1 and Table 16-2.
- Atrial or ventricular myocardium: Depolarization is sodium channel gated and repolarization is potassium channel dominated. To treat arrhythmias that originate from the atrial and ventricular myocardium, Na channel blockers (NCB), K channel blocker (KCB) or combinations thereof are often used in conjunction with BBs. The NCB used for treatment of arrhythmias in dogs are lidocaine (IV only) and mexiletine and rarely procainamide. The most important KCB is sotalol, which also has BB properties. The authors also use amiodarone, which is predominantly a KCB, but also has potent NCB and some CCB and BB activity. For drug dosages consult Table 16-1 and Table 16-2.

For optimal long-term management of most arrhythmias, a 24-hour Holter recording should be acquired in addition to the electocardiogram (ECG). Even though a correct diagnosis of an arrhythmia may be obtained by a short in-hospital ECG, in some patients with an intermittent arrhythmia, the 24-hour Holter recording is required to establish a definitive diagnosis.

The decision regarding how and when to treat an arrhythmia should be based on the clinical signs and urgency of intervention. Emergency management using intravenous drugs may be required before a 24-hour Holter recording can be obtained. Both diltiazem and esmolol are available in an IV formulation, allowing emergency treatment of excessively rapid supraventricular arrhythmias (SVAs), Lidocaine is the most important intravenous drug used for life-threatening ventricular arrhythmias.

Table 16-1 Agents for Rate Control/Abolishing Arrhythmias in Canine Patients with Supraventricular Arrhythmias

Drug	Oral administration	Intravenous administration	Indication
Diltiazem XR (Dilacor)	3-4 mg/kg BID		AF, AFl, AT OAVRT
Diltiazem (Cardizem)	0.5 mg/kg TID titrated up (max 1.5-2 mg/kg TID)	0.1-0.2 mg/kg bolus, then CRI 2-6 μg/kg/min	Acute AF, AFl, OAVRT
Atenolol (Tenormin)	0.25-1 mg/kg SID to BID		AFl, AT, OAVRT
Esmolol (Brevibloc)		50-100 μg/kg bolus (repeat up to max 500 μg/kg); 50-200 μg/kg/min CRI	Acute AF, AFl, AT or OAVRT
Sotalol (Betapace)	1-2.5 mg/kg BID		AF, AFl, AT
Digoxin (Lanoxin)	0.003-0.005 mg/kg BID Liquid suspension available for small dogs Max dose for Dobermans: 0.25 mg BID		AF
Procainamide (Procain)		10-15 mg/kg IV bolus slowly over 2 minutes, if needed start a CRI: 25-50 μg/kg/min	AT
Amiodarone (Cordarone)	10 mg/kg BID for 1 week (loading dose)* 5 mg/kg SID (maintenance dose)*		AF, AT
Lidocaine		2 mg/kg IV bolus, repeat if needed	AF if due to narcotics

*Recommended dose range in veterinary medicine is anecdotal and variable.
BID, Twice a day; *AF*, atrial fibrillation; *AFl*, atrial flutter, *AT*, atrial tachycardia, *OAVRT*, orthodromic atrioventricular reciprocating tachycardia; *TID*, three times a day; *CRI*, constant-rate infusion; *SID* once daily.

- The benefits of a 24-hour Holter recording include in-depth assessment of quantity and quality of the arrhythmia(s). The following parameters should be examined: Number of abnormal beats (supraventricular and or ventricular) relative to overall number of beats, duration and rate of runs of abnormal beats; the average hourly and daily heart rate, the amount of time when the heart rate is greater than 120 or lesser than 50 bpm as well as the presence and length of pauses. A diary kept by the client or hospital staff with the sleep/wakefulness activity or observed events such as syncope or excessive anxiety or panting help correlate ECG changes on the Holter with clinical signs. These parameters are vital for a baseline evaluation of a patient's arrhythmias and needs for antiarrhythmic therapy.
- If treatment is instituted, it is critical to obtain a repeat Holter recording after 1 or 2 weeks to determine if the drugs are efficacious at suppressing the abnormal rhythms, or possibly harmful by being proarrhythmic, that is causing ventricular arrhythmias or excessive pauses. This can only be established if a comparison to the pre-drug baseline is performed.
- If a Holter shows that a drug is effective, we recommend monitoring the progression of the arrhythmia by repeat Holter recordings every 6 to 12 months. If an animal experiences recurrent syncope during that time, an immediate repeat Holter is recommended.
- In animals that need to be stabilized immediately (no time for a baseline 24-hour Holter recording prior to intravenous antiarrhythmics), it is still advised to acquire a post-treatment Holter recording to evaluate drug efficacy and possible

Table 16-2 Agents for Rate Control/Abolishing Arrhythmias in Canine Patients with Ventricular Arrhythmias

Drug	Oral administration	Intravenous administration	Indication
Sotalol (Betapace)	0.5-2 mg/kg BID		VA, VT
Mexiletine (Mexitil)	4-8 mg/kg TID		VA, VT, Usually not effective as monotherapy
Amiodarone (Cordarone)	10 mg/kg BID for 1 week (loading dose)* 5 mg/kg SID (maintenance dose)*		Refractory VA, VT
Lidocaine		2 mg/kg IV bolus, repeat 3 times, if needed start a CRI: 30-80 μg/kg/min	Life-threatening VT
Procainamide		10-15 mg/kg IV bolus slowly over 2 minutes, if needed start a CRI: 25-50 μg/kg/min	Life-threatening VT
Atenolol (Tenormin)	0.25-1 mg/kg SID to BID		VA, VT, effective only in combination with mexiletine
Esmolol (Brevibloc)		50-100 μg/kg bolus, repeat up to max 500 μg/kg) if needed start a CRI: 50-200 μg/kg/min	Life-threatening VT

*Recommended dose range in veterinary medicine is anecdotal and variable.
BID, Twice daily; *VA*, ventricular arrhythmias; *VT*, ventricular tachycardia; *TID*, three times daily; *SID,* once daily; *CRI,* continuous-rate infusion.

toxicity once the dog is stabilized and receiving chronic oral antiarrhythmic therapy.

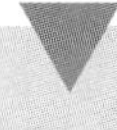

Supraventricular Arrhythmias

SVAs include rhythms that originate in the sinus node, atrial tissue and AV junction. Importantly, SVA must be differentiated from accelerated normal sinus rhythm. Physiologic sinus tachycardia can be caused by many conditions including febrile states, anemia, heart failure, adrenergic medications and anxiety. In these cases, management should foremost be focused on correcting the underlying cause or disease resulting in increased sympathetic tone.

- Because of the mechanism of action of antiarrhythmic drugs, it is useful to assess SVA as either AV node independent (does not need the AV node to sustain the rhythm) or AV node dependent (pathway requires the AV node to sustain the rhythm).
- An SVA is AV node independent, if the ECG contains P waves not conducted to the ventricle without termination of the SVA. Interventions such as vagal maneuvers or drugs that slow AV node conduction can help identify the underlying mechanism:
  - If the atrial activation rate is unchanged (PP interval the same) following the intervention, but the ventricular rate slows due to AV block, the SVA is likely AV node independent.
  - If the intervention results in abolishment of the SVA and restoration of a normal sinus rhythm (even if it is only transient), the arrhythmia is likely AV node dependent.
- Examples of AV node–independent rhythms include sinus node reentrant tachycardia, AF, AFL, and ectopic atrial tachycardia. These arrhythmias can be challenging to manage, since the antiarrhythmic drugs (NCB, KCB or combinations thereof) are often not very efficacious for suppression of these arrhythmias. If the abnormal rhythm cannot

be abolished with drugs, the secondary mode of treatment aims at controlling the ventricular response rate by slowing the AV node conduction with CCBs, BBs or digoxin.

- AV node–dependent SVAs include AV reentrant tachycardia (accessory pathway [AP] mediated) and AV nodal reentrant tachycardia. AV node–dependent arrhythmias can usually be treated with drugs that target the AV node (CCBs and BBs).

KEY POINT

To help guide treatment of SVAs, they should be characterized as AV node dependent or independent.

ATRIAL FIBRILLATION

- AF is one of the most commonly seen SVAs in veterinary practice. In dogs and cats, AF is usually a chronic arrhythmia associated with advanced stages of chronic AV valve insufficiency or cardiomyopathy. In those patients, the ventricular response rate is often markedly elevated, which contributes to the clinical signs of heart failure. AF can also occur in the absence of overt structural heart disease (lone or primary AF). In these cases, the ventricular response rate can be normal or only mildly elevated.

KEY POINT

The management of AF largely depends on the average heart rate. A baseline 24-hour Holter recording, acquired in the home environment is ideal to determine the average heart rate of a patient.

- The following flow chart (Figure 16-1) should serve to identify patients in need of treatment for AF and to decide which therapeutic approach might be best in each individual case.

Therapy

- AF is an AV node–independent arrhythmia, caused by multiple simultaneous intra-atrial reentrant circuits. Medical conversion of AF to sinus rhythm with drugs is very difficult and rarely achieved in

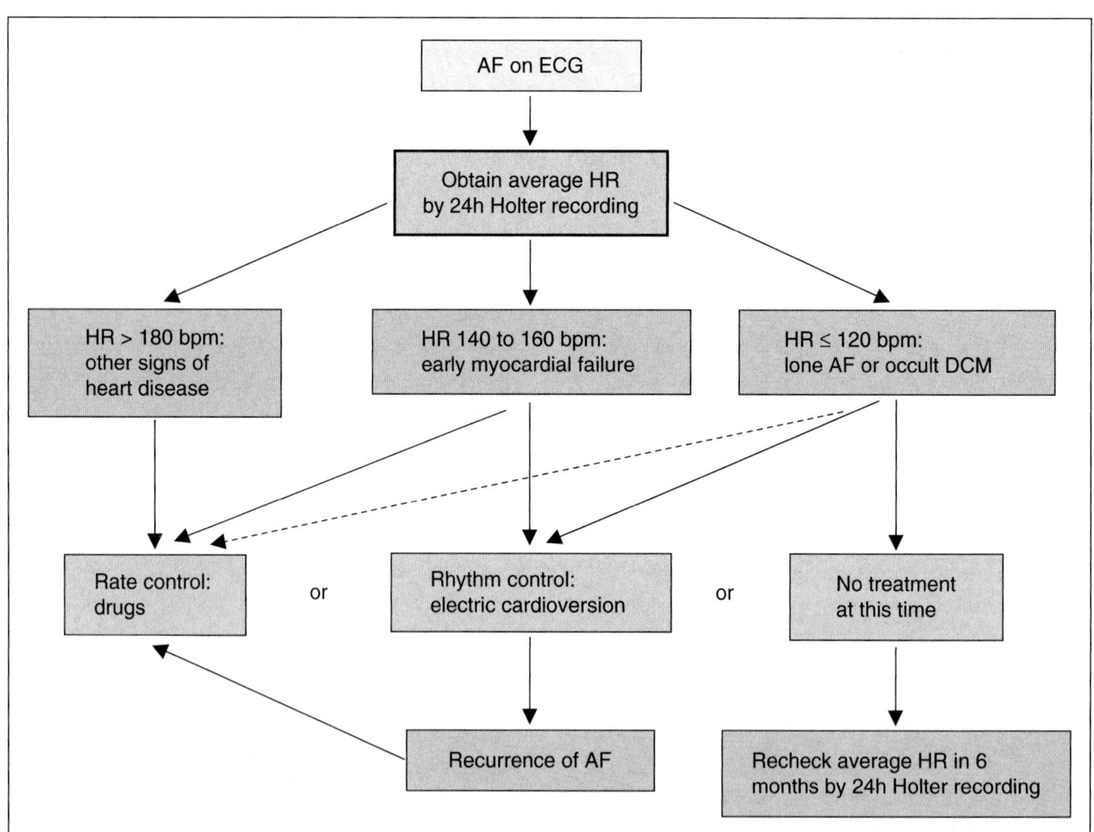

Figure 16-1. Flow chart describing the approach to treatment of atrial fibrillation *(AF)* based on the average heart rate *(HR)* of a patient as determined by a 24-hour Holter recording. *AF,* Atrial fibrillation; *HR,* heart rate; *bpm,* beats per minute; *DCM,* dilated cardiomyopathy.

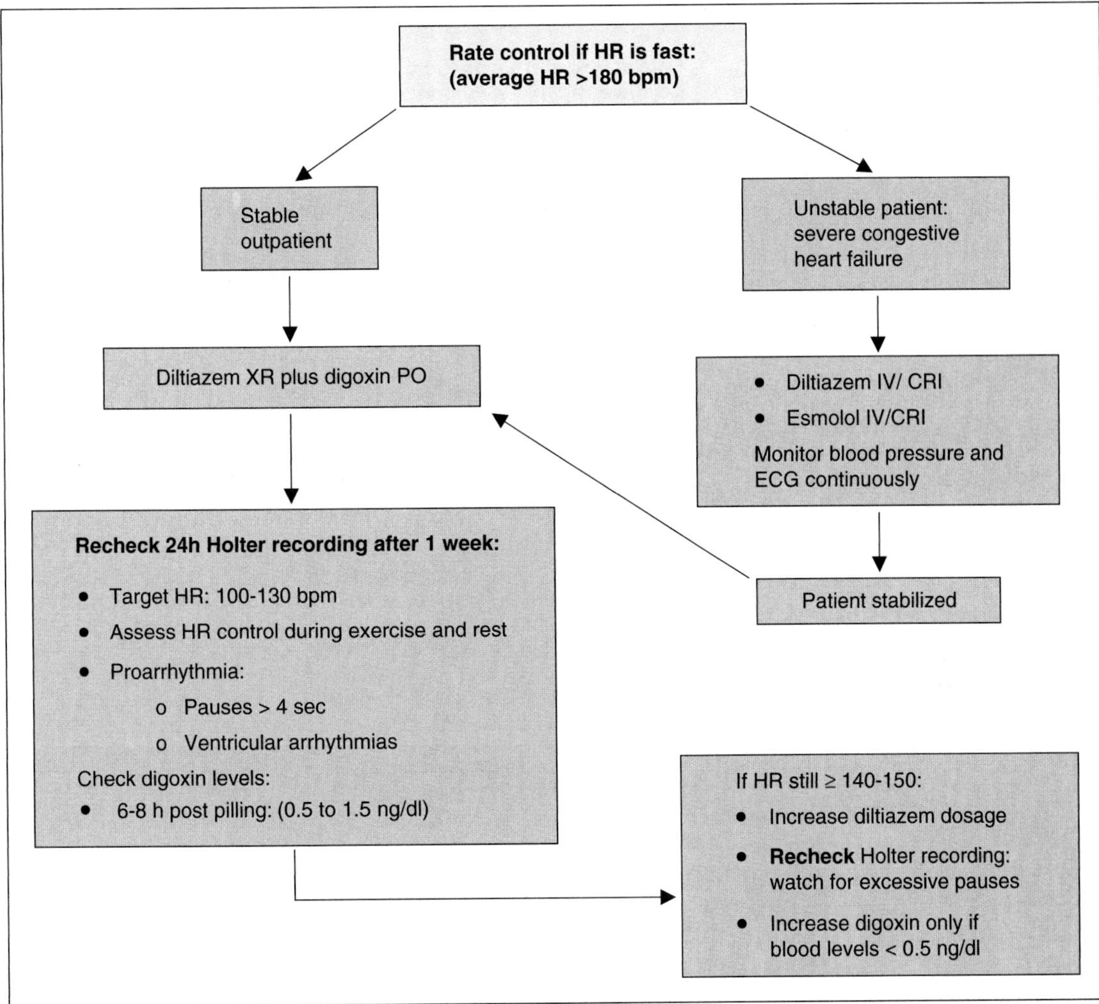

Figure 16-2. Management of dogs with AF with a fast heart rate (average heart rate > 180 bpm). *HR,* Heart rate; *bpm;* beats per minute; *CRI,* constant-rate infusion.

canine patients. In most cases, ventricular rate control via slowing of AV node conduction with diltiazem and or digoxin is the goal (drug dosages are listed in Table 16-1). The veterinary literature also cites atenolol as effective for rate control of AF. The authors do not have much personal experience with atenolol for this purpose. The reluctance to use atenolol for rate control stems in part from the concomitant degree of advanced myocardial failure in many patients with AF. In our experience diltiazem XR is very well tolerated even in dogs with severe systolic myocardial dysfunction.

- Dogs with normal cardiac function or only mild dysfunction and normal to moderately elevated ventricular response rates may be candidates for electric cardioversion of AF to sinus rhythm.
- Medical management varies with the initial average heart rate and overall condition of the dog (Figures 16-2 through 16-4). Treatment can be tailored to the patient based on the approximate average heart rate. The authors prioritize treatment according to three general categories of ventricular response rate: (1) fast (Figure 16-2: average heart rate faster than 180 bpm), (2) moderate (Figure 16-3: average heart rate 130 to 160 bpm) and (3) slow (Figure 16-4: heart rate around 100 bpm). The dosages for the drug listed in Figures 16-2, 16-3 and 16-4 are provided in Table 16-1.
- Treatment of AF in cats is challenging. There is usually significant underlying heart disease present, resulting in markedly enlarged atria and very rapid AF. Medical management for rate control with a target heart rate of 130 to 150 bpm may be achieved using either CCB or BB (for drug dosages for antiarrhythmic drugs in cats see Table 16-3).
- Occasionally, the administration of narcotics has been associated with the induction of AF in large dogs. This is likely caused by the increased vagal

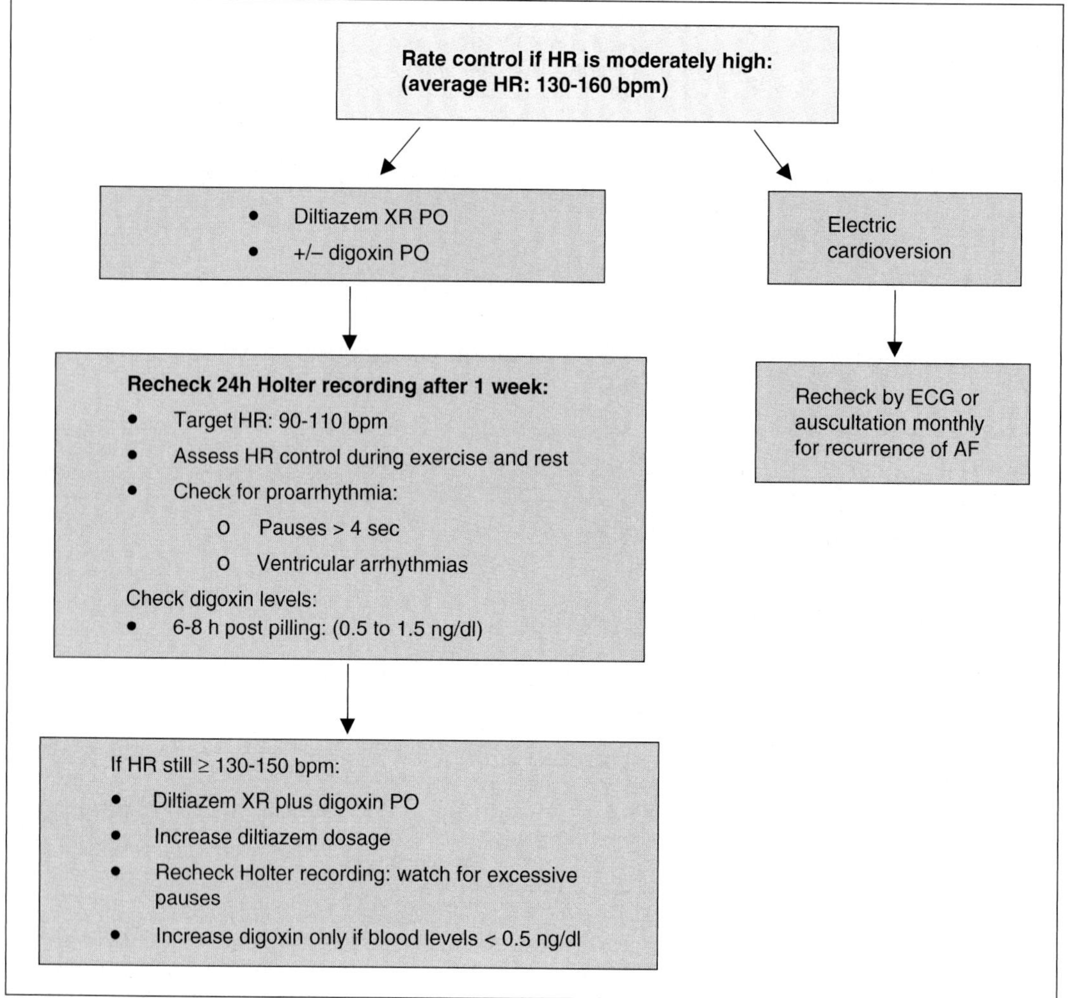

Figure 16-3. Management of dogs with AF with a moderately elevated average heart rate of 130 to 160 bpm. *HR,* Heart rate; *bpm,* beats per minute; *AF,* atrial fibrillation.

tone that occurs with narcotics. Treatment with 2 mg/kg **lidocaine** IV within 4 hours of onset has been demonstrated to restore sinus rhythm. Vagolytic drugs (atropine) should prevent onset or recurrence of AF in such cases.

> **KEY POINT**
>
> Digoxin monotherapy does not control the ventricular response rate adequately during times of excitement, stress or exercise. Thus, dogs with AF and moderate to fast heart rates will require combination therapy of digoxin with diltiazem or atenolol.

Electric Cardioversion (Rhythm Control)

In a subgroup of canine patients with mild structural heart disease or lone AF, electric cardioversion of AF to sinus rhythm can be achieved. The patients selected for this treatment are well compensated and the goal of cardioversion is to avoid structural or functional remodeling from chronic AF, even if the heart rate is slow. The rate of recurrence of AF after successful cardioversion is high and morbidity associated with repeat transthoracic cardioversions under general anesthesia make this management less practical. Pretreatment with sotalol, amiodarone or angiotensin-converting enzyme inhibitors may improve the chances of cardioversion and lessen the rate of recurrence of AF; however, no studies in veterinary medicine have proven these concepts.

Transthoracic Electrical Cardioversion Procedure

- Procedure requires a brief general anesthesia
- Fast Patch electrodes are recommended instead of hand-held paddles to optimize electrode position for cardioversion.
- Dog is shaved before application of the patch over the heart on both lateral sides of the thorax.

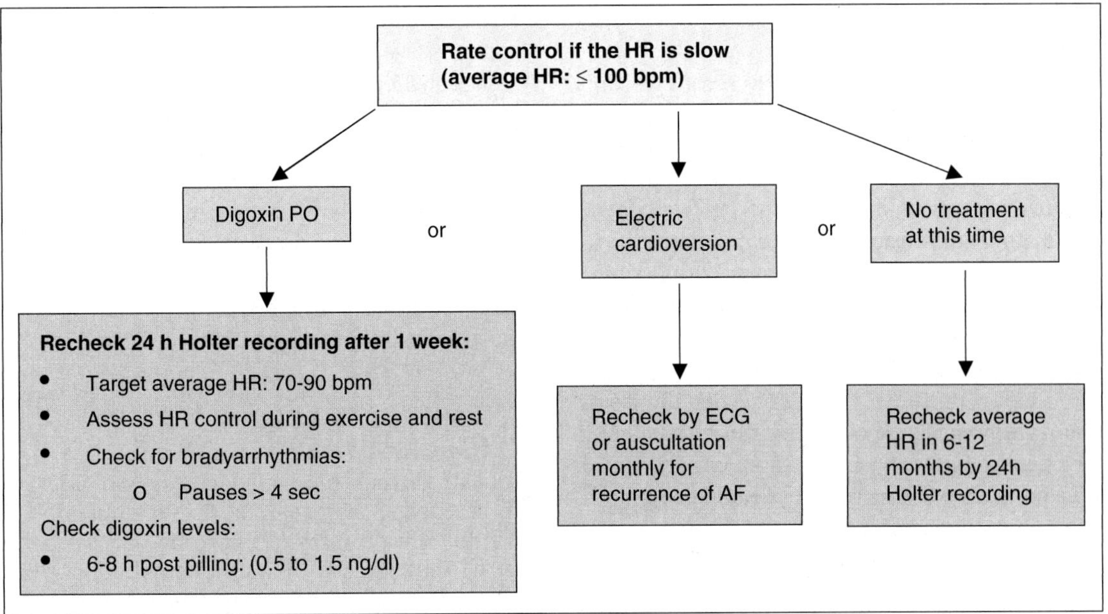

Figure 16-4. Management of dogs with AF with a low average heart rate (≤ 100 bpm). *HR*, Heart rate; *bpm*, beats per minute; *AF*, atrial fibrillation.

Table 16-3 Agents for Rate Control/Abolishing Arrhythmias in Feline Patients with Arrhythmias

Drug	Oral administration	Intravenous administration	Indication
Diltiazem XR (Dilacor®)	30-60 mg SID–BID (start with 30 mg SID)		AF, AT, accessory pathway
Diltiazem (Cardizem®)	10 mg/kg SID	0.1-0.2 mg/kg bolus, then CRI at 2-6 μg/kg/min	Acute AF, accessory pathway
Atenolol (Tenormin®)	6.25 mg-12.5mg SID–BID		AT, accessory pathway, VT
Esmolol (Brevibloc®)	NA	50-100 μg/kg bolus (repeat up to max 500 μg/kg); 50-200 μg/kg/min CRI	Acute AF, AT, accessory pathway, life-threatening VT
Sotalol (Betapace®)	⅛ of an 80 mg tablet BID*		VT
Procainamide (Procain®)	2-5 mg/kg BID–TID	10-15 mg/kg IV bolus slowly over 2 minutes or CRI at 25-50 μg/kg/min	AT, accessory pathway
Lidocaine	NA	0.25-1 mg/kg IV bolus (us with extreme caution in cats)	Life-threatening VT

*Recommended dosage range is anecdotal and variable.
SID, Once daily; *BID*, twice a day; *AF*, atrial fibrillation; *AT*, atrial tachycardia; *CRI*, continuous-rate infusion; *VT*, ventricular tachycardia; *NA*, not available.

- Dog is positioned in lateral recumbency to optimally "position" heart between the two patch electrodes.
- Defibrillator ECG cables need to record patient's ECG and synchronize to the R waves. With false synchronization to T waves (occurs if T wave is taller than the R wave) the cardioversion shock can induce VF!
- Using a monophasic defibrillator:
  - Start with 4 J/kg; If no cardioversion occurs, increase dose by 50 J and repeat until a maximum of 360 J.
- Using a biphasic defibrillator:
  - Start with 1 to 2 J/kg; If no cardioversion occurs, increase dose by 50 J and repeat until a max of 360 J.
- Short, transient runs of ventricular tachycardia (VT) or sinus pauses or AV block are common following electric cardioversion.

ATRIAL FLUTTER

- Atrial flutter (AFL) is relatively uncommon in veterinary patients. Theoretically, AFL could set the stage for development of AF due to the remodeling that occurs with continuous rapid activation of the atrial myocardium. In some patients AFL co-exists with AF on a 24-hour Holter, which might represent a transition phase to chronic AF. AFL is an AV node–independent intra-atrial macro-reentry rhythm. The atrial activation rate (PP interval) is 300 to 600 bpm. AFL is paroxysmal or chronic and can be associated with excessively high ventricular response rates. AV conduction usually changes between 1:1 and 3:1 or 2:1 due to variable degrees of AV block.
- A baseline 24-hour Holter is recommended to determine of the arrhythmia is chronic or paroxysmal. If it is chronic, drug therapy is indicated.
- If it is paroxysmal and infrequent, treatment may be postponed, but a reevaluation by Holter 6 months later should be performed to check for progression from paroxysmal to chronic AFL or presence of concurrent AF.

Drug Therapy

- Ideally, therapy is aimed at suppressing the atrial reentry circuit using sotalol, amiodarone or procainamide; however, abolishing the AFL with drugs is often unsuccessful; propafenone and flecainide are used in humans with AFL, but the authors have had little success in dogs with these drugs. The adequate dose for dogs has not been identified. Rate-control via slowing of the AV node with CCBs or BBs is used effectively in dogs (for drug dosages see Table 16-1). Digoxin monotherapy is ineffective for management of AFL.
- A post-drug 24-hour Holter should be obtained to determine if drugs are effective at suppressing the AFL or producing the desired AV block, thereby slowing the ventricular response adequately. It also allows survey for drug toxicity, manifest as bradycardia or pauses secondary to excessive AV block. Pauses, if they occur only during sleep or rest, are usually of no concern.

ECTOPIC ATRIAL TACHYCARDIA

- Atrial tachycardia (AT) occurs when ectopic foci in the atria develop the ability to fire rapidly on their own. It is an AV node–independent arrhythmia. Ectopic AT is often paroxysmal and may display a gradual onset and offset (warm-up and cool-down period) if the underlying mechanism involves abnormal automaticity. The heart rate can vary from 150 to 300 bpm and can cause anxiety or panting in affected dogs. In cats ectopic AT is rare.
- A baseline 24-hour Holter should be obtained to determine what percentage of time a dog is in AT, and how fast the heart rate is during the AT.

Therapy

- Ideally, suppression of the rapidly firing atrial focus is attempted by using sotalol, amiodarone or procainamide. In people, propafenone is used for treatment of AT, but we have not found these agents efficacious in our patients. In fact, targeting the abnormal rhythm directly with these drugs is often unsuccessful. Thus, as a second choice, therapy for AT should be aimed at slowing AV node conduction with CCBs or BBs to reduce the ventricular response. Digoxin is ineffective for management of AT.
- A post-drug 24-hour Holter should be obtained to determine if drugs are effective at suppressing the AT or producing the desired AV block, thus slowing the ventricular response adequately. The Holter also allows survey for excessive AV block; this may be undesired if it occurs other than during rest or sleep.

KEY POINT

Although amiodarone is a potent antiarrhythmic drug, its benefits must be balanced against its slow onset to action and adverse effects which include hepatic toxicity, gastrointestinal disturbances and blood dyscrasias in canine patients.

ATRIOVENTRICULAR NODAL REENTRANT TACHYCARDIA

- Atrioventricular nodal reentry tachycardia (AVNRT) is a form of micro-reentry within the AV node that gives rise to rapid, simultaneous activation of the ventricles and atria. AVNRT is AV node dependent, thus AV node slowing medication may terminate the arrhythmia. The prevalence in dogs is likely very low, but definitive diagnosis requires intracardiac mapping studies to prove dual AV node physiology.
- For treatment of AVNRT see the following discussion of treatment of atrioventricular reentrant tachycardia (AVRT).

ATRIOVENTRICULAR REENTRANT TACHYCARDIA

- AVRT is a macro-reentry arrhythmia whose circuit comprises the AV node as well as an AP that can conduct impulses from the atria to the ventricles directly, thereby bypassing the AV node and His-Purkinje system. Response to a vagal maneuver or intravenous drug challenge may be used to confirm its AV node–dependent properties. One-to-one AV association is a requisite of AVRT because the atria and ventricles are both integral parts of the arrhythmia circuit. If AV dissociation occurs spontaneously without termination of the SVA, AV reentrant tachycardia can be excluded.
- AVRT is a paroxysmal, intermittent SVA and 24-hour Holter may be required to make a definitive diagnosis of this SVA, as well as determine its clinical significance. Animals with AVRT may be asymptomatic, or present with syncope, episodic weakness or lethargy.
- In dogs the arrhythmia most commonly follows a pattern of orthodromic conduction through the AV node (from atria down to the ventricles) and retrograde over the AP back up to the atria, implying that the AP is only able to conduct in one direction (concealed conduction). This form is prevalent in Labrador Retrievers and termed *orthodromic AV reciprocating tachycardia* or *orthodromic AV reciprocating tachycardia.*
- Most APs in dogs do not allow conduction in the antegrade direction (concealed conduction) and are therefore not identifiable during normal sinus rhythm. In cats with AVRT however, the AP may conduct in both directions, such that ventricular pre-excitation is present during normal sinus rhythm. Pre-excitation occurs, when the atrial depolarization travels through both the AV node as well as the AP, which allows rapid, early activation of the ventricles. The ECG morphology of a P wave slurring directly into the upstroke of the QRS complex (delta wave) is a distinct feature of AP. Presence of delta waves may create the appearance of wide-complex tachycardia and thus resemble VT.

Therapy

- Treatment with oral diltiazem or atenolol is the first choice for suppression of AVRT or AVNRT in dogs and cats. For acute management intravenous diltiazem or esmolol is effective. For refractory cases in dogs sotalol, procainamide or amiodarone may be added, because they slow conduction the atria, APs and ventricles.
- To determine if antiarrhythmic therapy of intermittent AVRT or AVNRT is effective, a post-drug 24-hour Holter should be compared to the baseline 24-hour Holter. This Holter also allows to check for excessive AV block; this may be undesired if it occurs other than during rest or sleep.
- Some dogs with orthodromic AV reciprocating tachycardia display antegrade conduction over the AP (pre-excitation) and display a delta wave on surface ECG after antiarrhythmic drug administration.
- In severely affected dogs drug therapy may be ineffective. In such cases cure may be achieved using transvenous catheter ablation of the AP using radiofrequency energy. This procedure can only be performed at specialized electrophysiology laboratories, available at very few veterinary referral centers.

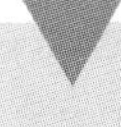

Bradyarrhythmias and Conduction Disturbances

The bradyarrhythmias that require treatment are usually due to sinus node dysfunction (e.g., sinus bradycardia or sick sinus syndrome), atrial conduction disturbances causing atrial standstill or AV node conduction abnormalities causing high grade second- or third-degree AV block. Ventricular conduction disturbances such as left and right bundle branch block as well as left anterior fascicular block do not warrant treatment, per se.

SINUS BRADYCARDIA

- Sinus bradycardia is diagnosed when the sinus node discharge rate is low (< 50 bpm) in an awake dog. Sinus bradycardia of 45 to 60 bpm during sleep is normal. Sinus bradycardia can exist in the form of a pronounced sinus arrhythmia or regular sinus bradycardia. This pathologic bradycardia often persists during excitement or exercise. The bradycardia is either primary, which is a form of sick sinus syndrome (see next section) or secondary to an underlying systemic disease or drug toxicity (e.g., narcotics or overdosing of BBs, CCBs, or digoxin).

- Secondary sinus bradycardia is usually caused by excessive vagal tone elicited by a systemic disease. Central nervous system disease (increased intracranial or intraocular pressure or head trauma), severe pain, or respiratory or gastrointestinal disease can all cause increased vagal tone and sinus bradycardia. A vagal maneuver (e.g., carotid sinus massage) can cause transient sinus bradycardia by the same mechanism of action. Correction of the underlying condition or discontinuation of drugs will usually resolve secondary sinus bradycardia.
- Clinical signs may be absent (incidental finding) or dogs may display weakness, exercise intolerance or syncope. A 24-hour Holter may be required to determine the severity of bradycardia and possible association of clinical signs with the slow heart rate. Mild exercise intolerance is often underrecognized by owners and mistakenly attributed to "old age."
- In cats, sinus rhythm at less than 120 bpm can be considered bradycardia, and heart rates below 100 bpm are often associated with lethargy or syncope in cats.

Treatment

- The decision to treat sinus bradycardia should be based on clinical signs and the degree of bradycardia. In patients experiencing syncope or episodic weakness, pacemaker therapy is indicated.
- In an animal with no clinical signs, sinus bradycardia may be "waited out" with close monitoring.
- If the animal appears unstable and pacemaker therapy is not an option, medical therapy aimed at abolishing high vagal tone can be attempted for temporary support. An atropine response test may help identify patients that would benefit from such medical management. Following injection of **atropine** 0.02 mg/kg (0.01 to 0.04) IM or IV, the baseline heart rate should increase by 50% to 100% within 5 to 10 minutes (initial worsening of AV block is a normal transient response). Patients experiencing at least a partial response to atropine may be candidates for medical management of sinus bradycardia. Treatment options include either a combination of a vagolytic drug (e.g., **probantheline bromide**: Pro-Banthine 0.25 to 0.5 mg/kg PO twice a day) and a sympathomimetic (e.g., **albuterol**: Proventil 0.02 to 0.05 mg/kg PO two to three times a day) or a phosphodiesterase inhibitor (e.g.,**theophylline**; Theo-Dur 20 mg/kg PO twice a day).
- In the authors' experience, erratic and poor efficacy as well as adverse effects such as anxiety, excessive panting, anorexia or gastrointestinal signs are significant disadvantages to these therapies; therefore, we usually do not prescribe these drugs in our clinic.

SICK SINUS SYNDROME

- The spontaneous sinus node discharge is either slower than normal (primary sinus bradycardia) or intermittently absent (sinus arrest or exit block from the sinus node). In the latter, there are pauses of various durations without P waves or an escape rhythm. The subsidiary pacemaker tissue (AV node and Purkinje fibers) is often also abnormal, resulting in inadequate escape rhythms, such that complete asystole (pauses) can last up to 10 seconds. Miniature Schnauzers, Cocker Spaniels, West Highland White Terriers and Dachshunds are over-represented. Doberman Pinschers are also reported to have syncope associated with long sinus pauses, suggestive of sick sinus syndrome (SSS).
- Clinical signs range from exercise intolerance and lethargy to syncope. Dogs with SSS manifest as primary sinus bradycardia typically show only mild exercise intolerance, which is often underrecognized by owners and mistakenly attributed to "old age." SSS may be incidentally diagnosed during a routine pre-anesthesia workup in a geriatric dog. If these dogs are treated with a pacemaker, owners often are delighted by the return of youth and energy in their "old dogs."
- Due to the intermittent nature of the sinus pauses in some cases, a 24-hour Holter is often necessary to definitively determine the cause of clinical signs.

Treatment

- Pacemaker therapy is indicated for syncopal or lethargic dogs with SSS. In dogs with intact AV node function, transvenous placement of a pacing lead in the right atrium or auricle can successfully abolish the sinus pauses. In dogs with concomitant AV node dysfunction, the lead should be placed in the right ventricle or dual chamber pacing performed.
- Some cases have brady-tachy syndrome, where in addition to the sinus pauses, supraventricular tachyarrhythmias (e.g., atrial tachycardia, flutter or fibrillation) are present. In such cases a 24-hour Holter should be obtained to determine

the clinical relevance of the SVA and requirement for antiarrhythmic therapy. Antiarrhythmic therapy may be necessary if the SVA persists post pacemaker implantation. In many cases, SVA spontaneously resolves once the long sinus pauses are prevented by the pacemaker.

- If the animal does not have syncope and shows either no or only mild clinical signs, medical management can be attempted (see medical treatment of sinus bradycardia).
- However, many of the mild forms of SSS tend to progress over weeks or months to the point of syncope, and pacemaker implantation will eventually be required.
- It is the authors' experience that medical management is ineffective in dogs with syncope and pacemaker therapy is always recommended.

ATRIAL STANDSTILL

- Atrial standstill occurs when the atrial myocardium is not able to depolarize, and P waves cannot be identified on the surface ECG. The two main causes are (1) persistent atrial standstill or "silent atrium" due to primary atrial muscle disease and (2) secondary atrial standstill caused by hyperkalemia (i.e., renal failure, ruptured bladder, Addisons' disease, or other electrolyte imbalances). Hyperkalemia alters atrial transmembrane resting potential and the atria become inexcitable at very high plasma K^+ levels. Atrial standstill is uncommon in dogs and exceedingly rare in cats.

Therapy

- If atrial muscle disease is causing atrial standstill, pacemaker therapy is required. Because the atria are structurally abnormal, the pacing lead has to be placed in the right ventricle. Unfortunately, the primary cardiac muscle disease progressively affects the ventricles. Within 1 to 2 years, ventricular myocardial dysfunction and significant AV valve regurgitation may develop and pacemaker failure may ensue due to lack of capture.
- For atrial standstill secondary to hyperkalemia, emergency therapy according to the severity of the hyperkalemia and bradycardia is required. Intravenous fluids are the primary treatment. This will lower potassium values by dilution and increased excretion. Acceptable fluids include normal saline, half-strength saline with 2.5% dextrose, or 5% dextrose in water. Alternatively, potassium can be lowered by promoting entry of K ions back into the intracellular space. The dextrose in fluid therapy will lead to insulin secretion that will drive potassium back into the cells. More aggressive therapy involves intravenous **sodium bicarbonate** (1 to 2 mEq/kg IV slowly over 20 minutes) to drive K back into the cell. Alternatively, slow intravenous administration of 0.5 U/kg of regular insulin coupled with 2 g of dextrose per unit of insulin can be administered. Monitoring for hypoglycemia post treatment is required. **Calcium gluconate** (0.5 to 1 ml/kg of a 10% solution) may be given by very slow intravenous administration for refractory cases of hyperkalemia. This is "cardioprotective" because the increased extracellular Ca^{2+} makes more sodium channels available for activation.

ATRIOVENTRICULAR (AV) CONDUCTION ABNORMALITIES

AV Block, First Degree

- Prolonged conduction time through the AV node, results in an increased PR interval of 0.13 second in dogs and 0.09 second in cats. There are normal P waves and QRS complexes, conducting at a 1:1 ratio. No treatment is required

AV Block, Second Degree

- There are normal P wave and QRS complexes with a constant PR interval, but intermittently P waves are not followed by QRS complexes. In Mobitz type I (Wenckebach) AV block, the PR interval gradually prolongs before a P wave is blocked. This form of second-degree AV block is less frequent in dogs. Mobitz type II AV block demonstrates a consistent PR interval prior to a blocked P wave. Mobitz type II AV block may represent a more advanced degree of conduction abnormality that occurs in the AV junction, His bundle, or below. Occasional single blocked P waves are of no clinical significance.
- In "high grade" second-degree AV block, there are several consecutive blocked P waves. Clinical signs depend on the length of ventricular asystole. In cases with intermittent high grade second-degree AV block, a 24-hour Holter may be required to make a definitive diagnosis. If clinical signs such as lethargy or syncope are observed, pacemaker therapy is indicated.

AV Block, Complete or Third Degree

- None of the P waves conduct through the AV node, thus the atrial and ventricular activities are independent. The atrial rate (PP interval) is faster than the ventricular (escape) rate differentiating complete AV block from AV dissociation due to accelerated idioventricular rhythms. The ventricular escape rhythm is usually regular and below 40 bpm, whereas a low AV junctional escape rhythm has a rate of 40 to 60 bpm in dogs. In cats with complete AV block the ventricular escape rhythm varies from 60 to 100 bpm.

- Complete AV block is a primary abnormality of the AV conducting system (AV node). However, it is important to evaluate the animal's electrolyte and acid-base status. Systemic diseases causing hyperkalemia such as Addison's disease or urethral obstruction can cause AV block that is reversible with normalization of K levels.
- In cats hyperthyroidism can cause significant AV node disease, which may or may not be reversible with normalization of thyroid levels. Third-degree AV block is often not as life threatening in cats as in dogs, and cats with collapse episodes may live for longer than 1 year without pacemaker implantation. They often succumb to other systemic diseases or structural heart disease rather than the actual bradyarrhythmia

Treatment of Complete AV Block

- If no underlying abnormalities are discovered, a permanent cardiac pacemaker is the only effective treatment. Ideally, pacing systems that allow sensing of P waves in the atria and subsequent pacing of the ventricles are used (i.e., dual-chamber or single lead atrial sensing-ventricular pacing systems).

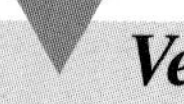

Ventricular Arrhythmias

General Remarks

Ventricular arrhythmias may occur in structurally normal hearts (hereditary arrhythmias) or may be a consequence of myocardial abnormalities associated with cardiomyopathy, significant valvular disease or myocarditis. To date, there is no medical therapy available that is known to prevent sudden death in animals afflicted with ventricular tachyarrhythmias. However, clinical signs such as syncope or episodic weakness can be alleviated in some animals with appropriate medical therapy. Clinically important ventricular arrhythmias are most commonly identified in certain breeds such as Boxers with arrhythmogenic right ventricular cardiomyopathy (ARVC), Doberman Pinschers and Great Danes with dilated cardiomyopathy (DCM), and German Shepherds with inherited ventricular arrhythmias. Dogs with congenital heart disease, such as severe subaortic or pulmonic stenosis are predisposed to development of ventricular arrhythmias, likely due to abnormal myocardial perfusion secondary to myocardial hypertrophy. These arrhythmias can be worse during exercise and may be exacerbated during cardiac catheterization for angiography or interventional therapy. Catheter contact with the endocardium can elicit ventricular arrhythmias and even cause VF.

Furthermore, significant ventricular arrhythmias can be seen in any dog hit by a car (traumatic myocarditis), large breed dogs with gastric torsion or dogs with neoplasia involving the myocardium. However, in many patients with ventricular arrhythmias a cause can not be identified.

TREATMENT OF VENTRICULAR TACHYCARDIA

- VT is recognized by abnormally wide and bizarre QRS complex morphology. P waves are present but may be hiding in the QRS-T complexes. AV dissociation occurs due to the accelerated ventricular rate as compared to the sinus rate. VT can be monomorphic (where each QRS complex is identical) or polymorphic (where the QRS complexes are constantly variable). Rapid, polymorphic VT is considered the most unstable arrhythmia, because it is most likely to degenerate into VF.
- From a treatment perspective it is also important to differentiate between "fast" VT (170 to 350 bpm) and "slow" VT (rate 80 to 160 bpm).
- Fast VT causes significantly reduced cardiac output and clinical signs depend on the duration of the episode of abnormal rhythm. Affected animals may experience syncope or weakness or sudden death, or no signs at all. It warrants antiarrhythmic therapy either to convert the arrhythmia to sinus rhythm or at least to slow down the rate of the VT or reduce the length of the runs.
- Slow VT may be unrelated to structural cardiac disease but associated with underlying systemic disease or can occur transiently after a gastric dilatation-volvulus or hit-by-car (traumatic myocarditis). It often does not require antiarrhythmic treatment. Instead supportive care and monitoring of the underlying condition is imperative; however, if affected animals show signs of hypotension or lethargy, then they may benefit from treatment of slow VT.

- A baseline 24-hour Holter is essential prior to initiation of therapy of VT to determine the percentage of ventricular ectopic beats and the duration and rate of runs of VT as well as the presence and length of pauses. A diary kept by the client or hospital staff documenting the activity of a dog and the exact time of observed syncope can help correlate ECG changes on the Holter with clinical signs.
- This information is critical both to institute suitable antiarrhythmic therapy and to assess drug efficacy by comparison of a post-treatment Holter to the baseline Holter.
- Cats with severe forms of cardiomyopathy, hyperthyroidism, sepsis, neoplasia, and severe electrolyte imbalances may develop ventricular arrhythmias. Clinical signs depend on duration and rate of the VT, but may include lethargy or syncope if the rate is > 250 bpm.

Acute Intravenous Antiarrhythmic Therapy (see Tables 16-2 and 16-3 for drug dosages)

- For treatment of acute, life-threatening VT intravenous lidocaine is the first choice. Up to 3 bolus injections can be repeated and if effective a continuous-rate infusion should be instituted. A lidocaine bolus can causes a transient drop in blood pressure and can lead to vomiting or seizures. If serum potassium levels are too low, lidocaine may not be effective. Lidocaine should be used judiciously for life-threatening VT in cats due to their low threshold for seizures with this drug.
- If the lidocaine is not successful at restoring sinus rhythm or slowing of the VT, then procainamide IV can be added or administered instead. Procainamide is given initially as a slow bolus, followed by a constant rate infusion. Procainamide can lead to hypotension, so careful monitoring of the patient during the infusion is recommended.
- Intravenous esmolol may be effective, especially in cases where high catecholamine levels may be contributing to the presence of ventricular arrhythmias. Also in dogs developing VT while undergoing an interventional procedure (i.e. balloon valvuloplasty for pulmonic stenosis), esmolol alone or in combination with lidocaine can be effective. Combination of esmolol with procainamide may cause a significant drop in cardiac output and hypotension. Esmolol may be safer to use than lidocaine in cats with acute life-threatening VT.
- The authors have limited experience with intravenous amiodarone for acute, refractory VT. We have not used it successfully, and it is very costly.

Chronic Oral Antiarrhythmic Therapy (see Tables 16-2 and 16-3 for drug dosages)

- The first-line oral antiarrhythmic drug for treatment of VT in most dogs is sotalol, the exception being German Shepherds, due to proarrhythmic effects in this specific breed.
- If a dog has very advanced myocardial systolic dysfunction (fractional shortening < 15%), then sotalol may not be tolerated due its beta-blocker effect.
- Alternatively, mexiletine in combination with atenolol is very effective, particularly in Boxers. The atenolol dosage can be started at the lower end, in case of poor myocardial function. A practical disadvantage of this treatment regimen is the frequency of drug administration (mexiletine is given every 8 hours).
- For refractory VT or recurrent syncope a combination of sotalol with mexiletine is often effective. These drugs should be initiated in a staggered protocol (usually sotalol first, mexiletine added after 2 days) to avoid side effects, such as AV block or inappetence. Because this is a treatment protocol for refractory arrhythmias, the patients often already are on sotalol or mexiletine, in which case addition of the second drug is usually well tolerated.
- Oral procainamide or atenolol monotherapy usually are both not efficacious for treatment of VT in dogs.
- As a last resort, oral amiodarone is effective for treatment of refractory VT. It has less negative inotropic effects than sotalol or atenolol, thus can be used in dogs with end-stage myocardial failure. But caution is advised when considering amiodarone therapy because of its adverse effects. Signs of toxicity include anorexia, vomiting, lethargy and hepatic enzyme elevation.
- Oral atenolol or sotalol may be effective for treatment for VT in cats.
- Amiodarone toxicity in dogs
    - A maintenance dosage of 200 mg PO every 24 hours is usually well tolerated but a maintenance dose of 400 mg every 24 hours is consistently associated with toxicity.
    - Monitoring of serial serum chemistries is recommended, because increases in liver enzyme activities usually precede the onset of clinical signs of amiodarone toxicity. Liver enzymes should be measured after 7 days of drug loading and once monthly during maintenance therapy. If after 3 months of maintenance therapy no

enzyme elevations develop, the time interval between testing may be increased to 2 months.
- Amiodarone hepatopathy is reversible after reduction of dosage or discontinuation of the drug. Overt clinical signs of toxicity resolve within a few days of stopping amiodarone. Hepatic enzyme activity gradually returns to normal within three months after amiodarone is discontinued or the dosage is reduced.
- Doberman Pinschers have a higher prevalence of inherent hepatopathies and thus the incidence amiodarone toxicity is possibly increased in this breed. Pre-existing liver enzyme elevations are a contraindication for amiodarone therapy in Doberman Pinschers, unless no other alternative is available.

- A post-treatment 24-hour Holter is essential both to check efficacy and assess possible proarrhythmic effects of the drugs. Worsening of VT following sotalol therapy has been documented both in Boxers and German Shepherds.

BREED-SPECIFIC ARRYHYTHMIAS

Arrhythmogenic Right Ventricular Cardiomyopathy in Boxers

- Ventricular arrhythmias and DCM, both manifestations of arrhythmogenic right ventricular cardiomyopathy (ARVC), are a common cause of morbidity and mortality in the Boxer. The clinical presentation of ARVC can be grouped into three categories: (1) isolated subclinical ventricular arrhythmias, (2) arrhythmia-associated syncope or sudden death with normal myocardial function, and (3) systolic myocardial failure with or without ventricular arrhythmias. ARVC is inherited in an autosomal dominant pattern in Boxers.
- The morphology of the VT in Boxers is characteristically positive in the ventrocaudal leads (leads II, III, and aVF) or a "left bundle branch block pattern," suggesting a right ventricular origin of the arrhythmia.
- Syncope is often the first clinical sign and usually, but not always, associated with rapid runs of VT. Boxers can have multiple syncopal episodes and recover. These episodes may be more common during exercise or stress.
- A subset of Boxers also has a form of sick sinus syndrome.
- Some Boxers also have SVAs including AF, especially if they have advanced stages of DCM and congestive heart failure.

Ventricular Tachycardia in Boxers with Arrhythmogenic Right Ventricular Cardiomyopathy (see Table 16-2 for drug dosages)

Chronic Oral Antiarrhythmic Therapy

- Due to the association of VT with ARVC and myocardial systolic dysfunction, it is recommended to obtain an echocardiogram before making specific antiarrhythmic drug recommendations.
- Sotalol is the treatment of choice for VT in Boxers, if the myocardial function is normal or only mildly decreased. If a Boxer has significantly reduced myocardial function sotalol administered at its most effective antiarrhythmic dosage may reduce contractility and lead to worsening of heart failure.
- In such cases mexiletine in combination with atenolol can be used. The atenolol dosage can be started at a lower dose, to limit the BB effect on myocardial contractility.
- For refractory VT and recurrent syncope the combination of sotalol with mexiletine is useful. If the dog is already receiving sotalol with inadequate success, addition of mexiletine is usually well tolerated.
- If VT persists or the dog does not tolerate sotalol or mexiletine/atenolol, amiodarone may be beneficial. However amiodarone hepatopathy may occur with long-term use. Monthly monitoring of liver enzyme activities is recommended.

Acute Intravenous Antiarrhythmic Therapy

- See under general section: Treatment of VT

Ventricular Arrhythmias and Dilated Cardiomyopathy in Doberman Pinschers

- Ventricular arrhythmias, syncope and sudden death associated with DCM are common in Doberman Pinschers. The DCM is characterized by a slowly progressive, clinically occult phase during which ventricular premature contractions first appear. This phase is followed by the development of left ventricular dysfunction and usually, progressively more severe ventricular tachyarrhythmias. The natural outcome in cardiomyopathic patients is usually either sudden death due to ventricular arrhythmias or end-stage congestive heart failure, often associated with AF. The incidence of sudden death prior to the onset of CHF is between 30% and 50%.

KEY POINTS

- VT in Doberman Pinschers has both monomorphic and polymorphic characteristics.
- Syncope or episodic weakness has been documented in Dobermans due to VT as well as bradyarrhythmias such as paradoxical sinus bradycardia and cardiac asystole. Unlike Boxers with ARVC, Doberman Pinschers with VT and DCM may die suddenly during their first syncopal episode.

Ventricular Tachycardia in Doberman Pinschers with Dilated Cardiomyopathy (see Table 16-2 for drug dosages)

Chronic Oral Antiarrhythmic Therapy

- For treatment of VT in Doberman Pinschers sotalol is effective. A combination of mexiletine with sotalol or atenolol may be more powerful. With both drug regimens monitoring by echocardiogram is recommended to check for worsening of myocardial function due to beta blockade. In cases with only moderate VT or significantly reduced myocardial function monotherapy with mexiletine may be beneficial, because mexiletine does not affect contractility.
- Amiodarone is also effective in Dobermans with significant VT and end-stage myocardial failure; however, in this particular breed careful monitoring of liver enzyme levels is imperative, because Dobermans have a high incidence of amiodarone toxicity (more details see under general section: Treatment of VT)

Acute Intravenous Antiarrhythmic Therapy

- See under general section: Treatment of VT

Inherited Ventricular Arrhythmias in Young German Shepherds

- Inherited ventricular arrhythmias and a propensity for sudden death occur in young German Shepherds. This disorder has a wide phenotypic spectrum in which some German Shepherds have very few ventricular premature complexes, and others have frequent, rapid (rates > 350 bpm) polymorphic VT and sudden death. Only dogs with VT die. Of German Shepherds with more than 10 runs of VT per 24 hours, approximately 50% die suddenly; however, this represents about 10% to 15% of the total affected populations studied. The prevalence of this disorder in the general German Shepherd population is unknown. Affected dogs have abnormal sympathetic innervation of the heart and ventricular arrhythmias may be initiated by early afterdepolarizations documented in the Purkinje fibers of these dogs.
- German Shepherds develop ventricular arrhythmias at 12 to 16 weeks of age, and the frequency and severity increase until 24 to 30 weeks of age. After that time, some dogs remain severely affected, whereas others show a progressive decline in the frequency of the arrhythmias. The dogs typically do not have syncope or other clinical signs. Most dogs have a low incidence of VT. If dogs reach the age of 18 months, the probability of sudden death declines markedly.

Therapy of German Shepherds with Ventricular Tachycardia (see Table 16-2 for drug dosages)

- Dogs with mild to moderate amounts of ventricular arrhythmias do not warrant antiarrhythmic therapy.
- In dogs at high risk of sudden death (> 10 runs/ 24 hours) based on a 24-hour Holter, antiarrhythmic therapy may be administered until the dog has "survived" the vulnerable time period.
- Intravenous lidocaine is effective in eliminating the ventricular arrhythmias acutely. However, the oral NCB mexiletine does not suppress the ventricular arrhythmias significantly. Sotalol monotherapy has proarrhythmic effects (i.e., causes increased numbers of runs of VT) in this specific breed, probably due to the action potential prolonging effects, which can exacerbate early afterdepolarization–induced triggered activity.
- The authors have found the combination therapy of mexiletine and sotalol to be beneficial in reducing the incidence and rate of VT in severely affected dogs; however, it is unknown if the risk of sudden death is reduced with this treatment.
- We have not tested amiodarone therapy in this breed. There is a poor response to procainamide.

VENTRICULAR ASYSTOLE

- Ventricular asystole is characterized by a complete absence of a ventricular rhythm. P waves may be present if AV block exists, but no QRS complexes are observed. Primary asystole occurs when the Purkinje fibers intrinsically fail to generate a ventricular depolarization. It is usually is preceded by a bradyarrhythmia due to complete heart block, sick sinus syndrome, or both.

Therapy

- Immediate external cardiac pacing with either transthoracic, transvenous or epicardial electrodes (temporary pacing lead) may be effective, if the asystole is the result of advanced complete AV bock. Permanent pacemaker therapy is indicated. During cardiopulmonary resuscitation epinephrine, isoproterenol or atropine can be administered intravenously, but little effect is to be expected.
- Secondary asystole occurs when noncardiac factors suppress the electrical conduction system, resulting in a failure to generate any electrical depolarization. Massive pulmonary embolus, hyperkalemia, hypothermia, untreated VF or VT that deteriorates to asystole, unsuccessful defibrillation or narcotic overdoses leading to respiratory failure can lead to secondary asystole. In such cases, the final common pathway is usually severe tissue hypoxia with metabolic acidosis.
- The prognosis is usually grave for secondary asystole, because external pacing is not effective in such cases.

VENTRICULAR FIBRILLATION

- No distinctive QRS complexes are identifiable on the ECG. Instead there is an irregularly undulating baseline of variable amplitude due to a rapid and chaotic activation of the ventricles. The sinus node is usually discharging regularly, but P waves are buried in the VF waveform. There is no mechanical contraction of the ventricles during VF; thus blood pressure drops to zero instantaneously. The rhythm cannot convert to sinus rhythm spontaneously and causes death within a few minutes due to lack of cardiac output. VT can degenerate to VF in any of the described scenarios of VT (previous section). VF can also occur secondary to systemic disease (i.e., severe hyperkalemia). Dogs with congenital heart disease predisposed to ventricular arrhythmias may develop VF during cardiac catheterization for angiography or interventional therapy due to "catheter irritation" of the myocardium.

Therapy

- Drug therapy is not effective for treatment of VF. Since there is no blood pressure or blood flow during VF, drugs administered in a peripheral vein will not reach the myocardium. Electric defibrillation is the only viable treatment option for VF.
- If VF occurs secondary to electrolyte imbalances or systemic disease, then the prognosis is usually grave, despite aggressive cardiopulmonary resuscitation efforts.
- Animals with a predisposition to ventricular arrhythmias or that fibrillate during an anesthetic procedure performed for catheter treatment of heart disease but that are otherwise relatively healthy can usually be treated successfully with electric defibrillation.
- VF has a grave prognosis if not corrected within the first 3 minutes of onset. Development of myocardial ischemia during VF contributes to worsening prognosis as time goes by. If VF has been present for 3 minutes or longer, cardiopulmonary resuscitation with chest compression should be performed briefly prior to defibrillation, to provide some blood flow to the myocardium and increase chances of successful defibrillation.

Transthoracic Electrical Defibrillation Procedure

- Dogs in VF become unconscious within 10 seconds due to the lack of blood flow to the brain.
- Defibrillation should be attempted using transthoracic hand-held paddles or "Fast Patch electrodes."
- Animals should be placed in dorsal recumbency and copious contact gel applied to the thorax if hand-held paddles are used. For optimal current flow, the chest is first shaved, but that may not be feasible in the interest of time. The dorsal recumbent position is safest for the operator but may not be optimal for defibrillation success in deep-chested dogs. If patch electrodes are available, the dogs can also be placed in lateral recumbency, which might allow the defibrillation electrodes to be closer to the heart.
- Defibrillator ECG cables or the hand-held paddles placed on the thorax should be used to ascertain presence of VF prior to defibrillation.
- Using a monophasic defibrillator:
  - Start with 6 J/kg
  - If VF persists, increase the dose by 50 J and repeat until a maximum of 360 J.
- Using a biphasic defibrillator:
  - Start with 3 J/kg
  - If VF persists, increase the dose by 50 J and repeat until a maximum of 360 J.
- Short, transient runs of VT or sinus pauses or AV block are common following defibrillation.

Frequently Asked Questions

What are idioventriucular rhythms and should they be treated?
Idioventricular rhythm is a form of ventricular arrhythmias characterized by a rate that is slow or comparable to the sinus rates (60 to 150 bpm in the dog, and > 100 bpm in cats). The ventricular rate usually remains within 10 to 15 bpm of the sinus rate and the cardiac rhythm "switches" back and forth between the two competing pacemaker sites. This arrhythmia may occur for several reasons including systemic diseases (e.g., anemia, splenic hemangiosarcoma), drugs (e.g., digoxin, opiods) and electrolyte abnormalities (e.g., hypokalemia). Generally, no clinical signs are associated with idioventricular rhythms. If clinical signs are present, they are often associated with the underlying process. Idioventricular rhythms usually do not require treatment. Management of the underlying cardiac disease or metabolic abnormality is required.

MANAGEMENT OF AF: RYTHYM CONTROL VERSUS RATE CONTROL

What should veterinarians do for the management of AF?
The answer is not straight forward and unfortunately, we are lacking appropriate clinical trials to answer this question satisfactorily; however, we do know it is important to slow the heart rate. What we do not know is if cardioversion is necessarily superior to rate control. The main advantages and disadvantages of rate control and cardioversion are summarized hereafter. They are intended to aid in clinical judgment and one must always consider a patient's individual needs.

What are the advantages of rate control?
Management is relatively simple because it can be achieved in the home environment with oral medication. Rate control successfully achieves improved left ventricular function, reduction in clinical signs, limited hospitalizations, and prevention of tachycardiomyopathy.

What are the disadvantages of rate control?
Heart rate control is not "perfect" as compared to sinus rhythm and side effects from antiarrhythmic medication can occur (gastrointestinal signs, hypotension, worsening of heart failure or arrhythmias). In addition, owner compliance and cost for lifelong therapy must be taken into consideration. If done properly, optimal rate control can only be achieved with periodic Holter recordings—which increases costs to the client.

What are the advantages of cardioversion (electrical or pharmacologic conversion)?
Cardioversion has similar advantages to adequate rate control in that tacycardiomyopathy is avoided, reduction in clinical signs and improved exercise tolerance can be achieved. Probably, the most important advantage is that the patient has a "normal" sinus rhythm which is physiologic compared to "slow" AF.

What are the disadvantages of cardioversion (electrical or pharmacologic conversion)?
The main disadvantages of electrical cardioversion are that it requires general anesthesia, risk of cardiac arrest from "shocking," hospitalization, and expensive equipment. Pharmacologic cardioversion's main disadvantage includes side effects from drug administration; owner compliance can be of concern due to the daily need to administer drugs. There is a risk of reoccurrence of AF even after successful cardioversion with either method of cardioversion.

Generally, in our clinic the majority of patients are treated with rate control (see Figures 16-1, 16-2, and 16-3) because the majority of our canine patients have advanced cardiac disease.

SUGGESTED READINGS

Basso C, Fox PR, Meurs KM, Towbin JA, Spier AW, Calabrese F, Maron BJ, Thiene G: Arrhythmogenic right ventricular cardiomyopathy causing sudden cardiac death in Boxer dogs: a new animal model of human disease, Circulation 109(9):1180-1185, 2004.

Fogors RN: The electrophysiology Study in the evaluation of supraventricular tachyarrhythmias. In Fogoros RN: Electrophysiologic testing, ed 3, Malden, Mass, 1998, Blackwell Science.

Gelzer RM, Kraus MS: Management of atrial fibrillation. Vet Clin North Am Small Anim Pract 34:1127-1144, 2004.

Gelzer ARM, Moise NS, Koller ML: Defibrillation of German shepherds with inherited ventricular arrhythmias and sudden death, J Vet Cardiol 7(2): 97-107, 2005.

Gelzer ARM, Kraus MS, Moise NS, Pariaut R, Charter ME, Renaud-Farrell S: Assessment of antiarrhythmic drug efficacy to control heart rate in dogs with atrial fibrillation using 24-hour ambulatory electrocardiographic (Holter) recordings, J Vet Intern Med 18(5):779, 2004.

Jacobs G, Calvert C, Kraus M: Hepatopathy in 4 dogs treated with amiodarone, J Vet Intern Med 14(1): 96-99, 2000.

Kraus MS, Moise NS, Rishniw M: Morphology of ventricular tachycardia in the Boxer and pace mapping comparison. J Vet Intern Med 16:153-158, 2002.

Kraus MS, Ridge LG, Gelzer ARM, Pariaut R, Moise NS, Calvert C: Toxicity in Doberman pinscher dogs with ventricular arrhythmias treated with amiodarone, J Vet Intern Med 19(3):407, 2005.

Meurs KM: Boxer dog cardiomyopathy: an update, et Clin North Am Small Anim Pract 34:1235-1244, 2004.

Meurs KM, Spier AW, Wright NA, et al: Comparison of the effects of four antiarrhythmic treatments for familial ventricular arrhythmias in Boxers, J Am Vet Med Assoc 221(4):522-527, 2002.

Moise NS, Gilmour RF Jr, Riccio ML, Flahive WF Jr: Diagnosis of inherited ventricular tachycardia in German shepherd dogs, J Am Vet Med Assoc 210(3): 403-410, 1997.

Moise NS: Diagnosis and management of canine arrhythmias. In Fox PR, Sisson D, Moise NS, eds: Textbook of canine and feline cardiology, ed 2, Philadelphia, 1999, WB Saunders.

CHAPTER 17

Cardiopulmonary Resuscitation

Steven G. Cole and Kenneth J. Drobatz

INTRODUCTION

Cardiopulmonary resuscitation (CPR) describes a set of techniques to provide circulatory and ventilatory support following cardiopulmonary arrest (CPA). CPR encompasses both basic life support and advanced life support. Basic life support includes the ABCs of resuscitation and involves establishing an airway, providing manual ventilation, and performing external chest compressions or internal cardiac compressions to generate blood flow. Advanced life support includes the Ds and Es of resuscitation, including drug therapy, defibrillation, and electrocardiogram (ECG) analysis during resuscitation. The goal of CPR is to maximize blood flow and oxygen delivery to the heart and brain until return of spontaneous circulation (ROSC) is achieved and the underlying cause of the arrest may be addressed.

- *CPA* is defined as the cessation of spontaneous circulation and ventilation. Causes of CPA include primary myocardial disease (although this is rare in veterinary patients), hypotension (secondary to hypovolemia, sepsis, or drug administration), hypoxemia (secondary to hypoventilation or lung disease), metabolic derangements (e.g., severe metabolic acidosis) or electrolyte abnormalities (e.g., hyperkalemia). It is important to recognize that these predisposing causes of arrest may be associated with either reversible or irreversible underlying disease processes.
- The prognosis for patients requiring CPR is guarded, and long-term survival is generally less than 10%. The likelihood of a successful outcome is improved when an arrest is rapidly recognized and a reversible cause is identified and addressed.
- CPR is most likely to be successful when the team is prepared, the techniques are practiced, communication is clear, and the resuscitation takes place in a well-equipped area within the hospital.

KEY POINT

CPR is a potentially lifesaving procedure that requires preparation, coordination, and communication to achieve optimal results.

BASIC LIFE SUPPORT

Airway

- Establishing an airway is the first step in performing basic life support. Orotracheal intubation is generally performed in a routine fashion, and this may be facilitated by the use of a laryngoscope and/or a stylet for the endotracheal tube. It is also helpful to have suction available if secretions or blood obscure visualization of the glottis. In situations where the glottis cannot be visualized, the larynx may be directly palpated and the endotracheal tube may be guided by feel.

- In rare situations, an emergency tracheostomy is required. This technique may be performed in less than 30 seconds after rapidly clipping and prepping the ventral cervical region. A midline incision is performed and sharp dissection is used to expose the trachea. Care is taken during dissection to remain on midline (between the sternohyothyroideus muscles) in order to avoid vascular structures. Once the trachea has been isolated, a transverse incision is made between cervical rings (approximately 50% of the diameter) and a cuffed tracheostomy tube is inserted. A standard endotracheal tube may also be used in this situation.
- Once an airway is in place, it is important to confirm correct tube placement. This may be done by direct visualization, cervical palpation, auscultation of lung sounds, and observing chest wall movement. The use of end-tidal carbon dioxide (CO_2) monitoring in this situation is also useful, as tracheal gas is always higher in CO_2 than esophageal gas. Once placement is confirmed, it is vital to secure the endotracheal tube, as inadvertent tube dislodgement is very common in an arrest situation.
- Problems during an arrest (i.e., unable to auscult lung sounds, chest wall not moving with ventilation) should prompt rapid reevaluation of endotracheal tube placement. It is also important to ensure that the cuff has been inflated, as this is often the source of problems. If airway problems have been ruled out, difficulty ventilating a patient during an arrest suggests severe pleural space, airway, or parenchymal disease.

Breathing

- Patients should be manually ventilated with 100% oxygen. Methods for providing positive pressure ventilation in an arrest situation include the use of an Ambu-bag or an anesthesia machine.
- Respiratory rate should be between 10 to 24 breaths/minute. It should be noted that excessive ventilation often occurs during CPR. It has been shown in animal models that increasing respiratory rates results in higher mean intrathoracic pressures, decreased myocardial perfusion pressure, and decreased survival.
- Normal chest wall motion should be observed and peak pressure of less than 20 cm H_2O should be maintained if possible. Problems with decreased compliance or diminished chest wall motion may include airway obstruction, severe parenchymal disease, or pleural space disease (e.g., pneumothorax, pleural effusion, diaphragmatic hernia, mass lesions).

Circulation

- Artificial circulation during CPR may be provided by performing external chest compressions or internal cardiac massage. The goal of either technique is to maximize blood flow to the coronary and cerebral vasculature.
- Myocardial perfusion pressure is the best predictor of ROSC in human patients and animal models of CPR, and it is represented by the following equation: MPP = aortic diastolic pressure − central venous pressure.
- Cerebral perfusion pressure drives cerebral blood flow and is represented by the following equation: CPP = Mean arterial pressure − Intracranial pressure.
- There are two theories describing the mechanism of blood flow during external chest compressions. The cardiac pump theory describes actual compression of the heart through the chest wall and is likely to occur in small patients (< 15 kg). The thoracic pump theory describes blood flow as a result of phasic increases in intrathoracic pressure and has been documented in larger animals (> 15 kg).
- External chest compressions should be performed with the patient in lateral recumbency. The chest may be compressed circumferentially or directly over the heart in small patients (< 15 kg) and at the widest point of the chest in larger patients (> 15 kg). The rate of chest compressions should be 100 to 120 per minute with a ratio of compression to relaxation of 50:50. While higher compression rates have been shown to generate greater cardiac output, it is difficult to sustain higher rates for extended periods of time during CPR. Compressions should be given with enough force to decrease the diameter of the chest wall by approximately 25% to 33%.
- Interposed abdominal compression (IAC) may be used to improve the efficacy of external chest compressions. With this technique, the abdomen is compressed during "diastole" (relaxation phase of chest compression) in order to increase the pressure gradient favoring blood return to the chest, thereby improving cardiac output, blood pressure, and myocardial and cerebral perfusion pressure.
- Even optimal external chest compression produces approximately 20% of normal cardiac output.

Open-chest CPR and internal cardiac compression may produce 100% of normal cardiac output, with dramatic increases in blood flow to the heart and brain. Indications for open-chest CPR include pleural space disease (e.g., pneumothorax, pleural effusions, diaphragmatic hernia), pericardial effusion, penetrating wounds, chest wall trauma, intraoperative arrests, hemoperitoneum, large dogs in which closed-chest compressions are unlikely to generate effective blood flow, or in prolonged resuscitations (> 2 to 5 min without ROSC).

- To perform open-chest CPR, the heart may be accessed via a left lateral thoracotomy (or transdiaphragmatically in patients undergoing abdominal surgery). Following a rapid clip and preparation of the left chest, an emergency thoracotomy may be performed in approximately 30 seconds. A skin incision is made in the fourth or fifth intercostal space and is extended through the chest wall musculature. Ventilation is temporarily suspended and the pleural space is accessed. A rib spreader is used to retract the ribs. Once the heart is exposed, the ventricles may be compressed with one or two hands depending upon the size of the patient. A rate of 100 to 120 compressions per minute is recommended. It is often easier to perform direct cardiac compression once an incision has been made in the pericardium (below the level of the phrenic nerve).
- Open-chest CPR allows for compression or cross-clamping of the descending aorta to direct blood flow to the heart and brain, and to avoid additional volume loss in cases of abdominal hemorrhage. In the absence of an atraumatic vascular clamp, the aorta may be manually compressed, or a Penrose drain or red rubber catheter may be tightened around the aorta. When appropriate, aortic flow may be gradually restored (over 5 to 10 minutes).
- Open-chest CPR requires that appropriate facilities and expertise be available for post-resuscitation care and management of the emergency thoracotomy.

KEY POINT

Basic life support measures are the basis for all resuscitation efforts. These techniques are easily learned and are effective in maintaining ventilation and artificial circulation in patients suffering CPA.

ADVANCED LIFE SUPPORT

Establishing Access for Drug and Fluid Therapy

- Rapid access to the circulation is vital in CPR. Central venous access (e.g., jugular vein) is ideal, as drug circulation times are significantly decreased when compared to peripheral sites. Because of the low-flow state that occurs during CPR, large flush volumes are necessary, especially when peripheral catheters are employed. Short, large bore catheters are ideal, as these provide the highest flow rates for drug and fluid administration.
- Surgical cutdown should be performed immediately if an initial attempt at percutaneous vascular access is not successful. Surgical cutdown involves making a skin incision adjacent and parallel to the long axis of the vein (usually jugular, cephalic, or saphenous) to be isolated. Blunt dissection with a hemostat is used to expose the vein, and an intravenous catheter is introduced. Cutdown catheters should be secured with suture and bandaged appropriately.
- Intraosseous (IO) access is an alternative to peripheral venous access, especially in small puppies, kittens, and exotic species. The intertrochanteric fossa of the femur, proximal humerus, and proximal tibia are readily accessible sites to obtain intraosseous access.
- Intratracheal (IT) administration is an excellent method to deliver drugs when intravenous access is not available. Most drugs used in CPR (with the exception of sodium bicarbonate) may be delivered by this route. When delivering drugs intratracheally, the dose of the drug is doubled, the medication is diluted to 2 to 5 ml (depending upon patient size), and the drug is delivered through a red rubber catheter placed through and beyond the tip of the endotracheal tube (at the level of the carina). Air may be used to flush the catheter.
- Intracardiac drug administration is not recommended in CPR, as there is a risk for inadvertent laceration of the lung or coronary vasculature, as well as the potential for intramyocardial drug administration (which may exacerbate arrhythmias or ischemia in the case of epinephrine).

Electrocardiography

- ECG monitoring is integral to providing advanced life support. The course of action taken during CPR depends upon the rhythm that is present, and changes in the rhythm during the course of an arrest often dictate changes in therapy (Figure 17-1).

- A retrospective study of veterinary patients undergoing CPR has shown that common initial arrest rhythms include pulseless electrical activity, asystole, ventricular fibrillation, and sinus bradycardia.
- Although ventricular fibrillation is most responsive to treatment (defibrillation), a recent study of veterinary patients surviving CPR found that asystole was the most common initial rhythm identified.

Drug Therapy

- See Table 17-1 for drug therapy guidelines
- **Intravenous fluids** may be administered in shock doses (90 ml/kg in dogs and 60 ml/kg in cats) to patients that are hypovolemic. Intravenous fluids may also be useful to help flush drugs from peripheral sites into the central circulation. It should be noted, however, that myocardial perfusion pressure may be reduced by significant increases in central venous pressure, and that bolus fluid therapy may be counterproductive in patients that are euvolemic or volume overloaded at the time of arrest.
- **Atropine** is a vagolytic drug that abolishes parasympathetic tone. It is indicated in patients with bradycardias (as may occur in vagal events), as well as in pulseless electrical activity and asystole. It should be noted that high doses of atropine may cause a profound tachycardia in patients with perfusing rhythms, and that the dose is often reduced by 50% to 75% in these situations. The dose of atropine is 0.04 mg/kg (dogs and cats, can be given IV, IT, IO). Atropine is available in a concentration of 0.54 mg/ml, and a shortcut dose is 1 ml/10 kg. The dose may be repeated at 5 minute intervals.
- **Epinephrine** is a potent alpha and beta catecholamine receptor agonist. Experimental studies have shown that it is the alpha (vasoconstrictor) effects rather than the beta (chronotropic/inotropic) effects that are most important in achieving ROSC. This is due to the increased peripheral resistance created by adrenergic stimulation and the resultant increase in aortic pressure. This increase in aortic pressure leads to an increase in myocardial perfusion pressure and increased likelihood of successful resuscitation. Epinephrine is indicated in all cardiac arrest situations. There are both high- and low-dose recommendations for epinephrine in CPR. The low dose (dogs and cats, 0.01 to 0.02 mg/kg) is favored in people, due, in part, to worse neurologic outcomes with initial high dose therapy. Conversely, high-dose epinephrine (dogs and cats, 0.1 to 0.2 mg/kg) has been shown to improve results in dog models of CPR. Epinephrine may be given IV, IT or IO, and a shortcut for high-dose epinephrine is 1 ml/10 kg, and the dose may be repeated at 5-minute intervals.
- **Vasopressin** is a noncatecholamine vasopressor drug that has recently been included in human CPR guidelines. Potential advantages of vasopressin (compared to epinephrine) include efficacy in the presence of acidosis, lack of potentially harmful beta effects, and a longer half-life. The role of vasopressin in CPR is still being investigated, however there is evidence that this drug may be equivalent to or even superior to epinephrine is some situations. The dose of vasopressin is 0.8 μ/kg (dogs and cats), and the dose may be repeated at 5 minute intervals.
- **Lidocaine** is indicated in ventricular fibrillation or pulseless ventricular tachycardia that is not responsive to initial defibrillation attempts. Like other antiarrhythmic drugs, lidocaine may increase the defibrillation threshold. Additionally, lidocaine must be used with care in the post-arrest period, as its use may suppress a functional ventricular escape rhythm. The dose of lidocaine is 2 mg/kg (dogs, IV, IO, IT), and a shortcut dose for the 2% (20 mg/ml) solution is 1 ml/10 kg.
- **Amiodarone** has been incorporated into human CPR guidelines, and has been favorably compared to lidocaine in ventricular fibrillation that is refractory to defibrillation. There is limited experience with amiodarone in the context of CPR in veterinary patients. The dose of amiodarone is 5 to 10 mg/kg (dogs, IV), and it is diluted in 5% dextrose prior to administration. Hypotension is a common occurrence during amiodarone administration.
- **Sodium bicarbonate** is not routinely recommended for use in all arrest situations. It is indicated, however, in patients with a preexisting acidosis, patients with hyperkalemia, and in prolonged (> 10 minute) arrests. The dose for sodium bicarbonate is 1 to 2 mEq/kg (dogs and cats, IV, IO). A shortcut dose is 1 ml/kg of a standard 1 mEq/ml solution. Sodium bicarbonate should not be given intratracheally, as this will inactivate surfactant and have deleterious effects on pulmonary function.
- **Calcium gluconate** is also not routinely recommended in all arrest situations, as its use may

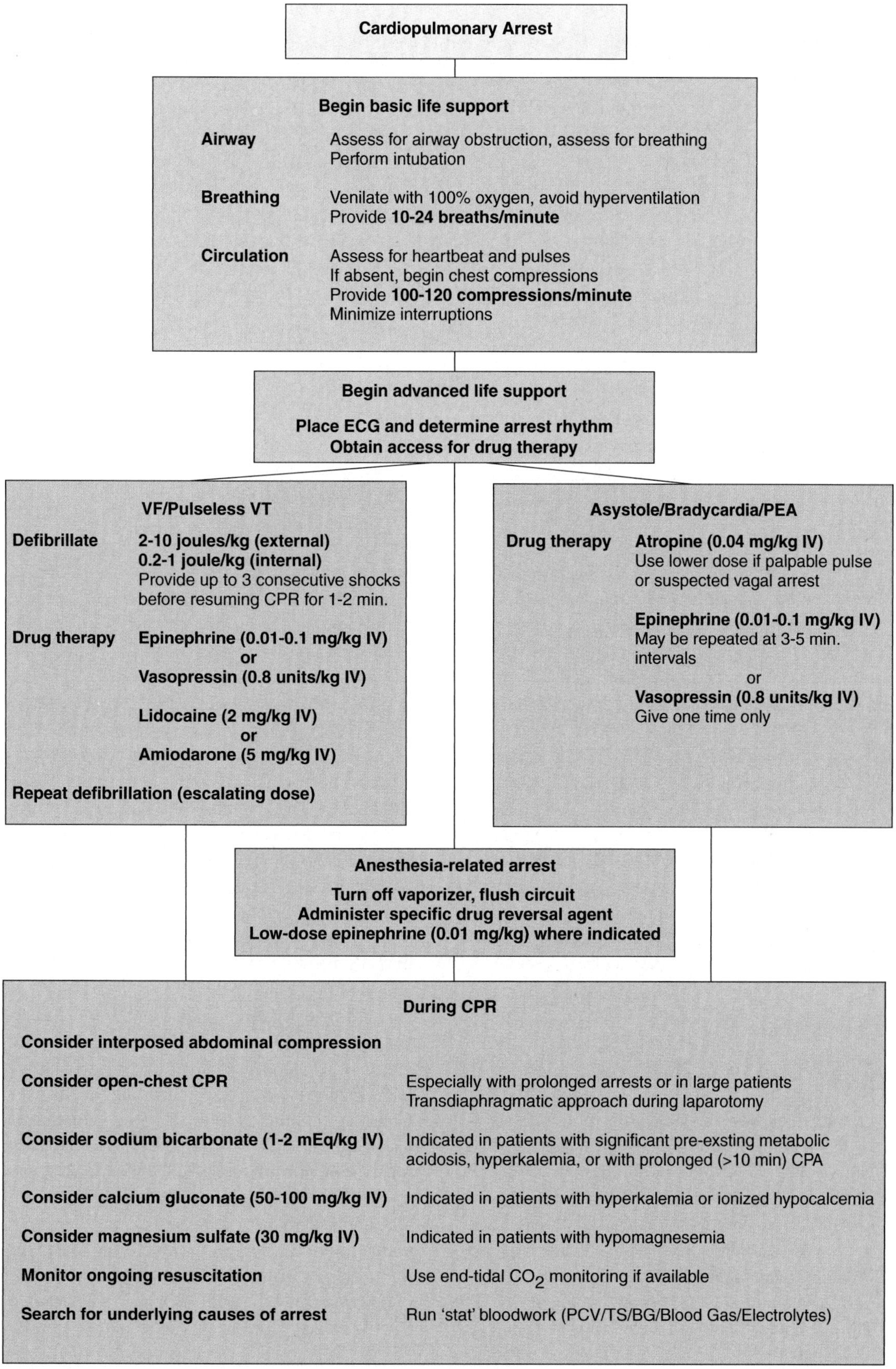

Cardiopulmonary Arrest

Begin basic life support

Airway — Assess for airway obstruction, assess for breathing
Perform intubation

Breathing — Venilate with 100% oxygen, avoid hyperventilation
Provide **10-24 breaths/minute**

Circulation — Assess for heartbeat and pulses
If absent, begin chest compressions
Provide **100-120 compressions/minute**
Minimize interruptions

Begin advanced life support

Place ECG and determine arrest rhythm
Obtain access for drug therapy

VF/Pulseless VT

Defibrillate — **2-10 joules/kg (external)**
0.2-1 joule/kg (internal)
Provide up to 3 consecutive shocks before resuming CPR for 1-2 min.

Drug therapy — **Epinephrine (0.01-0.1 mg/kg IV)**
or
Vasopressin (0.8 units/kg IV)

Lidocaine (2 mg/kg IV)
or
Amiodarone (5 mg/kg IV)

Repeat defibrillation (escalating dose)

Asystole/Bradycardia/PEA

Drug therapy — **Atropine (0.04 mg/kg IV)**
Use lower dose if palpable pulse or suspected vagal arrest

Epinephrine (0.01-0.1 mg/kg IV)
May be repeated at 3-5 min. intervals
or
Vasopressin (0.8 units/kg IV)
Give one time only

Anesthesia-related arrest

Turn off vaporizer, flush circuit
Administer specific drug reversal agent
Low-dose epinephrine (0.01 mg/kg) where indicated

During CPR

Consider interposed abdominal compression	
Consider open-chest CPR	Especially with prolonged arrests or in large patients Transdiaphragmatic approach during laparotomy
Consider sodium bicarbonate (1-2 mEq/kg IV)	Indicated in patients with significant pre-exsting metabolic acidosis, hyperkalemia, or with prolonged (>10 min) CPA
Consider calcium gluconate (50-100 mg/kg IV)	Indicated in patients with hyperkalemia or ionized hypocalcemia
Consider magnesium sulfate (30 mg/kg IV)	Indicated in patients with hypomagnesemia
Monitor ongoing resuscitation	Use end-tidal CO_2 monitoring if available
Search for underlying causes of arrest	Run 'stat' bloodwork (PCV/TS/BG/Blood Gas/Electrolytes)

Figure 17-1. Algorithm for performing CPR in veterinary patients. (Adapted from Cole SG, Otto CM, Hughes D: Cardiopulmonary cerebral resuscitation in small animals: a clinical practice review. Part II. J Vet Emerg Crit Care 13[1]:13-23, 2003.)

Table 17-1 Guidelines for Drug Therapy and Initial Defibrillator Settings (Monophasic Waveform Defibrillators) During CPR

	Weight (lb)	5	10	20	30	40	50	60	70	80	90	100
	Weight (kg)	2.5	5	10	15	20	25	30	35	40	45	50
Drug (conc.)	**Dose**	**ml**										
Epi low (1:10,000)	0.01 mg/kg	0.25	0.5	1	1.5	2	2.5	3	3.5	4	4.5	5
Epi high (1:1,000)	0.1 mg/kg	0.25	0.5	1	1.5	2	2.5	3	3.5	4	4.5	5
Atropine (0.54 mg/ml)	0.05 mg/kg	0.25	0.5	1	1.5	2	2.5	3	3.5	4	4.5	5
Lidocaine (20 mg/ml)	2 mg/kg	0.25	0.5	1	1.5	2	2.5	3	3.5	4	4.5	5
Sodium bicarbonate (1 mEq/ml)	1 mEq/kg	2.5	5	10	15	20	25	30	35	40	45	50
Calcium gluconate (100 mg/ml)	50 mg/kg	1	2.5	5	7.5	10	12.5	15	17.5	20	22.5	2.5
Magnesium sulfate (4 mEq/ml)	0.2 mEq/kg	0.1	0.25	0.5	0.75	1	1.25	1.5	1.75	2	2.25	2.5
Vasopressin (20 units/ml)	0.8 μ/kg	0.1	0.2	0.4	0.6	0.8	1	1.2	1.4	1.6	1.8	2
Amiodarone (50 mg/ml)	5 mg/kg	0.25	0.5	1	1.5	2	2.5	3	3.5	4	4.5	5
Naloxone (0.4 mg/ml)	0.04 mg/kg	0.25	0.5	1	1.5	2	2.5	3	3.5	4	4.5	5
Flumazenil (0.1 mg/ml)	0.02 mg/ml	0.5	1	2	3	4	5	6	7	8	9	10
External defibrillation	2-10 J/kg	20	30	50	100	200	200	200	300	300	300	360
Internal defibrillation	0.2-1 J/kg	2	3	5	10	20	20	20	30	30	30	50

Adapted from Cole SG, Otto CM, Hughes D: Cardiopulmonary cerebral resuscitation in small animals: a clinical practice review. Part II. J Vet Emerg Crit Care 13(1):13-23, 2003.

exacerbate ischemia-reperfusion injury. It is indicated in patients with hyperkalemia and in patients with known hypocalcemia. The dose of calcium gluconate is 50 to 100 mg/kg (dogs and cats, IV, IO)

- **Magnesium sulfate** is indicated in patients with known hypomagnesemia, and in rare ventricular arrhythmias (e.g. torsades de pointes). The dose of magnesium sulfate is 30 mg/kg (dogs and cats, IV, IO)

Defibrillation

- See Table 17-1 for defibrillation guidelines
- Electrical defibrillation is the only effective method to convert ventricular fibrillation to a perfusing rhythm. Defibrillation is also indicated in patients with pulseless ventricular tachycardia.
- The defibrillator must be used properly to minimize risks to members of the resuscitation team. It is strongly recommended that the patient be placed in lateral recumbency for both CPR and defibrillation. Attempting to defibrillate a patient in dorsal recumbency may allow the limbs to contact a team member. This may lead to the unintentional delivery of current to a staff member and a potentially harmful situation. Most defibrillators have attachments for an accessory flat paddle (often called a posterior paddle) that may be placed under the patient, with the handheld paddle placed over the heart on opposite sides of the chest wall.
- It is important to use large amounts of contact gel in order to prevent the current from "arcing" across the surface of the skin rather than being delivered through the chest. Arcing of current is inefficient, and may be potentially dangerous, especially if alcohol has been placed on the patient. Because of the risk of combustion during defibrillation, alcohol (to increase ECG contact) should not be used during CPR. ECG contact gel is a much safer alternative.
- Clear communication during defibrillation is also important to ensure safety. The operator must both inform the other resuscitation team members of an impending defibrillation attempt and confirm that no member of the team is in contact with the patient or table prior to delivering a shock. Because of this, a standard protocol is followed for each defibrillation. This protocol is as follows: (1) confirm ventricular fibrillation or pulseless ventricular tachycardia, (2) apply contact gel, (3) confirm current to be delivered and charge defibrillator, (4) halt ongoing CPR,

(5) call "Clear," (6) confirm that all personnel are clear of the patient (especially limbs) and table, (7) deliver current, (8) monitor success of defibrillation.

- The dose of energy for initial defibrillation is 3 to 5 J/kg. This corresponds to 10 to 15 J for a cat, 30 to 100 J for a small dog, 100 to 200 J for a medium dog, and 200 to 300 J for a large dog.
- If an initial shock is not successful, up to 2 additional shocks are given, increasing the energy delivered by 50%. If there is no conversion of the rhythm after a total of three shocks, CPR is resumed for 1 to 2 minutes before defibrillation is attempted again.

Monitoring CPR Efforts

- Patient monitoring during CPR can be difficult, and some standard techniques may be potentially misleading in an arrest situation.
- Palpation of femoral pulses during chest compression is an encouraging finding; however, the presence of pulses (and a discernible pulse pressure) does necessarily correspond to adequate arterial blood pressure or perfusion pressures. Direct arterial pressure measurement is ideal, although this is generally only feasible in patients with a previously placed arterial line.
- As mentioned above, ECG monitoring is vital during CPR, as this often dictates the type and timing of intervention. ECG findings must always be interpreted in the light of physical examination parameters. This is especially important when an apparent escape rhythm is present. The presence of auscultable heart sounds and, often, palpable pulses, indicates ROSC. Without these findings, the rhythm represents pulseless electrical activity and CPR should be continued.
- End-tidal CO_2 monitoring is an easily applied and extremely useful monitoring tool in CPR. If ventilation is constant, end-tidal CO_2 is linearly related to pulmonary blood flow and, by extension, cardiac output. As with myocardial perfusion pressure, higher end-tidal CO_2 during CPR has been shown to correlate with increased likelihood of successful resuscitation. Additionally, because end-tidal CO_2 is a surrogate marker for blood flow, marked increases in this parameter serves as a useful indicator of ROSC.
- Blood gas analysis may be misleading during CPR. Despite the low-flow state and global tissue ischemia that occurs, arterial blood gas results may appear relatively normal after equilibration with alveolar gas (especially with the hyperventilation that typically occurs during CPR). On the other hand, venous blood gas results reflect the metabolic and respiratory acidosis that characterizes the local tissue environment in the face of hypoperfusion and decreased clearance of metabolic byproducts. Because of this, venous blood gas results are more useful in the monitoring of CPR.

KEY POINT

Advanced life support techniques include the implementation of drug therapy and defibrillation. These interventions are based upon the circumstances unique to each arrest and provide options to augment the effectiveness of basic life support.

SPECIAL SITUATIONS

Anesthetic Arrests

- In general, anesthetic related arrests are rare; however, arrests that occur in conjunction with anesthesia are usually rapidly recognized, and some retrospective veterinary studies demonstrate that these patients are the most likely to be successfully resuscitated.
- Steps to take in an anesthetic related arrest include turning off gas anesthesia and flushing the anesthetic circuit, reversing injectable anesthetic agents with naloxone (for opioids) at 0.02 to 0.04 mg/kg (dogs and cats, IV), flumazenil (for benzodiazepines) at 0.02 to 0.04 mg/kg (dogs and cats, IV), or yohimbine/atipamenzole (for alpha-2 agonists) at 0.1 to 0.2 mg/kg (dogs and cats, IV) and instituting standard CPR.
- Immediate open-chest CPR should be performed in patients undergoing thoracotomy and should be considered in patients undergoing celiotomy (via a transdiaphragmatic approach).
- Possible underlying causes such as hypoventilation, hypoxemia, hypotension, or arrhythmias should be investigated and corrected immediately.

Vagal Events

- Vagal events, characterized by bradycardia, hypotension and collapse, may occur in critically ill patients, especially in conjunction with coughing, retching, vomiting, or straining to defecate. In extreme cases, bradycardia may be profound and lead to asystole.

- **Atropine** is the treatment of choice in patients with symptomatic bradycardia, and it should be noted that significant (although transient) tachycardia is often seen in patients with perfusing rhythms given a full arrest dose (dogs and cats, 0.04 mg/kg IV, IM, IT). Because of this, the atropine dose may be reduced to a fourth to half of the arrest dose (dogs and cats, 0.01 to 0.02 mg/kg IV, IM, IT) in patients with palpable pulses.
- Respiratory arrest may accompany these events, and prompt intubation and manual ventilation is indicated.
- Most patients suffering a witnessed vagal arrest respond remarkably well to prompt intubation, ventilation, and atropine administration. Full CPR should be instituted if no response to initial therapy occurs.

POST-RESUSCITATION CARE

Preventing Rearrest

- Many patients that are initially resuscitated suffer an additional episode of CPA within the first few hours, and often few minutes, following ROSC.
- A rapid search for underlying causes of the arrest must be undertaken, and these must be addressed immediately. Special emphasis should be placed on finding reversible disease processes, such as drug-induced hypotension, hypovolemia, hypoventilation, anemia, or electrolyte abnormalities, as these situations are most likely to result in successful outcomes when appropriately treated.

Cerebral Protection

- Cerebral ischemia (and subsequent reperfusion) may lead to long-term neurologic dysfunction in patients suffering CPA and subsequent resuscitation. This has led to the creation of the acronym *CPCR,* which stands for *cardiopulmonary cerebral resuscitation* and reflects the importance of neurologic outcome when assessing the success of resuscitation.
- Measures to limit progressive neurologic injury in post-CPA patients include head elevation to 30 degrees. This should be accomplished by elevating the entire chest, neck, and head to avoid acute kinking of the neck and possible jugular vein compression.
- **Mannitol** may be given at a dose of 0.25 to 1.0 gram/kg IV (dogs and cats) over 20 minutes to treat cerebral edema, improve cerebral microvascular flow, and to provide free radical scavenging effects.
- Ventilatory status should be evaluated (either by end-tidal CO_2, or ideally by blood gas analysis, and normocapnia should be maintained. This limits increases in intracranial pressure created by hypercapnia-induced cerebral vasodilation, as well as prevents hypocapnia-related cerebral vasoconstriction and diminished cerebral blood flow. Many patients that suffer protracted periods of CPA do not ventilate effectively in the immediate (< 24 hour) post-arrest period and require mechanical ventilation to maintain normocapnia.
- Induced hypothermia has been shown to be beneficial in improving neurologic outcome following CPR in human patients. Although this is difficult to translate to clinical veterinary patients, overzealous rewarming of mildly hypothermic patients is not recommended.

Intensive Care

- Patients resuscitated from CPA may suffer a range of post-resuscitation syndromes affecting multiple organ systems. The severity of these abnormalities is dependent on the duration of the arrest as well as the condition of the patient prior to the episode.
- In addition to neurologic dysfunction, post-arrest patients often have significant cardiovascular (arrhythmia, myocardial dysfunction, hypotension), renal (acute renal failure), and gastrointestinal (shock gut) sequelae. The low-flow state during CPA and CPR creates global ischemia followed by subsequent reperfusion and leads to systemic inflammation (systemic inflammatory response syndrome) and activation of the coagulation cascade and disseminated intravascular coagulation. There is also the possibility that CPR has created iatrogenic injury (rib fractures, pulmonary contusion) or has resulted in additional management concerns (post-thoracotomy or post-tracheostomy patients).
- Intensive monitoring and supportive care is required to address these conditions, as well as conditions underlying the arrest. It is not common for post-CPA patients to require pressor therapy, mechanical ventilation, or other advanced therapy to survive the post-arrest period and be discharged from the hospital.

KEY POINT

Post-resuscitation care is essential to the ultimate success of CPR. Intensive monitoring and supportive care is necessary to identify and address the underlying cause of CPA as well as to manage post-resuscitation syndromes.

Frequently Asked Questions

When should CPR not be performed?
The decision to perform CPR can be difficult, especially when this decision needs to be made in a crisis situation. Retrospective studies have shown that survival to discharge is generally less than 10% for patients suffering a full CPA. In general, the greatest chance for a successful outcome involves a patient in which a cause for the arrest can be rapidly identified and treated. This is not often the case for patients with advanced or multisystemic diseases. Although many of these patients can be initially resuscitated, survival to discharge is extraordinarily unlikely. Speaking to an owner about a resuscitation code (full CPR, limited CPR, or Do Not Resuscitate) is recommended in the instance that a critically ill patient with an advanced disease is admitted to the hospital. In this way, futile resuscitation efforts may be avoided, and appropriate end of life decisions may be made.

What is the neurologic outcome of veterinary patients surviving CPA?
As mentioned previously, the survival rate of patients suffering CPA is poor. Additionally, many veterinarians have concerns about the potential for neurologic dysfunction in patients that do survive to hospital discharge. Although this is a major concern in people that have received CPR, a recent retrospective study demonstrated that 16 of 18 veterinary patients that survived CPA were neurologically normal at the time of hospital discharge, and that 1 of the remaining 2 patients was normal within 2 months.

SUGGESTED READINGS

Cole SG, Otto CM, Hughes D: Cardiopulmonary cerebral resuscitation in small animals: a clinical practice review. Part I, J Vet Emerg Crit Care 12(4):261-267, 2002.

Cole SG, Otto CM, Hughes D: Cardiopulmonary cerebral resuscitation in small animals: a clinical practice review. Part II, J Vet Emerg Crit Care 13(1):13-23, 2002.

Kass PH, Haskins SC: Survival following cardiopulmonary resuscitation in dogs and cats, J Vet Emerg Crit Care 2(2):57-65, 1992.

Lehman TL, Manning AM: Postarrest syndrome and the respiratory and cardiovascular systems in postarrest patients, Compend Contin Ed Practic Vet 25(7):492-503,2003.

Lehman TL, Manning AM: Renal, central nervous, and gastrointestinal systems in postarrest patients, Compend Contin Ed Practic Vet 25(7):504-513, 2003.

Waldrop JE, Rozanski EA, Swanke ED, et al: Causes of cardiopulmonary arrest, resuscitation management, and functional outcome in dogs and cats surviving cardiopulmonary arrest, J Vet Emerg Crit Care 14(1):22-29, 2004.

Wingfield WE, Van Pelt DR: Respiratory and cardiopulmonary arrest in dogs and cats: 265 cases (1986-1991), J Am Vet Med Assoc 200(12):1993-1996, 1992.

CHAPTER 18

Emergency Management and Critical Care

Steven G. Cole and Kenneth J. Drobatz

INTRODUCTION

In general, cardiac emergencies may be divided into three groups:

Heart Failure

- Congestive heart failure (CHF) (commonly regarded as "backward" failure)
  - CHF patients generally present with respiratory signs (due to pleural effusion or pulmonary edema) or abdominal distension (due to ascites).
- Low output (commonly regarded as "forward" failure)
  - Animals with low-output heart failure most commonly have signs of weakness or collapse that are typically due to dilated cardiomyopathy or pericardial effusion.
  - The term *myocardial failure* is used to denote the presence of reduced myocardial contractility (e.g., dilated cardiomyopathy)

KEY POINT

It is important to remember that the ultimate cardiac emergency is cardiopulmonary arrest. The management of cardiopulmonary arrest and strategies for cardiopulmonary resuscitation in small animals are covered in a separate chapter.

Cardiac Rhythm Disturbances

- The most common cardiac arrhythmias causing emergent presentations are third-degree heart block and tachyarrhythmias. These animals generally present with low output failure and signs of weakness or collapse.

Thromboembolism

- Thromboembolic disease typically presents with acute dysfunction of the area of compromised blood supply. In cats with cardiomyopathy, this is most often the hind limbs due to an aortic saddle thrombus, although other limbs may also be affected. Pulmonary thromboembolism may be an acute cause of respiratory distress and low output heart failure in dogs with a variety of underlying diseases. Thromboembolic disease is also encountered in animals with infectious endocarditis.

ASSESSING CARDIOVASCULAR FUNCTION IN THE EMERGENCY PATIENT

Physical Examination

- Historical complaints that support a primary cardiac emergency are varied and include weakness, lethargy, collapse or syncope, as well as cough, tachypnea, or respiratory distress. Additional complaints such as anorexia, vomiting, or diarrhea are not uncommon, as primary cardiovascular problems may have wide-ranging effects on all major organ systems.

- Physical examination findings consistent with primary cardiac emergencies are variable depending upon the specific condition.
  - Mucous membranes may be pale secondary to vasoconstriction or cyanotic secondary to hypoxemia. Capillary refill time is commonly prolonged due to diminished cardiac output and hypoperfusion. Decreased tissue perfusion is more commonly seen in instances of low output failure vs. congestive failure.
  - The majority of cases of canine and feline heart failure are accompanied by an audible murmur or gallop. Diminished heart sounds occur in cases of pericardial or pleural effusion or severe myocardial failure.
  - Bradyarrhythmias or tachyarrhythmias are common, and are often associated with irregular rhythms and diminished pulse quality or pulse deficits.
  - Pulsus paradoxus, where pulse strength gets weaker on inspiration is detected in approximately 50% of cases of pericardial effusion.
  - Tachypnea and respiratory distress is often present. In cases of pulmonary edema, auscultation will commonly reveal harsh lung sounds or crackles. In cases of pleural effusion, lung sounds are commonly diminished ventrally.
  - Animals suffering from low output failure often have a low body temperature and depressed mentation.
  - Jugular pulses or distension is commonly detected in animals with right-sided heart failure.

Diagnostic Tests

- Diagnostic tests include electrocardiography (ECG), pulse oximetry, blood pressure measurement, chest radiographs and echocardiography.
- A lead II ECG is usually sufficient for the rapid diagnosis of most cardiac rhythm disturbances.
- Pulse oximetry provides a useful estimate of hemoglobin saturation and arterial oxygen content, findings that may be further evaluated by arterial blood gas analysis.
- Noninvasive blood pressure measurement may be accomplished via Doppler or oscillometric techniques, and reflects cardiac output and vasomotor tone. It is useful in the recognition of shock states and in monitoring therapeutic interventions.
- Chest radiography is the ideal method to assess size and shape of the cardiac silhouette, pulmonary vasculature, pulmonary parenchyma and pleural space. It represents the gold standard in documenting CHF in the form of pulmonary edema and/or pleural effusion.
- Echocardiography provides information about cardiac structure and function. It is typically used to confirm a suspected diagnosis, determine severity of disease, assess myocardial contractility, and detect intracardiac or proximal pulmonary artery thrombi. Echocardiography is particularly useful in assessing patients with pericardial effusion for cardiac neoplasia.

KEY POINT

Animals presenting with emergency problems related to heart disease are often not stable enough for prolonged diagnostic tests. Empiric therapy for the most likely cardiac problem based on signalment, history, physical examination, and chest radiographs is often performed. In many cases, appropriate therapy can be instituted without the need for an immediate echocardiographic exam.

EMERGENCY TREATMENT OF HEART FAILURE

- Treatment of heart failure involves the following:
  - Identification and remediation of underlying causes
  - Elimination of aggravating conditions (i.e., cardiac depressants, hypertension, arrhythmias)
  - Control of congestion
  - Improvement of myocardial contractility
  - Improvement of myocardial relaxation
  - Reduction of cardiac work
  - Reduction of pathologic remodeling and neurohormonal activation

Congestive Heart Failure

- CHF results from elevated cardiac filling pressures that cause pulmonary or systemic venous hypertension and extravasation of fluid into the interstitial space or a body cavity.
- The location of this fluid is dependent upon the failing ventricle (left-sided, right-sided, or biventricular failure) and the subsequent signs of CHF relates to the magnitude of the fluid accumulation.
- CHF is the result of many cardiac diseases including chronic valvular disease, cardiomyopathies, infectious endocarditis, myocarditis,

persistent arrhythmia, or congenital cardiovascular anomalies.

Left-Sided Congestive Heart Failure

- Left-sided congestive heart failure (LCHF) results from elevated left atrial pressure. Elevated left atrial pressure may result from mitral valve insufficiency, mitral valve stenosis, or systolic or diastolic dysfunction of the left ventricle. In dogs, LCHF causes pulmonary edema, whereas in cats it may be associated with both pulmonary edema and pleural effusion.
- Clinical signs
  - Clinical signs of LCHF failure result from pulmonary compromise and include tachypnea, respiratory distress, lethargy, and exercise intolerance. Dogs with pulmonary edema frequently have a cough, whereas a cough is rare in cats with heart failure.
  - Physical examination findings include harsh lung sounds and crackles in patients with pulmonary edema. Cats with pleural effusion usually have dull lung sounds in the ventral lung fields, especially when compared to the degree of respiratory effort. Severely compromised patients will present in respiratory distress, and cyanosis is not uncommon. Most patients with LCHF will be tachycardic and usually have abnormalities on auscultation such as a heart murmur, gallop rhythm, or an arrhythmia.

Diagnostics

- Confirmation of LCHF is made by obtaining chest radiographs to document the presence and severity of pulmonary edema or pleural effusion.
- In dogs, pulmonary edema tends to be most evident at the perihilar region, although all lung lobes may be affected in severe cases. Pulmonary edema in cats does not follow this pattern, and the location of affected lung tissue is variable. Pleural effusion in cats may be found either with or without concurrent pulmonary edema. Other changes supportive of LCHF include cardiomegaly, evidence of left atrial enlargement, and dilated pulmonary vasculature, particularly the pulmonary veins.
- ECG analysis may show a variety of changes, including prolongation of P wave duration (P-mitrale), increased R wave amplitude or duration, a left axis shift, bundle branch block, supraventricular or ventricular premature complexes or tachycardia, or atrial fibrillation.
- Echocardiography provides definitive information regarding the size of the cardiac chambers as well as indicators of systolic and diastolic cardiac function.
- Many patients that present with LCHF have severe respiratory distress and cannot tolerate a full diagnostic workup. Because of this, therapy is often instituted prior to obtaining radiographs or an echocardiogram. In these cases, the decision to treat for CHF is based on the history, clinical signs, and physical examination findings at the time of presentation. If access to a portable ultrasound machine is available, additional information may be obtained from a brief screening examination of the thorax for the presence of pleural effusion or grossly recognizable changes in cardiac structure (e.g., dilated left atrium, myocardial chamber dimension or wall thickness) or function (e.g., markedly diminished fractional shortening).

Treatment

- Emergency treatment of LCHF involves the use of diuretics, vasodilators, and in some cases, inotropic agents. Additionally, oxygen therapy is vital in patients with compromised pulmonary function, and some patients may benefit from the judicious use of anxiolytic drugs. Cats with significant pleural effusion require therapeutic thoracocentesis.

Diuretic Therapy

- The goal of diuretic therapy in the treatment of LCHF is to reduce the circulating blood volume, thereby reducing the preload of the left ventricle and left atrial pressure. The primary diuretic used in the acute management of CHF is furosemide.
- **Furosemide** may be administered intravenously, although the intramuscular route may be used in patients without vascular access.
- The dose is dependent upon the severity of clinical signs and patient response. In dogs, an initial dose of 2 to 6 mg/kg IV, IM, or SC may be followed by additional doses every 1 to 2 hours until the respiratory character improves. Following improvement, additional doses of 2 mg/kg are typically given at 6 to 12 hour intervals dependent on clinical status. Cats tend to be more sensitive to furosemide therapy, and initial doses of 1 to 2 mg/kg IV, IM, or SC every 1 to 2 hours followed by 1 to 2mg/kg every 8 to 12 hours are recommended following initial clinical response.
- Side effects of furosemide include dehydration, azotemia, hypokalemia, metabolic alkalosis, and, potentially, volume depletion.

Vasodilator Therapy

- Vasodilator therapy has two purposes. First, venodilation decreases preload by providing additional vascular capacitance. Second, arterial vasodilation reduces left ventricular afterload, thereby reducing myocardial work and promoting forward flow.
- **Sodium nitroprusside** (dogs; 2 to 10 mcg/kg/min constant-rate infusion [CRI]) increases the concentration of nitric oxide, a potent vasodilator, and is considered to be a balanced vasodilator providing both venous and arterial dilation. Combined with aggressive diuretic therapy, the use of sodium nitroprusside is very effective in resolving severe pulmonary edema. Because of its potency and the potential for excessive vasodilation and secondary hypotension, it is recommended that blood pressure be monitored closely during infusion.
  - In all cases, the initial dose should be at the low end of the range, and the dose increased based upon clinical response and blood pressure measurement. In general, mean arterial pressure should be maintained above 60 mm Hg, while systolic pressures should not be less than 90 mm Hg.
  - Sodium nitroprusside is light sensitive and may induce precipitation of co-administered IV drugs. Thus, it is ideally administered through a separate, light-protected IV set and catheter.
  - Long-term nitroprusside therapy is limited by the production of molecular cyanide, although toxic doses are not usually reached until 36 to 48 hours following onset of therapy.
- **Nitroglycerin ointment (2%)** is a commonly used venodilator in small animal emergency patients. The ointment is applied topically to a clipped area on either the pinna or inguinal region and is dosed according to body size. A ⅛-inch strip is used in cats and small dogs (< 10 kg), a ¼-inch strip in medium dogs (10 to 25 kg), and a ½-inch strip in large dogs (> 25 kg). The ointment may be applied every 12 hours for the first 24 to 36 hours of treatment and should be handled with gloves, as it may be absorbed transdermally.
  - Although the use of nitroglycerin ointment is common, it should be noted that topically applied therapy is limited in severe CHF, especially given the profound peripheral vasoconstriction that exists in these patients, and efficacy is questionable.
- **Hydralazine** (dogs: 0.5 to 1 mg/kg IV or PO every 12 hours) is an arterial dilator that causes a marked reduction in afterload and is useful in cases of severe mitral regurgitation. As with other arterial dilators, hydralazine may be associated with hypotension and reflex tachycardia in the face of decreased peripheral resistance.

Positive Inotropic Agents

- Positive inotropic agents are indicated in managing LCHF associated with systolic dysfunction of the left ventricle. These drugs are administered in conjunction with diuretic and vasodilator therapy. Dilated cardiomyopathy is the most common disease producing this condition; however, myocardial failure secondary to advanced chronic valvular disease, or end-stage forms of other cardiomyopathies may also result in severe systolic dysfunction.
  - **Dobutamine** (dogs, 2 to 15 mcg/kg/min CRI; cats, 1 to 5 mcg/kg/min CRI) is a beta-adrenergic sympathomimetic. Side effects of dobutamine may include tachycardia and ventricular arrhythmias. Cats may develop gastrointestinal or neurologic signs associated with administration.
  - **Dopamine** (dogs and cats, 2 to 8 mcg/kg/min CRI) should be used with caution, as it has alpha-adrenergic effects at higher doses and may cause deleterious vasoconstriction and tachycardia in the face of diminished myocardial function.
  - Additional options for inotropic support include phosphodiesterase inhibitors such as milrinone. **Milrinone** (dogs, 50 mcg/kg slow IV bolus followed by 0.40 to 0.75 mcg/kg/min CRI) is a drug that has both positive inotropic and vasodilatory properties, similar to a combination of dobutamine and sodium nitroprusside. Experience with clinical use in emergency patients is limited, but milrinone may be an effective agent for the short-term management of LCHF associated with systolic dysfunction.

Oxygen Therapy

- Oxygen therapy (40% to 60% fraction of inspired oxygen) helps to maintain the arterial oxygen content in the face of pulmonary dysfunction (in the form of ventilation-perfusion mismatch) induced by pulmonary edema. Oxygen therapy may also reduce pulmonary vascular resistance by ameliorating hypoxic pulmonary vasoconstriction.
  - An oxygen cage is often the most effective method to administer supplemental oxygen to patients with heart failure, although other alternatives (such as nasal, mask, flow-by, hood, or intratracheal oxygen supplementation) exist. Although an oxygen cage provides a quiet environment that can achieve high concentrations of oxygen, these concentrations decrease

rapidly when the cage is opened. Thus, an oxygen cage is less effective when patients require frequent treatments or physical examination.

- Patients should receive oxygen supplementation until their respiratory rate and effort have improved and/or objective measurements of pulmonary function (i.e., pulse oximetry or arterial blood gas) have returned to normal. If possible, the fraction of inspired oxygen should be tapered over 6 to 12 hours to allow the patient to adjust to breathing room air.
- For patients with fulminant LCHF and massive pulmonary edema, standard oxygen supplementation may not be sufficient to prevent either respiratory or ventilatory failure. In these cases, only early intubation and mechanical ventilation will provide the respiratory support necessary to sustain life. Mechanical ventilation is a significant commitment for both the owner and clinician; however, in many cases, mechanical ventilation may be weaned after only a short period (1 to 2 days) following aggressive medical management of CHF.
- The use of anxiolytic agents in the treatment of CHF is common in human medicine and may also be useful in veterinary patients. Low-dose **morphine** (dogs, 0.1 mg/kg IV every 4 to 6 hours as needed), **butorphanol** (dogs and cats, 0.1 to 0.2 mg/kg IV every 4 hours), **diazepam** or **midazolam** (dogs and cats, 0.1 to 0.3 mg/kg IV every 4 hours), or low doses of **acepromazine** (dogs and cats, 0.005 to 0.02 mg/kg IV every 6 to 8 hours) can be administered.

Therapeutic Thoracocentesis

- Cats with significant pleural effusions associated with LCHF experience significant benefit from therapeutic thoracocentesis. Some cats will tolerate the thoracocentesis with minimal restraint, although many cats require some degree of sedation (butorphanol [0.1 to 0.2 mg/kg] in combination with diazepam or midazolam [0.1 to 0.3 mg/kg]).
  - Thoracocentesis is generally performed between the seventh and ninth intercostal spaces at the level of the costochondral junction. The area is clipped and aseptically prepared prior to initiating the procedure. Thoracocentesis in cats is generally performed with a 21-gauge butterfly catheter attached to a three-way stopcock and a 10-ml or 20-ml syringe. In extremely obese cats, a 22-gauge needle and extension set is used in place of the butterfly catheter. In larger dogs, a 16- or 18-gauge catheter with a 60-ml syringe may be used.
  - The needle should be introduced just cranial to a rib to avoid the intercostal vessels and advanced into the pleural space. The needle should be redirected or the procedure terminated once lung tissue is felt at the tip of the needle or fluid is no longer able to be aspirated. Both sides of the chest should be aspirated as bilateral fluid accumulation is found in the majority of cats with pleural effusion secondary to CHF. It is not uncommon to remove 200 to 300 ml of fluid from the thorax of cats with severe pleural effusion.

Right-Sided Congestive Heart Failure

- Right-sided congestive heart failure (RCHF) is much less common in patients presenting to the emergency room. An exception is pericardial effusion and cardiac tamponade (see Pericardial Effusion below). RCHF results from elevated right atrial and central venous pressures. Conditions that may result in elevated central vencus pressure (CVP) include tricuspid valve insufficiency or stenosis, pulmonic valve insufficiency or stenosis, pulmonary hypertension, and right ventricular systolic or diastolic dysfunction.
- Clinical signs of RCHF are related to the presence of pleural effusion, ascites, or peripheral edema that results from increased right atrial pressure. Patients with large volume pleural effusion may present in respiratory distress and with dull lung sounds. Patients with ascites will present with a distended abdomen and may have respiratory compromise. Additional indications of RCHF are the presence of distended jugular veins and prominent jugular pulses, as well as the presence of a heart murmur (particularly with a maximal intensity at the left heart base or the right side of the chest). Other changes such as a split S_2 sound or gallop rhythm are variable dependent upon the underlying disease.
- Emergency therapy for RCHF consists of thoracocentesis for large volume pleural effusions (see previous section).
- In animals with tense ascites, abdominocentesis may be performed to reduce pressure on the diaphragm and improve ventilation. Abdominocentesis can be performed with equipment similar to thoracocentesis.
  - The procedure may be performed standing or with the patient in left lateral recumbency, which reduces the likelihood of lacerating the spleen. An area caudal to the umbilicus

is clipped and prepared aseptically, and the needle or catheter is induced on or just lateral to the midline. An alternative technique uses two or more short 16- to 18-gauge catheters placed just caudal and to either side of the umbilicus. The animal remains standing during the procedure and fluid is allowed to drain passively. Debate exists about the volume of fluid that can be removed safely from an animal with ascites. Most dogs will tolerate the removal of 50 to 100 ml/kg of ascites without untoward effects.

Pericardial Effusion

- Pericardial effusion typically results from an underlying neoplasia, such as hemangiosarcoma, heart base tumors, lymphoma, or mesothelioma. Other causes of pericardial effusion include inflammatory or infectious pericarditis, restrictive pericarditis, coagulopathy, atrial rupture secondary to chronic dilation, and blunt or penetrating thoracic trauma. Small volume pericardial effusions associated with CHF may also occur, and this phenomenon is relatively common in cats.
- Clinical signs result from cardiac tamponade and RCHF and may include abdominal distension from ascites, tachypnea from pleural effusion, weakness, lethargy, or collapse.
- Physical examination findings include tachycardia and dull heart sounds on auscultation. In some cases, pulsus paradoxus (decrement of pulse pressure pulse quality that occurs during the inspiratory phase of the respiratory cycle) may be recognized. Additional physical exam findings may include jugular distension and prominent jugular pulses, abdominal distension with a palpable fluid wave, and dull ventral lung sounds if pleural effusion is present. A depressed mentation and delayed capillary refill is suggestive of cardiovascular collapse and hypoperfusion in severe cases.
- Diagnostic test results consistent with pericardial effusion and cardiac tamponade include sinus tachycardia with diminished complex size on the ECG, with or without the presence of electrical alternans. Electrical alternans describes an alternation in the height of the R wave of the QRS complex, and results from beat to beat changes in the mean electrical axis as the heart moves within the fluid filled pericardium. Chest radiographs often demonstrate an enlarged cardiac silhouette, as well as distension of the caudal vena cava. Pleural effusion or evidence of metastatic lung disease may be present. The cardiac silhouette often has a classic "globoid" appearance; however, this may not be true in cases of acute pericardial effusion. A brief echocardiographic exam can generally confirm the presence of pericardial effusion.

KEY POINT

The differentiation of pericardial effusion from pleural effusion on echocardiographic exam can be challenging. Pericardial effusion is recognized by the circular appearance of hypoechoic fluid surrounding the heart. This fluid is bordered by the hyperechoic pericardium. Cardiac tamponade may be recognized as collapse of the right atrium, and in some cases, an underlying cause for the effusion is seen, such as a mass involving the right atrium or atrioventricular (AV) groove. In patients with pleural but not pericardial effusion, the fluid does not encircle the heart, and lung tissue as well as mediastinal tissue may be seen within the effusion.

- Although blood tests are not often a primary diagnostic tool in the diagnosis of pericardial effusion, documenting the presence of a coagulopathy is vital in the management of those patients in which this is a primary cause of the pericardial effusion. Additionally, it should be recognized that patients with more chronic pericardial effusions may develop hyponatremia and hyperkalemia. These pseudo-Addisonian electrolyte changes result from the enhanced antidiuretic hormone secretion and decreased renal perfusion that occurs secondary to decreased effective circulating volume in these patients. These abnormalities rapidly resolve with the resolution of cardiac tamponade.
- The emergency treatment of symptomatic pericardial effusion and cardiac tamponade involves volume expansion and pericardiocentesis.
  - Volume expansion using partial shock doses (30 to 45 ml/kg) of an isotonic crystalloid transiently increases right atrial pressure. This may improve stroke volume and cardiac output and often results in clinical improvement while steps are taken to perform pericardiocentesis.
  - Pericardiocentesis is the treatment of choice for the initial management of cardiac tamponade and is a life-saving procedure in many cases. To perform pericardiocentesis, the patient is placed in left lateral recumbency. Sedation may

be required in some patients, and conservative doses of an opioid in combination with a benzodiazepine are generally well tolerated. Other patients require only local anesthesia.

- An area from the third to the seventh intercostal spaces is clipped and prepared aseptically, and a local anesthetic is infiltrated at the fifth intercostal space at the level of the costochondral junction. A small stab incision is made in the skin, and a catheter is advanced through the chest wall, just cranial to the sixth rib. In large dogs, a 14-gauge, 12-cm over-the-needle catheter is used, whereas a 16-gauge, 8-cm over-the-needle catheter is used in smaller dogs. In very small dogs, or in cats, an 18-gauge, 2-inch over-the-needle catheter may be used.
- The catheter is slowly advanced toward the pericardium. Generally, the catheter may be felt as first the chest wall and then the pericardium is punctured. Entrance into the pericardium is accompanied by the presence of fluid flashing back into the catheter hub. This may be recognized sooner if a syringe is attached to the needle and a slight negative pressure is applied as it is advanced, or if the needle has been filled with sterile saline prior to the procedure.
- Once the pericardium has been punctured, the catheter is advanced off the stylet, and attached to an extension set with a three-way stopcock and syringe. The pericardial fluid is aspirated, and fluid should be immediately placed into an activated clotting time tube. This allows pericardial fluid, which should not clot, to be differentiated from peripheral blood, which should clot. As the pericardium is drained, additional samples should be obtained for fluid analysis and cytology.
- The ECG should be monitored during the procedure for the presence of ventricular arrhythmias that occur when the catheter contacts the epicardium. If present, these arrhythmias may be treated by slightly withdrawing the catheter or with an intravenous bolus of lidocaine (dogs, 2 mg/kg). The ECG is also useful to confirm the effectiveness of the procedure, as the heart rate often returns to the normal range and electrical alternans disappears as the heart is decompressed.
- Once fluid can no longer be aspirated, the catheter is withdrawn. Confirmation of a successful pericardiocentesis may be obtained with a brief recheck ultrasound. Following the procedure, the patient should be monitored for recurrent effusion. Further management of pericardial effusion involves a complete echocardiogram and the consideration of more definitive therapy such as a subtotal pericardectomy or a thoracoscopic pericardial window.

KEY POINT

In patients that are clinically stable, a complete echocardiographic examination is often performed prior to pericardiocentesis as the presence of effusion supplies useful echocardiographic contrast in the attempt to identify cardiac neoplasms.

Forward (Low-Output) Heart Failure

- Forward heart failure is the result of impaired myocardial function and results in diminished cardiac output and cardiogenic shock. Common causes of forward heart failure include dilated cardiomyopathy and myocardial failure secondary to end-stage chronic valvular disease, or doxorubicin toxicity. Significant tachyarrhythmias and bradyarrhythmias may also result in a form of forward heart failure.
- Clinical signs of cardiogenic shock include weakness, lethargy, and collapse. Respiratory signs may be seen if CHF is also present. Physical examination findings associated with forward heart failure include hypothermia, pallor, delayed capillary refill time, tachycardia, and poor pulse quality. Heart sounds may be diminished or a heart murmur and/or gallop rhythm may be heard. The presence of pulmonary edema or pleural effusion will produce characteristic changes on auscultation.
- The clinical diagnosis of forward heart failure is made by finding evidence of decreased myocardial function in combination with hypotension and clinical signs of hypoperfusion. Decreased systolic function is documented using echocardiography and is evidenced by diminished fractional shortening, increased left ventricular end-systolic dimension, increased E-point to septal separation, and decreased aortic and pulmonic flows. Chest radiographs may document the presence and severity of concurrent CHF, and a lead II ECG will help identify significant rhythm disturbances.
- Treatment of forward heart failure involves efforts to improve myocardial performance and cardiac output. This may be accomplished by ensuring

that adequate preload is present and by providing inotropic support.

- Clinical estimates of preload may be obtained by measuring left and right ventricular filling pressures.
  - Right ventricular filling pressures may be assessed by placing a central venous catheter and measuring the CVP. Normal CVP ranges between 0 and 8 cm H_2O, although wide variability exists between patients.
  - Left ventricular filling pressures may be assessed by placing a pulmonary artery catheter and measuring pulmonary capillary wedge (occlusion) pressures (PCWP). Normal PCWP ranges between 5 and 14 cm H_2O. In animals with low CVP or PCWP, judicious fluid therapy may be used to increase preload and cardiac output. If the CVP or PCWP is normal or high, fluid therapy is not likely to be of benefit and may precipitate CHF.
- Inotropic support is indicated in cases of cardiogenic shock secondary to myocardial systolic dysfunction.
  - **Dobutamine** (dogs, 2 to 15 mcg/kg/min; cats, 1 to 5 mcg/kg/min) is generally the first line agent in dogs due to its ability to increase contractility without significant increases in heart rate. Dobutamine may also be used in cats, although gastrointestinal and neurologic side effects usually limit utility.
  - **Dopamine** (dogs and cats, 2 to 8 mcg/kg/min) may also be used. Dopamine should be used with caution; however, as it has alpha-adrenergic effects at higher doses and may increase afterload and cause reductions in cardiac output. In patients with a pulmonary artery catheter, cardiac output may be obtained by the thermodilution method. Combined with measurements of direct arterial blood pressure and calculation of systemic vascular resistance, this allows for the most effective clinical assessment of hemodynamics and the response to therapy.
  - Oral **pimobendan** therapy (0.25mg PO every 12 hours) should be considered if intravenous therapy is not possible.

CARDIAC RHYTHM DISTURBANCES

- See Chapter 16, Treatment of Cardiac Arrhythmias and Conduction Disturbances, for further discussion.
- Cardiac arrhythmias are common in emergency patients and may be associated with alterations in autonomic tone or responsiveness, drug exposure, electrolyte abnormalities, impaired myocardial oxygen delivery, myocardial trauma or inflammation, and primary myocardial disease.
- In many situations, these cardiac rhythm disturbances represent the cardiac effects of a systemic disease and do not require specific treatment. In other cases, aggressive intervention is required to address unstable rhythms or life-threatening perfusion deficits.
- Physical examination findings consistent with a cardiac rhythm disturbance include bradycardia or tachycardia, an irregular rhythm on auscultation, and the identification of pulse deficits. Depressed mentation or collapse may also be encountered, and syncope may be observed in cases of acute, arrhythmia-induced decreases in cerebral perfusion.
- Confirmation of cardiac rhythm disturbances is achieved by ECG. Obtaining a lead II rhythm strip is often sufficient to diagnose most rhythm disturbances. However, a 6- or 10-lead ECG may be helpful to accurately identify and characterize complex arrhythmias.

KEY POINT

Cardiac rhythm disorders may be intermittent and may not be noted on a single lead II ECG. Detection of rhythm disorders sometimes requires 24-hour telemetric, Holter, or event monitoring.

Bradyarrhythmias

- Bradycardia is a relatively uncommon finding in patients presenting to the emergency room.
- Clinical signs associated with bradyarrhythmias include weakness, lethargy, depression, and syncope.
- Causes of symptomatic bradyarrhythmias in emergency patients include increased vagal tone, electrolyte abnormalities, hypothermia, drug toxicities, and significant disturbances of the cardiac conduction system.
- ECG rhythms seen in bradycardic patients include sinus bradycardia, atrial standstill, sinus arrest, and high-grade second- or third-degree AV block.

Sinus Bradycardia

- In emergency patients, sinus bradycardia is most often seen associated with increased vagal tone.

- Increased vagal tone may result from intra-abdominal or intrathoracic diseases, or from coughing, vomiting, retching, or straining to urinate or defecate. The Cushing reflex, which occurs secondary to head trauma or other causes of elevated intracranial pressure, also produces sinus bradycardia. In this situation, bradycardia is associated with hypertension that is produced by a massive discharge from the medullary vasomotor center.
- Other causes of sinus bradycardia include absolute or relative drug overdoses, especially of anesthetic agents such as opioids, benzodiazepines, or alpha-2 adrenergic agonists. Cardiac or vasoactive medications, including calcium channel blockers, beta-adrenergic blockers, digoxin, and cholinergic agents, may also produce sinus bradycardia either by increases in vagal tone or by reducing sympathetic tone.
- Sinus bradycardia may also be associated with hypothermia or severe hypoglycemia (blood glucose less than 50 mg/dl).
- Management of symptomatic sinus bradycardia generally centers on the identification and treatment of underlying factors. In cases of hypothermia or hypoglycemia, the heart rate and clinical signs often improve markedly once these factors are identified and addressed. Hypothermia is best managed by the use of an indirect heating method such as a warm air blanket. This may help minimize overheating or detrimental vasodilation that may occur with direct heat sources such as heating pads or hot water bottles. Intravenous fluids that have been warmed to body temperature are also appropriate in patients without contraindications to fluid therapy.
- Although neurologic signs usually predominate over bradycardia, symptomatic hypoglycemia may be treated with a bolus of 0.25 to 1 gram/kg of 50% dextrose that has been diluted 50:50 with 0.9% saline. Additional dextrose bolus therapy or a dextrose infusion may be necessary while causes of hypoglycemia (such as insulin overdose, hypoadrenocorticism, paraneoplastic syndrome, systemic inflammatory response syndrome, or sepsis) are investigated.
- Increased vagal tone secondary to intrathoracic disease, intra-abdominal disease, coughing, gagging, retching, or straining may cause severe sinus bradycardia that results in cardiovascular collapse or syncope. In these situations, immediate administration of a parasympatholytic agent is necessary. Due to its rapid onset of action and short half-life, atropine is preferred over other agents such as glycopyrrolate. Although the cardiac arrest dose of atropine is 0.04 mg/kg, lower doses (0.005 to 0.01 mg/kg) are often effective in patients with bradycardia, and these doses are less likely to be associated with rebound sinus tachycardia. Intravenous administration is ideal (rarely, a brief centrally induced exacerbation of bradycardia may occur with this route), although atropine may also be administered via intratracheal, intraosseous, or intramuscular routes. Along with atropine administration, efforts to identify and correct the underlying cause of the increased vagal tone are necessary.
- Atropine is also indicated in treating sinus bradycardia associated with anesthetic agents, as are measures to decrease the depth of anesthesia and to administer specific drug reversal agents. Opioids may be reversed with Naloxone (0.03 mg/kg IV, IM, or SQ) and benzodiazepines may be reversed with Flumazenil (0.03 mg/kg IV, IM, or SQ). Sinus bradycardia associated with the administration of parasympathomimetics is also atropine responsive. There are specific recommendations for the management of patients receiving overdoses of cardiac medications such as digoxin, calcium channel blockers or beta-adrenergic blockers. These guidelines are discussed later.

Second- and Third-Degree Atrioventricular Block

- High-grade second-degree AV block and third-degree AV block represent severe disruptions of the normal cardiac conduction system. Although structural heart diseases, such as myocardial fibrosis, inflammation, or infiltration, are thought to be responsible for most cases of severe AV block, these rhythms may also be seen in patients with systemic disease or drug toxicities. Drugs associated with second or third-degree AV block include digoxin, calcium channel blockers and beta-adrenergic blockers
- Most emergency patients with high-grade second and third-degree AV block will have clinical signs relating to decreased cardiac output such as lethargy, depressed mentation, and, commonly, syncope. Rarely, these rhythms will be documented in an otherwise asymptomatic patient. These asymptomatic patients (generally cats) often have third-degree AV block with a relatively high ventricular rate supporting an adequate cardiac output.
- Medical management of high-grade second- and third-degree AV block consists of initial

parasympatholytic therapy followed by sympathomimetic drugs.

- Initially, **atropine** may be given at the full vagolytic dose of 0.4 mg/kg IV. This is often effective in elevating the rate of discharge of the sinus node, but is only rarely effective in improving the AV block in these patients.
- Alternate therapy consists of beta-1 agonist drugs given in an effort to accelerate the ventricular escape rate. **Isoproterenol** (dogs, 0.04 to 0.08 mcg/kg/min) is commonly used in this manner, although this drug can cause hypotension secondary to vasodilation. An alternative drug is dopamine (dogs and cats, 2 to 8 mcg/kg/min) at the beta agonist dose. Dobutamine is another beta-1 agonist; however, it has less of a positive chronotropic effect than dopamine.
    - Beta-1 agonists are also indicated in the treatment of beta-adrenergic blocker overdose. Whereas these drugs may be effective in some cases, an alternative therapy involves the use of **glucagon** (dogs, 200 mcg/kg). A bolus of may increase cardiac rate and contractility. If a response is noted then glucagon may be continued (dogs, 150 mcg/kg/min CRI). Glucagon may be used in dogs with calcium channel blocker overdose at a similar dosage.
- When medical management is ineffective, artificial pacemaker therapy is indicated in the treatment of symptomatic AV block (see Chapter 21, Pacemaker Implantation).
- Temporary transthoracic or transvenous pacing are considered emergency treatment to stabilize a patient until diagnostic tests may be performed or definitive therapy may be planned. If no underlying cause, such as a drug overdose or toxicity, is identified, patients with symptomatic AV block require the placement of a permanent pacemaker.

Sinus Arrest

- The most common cause of symptomatic sinus arrest is sick sinus syndrome, a condition characterized by periods of supraventricular tachycardia interspersed with periods of sinus arrest. Although this condition may occur in a number of breeds, it is seen most often in Miniature Schnauzers. Management is similar to patients with symptomatic AV block.

Hyperkalemic Cardiotoxicity

- Although not a primary cardiac abnormality, hyperkalemic cardiotoxicity is a frequent cause of symptomatic bradycardia in emergency patients. This is most common in cats with urethral obstruction, but also occurs in cases of acute renal failure, uroperitoneum, hypoadrenocorticism, and reperfusion injury.
- Hyperkalemia produces a characteristic set of changes on the ECG, however, the concentration at which these changes are noted is variable. Changes rarely occur if K^+ is < 6 mmol/L. The sequence of changes involves tented/spiked T waves, flattening of the P waves, prolongation of the P-R interval, bradycardia, loss of P waves (atrial standstill), prolongation of the QRS complex, and finally merging of the QRS and T wave complexes to form a "sine wave" pattern.
- Ventricular arrhythmias, ventricular fibrillation, and asystole may also occur secondary to severe hyperkalemia.
- The management of life-threatening hyperkalemia involves three phases: immediate cardioprotection, redistribution of serum potassium, and removal of potassium from the body.
    - Immediate cardioprotection is achieved via the use of intravenous **calcium gluconate** (dogs and cats, 50 to 100 mg/kg as a slow [3 to 5 minute] IV bolus). Overly rapid administration results in worsening bradycardia and potentially severe ventricular arrhythmias. The onset of action of calcium gluconate is usually rapid (within 5 minutes). The duration of effect is limited, however, and hyperkalemic ECG changes will recur unless steps are taken to reduce the serum potassium level.
    - Serum potassium may be transiently lowered by redistribution into the intracellular space using **regular insulin** (dogs and cats, 0.25 μ/kg; accompanied by dextrose bolus of 0.5 g/kg to help prevent iatrogenic hypoglycemia). Dextrose supplementation is also added to ongoing intravenous fluid therapy for 6 to 12 hours to prevent a decrease in blood glucose later in the course of treatment.
        - An alternative or adjunct to regular insulin therapy is the use of **sodium bicarbonate** (dogs and cats, 1 to 2 mEq/kg given over 10 to 15 minutes).
    - Definitive management involves removing potassium from the body. This is generally accomplished by establishing urine flow (relieving urethral obstruction, placing a peritoneal drainage catheter) and fluid diuresis. If adequate urine flow is unable to be achieved, patients are considered candidates for either peritoneal dialysis or hemodialysis.

Tachyarrhythmias

- Tachyarrhythmias are common in emergency patients. Clinical signs associated with pathologic tachyarrhythmias include weakness, lethargy, and collapse. On rare occasions, tachyarrhythmias may result in sudden death. Causes of symptomatic tachyarrhythmias include increased sympathetic tone, toxicities, electrolyte abnormalities, myocardial disease or ischemia, and re-entrant circuits within the myocardium. While isolated or infrequent supraventricular or ventricular premature complexes are often seen in the emergency room, most symptomatic patients have sustained tachyarrhythmias. These rhythms include sinus tachycardia, supraventricular tachycardia (including atrial or junctional tachycardia, and atrial fibrillation), and ventricular tachycardia.

Sinus Tachycardia

- Sinus tachycardia is associated with increased sympathetic tone. Common causes of sinus tachycardia in emergency patients include hypovolemia, hypotension, anemia, hypoxemia, pain, stress, fear, and excitement. No specific treatment is usually required. Rather, the heart rate responds when the underlying cause of the tachycardia is identified and addressed.
- The use of beta-adrenergic blockers, such as **esmolol** (dogs and cats, 0.05 to 0.25 mg/kg IV, followed with by 50 to 200 μg/kg/min CRI) or **propanolol** (dogs and cats, slow IV boluses of 0.02 mg/kg up to 0.1 mg/kg), is indicated in cases of sinus tachycardia secondary to drug or toxin exposures, or in cases where all other underlying causes of tachycardia (hypovolemia, hypoxemia, anxiety) have been addressed. Side effects of beta-adrenergic blockers include bradycardia, negative inotropy, and hypotension.

Supraventricular Tachycardia

- Supraventricular tachycardias may be atrial or junctional in origin. Atrial fibrillation is also considered to be an atrial tachycardia. Junctional tachycardias originate from within the AV node or involve re-entrant circuits within the AV node. Supraventricular tachycardias are also known as *narrow-complex tachycardias,* as the QRS complex resembles normal sinus complexes. In rare instances, a wide-complex tachycardia may result from a supraventricular focus due to the presence of a bundle branch block in the specialized conduction system.
- Supraventricular tachycardia results from abnormalities within the atrial or junctional myocardial tissue. This may occur due to grossly identifiable diseases, such as atrial dilation in the presence of elevated filling pressures or volume overload, myocardial fibrosis in the presence of cardiomyopathy, or infiltrative diseases such as cardiac neoplasia. Other conditions, including most patients with re-entrant circuits, cause supraventricular tachycardia in a heart that appears to be structurally normal. This is also the case in patients where supraventricular is due to electrolyte abnormalities or pharmacologic causes. Common agents that can result in supraventricular tachycardia include digoxin toxicity, caffeine, and amphetamines or other illicit drugs.
- Patients with supraventricular tachycardia usually present with symptoms such as weakness, lethargy, or collapse. Pulse quality is variable, but is often diminished. In cases of stimulant toxicosis, supraventricular tachycardia may be associated with excitement, hyperesthesia, or seizure activity.
- Treatment of supraventricular tachycardia involves attempts to identify and specifically treat any underlying cause of the tachycardia, such as an electrolyte abnormality or digoxin overdose. Additionally, variations in sympathetic tone may affect conduction through the AV node, and causes of increased sympathetic tone should be investigated. If no underlying cause of the tachycardia can be determined, a vagal maneuver may be attempted.
  - Vagal maneuvers include firm ocular pressure and carotid massage and are undertaken in an attempt to slow conduction through the AV node. In some instances, vagal maneuvers may temporarily terminate a supraventricular tachycardia.
- Pharmacologic therapy of supraventricular tachycardia in an emergency situation involves the use of injectable anti-arrhythmic agents. Initial choices for anti-arrhythmic therapy include beta adrenergic blockers, which limit the rate of spontaneous depolarization in ectopic pacemakers, and calcium channel blockers, which slow conduction through the AV node. Both classes of drug have potent negative chronotropic effects, and may also have profound negative inotropic properties. These negative inotropic effects are more pronounced when the drugs are given rapidly, in high doses, or in combination with other agents that impair contractility. This consideration is especially important in patients with significant structural heart disease and limited cardiovascular reserve.

- **Esmolol** (see dose listed under Sinus Tachycardia) is generally preferred to other beta-blocking agents, such as propanolol, due to its short half-life that allows rapid titration of effect.
- The use of a calcium channel blocker is an alternative to beta-blocking agents. **Diltiazem** (dogs and cats, 0.1 to 0.25 mg/kg and followed by 2 to 5 mcg/kg/min CRI) has a less pronounced negative inotropic effect than equivalent doses of esmolol.

- Other choices for anti-arrhythmic therapy of supraventricular tachycardia include procainamide and amiodarone.
  - **Procainamide** (dogs, 6 to 8 mg/kg, followed by 25 to 50 mcg/kg/min CRI) is a fast sodium channel blocker, and can be used for both supraventricular and ventricular arrhythmias.
  - **Amiodarone** (dogs, slow (20 to 30 minute) bolus of 5 to 10 mg/kg diluted in 5% dextrose in water) acts to prolong the action potential. Amiodarone may cause significant hypotension, vasodilation and pruritis during IV administration, and long-term use may be associated with hepatic dysfunction in dogs.

Ventricular Tachycardia

- Ventricular arrhythmias are very common in emergency patients, and ventricular complexes are recognized by a wide and bizarre QRS morphology. In many cases, such as isolated ventricular premature complexes, these rhythm disturbances do not require treatment. However, treatment is recommended if there are frequent or multifocal ventricular premature complexes, if the coupling interval is very rapid creating an R-on-T morphology, if there is sustained ventricular tachycardia (rates greater than 160 bpm), or if there are clinical or hemodynamic sequelae.
  - An accelerated idioventricular rhythm is very common in patients with noncardiac disease. This rhythm is recognized as a regular, monomorphic ventricular rhythm that is very similar in rate to the underlying sinus rhythm, and fusion complexes may be recognized during transitions between the ventricular and sinus rhythm. In general, this rhythm does not produce significant hemodynamic abnormalities and does not require therapy.
- Ventricular tachycardias result from abnormalities within the ventricular myocardium and occur due to abnormal automaticity, triggered activity, or re-entrant circuits. Ventricular arrhythmias may occur due to primary cardiac disease, such as dilated cardiomyopathy, arrhythmogenic cardiomyopathy, hypertrophic cardiomyopathy, chronic valvular diasease, aortic or pulmonic stenosis, myocarditis, or cardiac neoplasia. Ventricular arrhythmias may also be seen in a variety of noncardiac conditions, especially in patients with elevated sympathetic tone or inflammatory mediators, and with electrolyte disturbances such as hypocalcemia and hypokalemia.
- As with supraventricular tachycardia, long-standing ventricular tachycardia may produce myocardial failure in patients with otherwise normal hearts. This tachycardia-induced cardiomyopathy results in chamber dilation and diminished systolic function, and can result in CHF.
- Patients with symptomatic ventricular tachycardia usually present with symptoms such as weakness, lethargy, or collapse. Paroxsysmal ventricular tachycardia may result in syncope or episodes of near-syncope.
- Treatment of ventricular tachycardia involves attempts to identify and specifically treat any underlying cause of the tachycardia.
  - In many patients, ventricular arrhythmias respond to interventions such as fluid resuscitation in hypovolemic patients, the administration of blood products in anemic animals, the implementation of oxygen therapy in hypoxemic patients, and the use of analgesics in painful patients.
- Pharmacologic therapy of ventricular tachycardia in an emergency situation involves the use of injectable anti-arrhythmic agents. Initial choices for anti-arrhythmic therapy include class I agents such as lidocaine or procainamide. Alternatives include beta-adrenergic blockers, or class III agents such as amiodarone.
  - **Lidocaine** (dogs, 2 mg/kg IV bolus up to 8 mg/kg and followed by 25 to 80 mcg/kg/min CRI) is generally a first line choice in dogs. Cats are much more likely to develop adverse effects (gastrointestinal signs, neurologic signs including seizures) and the dose is significantly decreased to prevent these signs (cats, 0.25 to 0.5 mg/kg IV bolus followed by 10 to 20 mcg/kg/min CRI).
  - **Procainamide** (dogs, 8 to 15 mg/kg slow IV bolus followed by 25 to 50 mcg/kg/min) may also be used to treat ventricular tachycardia. Rapid administration may cause significant hypotension.
  - **Esmolol** (see dose listed under sinus tachycardia) is generally preferred to other beta blockers due to its short half-life. As with procainamide,

esmolol may cause hypotension, which is secondary to potent negative inotropic effects.
  - **Amiodarone** (see dose under supraventricular tachycardia) may also be used for the treatment symptomatic ventricular tachycardia, however vasodilation and systemic hypotension are common during administration in dogs.
- As mentioned previously, in rare cases, a wide-complex tachycardia may result from a supraventricular focus due to the presence of a bundle branch block in the specialized conduction system. Lidocaine is unlikely to be effective, whereas procainamide, beta blockers, or calcium channel blockers are more likely to be useful in the diagnosis and management of these patients.

> **KEY POINT**
>
> The morphology of ventricular premature complexes and ventricular escape beats is identical. The use of anti-arrhythmics in a patient with ventricular escapes may cause suppression of the escape rhythm with disastrous consequences.

THROMBOEMBOLIC DISEASE

- See Chapter 8 for additional discussion.
- Cardiac emergencies associated with thromboembolic disease may either be the cause or the result of severe cardiac disease. Massive pulmonary thromboembolism may cause heart disease by significantly increasing right ventricular afterload. This results in severe pulmonary hypertension, and may precipitate acute right-sided heart failure and cardiogenic shock. This occurs more commonly in dogs than cats and is generally associated with an underlying hypercoagulable state that results in pathologic clot formation. Conditions associated with pulmonary thromboembolism include hyperadrenocorticism, immune-mediated hemolytic anemia, sepsis, disseminated intravascular coagulation, protein losing nephropathy and enteropathy, and neoplasia.
- More commonly, emergency patients present with thromboembolic disease resulting from cardiac disease. This is especially common in cats with cardiomyopathy and associated left atrial enlargement. These patients are prone to the development of blood clots that subsequently embolize the systemic arterial tree. This condition, known as *feline aortic thromboembolism,* often causes acute limb paresis secondary to obstruction of arterial blood flow and subsequent tissue ischemia.
- Cats most commonly present with paraparesis, but may also present with unilateral hindlimb paresis or forelimb paresis. Cats may also embolize other organs, such as the brain, kidneys, or gastrointestinal tract. CHF may be present, although arterial embolization may occur alone. All cats benefit from analgesia and from treatment of any concurrent heart failure while in the emergency room. Thrombolytic agents such as streptokinase or tissue plasminogen activator may accelerate clot dissolution, however their use has not provided definitive evidence of benefit in clinical trials. In addition, these agents may cause significant complications including severe hemorrhage and fatal reperfusion syndromes.
- Conservative therapy involves the provision of supportive care and analgesia and some cats will re-establish arterial blood flow and regain function in ischemic limbs within 2 to 3 days.
  - Analgesia in the form of **fentanyl** (cats, 2 to 5 μg/kg/hr CRI for 12 to 18 hours as a fentanyl patch takes effect), **butorphanol** (cats, 0.1 to 0.2 mg/kg IV every 4 to 6 hours), or **buprenorphine** (cats, 0.005 to 0.015 mg/kg IV every 6 to 8 hours) is used. Other opioids such as hydromorphone, oxymorphone, or morphine may also be used.
  - Anticoagulation with unfractionated or low-molecular-weight heparin may be useful to help reduce clot propagation, and is generally well tolerated by cats. **Unfractionated heparin** (cats, 150 to 250 μg/kg SQ every 6 to 8 hours or as a CRI of 20 to 50 μg/kg/hr at a low fluid rate) or **low-molecular-weight heparin** (e.g., dalteparin, cats, 100 to 150 μg/kg SQ every 12 to 24 hours) is used. Unfractionated heparin will cause prolongation of the PTT, and a clinical target is to achieve a PTT 1.5 to 2.5 times the normal value. Low-molecular-weight heparin activity is typically monitored via a factor Xa assay that is not readily available to veterinarians. However, the PTT will be prolonged in patients at risk for hemorrhage secondary to low-molecular-weight heparin administration. All heparinized patients should be monitored for signs of clinical bleeding and should not have jugular venipuncture or cystocentesis performed. In addition, all cats that present to the emergency room with feline aortic thromboembolism should be monitored for hyperkalemia, azotemia, hypotension, cardiac arrhythmias and signs of cardiovascular collapse that may accompany reperfusion injury.

Frequently Asked Questions

Why don't animals with pericardial effusion present with LCHF and pulmonary edema?

Pericardial effusion results in preload reduction to the heart. The pressure that develops around the heart due to effusion prevents the heart chambers from being able to accommodate venous return to the heart. This effect is most pronounced on the right side because it is the "low pressure" side of the heart. Therefore, with severe pericardial effusion, the right side cannot fill adequately because the pericardial fluid accumulation compresses that side more readily than the left side, and right-sided heart failure develops.

What is the purpose of oxygen supplementation and sedative drugs in the treatment of CHF with pulmonary edema?

When an animal develops severe pulmonary edema, hypoxemia can result. The fluid accumulation within the lung and the hypoxemia stimulate ventilation. The hypoxemia and the fluid accumulation within the lung cause anxiety and decreased lung compliance of the lung, resulting in tachycardia, increased work of breathing due to poor lung compliance, and increased oxygen demand. Oxygen helps relieve the hypoxemia which can in turn decrease anxiety helping slow the heart down. Sedative drugs help relieve anxiety which decreases another stimulus for tachycardia. This combination of therapies will ultimately increase oxygenation of the blood, slow the heart rate, and decrease oxygen demand by the respiratory muscles, all of which are favorable for an ailing heart.

SUGGESTED READINDS

Bonagura JD: Electrical alternans associated with pericardial effusion in the dog, J Am Vet Med Assoc 178(6):574-579, 1981.

Cote E: Cardiogenic shock and cardiac arrest, Vet Clin North Am 31(6):1129-1146, 2001.

DeFrancesco TC, Hansen BD, Atkins CE, et al. Noninvasive transthoracic temporary cardiac pacing in dogs, J Vet Intern Med 17(5)663-667, 2003.

Kittleson MD: Management of heart failure. In Kittleson MD, Kienle RD, eds: Small animal cardiovascular medicine, St Louis, 1998, Mosby.

Laste NL: Cardiovascular pharmacotherapy: hemodynamic drugs and antiarrhythmic agents, Vet Clin North Am 31(6):1231-1252, 2001.

Moise NS: Diagnosis and management of canine arrhythmias. In Fox PR, Sisson D, Moise NS, eds: Textbook of canine and feline cardiology: principles and clinical practice, ed 2, Philadelphia, 1999, WB Saunders.

Moise NS: Diagnosis and management of feline arrhythmias. In Fox PR, Sisson D, Moise NS, eds: Textbook of canine and feline cardiology: principles and clinical practice, ed 2, Philadelphia, 1999,WB Saunders.

Smith SA, Tobias AH, Jacob KA, et al. Arterial thromboembolism in cats: acute crisis in 127 cases (1992-2001) and long-term management with low-dose aspirin in 24 cases, J Vet Intern Med 17:73-83, 2003.

CHAPTER 19

Anesthesia of the Cardiac Patient

Thomas K. Day

INTRODUCTION

Anesthesia of the patient with heart disease can be a challenge. Most veterinary patients with heart disease that are presented for sedation or anesthesia do not have clinical signs of heart failure. Anesthetic protocols that are routinely used for normal patients without heart disease can result in acute decompensation in patients with heart disease. Differences between dogs and cats in the response to anesthetic and analgesic drugs can compound the complex nature of cardiac anesthesia. In addition, most patients with heart disease may be treated with a variety of cardiac drugs that may interact with anesthetic drugs. This chapter provides a general view of anesthetic drugs that are indicated and contraindicated in dogs and cats with heart disease. Anesthetic considerations for specific cardiac diseases are also presented.

KEY POINT

Suggested anesthetic protocols for dogs and cats are presented based on the functional classes of heart failure.

GENERAL PRINCIPLES

- The veterinary anesthetist must understand and recognize several factors to provide safe and effective sedation or anesthesia, including the hemodynamic changes produced by heart disease, the possible interactions between cardiac and anesthetic drugs, the presence of arrhythmias, and the potential for anesthetic drugs to predispose to the production of arrhythmias.
- Knowledge of the length of sedation or anesthesia that is desired and recognition of the need for analgesia are also important.
- Virtually all anesthetic drugs directly depress cardiac function, alter vascular tone, or modify normal cardiovascular regulatory mechanisms.
- One "magic bullet" anesthetic protocol that will safely anesthetize any dog or cat with heart disease does not exist.
- Each patient and each etiology of cardiac disease should be considered on an individual basis to provide the safest sedation, analgesic or anesthetic protocol.

KEY POINT

The general rule of thumb is to devise an anesthetic plan that provides minimal cardiopulmonary depression and returns the patient to preanesthetic status as soon and as safely as possible.

PREANESTHETIC CONSIDERATIONS

Diagnosis of the Etiology of Heart Disease

- The decision on which sedation or anesthetic protocol to administer to a patient with heart disease should be made primarily on the specific etiology.

Table 19-1 Classification of Physical Status for Anesthetized Patients

ASA Category	Description of Physical Status	Example
I	Normal, healthy	No cardiac disease, elective surgery (spay, castration)
II	Mild systemic disease	Compensated heart disease (no cardiac medications), fracture without shock
III	Severe systemic disease	Compensated heart disease (cardiac medications), anemia, fever, compensated renal disease, dehydration
IV	Severe systemic disease and a constant threat to life	Decompensated heart disease, electrolyte imbalance, uncontrolled internal hemorrhage
V	Moribund patient not expected to live with or without surgery	Decompensated heart disease refractory to cardiac drugs, terminal malignancy

Adapted by the American Society of Anesthesiologists.

Once the etiology of heart disease has been determined, specific recommendations can be provided on the choice of sedation or anesthesia.

Functional Classification of Heart Failure

- Three functional classifications of heart failure are based on clinical signs. The decision on whether or not to immediately sedate or anesthetize a patient with heart disease should begin with placing the patient in one of the three classifications.
- The first classification describes the asymptomatic patient that has confirmed heart disease, yet is not exhibiting clinical signs of heart failure. Patients that fulfill criteria for this classification of heart failure can be safely anesthetized without further stabilization.
- The second classification describes when mild to moderate clinical signs of heart failure are evident at rest or with mild exercise. Stabilization of clinical signs and the lack of clinical signs for several days with drug therapy are recommended prior to sedation or anesthesia. Patients with this classification of heart failure that require life-saving, emergency surgery should have cardiac drug therapy instituted immediately by parenteral administration and clinical signs controlled as much as possible prior to anesthesia. Continuous and aggressive monitoring will be required for this classification of patient during and immediately after sedation or anesthesia. Cardiac drug therapy should continue during anesthesia and surgery and in the immediate postoperative period.
- The third classification describes when advanced clinical signs of heart failure are immediately obvious. Patients severely affected can present in cardiogenic shock, and death or severe debilitation is likely without therapy.

KEY POINTS

- Anesthesia is contraindicated in this third category of patients until clinical signs are immediately stabilized with aggressive drug therapy.
- Clients should be advised of the increased risk of death or severe debilitation during or immediately after anesthesia if patients in this third category of heart failure are anesthetized following aggressive cardiac drug therapy.

Anesthetic Risk Classification

- The anesthetic risk of a patient can be determined based on physical status.
- Five categories of physical status have been developed for veterinary patients and parallel the classification scheme adopted in human medicine by the American Society of Anesthesiologists (ASA) (Table 19-1).
- Most clinically stable cardiac patients will be ASA II or III, depending on the presence of any other underlying disorders.

KEY POINTS

- Unstable patients with clinical signs of cardiac decompensation and heart failure that fulfill the criteria of ASA IV should not be anesthetized until the cardiac disease has been stabilized.
- There may be patients that present in the ASA V category, especially patients with a long history of heart disease that is currently refractory to all cardiac drugs. Stabilization of the signs of heart failure may not be possible, and death during anesthesia is likely.

Preanesthetic Diagnostic Evaluation and Laboratory Tests

- The patient with heart disease should have a complete diagnostic cardiac evaluation.
- All patients should have the following diagnostic and laboratory tests prior to sedation or anesthesia:

Physical Examination

- Particular attention should be paid to thoracic auscultation of the heart and lungs. The character of the peripheral pulse, jugular veins, mucous membranes, and capillary refill time should be noted and the peripheral pulse should be palpated simultaneously with thoracic auscultation of the heart sounds to detect pulse deficits.

Additional Tests

- Thoracic radiography and an electrocardiogram (ECG) should be performed as well. If a complete cardiac diagnostic evaluation has been performed less than 1 to 2 weeks previous to anesthesia, and the patient's physical status has not changed, a physical examination and electrocardiogram are the only diagnostic tests that require repetition. Complete blood count and serum chemistries should be performed at the discretion of the veterinarian, with particular attention to renal values and electrolytes.

CARDIAC DRUGS AND POTENTIAL ANESTHETIC DRUG INTERACTIONS

Diuretics

- The loop diuretic, furosemide, is the most commonly used diuretic in patients with heart disease. The most common electrolyte disturbance produced by furosemide is hypokalemia. Hypokalemia can result in tachyarrhythmias or predispose to digoxin toxicity. Furosemide may promote dehydration and predispose the patient to hypotension during sedation or anesthesia.
- The potassium sparing diuretic, spironolactone, can result in hyperkalemia if used alone for extended periods of time. Hyperkalemia may result in arrhythmias, with equal likelihood of tachyarrhythmias or bradyarrhythmias.
- The thiazide diuretic, chlorothiazide, has similar side effects as the loop diuretics with chronic use. Hypokalemia and hypomagnesemia may produce or predispose to tachyarrhythmias.

Angiotensin-Converting Enzyme Inhibitors

- Enalapril and benazepril are the most commonly used angiotensin-converting enyme inhibitors (ACEIs). Each results in arterial vasodilation that can be enhanced by acepromazine, isoflurane, and sevoflurane predisposing to arterial hypotension. Arterial blood pressure should be monitored closely during sedation protocols involving acepromazine and during isoflurane and sevoflurane anesthesia.

KEY POINT

All patients receiving ACEIs should be monitored with direct or indirect blood pressure during inhalation anesthesia.

Digitalis Glycosides

- A common side effect of digoxin administration is ventricular arrhythmias. There is the possibility of an increase in arrhythmogenesis with concurrent use of sympathomimetics (dopamine, dobutamine, norepinephrine, epinephrine) during anesthesia. Isoflurane, sevoflurane and opioids have not been associated with increased incidence of arrhythmias secondary to digitalis.
- Hypokalemia, most commonly caused by chronic use of loop diuretics, can exacerbate digitalis toxicity. Acute onset of hypokalemia can occur during anesthesia as a result of hyperventilation (hypocarbia and concurrent respiratory alkalosis) and can exacerbate preexisting hypokalemia caused by diuretics.

KEY POINT

Always obtain a blood digitalis level prior to anesthesia.

Vasodilators

- Hydralazine is an arteriodilator that can cause reflex tachycardia and fluid and water retention. Tachycardia secondary to use of sympathomimetics (dopamine, dobutamine, norepinephrine, epinephrine) during anesthesia can be exacerbated with the use of hydralazine. Fluid administration must be minimized and monitored closely. Acepromazine, isoflurane and sevoflurane may exacerbate arteriodilation and predispose to arterial hypotension.

- Prazosin causes arterial and venodilation by alpha-1 adrenergic blockade. Acepromazine is contraindicated, as arteriodilation may be excessive and produce severe hypotension. Isoflurane may exacerbate arteriodilation and may predispose to arterial hypotension.

Calcium Channel Blockers

- Diltiazem is used to treat supraventricular arrhythmias and to improve diastolic function in cats with hypertrophic cardiomyopathy (HCM). Potential side effects include vasodilation, bradycardia, and decreased myocardial contractility. Concurrent use of acepromazine, isoflurane, and sevoflurane may exacerbate vasodilation and produce hypotension. Concurrent use of opioids and inhalation anesthetics (isoflurane and sevoflurane) may exacerbate bradycardia. Decreased myocardial contractility may be exacerbated by propofol.

Antiarrhythmic Agents

- The beta-adrenergic blocking agents propranolol and atenolol are commonly used to treat arrhythmias in dogs and cats and for treatment of HCM in cats. Potential side effects include bradycardia and decreased myocardial contractile function. Bradycardia may be exacerbated with use of opioids and inhalation anesthetics. Decreased myocardial contractility may cause hypotension during anesthesia, may be less responsive to sympathomimetics (dopamine and dobutamine), and may be exacerbated by propofol.

Class I Antiarrhythmic Agents

- Procainamide and tocainide can have side effects include decreased myocardial contractility and possible bradycardia. Decreased myocardial contractility may be exacerbated by propofol.

Nonsteroidal Anti-Inflammatory Drugs

- Cats with heart disease may be prescribed aspirin to potentially prevent thromboembolic disease. Aspirin impairs platelet function. Acepromazine should be avoided in cats receiving aspirin that are presented for surgery, as acepromazine also impairs platelet function. Clopidogrel (Plavix) may be used in the future and will likely have the same anesthetic concerns (impaired platelet function) as aspirin.

Combination Drug Therapy

- Most patients with heart disease are commonly administered more than one cardiac drug. The potential side effects of each drug must first be considered individually. Potential side effects of the combination of drugs should be considered next. The addition of anesthetic drugs may introduce a greater possibility of side effects. For example, a dog with compensated mitral insufficiency could have been prescribed digoxin, furosemide, and enalapril. There is a great potential for hypotension produced by excessive arteriodilation, bradycardia, or decreased myocardial contractility based on the combined side effects of each drug. Isoflurane and sevoflurane, which minimally decrease myocardial contractility and cardiac output, could produce severe hypotension in this patient secondary to peripheral vasodilation. Inhalation anesthesia should not be considered the primary anesthetic of choice in this dog.

ANESTHETIC DRUG SELECTION AND SUPPORTIVE CARE

Choice of either Sedation or General Anesthesia

- The definition of general anesthesia is the administration of injectable anesthetics, inhalation anesthetics, or a combination to produce hypnosis (sleep), analgesia, and muscle relaxation. General anesthesia is not solely produced by the administration of inhalation anesthetics. Many useful and safe general anesthetic protocols for cardiac patients are combinations of injectable anesthetic agents.

Oxygenation and Ventilatory Support

- All cardiac patients that are sedated or anesthetized should have oxygen administered in some form. Sedated patients should have oxygen delivered by mask at an insufflation rate of no less than 5 L/min. All intubated patients should be attached to an anesthetic machine to deliver 100% oxygen, regardless of whether or not an inhalation anesthetic is delivered.
- All cardiac patients anesthetized and maintained on isoflurane, sevoflurane or using injectable anesthetics should have ventilatory support provided. Isoflurane and sevoflurane are both potent respiratory depressants and can predispose the patient to hypoxemia or hypercarbia. Hypoxemia

and hypercarbia can result in the production or worsening of arrhythmias. All intubated patients should also have ventilation supported. The general rule is that four to six breaths should be delivered each minute. Expired carbon dioxide can be monitored with a capnometer (see Monitoring) to ensure adequate ventilation.

Anesthetic Drugs that are Contraindicated in Patients with Cardiac Disease

- The following sedatives and anesthetic drugs are contraindicated in patients with heart disease, regardless of the etiology. The benefits of convenience, effectiveness, or ease of administration and lower cost do not justify the use of these drugs because of the profound cardiopulmonary depression, the increased possibility of arrhythmia production, or the length of recovery time.

Alpha-2 Adrenergic Drugs

- Xylazine and medetomidine are potent respiratory and cardiac depressants. Decreased heart rate is usually responsive to anticholinergics. Xylazine can also decrease heart rate by a central mechanism of decreased sympathetic outflow that will not be responsive to anticholinergics. Xylazine decreases myocardial contractility, resulting in decreased cardiac output and hypotension. Medetomidine results in intense vasoconstriction and decreased cardiac output. Decreased heart rate is usually a result of intense vasoconstriction. Administration of an anticholinergic will greatly increase cardiac work.

Barbiturates

- Pentobarbital has a duration of action of approximately 45 to 60 minutes and results in prolonged recoveries. Pentobarbital is also a potent respiratory and cardiovascular depressant at dosages used for general anesthesia.
- Amobarbital (intermediate duration) and phenobarbital (long duration of action) are barbiturates with an extremely long duration of action and have cardiopulmonary effects inappropriate for use as anesthetics or sedatives in cardiac patients.

Inhalation Anesthetics

- Halothane is not used commonly, but is still available to some extent. Halothane is the most potent negative inotrope of the inhalation anesthetics and it predisposes the myocardium to the production of arrhythmias, especially ventricular arrhythmias. Halothane should not be used in a dog or cat with cardiac disease.
- Methoxyflurane is of more historical significance than is used in practice. The effects on inotropy and the possibility for arrhythmias fall between those of isoflurane, sevoflurane (discussed later) and halothane. Methoxyflurane is more likely to produce a prolonged recovery.
- Mask induction with isoflurane or sevoflurane is not recommended in cardiac patients. Most animals become very excited during mask induction, even with adequate preanesthetic medication, which could predispose to arrhythmias and increased myocardial work secondary to the stress response. Isoflurane has a very pungent odor and may result in laryngospasm, especially in cats, though sevoflurane is less pungent. Environmental contamination with isoflurane and sevoflurane administered by mask is a very important consideration for the safety of all personnel.

ANESTHETIC DRUGS THAT SHOULD BE USED WITH CAUTION

Preanesthetic Medication

Tranquilizers

- The phenothiazine, acepromazine, is considered a major tranquilizer owing to the high reliability of producing mental calming. It is also the most commonly used tranquilizer in small animals. The primary cardiovascular effect is peripheral vasodilation, with minimal effects on contractility and respiration. Hypotension can occur, and is primarily treated with intravenous fluids and, in severe cases, peripheral vasoconstriction agents (phenylephrine, norepinephrine). The sedative and cardiovascular effects are of long duration (4 to 6 hours), though the effects are not reversible. Acepromazine can be used effectively and safely at very low dosages in otherwise healthy cardiac patients

Anticholinergics

- Atropine and glycopyrrolate are primary used to maintain heart rate during anesthesia or sedation and are generally not recommended unless used with anesthetic drugs that are likely to lower heart rate (opioids) through increased parasympathetic tone. The potential side effects include the production of tachyarrhythmias (ventricular or supraventricular). The increase in myocardial oxygen consumption produced by an increase in heart rate above normal values may predispose the patient with heart disease to focal ischemia and the possibility of arrhythmias. There is little difference between atropine and glycopyrrolate in the effectiveness of producing an increase in heart rate, though glycopyrrolate will likely have a longer duration.

Intravenous Induction Agents

Thiobarbiturates

- Thiopental can be used safely in cardiac patients, though it is not recommended in patients with pre-existing arrhythmias. Thiopental can produce transient ventricular arrhythmias by sensitizing the heart to catecholamines. Transient decrease in blood pressure as a result of decreased contractility. Can be used effectively and safely in otherwise healthy cardiac patients at very low dosages following adequate preanesthetic medication.

Propofol

- Propofol has cardiovascular effects similar to thiopental, though the likelihood of arrhythmia production is less. Apnea can be profound, and is closely related to speed of injection. Propofol is rapidly redistributed, resulting in very rapid recovery.

Dissociatives

- Ketamine and the combination of tiletamine and zolazepam are usually very safe and effective in cardiac patients. Transient increases in heart rate can predispose to arrhythmias and are not recommended in patients with pre-existing arrhythmias. Increased heart rate is less severe if administered after preanesthetic medication. Ketamine should not be used as the sole anesthetic agent in cats with HCM. Acute fulminate congestive heart failure has been reported in cats with HCM administered ketamine and combinations of ketamine/diazepam as sole anesthetic.

Inhalation Anesthetics

- Inhalation anesthetics used as the sole anesthetic agent to induce (mask induction) and maintain anesthesia must be used with extreme caution. Both isoflurane and sevoflurane are potent vasodilators that could lead to hypotension and increased cardiac work. Both isoflurane and sevoflurane are potent respiratory depressants.

USEFUL ANESTHETIC DRUGS

Preanesthetic Medication

- The benefits of preanesthetic medication in patients with heart disease include reducing preoperative anxiety and stress, providing preemptive analgesia, lowering the requirement of intravenous induction agents and inhalation anesthetics, and ensuring a smooth recovery. Preanesthetic medication can be administered intramuscularly, subcutaneously, or intravenously. In most cardiac patients, the author recommends intramuscular administration of preanesthetic medications.

Tranquilizers

Benzodiazepines

- Diazepam and midazolam are considered minor tranquilizers because when used alone, benzodiazepines do not produce profound sedation in the normally mentated patient. Benzodiazepines may produce a profound effect on patients with advanced age or disease. The most common use is in combination with an opioid (neuroleptanalgesia). Both drugs minimally depress cardiopulmonary function. Both diazepam and midazolam are effectively absorbed after intramuscular administration, though diazepam may produce more pain on injection (propylene glycol based). Clinical effects of midazolam compared with diazepam are identical in dogs and cats, though midazolam is more expensive. The benzodiazepine antagonist, flumazenil, is available, though the effects of benzodiazepines rarely require antagonism.

Opioids

- The primary use of opioids in veterinary anesthesia is to provide analgesia. Most opioids do not possess profound sedative effects when administered alone; however, when used in combination with tranquilizers for neuroleptanalgesia (see following), adequate sedation can be achieved. Opioids do not affect myocardial contractility or vascular tone, which makes them very attractive for use in patients with heart disease. All effects produced by opioids can be antagonized by administration of naloxone, though repeat administration will likely be required as naloxone has a very short duration of action.

Morphine

- Minimal sedation is produced when used alone in normal patients, though profound sedation can occur in compromised patients. Primary side effects are vomiting and bradycardia. Bradycardia is usually anticholinergic responsive. Depression of respiration is dose dependent.

Hydromorphone and Oxymorphone

- Opioid agonists have similar clinical effects and are 10 times more potent analgesia compared with morphine. Usually more effective than morphine in producing sedation when used alone, though even more effective in a neuroleptanalgesic combination. Potential for decreased heart rate (parasympathomimetic). Less respiratory depression than with morphine. Vomiting likely, though less likely compared with morphine. Can also be used as an induction agent in compromised patients.

Butorphanol

- Opioid agonist/antagonist that is usually less effective than oxymorphone or hydromorphone in producing sedation alone or in a neuroleptanalgesic combination. There is minimal cardiopulmonary depression, and it is unlikely to produce bradycardia. A"ceiling effect" occurs regarding sedation and analgesia. This means that higher doses beyond the recommended maximum dose (approximately 0.8 mg/kg) do not produce more sedation or analgesia. Vomiting is a rare side effect. Very poor analgesic for moderate to severe pain.

Buprenorphine

- Buprenorphine is a partial opioid agonist that is 20 times more potent in producing analgesia when compared with morphine. It is generally a poor sedative when used alone, though slightly more effective in a neuroleptanalgesia combination. There is minimal cardiopulmonary depression and a ceiling effect occurs similar to butorphanol. The onset of action is 20 to 30 minutes and there is a long duration of effect. Repeat injections of naloxone are required to maintain antagonism of effects, if required.

Fentanyl

- Fentanyl is an opioid agonist that is 100 times more potent in producing analgesia when compared with morphine. The onset of action is very rapid and it can be used as an intravenous induction agent in dogs. The duration of action is extremely short, making fentanyl an ideal agent for a continuous-rate infusion (CRI) to maintain general anesthesia. Bradycardia is more likely to occur and responds to anticholinergic administration (preferred) or a decrease in the rate of infusion.

Neuroleptanalgesia

- *Neuroleptanalgesia* is defined as the effect produced by the combination of a tranquilizer and an opioid. The neuroleptanalgesia combinations that are recommended for patients with heart disease include any combination of a benzodiazepine and an opioid. Intravenous or intramuscular administration may be used to produce an effect.

Opioid-Diazepam Combinations

- The preferred neuroleptanalgesia for patients with heart disease is the combination of an opioid with a benzodiazepine. The most reliable sedation occurs with an opioid agonist (morphine, hydromorphone/oxymorphone, fentanyl) compared to opioid agonist/antagonist (butorphanol) and partial opioid agonist (buprenorphine) combinations. Intramuscular administration produces effects within 15 minutes. Panting is a prominent feature when opioid agonists are used in dogs (not cats), and respiratory depression can be pronounced. Bradycardia is more likely with opioid agonist combinations, and is responsive to anticholinergics.

KEY POINT

A neuroleptanalgesia combination using acepromazine will produce the most profound sedative effect; however, acepromazine has a long duration of effect, including the effect of vasodilation, and has no reversal agent. The clinician must weigh the risks and benefits of using acepromazine.

INTRAVENOUS INDUCTION AGENTS

Barbiturates

- Thiopental can be used safely and reliably in patients with cardiac disease. Rapid induction and recovery follow a single intravenous dose as a result of rapid redistribution to lean tissue. Cumulative effects occur if more than one intravenous dose is administered, which will result in prolonged recovery. Transient decreases in blood pressure occur as a result of decreased contractility. Apnea can be prominent, and may be partly related to speed of induction. Thiopental can be used effectively and safely in otherwise healthy patients at very low dosages following adequate preanesthetic medication.

Dissociatives

- Ketamine is used commonly as an induction agent in patients with heart disease but should not be used alone. Always combine ketamine with diazepam or midazolam to minimize adverse effects of rigidity and possible seizures. Induction with ketamine and diazepam results in a rapid induction of anesthesia. The combination will increase heart rate, maintain arterial blood pressure, and have minimal effects on respiration, though apnea has been reported with ketamine-diazepam combination. Potential side effects include myoclonus activity and rough recovery. Cats with HCM should not be administered ketamine or ketamine-diazepam as sole agents. Administration of ketamine or ketamine-diazepam after neuroleptanalgesia may decrease untoward cardiovascular effects related to dissociatives.

Tiletamine and Zolazepam

- The effects are similar to ketamine-diazepam when administered as an intravenous bolus for induction. There is less myoclonus activity and a generally smoother induction. There are longer and potentially rougher recoveries than ketamine-diazepam when used as a sole agent without preanesthetic medication. Preanesthetic medication is highly recommended prior to use of tiletamine-zolazepam. Higher doses will be required if no preanesthetic medication is administered, and there is a potential for longer recoveries. There are likely the same considerations in cats with HCM as with ketamine combinations.

Nonbarbiturates

Propofol

- Propofol is classified as a phenolic compound unrelated to opioids, barbiturates, or steroid anesthetics. Propofol induction is characterized as a very rapid and smooth induction with a very rapid and smooth recovery. Noncumulative effects make propofol an ideal drug for constant rate infusions. Transient decreases in arterial blood pressure occur and are produced by a decrease in myocardial contractility. A reflex increase in heart rate is likely. Apnea can be profound, and is closely associated with speed of injection. Use of preanesthetic medication greatly reduces the dose of propofol required for induction of anesthesia, and reduces the possibility of decreases in blood pressure.

Etomidate

- Etomidate is an imidazole derivative unrelated to barbiturates and opioids. Etomidate induction is characterized as a very rapid induction with a very rapid and smooth recovery. Induction with etomidate results in a much less desirable induction and recovery if administered alone without preanesthetic medication. Severe myoclonus activity can occur when used alone. Minimal cardiopulmonary depression and minimal effect on cardiac electrical activity makes etomidate an ideal intravenous induction agent for the less stable patient with heart disease after appropriate preanesthetic medication. Etomidate is prepared in a propylene glycol base and has a high osmolality. Intermittent bolus or constant rate infusion is not recommended owing to possibility of acute red blood cell lysis.

MAINTENANCE OF ANESTHESIA

Inhalation Anesthetics

Isoflurane and Sevoflurane

- Each inhalation anesthetic has a very similar clinical effect of rapid induction and recovery. Minimal effects on cardiac rhythm and contractility result in minimal decreases in cardiac output. The main cardiovascular effect is dose-dependent peripheral vasodilation, which is the primary mechanism of hypotension induced by isoflurane and sevoflurane. A general rule is to administer the lowest effective concentration of isoflurane or sevoflurane that will maintain a surgical depth of anesthesia. The use of preanesthetic medications and intravenous induction agents is highly recommended, and will lower the amount of isoflurane necessary to maintain a surgical depth of anesthesia. Each are potent respiratory depressants that can be additive with opioids, and manual ventilation is mandatory to prevent hypoxemia and hypercarbia.

Nitrous Oxide

- Nitrous oxide used in combination with oxygen cannot alone produce anesthesia. Therefore, it is used as an adjunct to inhalation anesthesia only. Use of nitrous oxide can lower the inhalation anesthetic requirement. Safety considerations (life threatening hypoxemia) prevent widespread use of nitrous oxide.

KEY POINT

Only experienced anesthetists should use nitrous oxide.

INJECTABLE GENERAL ANESTHESIA

- Injectable anesthetics can be used to maintain a surgical plane of general anesthesia. The definition of general anesthesia is the production of sleep, muscle relaxation, and analgesia. All three criteria can be met effectively and safely with injectable anesthetics. Specific examples will be offered at the end of the chapter, though general concepts of using all injectable agents are offered below.

Preanesthetic Medication and Propofol

- The neuroleptanalgesic combination of an opioid and a benzodiazepine is administered intramuscularly.
- Induction and CRI of propofol with an initial induction dose of 1 to 5 mg/kg, IV followed by a CRI administered by syringe pump or drip at a rate of 0.14 to 0.4 mg/kg/min, IV, depending on other anesthetic drugs used as preanesthetic medication and the achieved effect. Higher infusion rates are required to maintain surgical plane of anesthesia and to maintain an endotracheal tube.
- Intermittent boluses of propofol can be used instead of a CRI. Administer propofol by slow bolus at a dosage of 0.5 to 1.0 mg/kg, IV following initial induction dose, depending on other anesthetic drugs used as preanesthetic medication.

Preanesthetic Medication and Ketamine-Diazepam

- The neuroleptanalgesic combination of an opioid and a benzodiazepine is administered intramuscularly.
- The induction dose of ketamine and diazepam is 1 ml/10 kg of a 50:50 mixture. Generally, one fourth to one third of the initial induction dose can be administered as an intermittent bolus, depending on other anesthetic drugs used as preanesthetic medication.

SPECIES DIFFERENCES (DOG VS. CAT) IN ANESTHETIC DRUG EFFECTS

Tranquilizers

- Compared with dogs, cats are less responsive to the mental calming effects of an equivalent dose of acepromazine when used alone.

Opioids

- Cats are more likely to become excited from the effects of opioids and, at times, to neuroleptanalgesic combinations of diazepam and an opioid.
- Cats do not have as profound sedative effects from neuroleptanalgesic combinations. Some dogs become laterally recumbent after certain neuroleptanalgesic combinations, whereas cats rarely respond in the same manner. The general rule is that an effective neuroleptanalgesia in cats occurs when the cat assumes sternal recumbency, is very amenable to mild restraint and has mydriasis.
- Vomiting occurs less frequently in cats.
- Dogs develop miosis when an opioid is administered and cats develop mydriasis.

Dissociatives

- The dissociatives are the primary class of anesthetic drugs recommended for chemical restraint in cats. The dissociatives are used primarily as intravenous induction agents in dogs. Ketamine should never be used as a sole anesthetic in the dog. Ketamine can be used alone in the cat, though muscle rigidity and salivation can be profound.
- Tiletamine and zolazepam are metabolized differently in cats and dogs, which can explain the general recovery characteristics. Tiletamine is metabolized at a more rapid rate than zolazepam in cats, and recoveries tend to be smooth. The reverse occurs in dogs, where zolazepam is metabolized at a more rapid rate, and recoveries tend to be rough. Use alone with extreme caution in cats with HCM. Anecdotal reports of pulmonary edema have been reported in cats.

Propofol

- There is evidence that multiple exposures (consecutive days) of cats to propofol can result in oxidative injury to feline red blood cells. One anesthetic episode of propofol (induction, CRI, or intermittent boluses) will not produce oxidative injury to feline red blood cells. Propofol should not be used as an anesthetic technique for consecutive, multiple use therapy as in radiation therapy or bandage care in cats.

ADJUNCT TECHNIQUES

Local and Regional Anesthesia/Analgesia

- Local and regional anesthesia/analgesia techniques are highly effective at reducing the amount of inhalation anesthetic required to maintain anesthesia. Many techniques are available and the specific technique is dependent upon the location of the surgical procedure. Please refer to specific anesthesia and analgesia texts for description of the available techniques.

Local Anesthetic Drugs

- Lidocaine (2%) and bupivacaine (0.25%) are the most commonly used local anesthetics. Lidocaine has a rapid onset (5 minutes) and short duration (60 minutes) of action. Bupivacaine has a longer onset (15 to 20 minutes) and duration (2 to 4 hours) of action. All nerve types are blocked with local anesthetics. Therefore, regional analgesia techniques such as lumbosacral anesthesia will result in temporary rear limb paralysis.

Opioids

- Morphine can be used in lumbosacral epidural techniques for prolonged analgesia. However, morphine should not be used alone to provide surgical anesthesia, as morphine blocks nerves that conduct pain pathways only and is meant for postoperative analgesia. The onset of action is up to one hour and analgesia has been reported to be up to 12 to 24 hours. Movement of limbs is maintained, as motor nerves are not affected by morphine.

Infiltration Techniques

- Lidocaine (2%) can be infiltrated subcutaneously to a maximum dose of 10 mg/kg in dogs and cats. Lidocaine can be diluted to 1% to obtain more total volume to block a larger area. Bupivacaine is not recommended as a sole agent for infiltration due to a long onset of action.

REGIONAL TECHNIQUES

Lumbosacral Epidural—Dogs

- Anesthesia and/or analgesia is produced caudal to the umbilicus.
- **Morphine** used as a sole agent—0.1 ml/kg diluted with 1 ml/4.5 kg sterile saline. A morphine epidural must be administered prior to the surgical procedure. Analgesia effects should be expected primarily during the postoperative period and should not be relied upon during surgery.
- **Lidocaine (2%)** used as a sole agent is administered at 1 ml/4.5 kg prior to surgery. Minimal residual analgesia occurs following surgery due to the short duration of action.
- **Bupivicaine (0.25%)** used as a sole agent is not recommended for surgery, unless 15 to 20 minutes of time is allotted prior to surgery to permit maximum effect of bupivacaine. A dose of 1 ml/4.5 kg is administered.
- A combination of **morphine, lidocaine (2%), and bupivacaine (0.5%)** can be used to provide immediate and postoperative analgesia. Morphine (0.1 mg/kg) is diluted with a 50:50 mixture of lidocaine (2%) and bupivacaine (0.5%) at a dose of 1 ml/4.5 kg. The end concentration of bupivacaine is 0.25% as 0.5% bupivacaine is contraindicated in the epidural space.
- Occasionally, an epidural technique in dogs results in appearance of cerebrospinal fluid in the spinal needle. There is no cerebrospinal fluid within the epidural space; therefore, the spinal needle has entered the subarachnoid space. The anesthetist can either remove the spinal needle and attempt the procedure again, or half of the agents can be administered in the subarachnoid space. Administration of local anesthesia in the subarachnoid space is called *spinal anesthesia.*
- A common complication of epidural anesthesia is inadvertent needle puncture of a blood vessel. The local anesthetic combination should not be administered if blood enters the spinal needle.

Lumbosacral Epidural—Cats

- A major anatomical difference in cats compared to dogs is that the spinal cord terminates in the sacral vertebral segments in cats compared to the caudal lumbar (L4-5) in dogs. Epidural techniques are more difficult in cats and the chance of entering the subarachnoid space is more likely in cats. Administer half of the volume of local anesthetic if cerebrospinal fluid is obtained in the spinal needle. Administration of local anesthesia in the subarachnoid space is called spinal anesthesia. There is also the possibility of spinal cord injury in cats.
- The combinations of local anesthetics and opioids used in dogs are the same for cats.

Intercostal Nerve Blocks

- Regional anesthesia for a lateral thoracotomy can be obtained by placing the local anesthetic at the dorsal most aspect of the intercostal nerves at the site of incision and two intercostals spaces cranial and caudal. The maximum dose of lidocaine (10 mg/kg) should not be exceeded.

Intrapleural Analgesia

- Regional anesthesia for a lateral thoracotomy can be obtained by placing the local anesthetic within the pleural space after surgery. **Bupivacaine** (0.25%; 1.5 mg/kg undiluted) is administered through a thoracostomy tube or by a pleurocentesis puncture and the patient is then placed surgery side down for 15 to 20 minutes to permit the adequate onset of action of bupivacaine.

> **KEY POINT**
>
> Intrapleural administration of bupivacaine is painful and should be administered with extreme caution in conscious patients.

Nondepolarizing Muscle Relaxant Drugs

- Nondepolarizing muscle relaxants drugs (NMRDs) block effects of acetylcholine at the neuromuscular junction resulting in complete paralysis. Use of NMRDs is reserved for specific instances during anesthesia and surgery when the patient has poor blood pressure and there is gross purposeful movement. The NMRDs will permit lack of movement to complete the procedure. Ventilatory support and use of anesthetic drugs to produce sleep are mandatory when using NMRDs.
- **Atracurium** (0.25 mg/kg, IV initially and 0.1 mg/kg, IV for repeated administration) is a short-acting NMRD with a duration of action (20 to 25 minutes). Atracurium is metabolized by Hoffman degradation in the plasma and does not require hepatic metabolism or renal excretion. Hypothermia and acidosis will prolong the effect of atracurium.
- **Pancuronium** (0.02 to 0.04 mg/kg, IV initially and 0.01 to 0.02 mg/kg, IV for repeated administration) has a longer duration of action (30 to 40 minutes). Hepatic metabolism and renal excretion is required for elimination. A mild increase in heart rate can occur after initial administration due to parasympatholytic action.
- Reversal of NMRDs is accomplished with neostigmine (0.02 mg/kg, IV) and atropine (0.02 mg/kg, IV) combined in the same syringe. Occasionally, a second dose is required using half of the original dose of both neostigmine and atropine.

MONITORING AND SUPPORTIVE CARE DURING SEDATION AND ANESTHESIA

- There are two aspects of monitoring during anesthesia: anesthetic depth and cardiopulmonary parameters. Anesthetic depth is best monitored by assessment of jaw tone. An adequately anesthetized patient has moderate jaw tone. A deeply anesthetized patient has extremely loose or no jaw tone. The only true sign of inadequate anesthetic depth is gross, purposeful movement. Heart rate, respiratory rate and jaw tone can all increase prior to movement and should be monitored continuously. The use of monitoring devices to assess cardiopulmonary parameters is highly dependent upon several factors including the severity of cardiac disease, the length of anesthesia, and the procedure being performed. Minimal equipment will be required for sedation and short procedures compared to anesthesia for major surgical procedures, both cardiac and noncardiac. The physical parameters of heart rate, respiratory rate, mucous membrane color, capillary refill time, and pulse character should be monitored at regular intervals of no more than 5 minutes during anesthesia and sedation of any duration, even if monitoring equipment is used.

> **KEY POINT**
>
> There is no accurate method to determine inadequate anesthetic depth when using NMRDs (see later).

Noninvasive Monitoring

Electrocardiography

- Continuous ECG monitoring should be performed in all patients with heart disease during sedation and anesthesia of any duration. The decision to continue ECG monitoring during the postoperative period should be determined based on the procedure and the status of the patient.

Arterial Blood Pressure Measurement

- Indirect methods are less accurate than direct measurements (see later). However, monitoring the trends of indirect arterial blood pressure can provide valuable information. The two indirect methods are Doppler ultrasound and oscillometric.

Doppler Ultrasound Method

- Systolic arterial blood pressure can be consistently obtained using the Doppler method, and diastolic values can be determined in some patients. Doppler is easier to perform in small dogs and cats. Accuracy of obtained values is highly dependent on several factors (cuff size, skin thickness, contact of crystal, positioning of limb, vasoconstriction); therefore, trends in blood pressure are monitored. The advantage of Doppler ultrasound is that active arterial blood flow can be heard at all times.

KEY POINT

Do not make therapeutic decisions regarding fluid therapy solely on any indirect method of blood pressure monitoring, especially in cats and small dogs.

Oscillometric Method

- Systolic, diastolic, and mean arterial blood pressure and heart rate are determined. Systolic pressure is the most accurate, though values can be underestimated. Accuracy of obtained values is highly dependent on several factors (cuff size, skin thickness, contact or positioning of cuff in relation to the artery, choice of artery, positioning of limb, vasoconstriction); therefore, trends in blood pressure are monitored. Oscillometric blood pressure monitoring is extremely inaccurate in small dogs, cats, and animals in states of hypotension, despite advances in technology.

Pulse Oximetry

- Pulse oximetry provides indirect determination of arterial oxygenation. Active pulsation of an arterial bed is required to determine oxygenation. Pulse oximetry is inaccurate in states of hypotension and peripheral vasoconstriction (hypothermia, pain). It is most accurate when placed on the tongue; therefore, heavy sedation or general anesthesia is required.

Capnometry

- Capnometry determines the partial pressure of exhaled carbon dioxide, which is closely related to arterial partial pressure of carbon dioxide. It indirectly provides information on cardiac output. Exhaled carbon dioxide is dependent upon adequate perfusion of the lungs (delivery of carbon dioxide to the lungs). Hypoventilation (increased partial pressure of carbon dioxide in arterial blood) can be detected on a breath-by-breath basis. Capnometry requires intubation in most cases for the most accurate values, though tight-fitting facemasks can provide the environment to obtain information on ventilatory status.

Invasive Monitoring

- The more invasive and complicated surgical procedures should incur more invasive monitoring techniques. Whereas the noninvasive techniques can provide general trends, invasive monitoring can provide more accurate data concerning cardiovascular function. Direct monitoring is less likely to provide false negative values and is less likely to fail during anesthesia.

Direct Arterial Blood Pressure Measurement

- A catheter placed in a peripheral artery (dorsal pedal most common). Requires fairly expensive equipment, though refurbished units are affordable and very useful. Technically more difficult to place a catheter in a peripheral artery.

KEY POINT

The advent of affordable, refurbished monitoring devices allows veterinarians to provide the ability to perform invasive, accurate blood pressure monitoring.

Central Venous Pressure

- The central venous pressure (CVP) monitors right heart function and is the most clinically reliable indicator of intravascular volume. CVP uses a properly placed jugular catheter with the tip within the thoracic cavity. Inexpensive equipment (manometers) can be used to measure central venous pressure, though the same device used to monitor direct arterial blood pressure can be used to monitor CVP. CVP can be a valuable tool during anesthesia or in the postoperative period to detect early cardiac failure or fluid overload.

Arterial and Venous Blood Gas

- Arterial blood gas monitoring provides information on ventilation ($PaCO_2$) and oxygenation (PaO_2). Venous blood gas monitoring from a central vein (jugular, cranial vena cava, pulmonary artery) provides indirect information on perfusion of tissues and cardiac output. Arterial and venous blood gas monitoring combined with cardiac output information can be used to calculate oxygen delivery variables (see later). Devices used for blood gas analysis are affordable and are commonly being used in clinical practice.

Box 19-1 Cardiovascular Equations

$$DO_2 = CO \times CaO_2$$
$$CO = HR \times SV$$
$$CaO_2 = (Hb \times SaO_2 \times 1.39) + (PaO_2 \times 0.003)$$
$$ABP = CO \times SVR$$

DO_2, Delivery of oxygen; *CO,* cardiac output; *HR,* heart rate; *SV,* strove volume; *CaO_2,* content of oxygen in arterial blood; *SaO_2,* saturation of oxygen in arterial blood; *1.39,* constant that describes the number of milliliters of oxygen in 100 ml of blood; *PaO_2,* partial pressure of oxygen in arterial blood; *0.003,* percentage of oxygen dissolved in plasma (0.3%) expressed as a decimal; *ABP,* arterial blood pressure; *SVR,* systemic vascular resistance.

Advanced Cardiovascular Monitoring—Cardiac Output

- Cardiac output monitoring requires pulmonary artery catheterization to obtain cardiovascular values that can provide information regarding ventricular function. (Box 19-1). Cardiac output computers remain extremely high-cost expenditures.

KEY POINTS

- Cardiac output is not synonymous with arterial blood pressure. Please note in Box 19-1 that cardiac output is a determinant of the calculation for blood pressure.
- An advance in cardiac output monitoring that may become clinically available for dogs and cats is lithium dilution cardiac output.

Fluid Therapy

- Most patients with heart disease that are anesthetized with inhalation anesthetics will require intravenous fluid support. The fluid of choice for the patient with heart disease is usually a sodium-restricted crystalloid fluid (0.45% NaCl/2.5% dextrose or 0.45% NaCl). The rate of fluid therapy administration, however, is far more important than the type of fluid administered. The rate should be less than the recommended fluid rate during anesthesia of normal, healthy patients (10 ml/kg/hr). A general rule would be to decrease the fluid rate to approximately one fourth to one third of the rate for a normal patient, yielding a rate of 2 to 3 ml/kg/h. Less stable patients with heart disease and those patients anesthetized for emergency surgery that present with signs of heart failure should have CVP measured to aid in monitoring fluid therapy. Colloid fluids should be used with caution in patients with heart disease, especially if a bolus of colloids is to be administered.

AFTERCARE

Basic Nursing Care

- Maintain body temperature using external warming devices such as warm water bottle, incubators or other devices that will raise the external temperature.
- Reduce stress and anxiety by providing a quiet, dry, and comfortable environment.

Oxygen Therapy

- Some patients may require oxygen by facemask, nasal cannula, oxygen cage, or incubator until completely recovered from anesthesia or sedation to maximize oxygen delivery parameters.

Electrocardiographic Monitoring

- Monitor cardiac rate and rhythm continuously until the patient is completely recovered from anesthesia or sedation. Some anesthetic drugs (ketamine and inhalation anesthetics) can predispose to cardiac arrhythmias.

Cardiovascular Monitoring

- The decision to monitor blood pressure and CVP should be determined by the severity of heart disease, stability of the patient, the reason for surgical intervention and the cardiovascular status during anesthesia and surgery. Some patients will not require further monitoring while some patients, such as a dog with dilated cardiomyopathy undergoing surgery to correct gastric dilatation-volvulus, may require all available monitoring. Invasive postoperative monitoring may be required in some patients.

ANALGESIA

- Always provide analgesia if an invasive procedure or surgery was performed. Preemptive analgesia should be practiced at all times. Preemptive analgesia is defined as analgesic techniques that are applied prior to surgical stimulation. Incorporating analgesic agents (opioids) in the preanesthetic medication is the easiest method of preemptive analgesia. Analgesia should be performed on a predetermined schedule (intermittent administration) or by continuous administration techniques for at least 12 to 24 hours after surgery.

Opioid Analgesia Techniques

Transdermal Fentanyl

- Transdermal fentanyl is very effective in providing postoperative analgesia. Transdermal fentanyl patches are available in two sizes based on the delivery of fentanyl: 25 and 50 μg/hr. Patches should be applied 12 to 24 hours prior to surgery for dogs and 8 to 12 hours prior to surgery in cats.
- The weight of the dog will determine which patch or patches to be applied. Dogs weighing less than 3 kg can have half of a 25 μg/hr applied by using the protective plastic portion of the patch to partially expose only half of the patch. Dogs weighing between 3 and 10 kg can have 25 μg/hr applied. Dogs weighing 10 to 20 kg can have a 50 μg/hr patch applied. Dogs weighing 20 to 30 kg will require 75 μg/hr (one each of a 25 and 50 μg/hr patch) applied simultaneously. Finally, dogs weighing more than 30 kg will require 100 μg/hr (two 50 μg/hr patches) applied simultaneously.
- Cats weighing less than 3 kg can have half of a 25 μg/hr applied as described previously using the protective plastic portion of the patch to expose only half of the patch. Cats weighing greater than 3 kg can have an entire 25 μg/hr patch applied.

Continuous Rate Infusion of Opioids and Opioid Combinations

- Opioids alone or in combination with the local anesthetic lidocaine and the dissociative drug ketamine can be used to provide analgesia in the postoperative period in dogs and cats. Many combinations exist and it is the decision of the clinician as to which CRI to administer. Decisions can be made based on severity of postoperative pain and experience of the clinician.

Opioids

- Both morphine and fentanyl can be used alone to provide postoperative analgesia. The administration rate of morphine is 0.12 mg/kg/hr and the rate of fentanyl is 2 to 10 μg/kg/hr.

Opioid Combinations—Dogs

Morphine-Lidocaine-Ketamine

- The following drugs are administered to a 1-L bag of 0.45% NaCl or 0.45% NaCl and 2.5% dextrose: morphine (15 mg/ml; 1.8 ml), lidocaine (2%; 20 mg/ml; 15 ml), ketamine (100 mg/ml; 0.6 ml). The initial intraoperative administration is typically the anesthesia rate of fluids (10 ml/kg/hr). However, many cardiac patients will require a limited rate of fluids (2.5 ml/kg/hr) that may delay the onset of action of this combination. The postoperative administration rate will be 2.5 ml/kg/hr regardless of the intraoperative administration rate.

Fentanyl-Lidocaine-Ketamine

- The following drugs are administered to a 1-L bag of 0.45% NaCl or 0.45% NaCl and 2.5% dextrose: lidocaine (2%; 20 mg/ml; 15 ml) and ketamine (100 mg/ml; 0.6 ml) are prepared as above. The volume of fentanyl (50 μg/ml) will vary based on the rate of fluid administration. A volume to provide a CRI of 3 μg/kg/hr should be prepared for intraoperative and postoperative administration. The fluid rates are similar to those used for morphine-lidocaine-ketamine preparations.

Opioid Combinations—Cats

- Continuous rate infusions of opioid combinations for cats are prepared and administered differently than for dogs. Cats tend to be more likely to have side effects from lidocaine. Therefore, lidocaine is not used in the combinations. Cats can become excited or dysphoric from the opioid combinations. Tranquilizers such as acepromazine (0.025 mg/kg, IV) can be used to decrease any side effects caused by opioids.

KEY POINT

Opioid agonists should not be avoided because of possible side effects of excitement or dysphoria in cats.

Morphine-Ketamine

- The following drugs are administered to a 1-L bag of 0.45% NaCl or 0.45% NaCl and 2.5% dextrose: morphine (15 mg/ml; 1.8 ml) and ketamine (100 mg/ml; 0.6 ml). The initial intraoperative administration is typically the anesthesia rate of fluids (10 ml/kg/hr). However, many cardiac patients will require a limited rate of fluids (2.5 ml/kg/hr) that may delay the onset of action of this combination. The postoperative administration rate will be 2.5 ml/kg/hr regardless of the intraoperative administration rate.

Fentanyl-Ketamine

- Ketamine (100 mg/ml; 0.6 ml) is added to a 1-L bag of 0.45% NaCl or 0.45% NaCl and 2.5% dextrose. The volume of fentanyl (50 μg/ml) will vary based on the rate of fluid administration. A volume to provide a CRI of 3 μg/kg/hr should be prepared for intraoperative and postoperative administration. The fluid rates are similar to those used for morphine-ketamine preparations.

ANESTHETIC CONSIDERATIONS FOR SPECIFIC CARDIAC DISEASES AND RECOMMENDED ANESTHETIC PROTOCOLS

Recommended for All Patients

- Preoxygenation with 5 L/min oxygen via facemask or "blow by" method prior to induction of anesthesia is used to maximize arterial oxygenation and oxygen delivery prior to administration of induction drugs. ECG monitoring prior to induction of anesthesia is also recommended. Ventilatory support should be provided to all patients maintained with inhalation anesthesia to reduce adverse effects of hypoventilation.

ANESTHETICS PROTOCOLS IN DOGS AND CATS

- The choice of anesthetic protocol should be based on the ASA classification (see p. 357) and not the specific cardiac disease. There are several differences to be noted regarding specific cardiac diseases, anesthetic drug effects and cardiovascular support. Therefore, a short discussion of the specific cardiac disease will be followed with the choice of anesthetic protocol based on the ASA classification. Anesthetic techniques (including injectable techniques) for medical and minor surgical procedures will be discussed followed by techniques for major surgical procedures within each ASA classification.

Common Cardiac Diseases and Anesthesia Techniques for Dogs

Mitral Valve Insufficiency

- Mild arterial vasodilation from anesthetic drugs can result in a decrease in the regurgitant fraction across the mitral valve and maximum cardiac output.
- Supraventricular and ventricular arrhythmias are common sequelae to mitral regurgitation and the ECG should be monitored at all times. Extremes in heart rate (bradycardia or tachycardia) can result in decreased cardiac output.

Dilated Cardiomyopathy

- Inotropic support with dobutamine or dopamine is recommended for any major surgery regardless of ASA status. Tachycardia may predispose to ventricular arrhythmias and the judicious use of atropine or glycopyrrolate is not recommended. Mild arterial vasodilation can maximize cardiac output.

Congenital Defects

Aortic and Pulmonic Stenosis

- Cardiac output is highly dependent upon heart rate and inotropic agents contribute little to no increase in cardiac output. Tachycardia may predispose to ventricular arrhythmias and the judicious use of atropine or glycopyrrolate is not recommended. The dose of atropine or glycopyrrolate should be decreased by half. Bradycardia can result in severe decreases in cardiac output.

Patent Ductus Arteriosus and Ventricular Septal Defect

- Pulmonary over circulation results in a rapid uptake of inhalation anesthetic and a more rapid inhalation anesthetic induction. There may be a delay in distribution of intravenous anesthetics, though a clinical effect is likely not evident. Mild arterial vasodilation may reduce the amount of blood flow across the patent ductus arteriosus or the ventricular septal defect.

ASA II Patients: Medical Procedure or Minor, Minimally Invasive Surgical Procedures

Injectable Anesthesia Technique

- The preanesthetic medication of choice would be a neuroleptanalgesic combination of **acepromazine** (0.025 mg/kg, IM) and **butorphanol** (0.4 mg/kg, IM). Prophylactic use of atropine is not recommended to minimize production of tachyarrhythmias.
- Induction can be achieved using **ketamine-diazepam** (1 ml/10 kg of a 50:50 mixture, IV) and anesthesia can be maintained using intermittent boluses of a third to a fourth the initial dose of ketamine-diazepam if additional anesthesia time is required. Alternatively, induction and maintenance of anesthesia can be achieved using **propofol** (2 to 6 mg/kg, IV) for induction followed by either CRI (0.14 to 0.4 mg/kg/min) or intermittent bolus (0.5 to 1.0 mg/kg, IV).

- Physical parameters, ECG, and Doppler blood pressure can be used for monitoring during the procedure.

Inhalation Anesthesia Technique

- Preanesthetic medication and induction as previously described above. Ketamine-diazepam is preferred over propofol due to a longer duration of action, which will require less inhalation anesthetic.
- Isoflurane or sevoflurane in oxygen at the lowest effective dose can be used to maintain anesthesia, using opioids intraoperatively as needed. Ventilation should be provided at all times during anesthesia and surgery.
- Physical parameters, ECG, Doppler blood pressure, and capnometry can be used for monitoring during the procedure.

> **KEY POINT**
>
> Potent opioid agonists are usually not required for these types of minor procedures.

ASA II Patients: Major Surgery

- An injectable anesthesia technique to maintain anesthesia is usually not required as these patients are considered very stable prior to anesthesia and surgery and should be able to tolerate inhalation anesthetics as the primary technique to maintain anesthesia.

Inhalation Anesthesia Technique

- A neuroleptanalgesic combination of **acepromazine** (0.025 mg/kg, IM) and **hydromorphone** (0.2 mg/kg, IM) can be used for preanesthetic medication. **Atropine** (0.22 mg/kg, IM) is recommended for smaller dogs (< 5 kg) only.

> **KEY POINTS**
>
> - Potent opioid agonists are preferred over opioid agonist/antagonists to provide adequate preemptive analgesia.
> - **Ketamine-diazepam** (1 ml/10 kg of a 50:50 mixture, IV) is preferred to induce anesthesia over **propofol** (2 to 6 mg/kg, IV) due to a longer duration of action that will initially reduce the dose of inhalation anesthetic.
> - Adjuncts to general anesthesia can be used to minimize use of inhalation anesthetics.

> A CRI of morphine-lidocaine-ketamine or fentanyl-lidocaine-ketamine should commence at the beginning of surgery at the anesthetic rate of fluid administration (10 ml/kg/hr). An epidural injection of a combination of lidocaine-bupivacaine-morphine analgesia should be administered prior to the beginning of surgery for all abdominal procedures. Other local anesthetic techniques can be dictated by the location of surgery. An intermittent bolus of opioid agonists may also be necessary during surgery. NMRDs can be used if blood pressure is low and the patient is not adequately anesthetized. Pancuronium (0.02 to 0.04 mg/kg, IV) has a longer duration of action than atracurium (0.25 mg/kg, IV). Ventilation should be provided at all times during anesthesia and surgery.

ASA III or IV Patients: Medical Procedure or Minor, Minimally Invasive Surgical Procedures

Injectable Anesthesia Technique

- A neuroleptanalgesic combination of **diazepam** (0.4 mg/kg, IM) and **butorphanol** (0.4 mg/kg, IM) is administered as the preanesthetic medication. Atropine is not recommended to minimize production of tachyarrhythmias.
- Induction can be achieved using **ketamine-diazepam** (1 ml/10 kg of a 50:50 mixture, IV) and anesthesia can be maintained using intermittent boluses of a third to a fourth the initial dose of ketamine-diazepam if additional anesthesia time is required. Alternatively, induction and maintenance of anesthesia can be achieved using **propofol** (2 to 6 mg/kg, IV) for induction followed by either CRI (0.14 to 0.4 mg/kg/min) of intermittent bolus (0.5 to 1.0 mg/kg, IV). **Etomidate** (1 to 2 mg/kg, IV) should be used as the induction agent if cardiac arrhythmias are present. Endotracheal intubation may be necessary, but is not required. Supplemental oxygen should be administered with this technique.
- Physical parameters, ECG, and Doppler blood pressure can be used for monitoring during the procedure.

> **KEY POINT**
>
> An inhalation anesthetic technique for a medical or minor surgical procedure is not indicated for ASA III-IV cardiac patients.

ASA III or IV Patients: Major Surgery

- An injectable anesthetic technique using low-dose inhalation, only if necessary, is recommended over a technique that relies on an inhalation anesthetic to maintain anesthesia.

KEY POINTS

- Anesthesia of ASA III or IV patients for major surgery will require intensive monitoring of anesthesia, cardiovascular parameters, and the patient.
- Neuroleptanalgesic combination of **diazepam** (0.2 mg/kg, IV) and fentanyl (1 μg/kg, IV) should be administered as preanesthetic medication. **Atropine** (0.22 mg/kg, IV) may be necessary if bradycardia occurs.
- **Fentanyl** (5 to 10 μg/kg) is recommended for induction of anesthesia. Induction with fentanyl is not considered a rapid induction and may take 30 to 60 seconds or more. Alternative induction with **etomidate** (1 to 2 mg/kg, IV) should be administered for induction if arrhythmias are present.
- A CRI of **fentanyl** (5 to 10 μg/kg/hr) administered by a dedicated syringe pump is recommended to maintain a surgical plane of anesthesia.
- Ventilation should be provided at all times during anesthesia and surgery. Lidocaine and ketamine can be administered for analgesia in a separate bag of fluids. Epidural analgesia for abdominal procedures is recommended. Other local anesthetic techniques are dictated by the location of surgery. NMRDs can be used if blood pressure is low and the patient is not adequately anesthetized. Pancuronium (0.02 to 0.04 mg/kg, IV) has a longer duration of action than atracurium (0.25 mg/kg, IV).
- Blood pressure (direct is preferred over indirect methods), ECG, capnometry, pulse oximetry, and physical parameters are continuously monitored.

CANINE PERICARDIAL DISEASE: PERICARDIOCENTESIS

ASA I or II Dogs that Require Pericardiocentesis

- Dogs not showing signs of pericardial tamponade may only require only an infiltration of local anesthetic (lidocaine) in the skin and intercostals musculature at the site of needle puncture for pericardiocentesis.
- Sedation techniques for dogs not compliant to local anesthesia only include a neuroleptanalgesia combination of **diazepam** (0.2 mg/kg, IV) and **hydromorphone** (0.2 mg/kg, IV). Atropine should only be used if bradycardia occurs.

ASA IV Dogs—Emergency Pericardiocentesis

- Dogs that require an emergency pericardiocentesis typically present with signs of collapse, right heart failure and/or ventricular arrhythmias all related to pericardial tamponade. Most dogs will require only an infiltration of local anesthetic (lidocaine) in the skin and intercostals musculature at the site of needle puncture for pericardiocentesis. Occasionally, dogs will require sedation in addition to local anesthesia. The neuroleptanalgesia combination of **diazepam** (0.2 mg/kg, IV) and **butorphanol** (0.2 mg/kg, IV) is recommended. Cardiac output is highly dependent on heart rate during pericardial tamponade and butorphanol is least likely to decrease heart rate. Atropine is not recommended. An induction agent may be necessary in addition to sedation in some instances. **Etomidate** (1 to 2 mg/kg, IV) is the drug of choice as there are minimal to no cardiopulmonary effects.

COMMON CARDIAC DISEASES AND ANESTHESIA TECHNIQUES FOR CATS

Hypertrophic Cardiomyopathy

- The most common cardiac disease in cats is hypertrophic cardiomyopathy (HCM). Hypertrophic cardiomyopathy is characterized primarily as diastolic dysfunction with normal ventricular contraction. Increases in heart rate and ventricular tachyarrhythmias caused by anesthetic drugs are best avoided.

ASA I and II Cats with HCM: Medical Procedure or Minor, Minimally Invasive Surgical Procedures

Injectable Anesthesia Technique

- A neuroleptanalgesic combination of **acepromazine** (0.025 mg/kg, IM) and **hydromorphone** (0.2 mg/kg, IM) is administered as preanesthetic medication. **Ketamine** (6 to 10 mg/kg, IM) is administered 10 to 15 minutes after the neuroleptanalgesic combination. This three drug combination may be all that is required to perform the procedure.

- **Propofol** (1 to 3 mg/kg, IV) can be administered if additional anesthesia is required. Propofol administered as either a CRI (0.14 to 0.4 mg/kg/min) of intermittent bolus (0.5 mg/kg, IV) can be used for longer procedures.
- Physical parameters, ECG, and Doppler blood pressure can be used for monitoring during the procedure.

Inhalation Anesthesia Technique

- Preanesthetic medication and induction done as previously described previously.
- Isoflurane or sevoflurane in oxygen is administered at the lowest effective dose.
- The three drug preanesthetic will greatly reduce inhalation anesthetic requirement.

KEY POINTS

- Ventilation will be required during surgery in all cats that receive the three drug preanesthetic combinations and inhalation anesthesia.
- Physical parameters, ECG, Doppler blood pressure, and capnometry can be monitored during the procedure.

ASA II Patients: Major Surgery

- Injectable anesthesia technique is usually not required as patients are considered very stable prior to anesthesia and surgery and should be able to tolerate inhalation anesthetics as the primary technique to maintain anesthesia.

Inhalation anesthesia Technique

- A neuroleptanalgesic combination of **acepromazine** (0.025 mg/kg, IM) and **hydromorphone** (0.2 mg/kg, IM) is followed in 10 to 15 minutes by **ketamine** (6 to 10 mg/kg, IM) for preanesthetic medication.

KEY POINTS

- Potent opioid agonists are preferred over opioid agonist/antagonists to provide adequate preemptive analgesia.
- Some cats may be able to be intubated without use of an induction agent. **Propofol** (1 to 2 mg/kg, IV) can be used to effect to permit intubation.
- Ventilation should be provided at all times during anesthesia and surgery. A CRI of morphine-ketamine is recommended to provide analgesia and minimize use of inhalation anesthetics.
- Lumbosacral epidural analgesia for abdominal procedures is recommended.
- NMRDs can be used if blood pressure is low and the patient is not adequately anesthetized. **Pancuronium** (0.02 to 0.04 mg/kg, IV) has a longer duration of action than **atracurium** (0.25 mg/kg, IV).

ASA III or IV patients: Medical Procedure or Minor, Minimally Invasive Surgical Procedures

Injectable Anesthesia Technique

- A neuroleptanalgesic combination of **diazepam** (0.2 mg/kg, IV) and **hydromorphone** (0.2 mg/kg, IV) is administered as preanesthetic medication.
- Use of an induction agent may not be necessary following the neuroleptanalgesic combination. **Propofol** (2 to 4 mg/kg, IV) may be used if needed. Propofol administered as either a CRI (0.14 to 0.4 mg/kg/min) or intermittent bolus (0.5 to 1.0 mg/kg, IV) can be used if additional time is required. **Etomidate** (1 to 2 mg/kg, IV) should be used as the induction agent if cardiac arrhythmias are present. Endotracheal intubation may be necessary, but is not required. Supplemental oxygen should be administered with this technique.
- Physical parameters, ECG, and Doppler blood pressure can be monitored during the procedure.

KEY POINT

An inhalation anesthetic technique for a medical or minor surgical procedure is not indicated for ASA III-IV cardiac patients.

ASA III or IV Patients: Major Surgery

- An injectable anesthetic technique using low dose inhalation, only if necessary, is recommended over a technique that relies on an inhalation anesthetic to maintain anesthesia.

KEY POINTS

- Anesthesia of ASA III or IV patients for major surgery will require intensive monitoring of anesthesia and the patient.
- A neuroleptanalgesic combination of **diazepam** (0.2 mg/kg, IM) and **hydromorphone** (0.2 mg/kg, IM) is followed in 10 to 15 minutes by **ketamine** (6 to 10 mg/kg) for preanesthetic medication.

- **Propofol** (2 to 4 mg/kg, IV) may be used if needed. **Etomidate** (1 to 2 mg/kg, IV) should be used as the induction agent if cardiac arrhythmias are present.
- A CRI of **fentanyl** (3 to 5 μg/kg/hr) administered by a dedicated syringe pump is recommended to maintain a surgical plane of anesthesia.
- Ventilation should be provided at all times during anesthesia and surgery. Ketamine can be administered for analgesia in a separate 1-L bag of fluids. Epidural analgesia for abdominal procedures is recommended.
- NMRDs can be used if blood pressure is low and the patient is not adequately anesthetized. **Pancuronium** (0.02 to 0.04 mg/kg, IV) has a longer duration of action than **atracurium** (0.25 mg/kg, IV).
- Blood pressure (direct is preferred over indirect methods), ECG, capnometry, pulse oximetry, and physical parameters should be monitored during surgery.

Frequently Asked Questions

Why should isoflurane and sevoflurane be used with caution to maintain anesthesia in patients with cardiac disease?

Isoflurane can certainly support cardiac output and heart rate, but it is a potent arterial vasodilator. Severe hypoperfusion and hypotension can occur during anesthesia if isoflurane or sevoflurane is used as the sole anesthetic agent to maintain anesthesia. Hypoperfusion and hypotension can be worse if the dog or cat is receiving an ACEI drug such as enalapril or benazapril. The less isoflurane or sevoflurane used, the less likely it is that adverse cardiovascular effects will occur.

Why are the main differences in the clinical effects of opioids in dogs and cats important?

We learned long ago in our profession that cats were not small dogs. The extreme popularity of opioids for anesthesia in dogs, and the advent of advanced analgesia techniques including CRIs of opioids, has led to the extension of opioid use to the feline species. However, many clinicians have been disappointed because cats do not respond in the same way to the drugs as dogs, and opioids are a possible detriment to cats. Opioid use in cats is essential to prevent the untoward effects of higher doses of ketamine in cats with HCM. Opioids are extremely safe in cats with HCM, as the myocardial contractility is not affected, and the heart rate is reduced. The most effective use of opioids in cats is with the concurrent use of tranquilizers. The more potent the tranquilizer, the better the clinical effect. Cats administered acepromazine with the opioid are better sedated than when a benzodiazepine is administered. The combination of a benzodiazepine and opioid in a cat could result in excitement. Clinicians should realize that cats will not be as heavily sedated (compared with dogs), and recoveries could be rough as well. Overall, the safety of opioids should outweigh these concerns.

What would be the most important cardiopulmonary side effect of anesthesia for the patient with cardiac disease?

By far, the most important aspect of anesthetizing a dog or cat with heart disease is respiratory depression. The opioids, dissociatives, and the inhalation anesthetics are all respiratory depressants. Severe respiratory depression will occur if all three of these anesthetic classes of drugs are used in the same anesthetic protocol. The most common cause of anesthetic death is respiratory arrest. Dogs and cats with cardiac disease undergoing anesthesia should have ventilation maintained either manually or with an anesthesia ventilator to eliminate the effects of respiratory depression. Monitoring with techniques such as capnometry and pulse oximetry will lead to early diagnosis and treatment of respiratory depression. The use of the nondepolarizing muscle relaxants dictates the use of ventilation.

SUGGESTED READINGS

Cornick-Seahorn JL: Anesthetic management of patients with cardiovascular disease, Comp Cont Ed 16:1121, 1994.

Day TK: Intravenous anesthetic techniques for emergency and critical care procedures. In Bonagura JD, ed: Kirk's current veterinary therapy XIII. Philadelphia, 2000, WB Saunders.

Drugs used for preanesthetic medication. In Muir WW, Hubbell JAE, Skarda RT, Bednarski RM, eds: Handbook of veterinary anesthesia, ed 4, St Louis, 2007, Mosby.

General anesthesia. In McKelvey D, Hollingshead KW, eds: Veterinary anesthesia and analgesia, ed 3, St Louis, 2003, Mosby.

Hellyer PW: Anesthesia in patients with cardiovascular disease. In Kirk RW, Bonagura JD, eds: Current veterinary therapy XI, Philadelphia, 1992, WB Saunders.

Ilkiw JE: Anaesthesia and disease. In Hall LW, Taylor PM, eds: Anaesthesia of the cat, London, 1994, Baillière Tindall.

Injectable anesthetics. In Thurmon JC, Tranquilli WJ, Benson GJ, eds: Lumb and Jones' veterinary anesthesia, ed 3, Baltimore, 1996, Williams & Wilkins.

Mason DE, Hubbell JAE: Anesthesia and the heart. In Fox PR, Sisson D, Moise NS, eds: Textbook of canine and feline cardiology, Philadelphia, 1999, WB Saunders.

Paddleford RR, Harvey RC: Anesthesia for selected diseases: cardiovascular dysfunction. In Thurmon JC, Tranquilli WJ, Benson GJ, eds: Lumb and Jones' veterinary anesthesia, ed 3, Baltimore, 1996, Williams & Wilkins.

Preanesthetics and anesthetic adjuncts. In Thurmon JC, Tranquilli WJ, Benson GJ, eds: Lumb and Jones' veterinary anesthesia, ed 3, Baltimore, 1996, Williams & Wilkins.

CHAPTER 20

Cardiac Surgery

E. Christopher Orton

INTRODUCTION

Cardiac surgery is increasingly an option for management of congenital and acquired cardiac conditions in small animals. Some cardiac surgeries are widely available, whereas open cardiac repairs that require cardiopulmonary bypass (CPB) are currently only performed at a few regional centers. Some cardiac surgeries are performed with curative intent, whereas others are considered palliative only. Cardiac surgeries include closed cardiac surgeries, cardiac surgeries performed during inflow occlusion, and cardiac surgeries performed under CPB.

CLOSED CARDIAC SURGERY

Patent Ductus Arteriosus Ligation

With few exceptions, closure of patent ductus arteriosus (PDA) is indicated in all small animals with this defect. Closure can be accomplished by catheter-based occlusion methods or surgical ligation. Although each has theoretical advantages, both approaches are successful in the hands of an experienced operator and neither approach should be regarded as always superior or preferred. Choosing an approach depends on several factors, including client preference, availability of equipment and expertise, and urgency of the procedure. PDA closure is curative when performed early in life before the onset of severe ventricular remodeling, systolic dysfunction, or functional mitral regurgitation (MR). Surgical ligation of PDA can be accomplished with little or no operative mortality when performed by experienced surgeons.

PDA ligation is undertaken through a left fourth thoracotomy in the dog and a left fifth thoracotomy in a cat (Figure 20-1). The most frequent surgical complication is hemorrhage during ductus dissection. If significant hemorrhage occurs during dissection, the ductus should be closed with pledget-buttressed mattress sutures with or without division of the ductus.

Pulmonic and Aortic Valve Dilation

Pulmonic stenosis (PS) and subvalvular aortic stenosis (SAS) are relatively common congenital heart defects in dogs. Despite the relative importance of PS, the natural history of untreated PS in dogs is not well documented. Dogs with moderate PS may tolerate the defect relatively well for many years. Transpulmonic pressure gradients > 100 mm Hg are considered an indication for intervention, especially if animals are exhibiting activity intolerance, syncope, or have concurrent tricuspid regurgitation. The natural history of untreated SAS in dogs is better understood. Dogs with transaortic pressure gradients >80 mm Hg are known to be at risk for sudden cardiac death early in life. Gradient reduction by valve dilation is assumed, but not proven, to be palliative for dogs with PS. Valve dilation for SAS does not result in sustained decreases in transaortic pressure gradients. Current evidence suggests

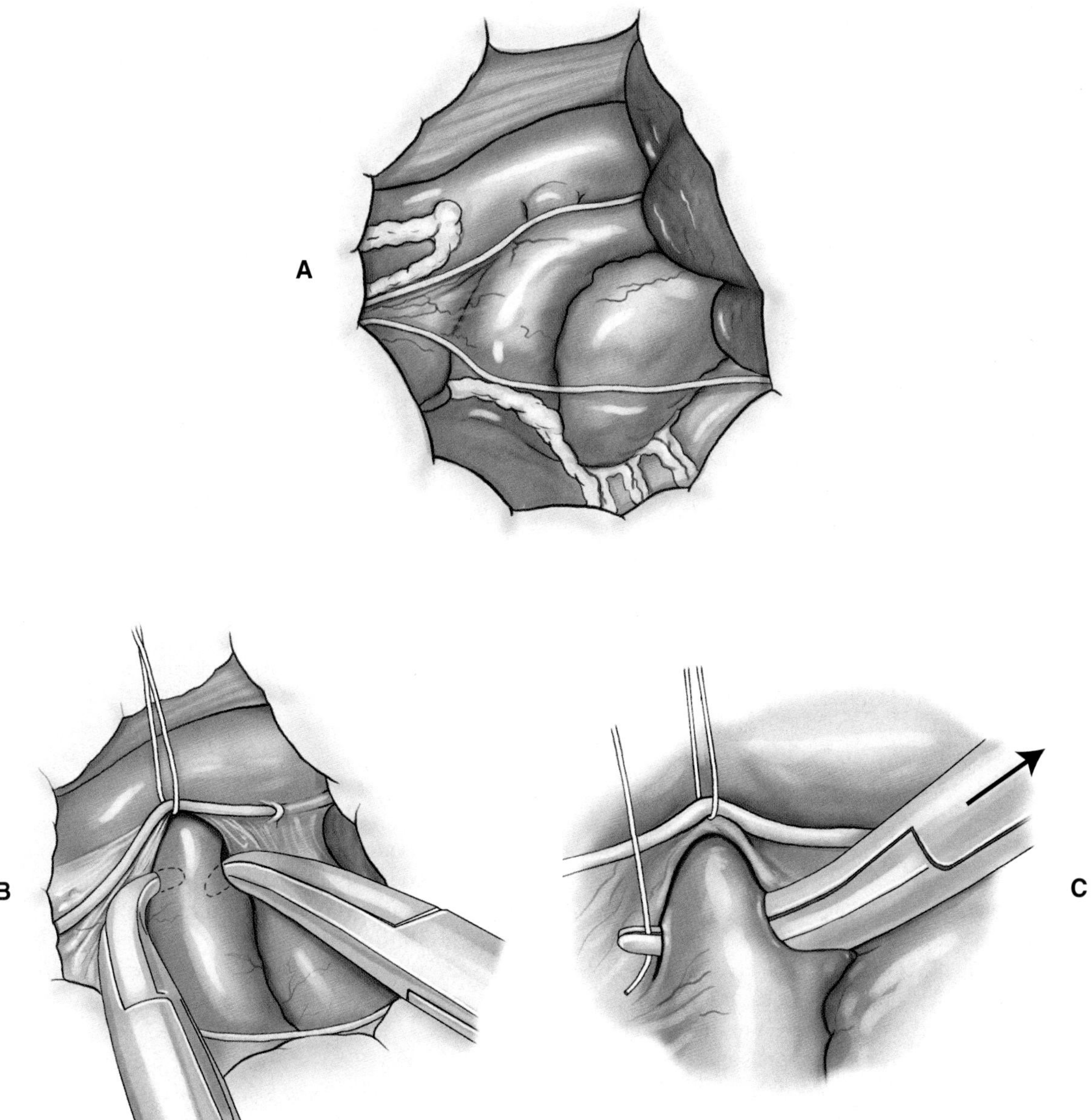

Figure 20-1. PDA ligation. The vagus nerve courses over the ductus arteriosus and serves as an anatomic landmark for identification of the ductus arteriosus **(A)**. The vagus nerve is isolated at the level of the ductus and gently retracted with one or two sutures **(B)**. Occasionally a persistent left cranial vena cava may overlie the ductus arteriosus. In this case, the vein should be carefully isolated and retracted with the vagus nerve. The ductus arteriosus is isolated by blunt dissection without opening the pericardium. Dissection of the caudal aspect of the ductus is accomplished by passing right-angled forceps behind the ductus parallel to the transverse plane. Dissection of the cranial aspect of the ductus is accomplished by angling the forceps caudally at approximately a 45-degree angle. Dissection is completed by passing the forceps medial to ductus from a caudal to cranial direction **(C)**. Two heavy silk ligatures are passed around the ductus by grasping the ligature with right-angled forceps. The ductus arteriosus is closed by slowly tightening and tying the ligature.

little or no palliative benefit from valve dilation or surgical treatment of SAS.

Catheter-based balloon valvuloplasty is preferred to surgical valve dilation of PS because it as a less invasive. Surgical valve dilation of PS is indicated for animals that fail balloon-catheter placement across the PS, or when equipment for cardiac catheterization is not available. Surgical valve dilation of PS is performed through a left fourth thoracotomy (Figure 20-2).

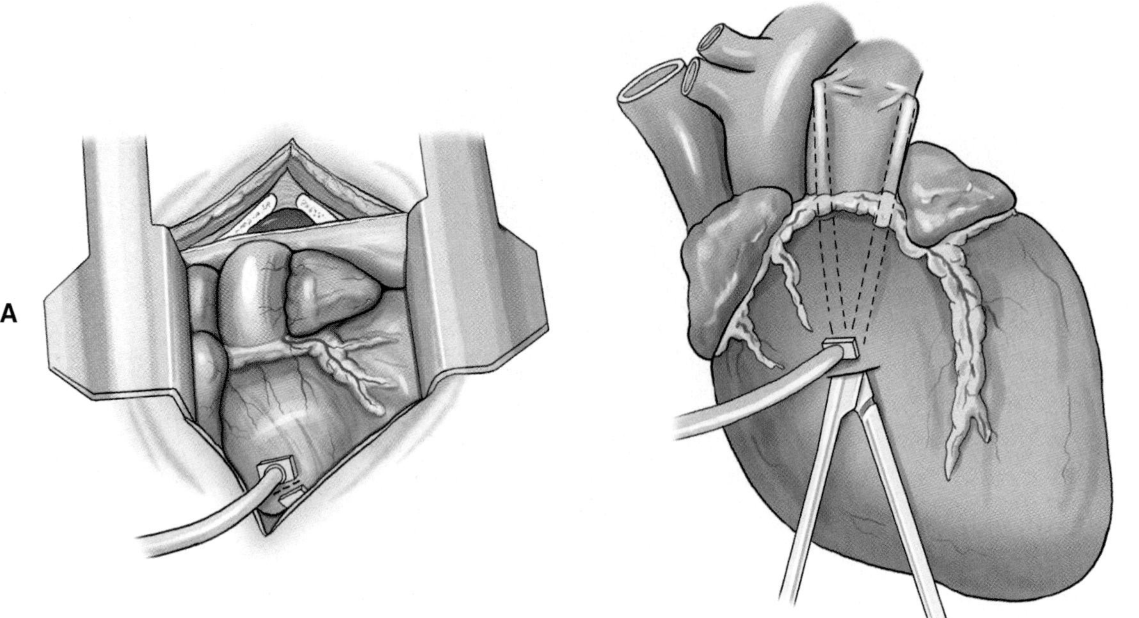

Figure 20-2. Pulmonary valve dilation. The pericardium over the right outflow tract is opened and sutured to the thoracotomy incision. A buttressed mattress suture is placed in the right ventricular outflow tract and passed through a tourniquet **(A)**. A stab incision is made in the ventricle within the confines of the mattress suture. A dilating instrument is passed into the right ventricular outflow tract and across the pulmonic valve **(B)**. The pulmonic valve is dilated several times. The ventricular incision is closed by tying the mattress suture.

Pulmonary Artery Banding

Pulmonary artery banding is a palliative surgery for ventricular septal defect (VSD) that consists of placement of a constricting band around the pulmonary artery. The intent is a measurable increase in right ventricular systolic pressure that thereby decreases the driving pressure gradient for shunt flow across the defect. The procedure provides protection against both progressive heart failure and pulmonary hypertension, and is a viable option for both cats and dogs with hemodynamically significant VSD. Diagnostic parameters that suggest hemodynamically significant VSD include radiographic evidence of pulmonary over circulation, echocardiographic evidence of left ventricular dilation (increased left ventricular diastolic diameter, left ventricular diastolic volume [index > 150 ml/m^2], Doppler-measured shunt flow velocity < 3.5 m/sec, or pulmonic ejection velocity > 2.5 m/sec. Evidence of progressive pulmonary hypertension based on Doppler echocardiography or direct catheter measurement is also a reason to consider surgery. Long term palliation of VSD is possible with this procedure. Possible complications of pulmonary artery banding include acute over tightening of the band or late-term progressive constriction of the band leading to reversal of shunt flow. Worsening of concurrent tricuspid regurgitation is also a possible adverse outcome.

Pulmonary artery banding is performed through a left fourth thoracotomy (Figure 20-3). The appropriate degree of pulmonic constriction is based on pulmonary artery pressure distal to the band and systemic arterial pressures. Pulmonary artery pressure is measured intraoperatively by a catheter introduced through a small purse-string suture in the pulmonary artery. Optimal banding is where pulmonary artery pressure distal to the band is decreased to less than 30 mm Hg (assuming significant pulmonary vascular remodeling is not present), and when the increase in systemic arterial pressure just begins to plateau. As a general rule, optimal banding requires a two-thirds reduction in the diameter of the pulmonary artery although this will vary depending on the degree of pulmonary artery dilation.

Systemic–to–Pulmonary Artery Shunt

Creation of a systemic–to–pulmonary artery shunt is a palliative surgery for tetralogy of Fallot. The functional goal of a systemic–to–pulmonary artery shunt

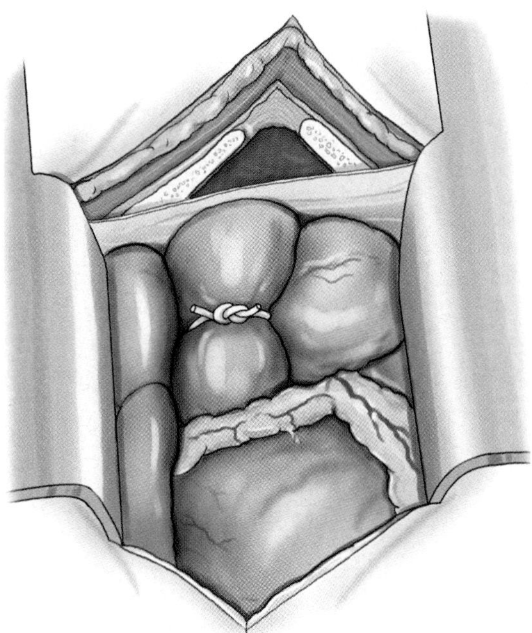

Figure 20-3. Pulmonary artery banding. The pericardium is opened and sutured to the thoracotomy incision. The pulmonary artery is separated from the aorta by sharp and blunt dissection. A large cotton or Teflon tape is passed around the pulmonary artery just distal to the pulmonic valve. The tape is tightened to reduce circumference of the pulmonary artery.

is to increase pulmonary blood flow without creating an overwhelming left-to-right shunt. The desired result is a measured increase in pulmonary blood flow that lessens hypoxemia by lessening the shunt-to-pulmonary flow ratio. Systemic–to–pulmonary shunt is indicated for animals that have resting cyanosis, debilitating activity intolerance or persistent polycythemia (polycythemia vera > 70%) that requires frequent phlebotomy. Most veterinary experience is based on various modifications of the classic Blalock-Taussig shunt. The original Blalock-Taussig shunt consisted of dividing the left subclavian artery and performing an end-to-side anastomosis of the distal end of the divided artery to the pulmonary artery. In animals, the left subclavian artery generally does not have sufficient length to reach the pulmonary artery without kinking. Several modifications of the classic procedure have been devised including a synthetic vascular graft matched in size to the subclavian artery, harvesting the left subclavian artery as a free autogenous graft, or using autogenous jugular vein. Animals can receive significant palliation from any of the previous methods so long as pulmonary blood flow is increased to an appropriate degree.

A modified Blalock-Taussig shunt is performed through a left fourth thoracotomy (Figure 20-4). A continuous thrill should be palpable on the pulmonary artery and hypoxemia should be lessened immediately after surgery.

Pericardiectomy

Pericardial disease can result from neoplasia, bacterial or mycotic infection, foreign body, or idiopathic causes. Pericardial disease can take the form of acute or chronic pericardial effusion, constrictive pericarditis, or constrictive-effusive pericarditis. These conditions can result in pathophysiologic syndromes of acute cardiac tamponade, chronic cardiac tamponade, or pericardial constriction. Pericardiectomy is indicated for the management of chronic pericardial effusions, particularly when the effusion recurs after pericardiocentesis. Pericardiectomy is either palliative or curative depending on the underlying cause of pericardial effusion. Pericardiectomy is the only viable treatment for animals with constrictive or constrictive-effusive pericarditis.

Pericardiectomy can be performed via either a right or left thoracotomy, or a median sternotomy. Median sternotomy has the advantages of providing access to both ventricles and requiring less cardiac manipulation, and thus is preferred by many surgeons (Figure 20-5). Excision of the pericardium ventral to the phrenic nerves (i.e., subphrenic pericardiectomy) is adequate in most cases. In animals with constrictive pericarditis, the pericardium may have to be separated from the epicardium by blunt and sharp dissection. Additionally, epicardial decortication may be necessary to relieve constrictive physiology in animals with pericarditis. Epicardial decortication entails careful separation of a fibrous layer from the myocardium by sharp dissection. Decortication should not be attempted over the atria or portions of the ventricles containing major coronary vessels.

Atrial Appendectomy

Atrial appendectomy is occasionally indicated for palliative removal of a right atrial hemangiosarcoma or for thrombosis of the right or left atrial appendage associated with atrial fibrillation. In the case of hemangiosarcoma, atrial appendectomy is often combined with pericardiectomy and is performed via a median sternotomy. Atrial appendectomy for atrial thrombosis is performed via fifth thoracotomy on the right or left side (Figure 20-6).

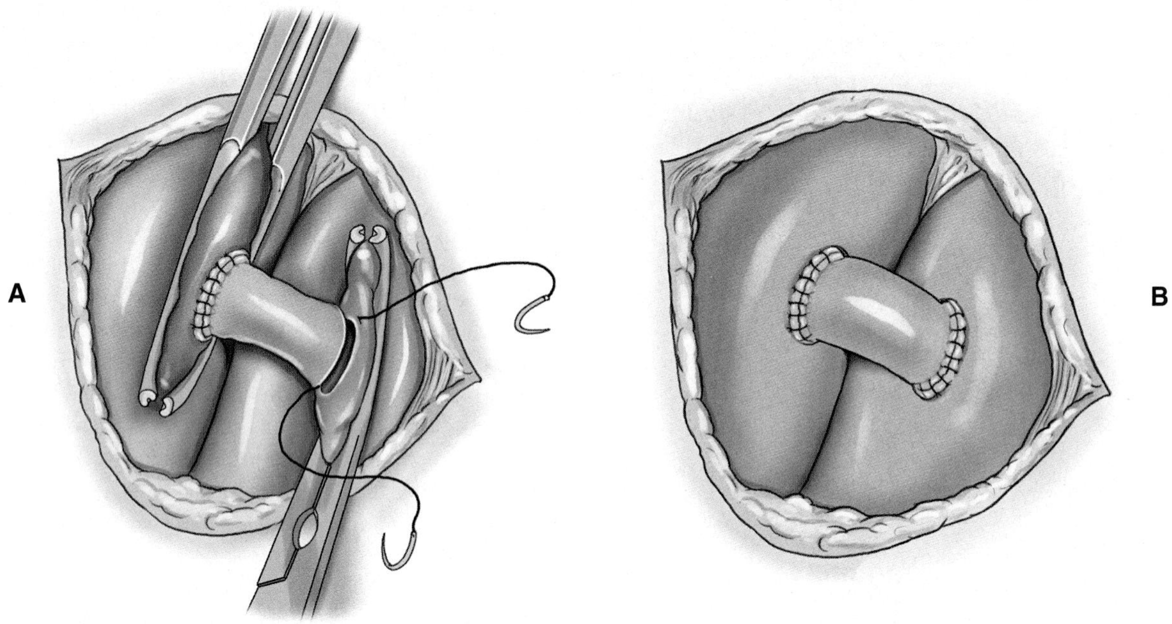

Figure 20-4. Systemic–to–pulmonary artery shunt. The pericardium is opened and sutured to the thoracotomy incision. Tangential vascular clamps are placed on the pulmonary artery and ascending aorta, and incisions are made in each vessel **(A)**. The autogenous or synthetic graft is interposed between the aorta and pulmonary artery by two end-to-side anastomosis using simple continuous suture patterns with polypropylene or polytetrafluoroethylene suture. The vascular clamps on the pulmonary artery and aorta are released **(B)**.

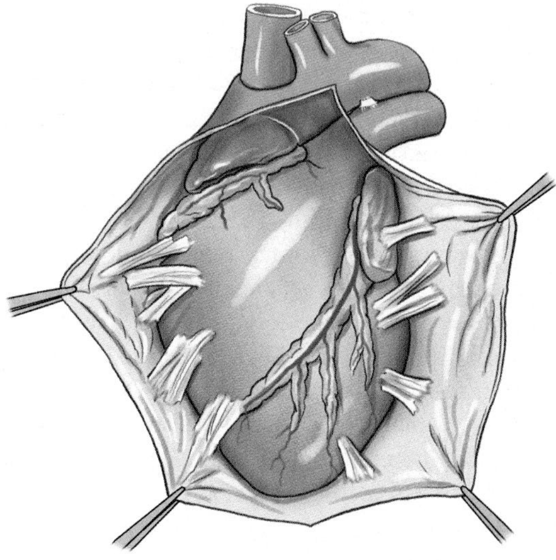

Figure 20-5. Pericardiectomy. Pericardiectomy may be performed via median sternotomy to provide access to both ventricles without extensive cardiac manipulation. In animals with constrictive pericarditis, adhesions may be present between the pericardium and epicardium.

CARDIAC SURGERY WITH INFLOW OCCLUSION

Inflow occlusion is a strategy for performing open cardiac surgery that entails brief cessation of venous flow to the heart and complete circulatory arrest. It is indicated for cardiac surgeries that require only a limited period when the heart is open. Its principal advantages are its simplicity, lack of need for specialized equipment, and minimal cardiopulmonary, metabolic, and hematologic derangements after surgery. The principal disadvantages of inflow occlusion are the limited time available to perform cardiac surgery, motion of the surgical field, and the unavailability a fall back or rescue strategy should something delay completion of surgery. As a result, cardiac surgery performed during inflow occlusion must be meticulously planned and flawlessly executed.

Circulatory arrest in a normothermic patient should be 2 minutes or less to minimize the risk of cerebral injury and ventricular fibrillation. Circulatory arrest time can be extended up to 4 minutes with mild whole body hypothermia (32° to 34° C) however the risk for ventricular fibrillation increases. Mild hypothermia is achieved readily in small animals by avoiding measures to keep the animal warm with or without surface cooling with ice packs depending on the size of the animal. Inflow occlusion requires careful and balanced anesthetic techniques that minimize inhalation anesthetic agents. Animals should be well ventilated, and acid-base balance should be optimized prior to inflow occlusion. Ventilation is discontinued during inflow occlusion and immediately resumed

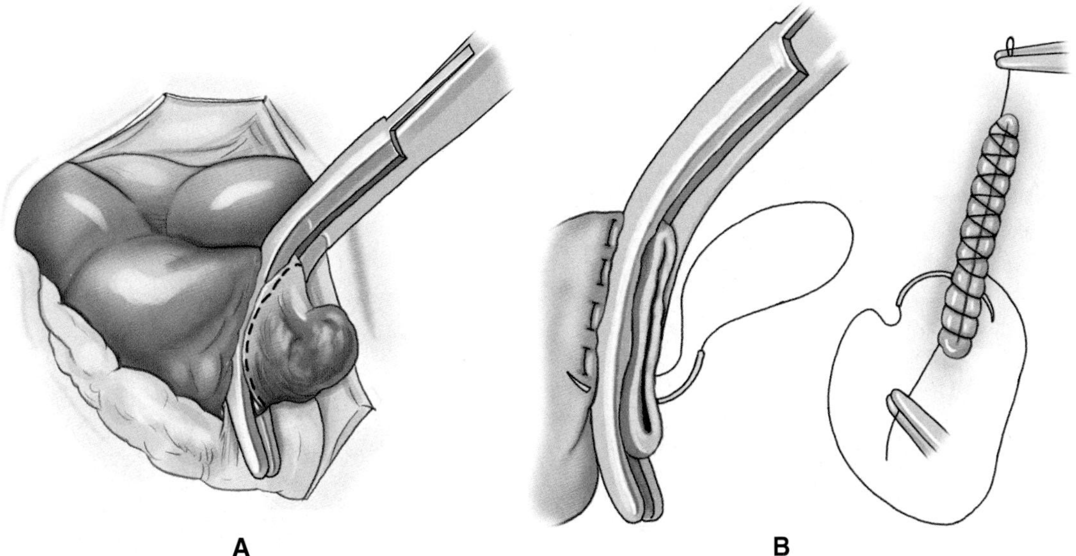

Figure 20-6. Atrial appendectomy. Excision of the atrial appendage is accomplished by placing a continuous mattress suture pattern across the base of the atrial appendage with the aid of a vascular clamp **(A)**. The atrial appendage is excised and the atriotomy incision is over sewn with a continuous suture pattern **(B)**.

upon release of inflow occlusion. Drugs and equipment for full cardiac resuscitation must be immediately available after inflow occlusion. Gentle cardiac massage may be necessary after inflow occlusion to reestablish cardiac function. Digital occlusion of the descending aorta during this period helps direct cardiac output to the heart and brain.

Inflow occlusion can be accomplished from a left or right fifth thoracotomy, or a median sternotomy depending on the cardiac surgery being performed. Direct access to the cranial and caudal vena cava and azygous vein for inflow occlusion is obtained readily from a right thoracotomy or median sternotomy. The vena cavae and azygous vein are accessed by dissecting through the mediastinum from a left thoracotomy. Tape tourniquets are passed around the vena cavae and azygous vein for inflow occlusion. The right phrenic nerve should be excluded from the tourniquets to avoid nerve injury.

Pulmonary Patch-Graft

Pulmonary patch-graft can be considered for dogs with severe PS who are exhibiting activity intolerance or are considered at risk for developing heart failure or sudden cardiac death. Because of the risk associated with this surgery, the threshold for performing this surgery should be fairly high. Pulmonic patch-graft generally is undertaken in dogs who have failed to be adequately palliated by less invasive balloon-dilation valvuloplasty. Dogs with severe PS characterized by valve dysplasia or dynamic outflow obstruction, or both, are more likely to require a patch-graft. Several surgical techniques for applying a patch-graft to the right ventricular outflow tract during brief inflow occlusion have been described. All techniques are plagued by relatively high operative risk and inconsistent results, even in the hands of experienced surgeons. (Alternatively, pulmonic patch-graft can be accomplished with the aid of CPB, which reduces operative risk and allows for more deliberate placement of the graft, thereby enhancing the effectiveness of the procedure.) A well-executed patch-graft generally results in more effective and more sustained pressure gradient reduction compared to valve dilation techniques. Occasionally dogs will develop right-sided congestive heart failure as a late sequela to pulmonary patch-graft despite good pressure gradient reduction. The cause of this late failure is not entirely clear and may be multifactorial. Contributing causes could include tricuspid regurgitation, right ventricular systolic dysfunction, and pulmonic insufficiency. Pulmonic insufficiency is an expected consequence of the patch-graft procedure and may be less tolerated than previously thought. English bulldogs and boxers with PS must be evaluated for the presence of an anomalous left coronary artery. If present, this anomaly precludes pulmonic patch-graft.

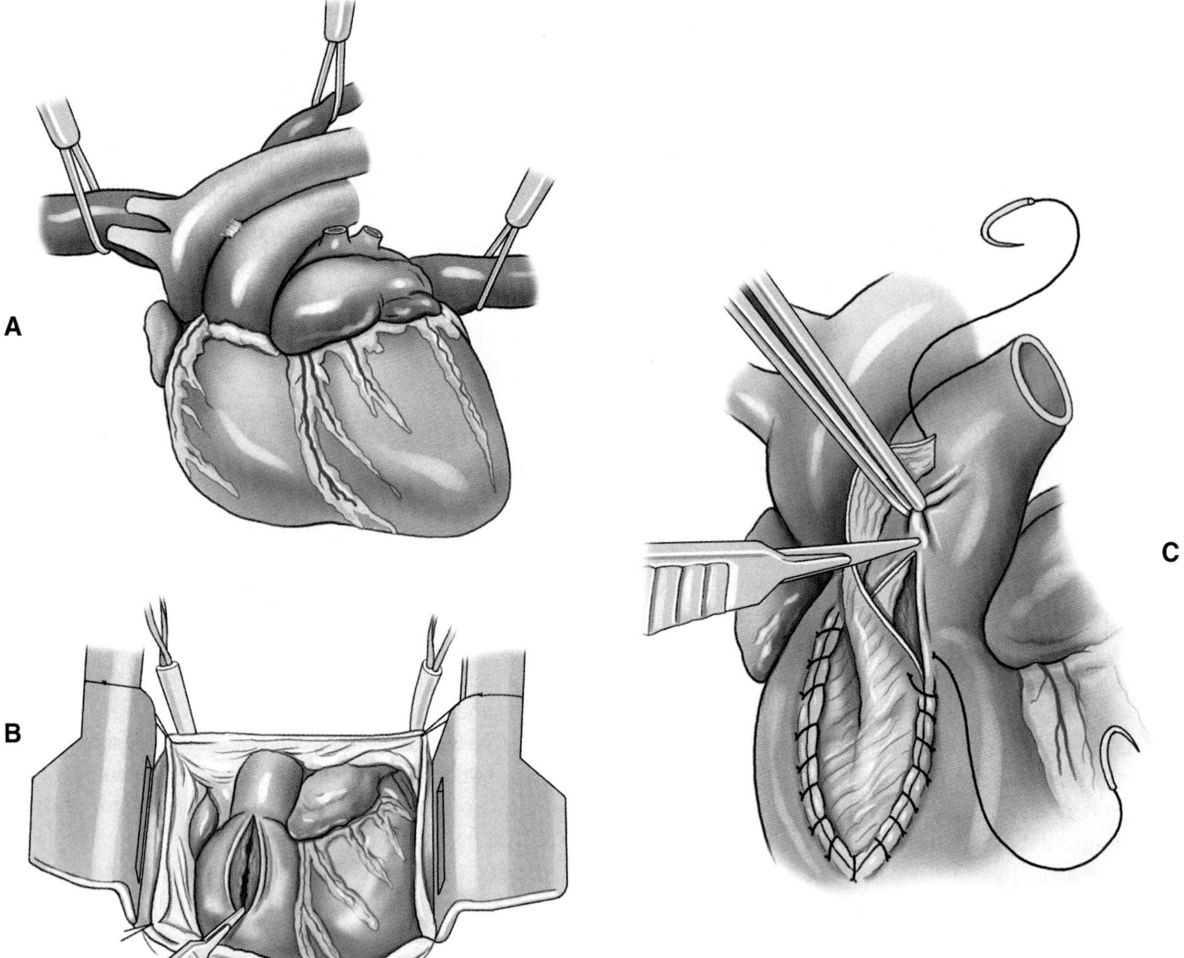

Figure 20-7. Pulmonary patch graft. Tape tourniquets are passed around the vena cavae and azygous vein for inflow occlusion **(A)**. Access to the azygous vein is obtained by dissecting dorsal to the descending aorta. A partial-thickness incision is made in the right ventricular outflow tract **(B)**. An oval expanded polytetrafluoroethylene (ePTFE) patch-graft is sutured to the ventriculotomy incision and the cranial aspect of the pulmonary artery **(C)**. After initiation of venous inflow occlusion, an incision is made in the pulmonary artery beneath the patch and extended full thickness across the pulmonic valve annulus and previously made partial-thickness incision in the right ventricular outflow tract. The unsutured portion of the patch graft is closed with a tangential vascular clamp to minimize circulatory arrest time. Inflow occlusion is discontinued and the heart is resuscitated as necessary. The unsutured portion of the patch graft is then closed and the vascular clamp removed.

Patch-graft correction of the PS by inflow occlusion is performed through a left fifth thoracotomy (Figure 20-7).

Cor Triatriatum Repair

Cor triatriatum is an uncommon congenital defect in companion animals that results from persistence of an embryonic membrane that divides the atrium into two chambers. The separation can occur in either the right (cor triatriatum dexter) or left atrium (cor triatriatum sinister).

Surgical correction of cor triatriatum dexter is by membranectomy through a right atriotomy during brief inflow occlusion. The surgery is performed via a right fifth thoracotomy. Tapes are placed around the cranial and caudal vena cavae and azygous vein for inflow occlusion. The pericardium is opened ventral to the phrenic nerve. The location of the membrane is often apparent by an indentation in the atrial wall. Stay sutures are placed in the lateral atrial wall to control the atriotomy incision during inflow occlusion. The atrium is opened transversely across the defect during inflow occlusion. The abnormal membrane is excised. A tangential vascular clamp is used to close the atriotomy as inflow occlusion is discontinued. Venous blood should flow from the atriotomy as the clamp is placed to remove air from the heart.

The atriotomy is closed with a continuous horizontal mattress pattern over sewn with a simple continuous pattern.

Successful surgical correction of cor triatriatum sinister with resolution of pulmonary edema by closed dilation of the atrial septum is reported in a cat.

Intracardiac Masses and Foreign Bodies

Intracardiac masses can include benign and malignant neoplasias, atrial or ventricular thrombus, and penetrating foreign bodies. These intracardiac masses and foreign bodies can, under certain circumstances, be removed from the heart with the aid of inflow occlusion. Most cardiac neoplasia in dogs is malignant and attempts at surgical excision of these tumors is rarely rewarding. Myxomas are an exception to this general rule. These benign pediculated cardiac tumors can become large enough to obstruct cardiac flow and are amendable to excision during inflow occlusion. Intracardiac thrombus should be considered for surgical removal when it is not associated with severe underlying cardiomyopathy. Penetrating foreign bodies such as pellets or bullets should be removed if they lodge within a cardiac chamber. Frequently these foreign bodies are surrounded by large amounts of hair that cause complications if not removed. Whenever possible intracardiac masses should be approached via an atriotomy rather than a ventriculotomy. An exception would be a large myxoma in the right ventricular outflow tract.

CARDIAC SURGERY WITH CARDIOPULMONARY BYPASS

CPB is a procedure that provides flow of oxygenated blood to the patient by diverting flow away from the heart and lungs through an extracorporeal circuit. CPB provides a motionless and bloodless operative field, and time to perform complex cardiac repairs. The disadvantages of CPB are its cost and considerable associated cardiopulmonary, metabolic, hematologic, and systemic inflammatory derangements.

CPB is performed by a team consisting of the surgeon, perfusionist, anesthesiologist, and their assistants. A principal role of the surgical team is to perform a series of cannulations to connect the animal to the CPB circuit. Prior to cannulation the patient is completely anticoagulated with sodium heparin (300 units/kg IV). Arterial cannulation for the return of oxygenated blood to the patient is accomplished via a single cannula placed in a femoral artery. Blood is diverted from the right heart to the CBP circuit by means of venous cannulae. Venous cannulation is accomplished by one of two strategies depending on the cardiac approach. Bicaval venous cannulation utilizes two angled cannulae, one in each vena cava, and is required whenever the cardiac approach is through the right atrium. Atriocaval cannulation utilizes a single two-stage cannula introduced into the right atrium and caudal vena cava via the right atrial appendage. Lastly, a cannula is placed in the ascending aorta for administration of cardioplegia solution and to vent the left heart during discontinuation of CBP. During the open cardiac repair, the aorta is cross-clamped and cardioplegia solution is administered to arrest and cool the myocardium.

Ventricular Septal Defect Repair

Definitive repair of VSD in dogs can be undertaken with the aid of CPB. Indications are the same as described for pulmonary artery banding. Definitive VSD repair, like PDA closure, is curative so long as it is undertaken before severe myocardial dysfunction or pulmonary hypertension develop.

Open repair of perimembranous VSD is accomplished through a right fifth thoracotomy. Venous cannulation is bicaval to allow complete isolation of the right atrium. The defect is approached through a right atriotomy. The septal leaflet of the tricuspid valve is retracted to expose the defect. The defect is closed with a Dacron or polytetrafluoroethylene (PTFE) patch secured with pledget-buttressed mattress sutures. Mattress sutures should be placed with partial thickness bites from the right side to avoid injury to atrioventricular conduction.

Atrial and Atrioventricular Septal Defect Repair

Various forms of atrial septal defect and atrioventricular septal defect have been described in small animals. As with VSD, surgical closure of atrial septal defect can be undertaken with the aid of CPB with curative intent. Indications for surgery include cardiomegaly, the size defect on echocardiography, pulmonary overcirculation on radiographs, hepatic venous congestion on ultrasound, and a Doppler-measured transatrial septal flow velocity > 0.45 m/sec. Surgical correction of atrial septal defect under CBP is similar to that of VSD and has been described.

Tetralogy of Fallot Repair

Definitive repair of tetralogy of Fallot under CPB can be undertaken in dogs with curative intent. Indications for surgery are the same as described previously for systemic–to–pulmonary artery shunt.

The repair is accomplished via a median sternotomy and involves closure of the VSD and correction of PS via a right ventriculotomy.

Double-Chambered Right Ventricle Repair

Double-chambered right ventricle (DCRV) is an uncommon congenital heart defect of dogs characterized by a fibromuscular diaphragm at the junction of the inflow and outflow portions of the right ventricle. The defect obstructs flow through the mid-portion of the ventricle and causes hypertrophy of the proximal portion of the right ventricle giving it a "double-chambered" appearance. The pathophysiology and natural history of DCRV are presumed to be similar to PS. Indications for surgery are essentially the same as for PS although dogs with DCRV may tolerate less of a pressure gradient compared to dogs with PS.

Surgical correction for DCRV is undertaken with CPB and has been described. The pulmonic valve is preserved. Surgical correction can be expected to improve exercise capacity and reduce the risk of developing heart failure.

Mitral Valve Replacement

MR is the most common cause of cardiac disability and death in dogs. Causes of MR include degenerative mitral valve disease, congenital mitral valve dysplasia, and functional MR secondary to dilated cardiomyopathy. Mitral valve replacement can be performed in dogs to correct severe MR secondary to acquired mitral valve disease or congenital mitral dysplasia. Indications for considering mitral valve replacement are diuretic-dependent congestive heart failure or severe left ventricular or atrial dilation (left ventricular diastolic volume index > 180 ml/m^2), or both. Relative contraindications for mitral valve surgery are very severe left ventricular dilation (> 300 ml/m^2), or severe secondary systolic dysfunction (> 90 ml/m^2). Atrial fibrillation is not a contraindication for surgery, but it does complicate the management after surgery. Serious systemic or noncardiac diseases are strong contraindications for the surgery.

Mitral valve replacement is currently the preferred surgical option for most dogs with severe MR and heart failure. The advantages of mitral valve replacement are perfect correction of MR and a lower operative death. Disadvantages of mitral valve replacement are the need for a prosthesis (expense, limitations on patient size) and for anticoagulation therapy after surgery. The estimated chance of surviving mitral valve replacement is 60% to 90% depending on the patient. Options for mitral valve replacement are mechanical valves or glutaraldehyde-fixed tissue valves. Glutaraldehyde-fixed tissue valves include porcine aortic valves and bovine pericardial valves. Mechanical valves have infinite durability, but require lifelong anticoagulation therapy to prevent valve thrombosis. Despite low operative mortality and excellent short-term results, valve replacement with mechanical prostheses is not recommended in dogs because of a high incidence of late-term thrombosis despite anticoagulation therapy. Tissue valves have a finite lifespan (about 7 to 15 years in human patients), but are less susceptible to thrombosis, and thrombosis is less catastrophic when it occurs. Other mechanisms of tissue valve prosthetic failure are structural tearing of leaflets, leaflet calcification, or an exuberant inflammatory response known as pannus. Anticoagulation therapy with warfarin is required for 3 months after valve replacement with a tissue valve. Atrial fibrillation occurs in about 20% of human patients undergoing mitral valve surgery and this sequela has been observed in dogs undergoing valve replacement as well. Adminstration of amiodarone 10 days before and after surgery decreases the risk of developing atrial fibrillation after mitral valve surgery and is currently recommended for dogs. Dogs that develop atrial fibrillation or flutter after valve replacement should undergo pharmacologic or electrical cardioversion if the arrhythmia persists for more than 6 weeks after surgery. Dogs with chronic atrial fibrillation at the time of mitral valve replacement should undergo prophylactic left atrial appendectomy to decrease the risk of atrial thrombosis after surgery. While the long-term durability of glutaraldehyde-fixed tissue valves in dogs has not been established, the short-term results have been encouraging. The procedure is limited to dogs with a lean body weight of about 10 kg by the size of the smallest available valve prosthesis (19 mm). Mitral valve replacement is considered a palliative therapy in that the consequences of a diseased native valve are substituted by the inherent management and potential complications of a valve prosthesis. That said, successful mitral valve replacement generally reverses congestive heart failure so long as secondary changes in the myocardium are not too advanced at the time of surgery. Mitral valve replacement can be expected to remain curative for heart failure so long as the prosthesis remains functional.

Surgical procedure for mitral valve replacement under CPB in the dog has been described.

Mitral Valve Repair

Mitral valve repair can be undertaken for dogs with moderate to severe MR caused by acquired degenerative mitral valve disease. Dogs with congenital mitral valve dysplasia are sometimes amendable to valve repair. The principle advantages of mitral valve repair are the avoidance of anticoagulation after surgery and the lack of a need for an expensive prosthesis. The disadvantages of mitral valve repair are a less predictable outcome compared to valve replacement and a higher operative death rate. The later is directly related to the difficulty in achieving perfect correction of MR when the valve is repaired. Mitral valve repair is best undertaken in dogs that have structural defects isolated to one valve leaflet before the onset of congestive heart failure. Most dogs are beyond mitral valve repair by the time they are in severe heart failure. Because of the inherent difficulty of mitral repair, the estimated chance of success is 60% to 75% depending on patient size, age, duration of heart failure, severity of left ventricular dilation, and degree of secondary systolic dysfunction.

Mitral valve repair employs a variety of surgical techniques to address the fundamental causes of MR. Surgical techniques for mitral valve repair in the dog have been described.

Tricuspid Valve Replacement

Congenital tricuspid dysplasia is a malformation of the tricuspid valve that occurs in several large breeds of dog including Labrador retrievers, Golden retrievers, and German shepherds. Tricuspid regurgitation is the most common hemodynamic manifestation, although tricuspid stenosis is possible. Tricuspid valve replacement can be considered for dogs with severe tricuspid regurgitation due to congenital tricuspid dysplasia. Tricuspid valve replacement must be undertaken sooner during the course of disease than mitral valve replacement. General indications for tricuspid valve replacement are severe tricuspid regurgitation resulting in severe or progressive cardiomegaly or hepatic venous enlargement, or both. Dogs with medically refractory congestive heart failure should not undergo tricuspid valve replacement. Atrial fibrillation is a complicating factor, but not an contraindication for surgery. The estimated chance of surviving surgery is 70% to 90% depending on the case. As with mitral valve replacement, glutaraldehyde-fixed tissue valves are currently recommended over mechanical valves. Three months of anticoagulation therapy is required after tricuspid valve replacement with a tissue valve. Expected outcome is similar to dogs undergoing mitral valve replacement. Dramatic reductions in heart size and resolution of heart failure can be expected so long as the valve prosthesis remains functional.

Tricuspid valve replacement is performed via a right fifth thoracotomy. Bicaval venous cannulation is utilized to isolate the right atrium. Approach to the tricuspid valve is through the right atrium. Surgical technique for tricuspid valve replacement is similar to mitral valve replacement.

SUGGESTED READINGS

Bureau S, Monnet E, Orton EC: Evaluation of survival rate and prognostic indicators for surgical treatment of left-to-right patent ductus arteriosus in dogs: 52 cases (1995-2003), J Am Vet Med Assoc 227:1794, 2005.

Griffiths LG, Boon J, Orton EC: Evaluation of techniques and outcomes of mitral valve repair in dogs, J Am Vet Med Assoc 224:1941-1945, 2004.

Kienle RD, Thomas WP, Pion DP: The natural history of canine congenital subaortic stenosis, J Vet Intern Med 8:423,1994.

Linn KA, Orton EC: Closed transventricular valve dilation of subvalvular aortic stenosis in dogs, Vet Surg 21:441, 1992.

Martin J, Orton EC, Boon J, et al: Surgical correction of double-chambered right ventricle in dogs, J Am Vet Med Assoc 220:770-774, 2002.

Meurs KM, Lehmkuhl LB, Bonagura JD: Survival times in dogs with severe subvalvular aortic stenosis treated with balloon valvuloplasty or atenolol, J Am Vet Med Assoc 227:420, 2005.

Monnet E, Orton EC, Gaynor J, et al: Partial atrioventricular septal defect: diagnosis and surgical repair in two dogs, J Am Vet Med Assoc 211:569-572, 1997.

Orton EC, Hackett TA, Mama K, Boon JA: Technique and outcome of mitral valve replacement in dogs, J Am Vet Med Assoc 226:1508-1511, 2005.

Orton EC, Mama K, Hellyer P, Hackett TB: Open surgical repair of tetralogy of Fallot in two dogs, J Am Vet Med Assoc 219:1089-1093, 2001.

Orton EC, Herndon GD, Boon J, et al: Intermediate-term outcome in dogs with subvalvular aortic stenosis: influence of open surgical correction, J Am Vet Med Assoc 216:364, 2000.

Wander KW, Monnet E, Orton EC: Surgical correction of cor triatriatum sinister in a kitten, J Am Anim Hosp Assoc 34:383, 1998.

CHAPTER 21

Pacemaker Therapy

Janice McIntosh Bright

"It struck me how easily excitable the myocardium is. You just touch it and it gives you a run of extra beats—so why should the heart that is so sensitive...die because there's nothing there to stimulate the chest?"

PAUL M. ZOLL, INVENTOR OF THE FIRST CLINICALLY SUCCESSFUL EXTERNAL PACEMAKER (JEFFREY K: PACE 22:1713;1999)

INTRODUCTION

Pacemaker therapy has become a common method of treating symptomatic bradycardia in dogs and cats. Pharmacologic therapy may provide temporary chronotropic support for patients with bradycardia, but successful long-term management usually requires implantation of a permanent pacemaker. The ultimate objective of cardiac pacing is to normalize cardiac function by providing optimal heart rate and rhythm chronically.

INDICATIONS FOR PACING

- Permanent pacemaker implantation is indicated for treatment of patients with chronic symptomatic bradyarrhythmias. In dogs the most frequent clinical manifestations of bradycardia are syncope, collapse, exercise intolerance, and/or lethargy. Less commonly, bradyarrhythmia results in congestive heart failure or seizures. In cats the most frequent complaint associated with bradycardia is syncope.
- The most common bradyarrhythmia necessitating pacemaker therapy in dogs and cats is advanced (high-grade second- or third-degree) atrioventricular (AV) block. Antibradycardia pacing is also indicated in dogs with sinus node dysfunction (sick sinus syndrome) and permanent atrial standstill. Less often permanent pacing is used to prevent vasovagal syncope.
- Whereas most dogs needing pacemaker therapy have little to no underlying structural heart disease, many cats have AV conduction block associated with underlying myocardial disease.

PRE-IMPLANTATION EVALUATION

- A standard electrocardiogram (ECG) should be obtained for definitive diagnosis of the arrhythmia. Occasionally, serial ECGs are needed to confirm an intermittent bradycardia. If it is unclear whether a patient's clinical signs are due to bradyarrhythmia, correlation of the clinical signs with arrhythmia should be obtained using some form of ambulatory ECG monitoring (Holter monitoring or event recording). Ambulatory ECG monitoring allows the ECG to be recorded over a longer period of time, either continuously for 24 to 48 hours (Holter monitoring) or intermittently during weeks to months (event recording).
- After confirming that an indication for permanent cardiac pacing exists, the most appropriate pacing system and pacing mode for the patient should be determined. Factors to be considered for this determination include: (1) specific underlying rhythm disturbance, (2) overall physical condition, (3) nature of any associated medical problems, and (4) exercise requirements of the patient.

- Therefore, all patients needing implantation of a permanent pacemaker should receive a thorough medical and cardiovascular evaluation prior to implantation to identify presence and severity of structural heart diseases or noncardiac diseases. Certain co-existing conditions may require additional medical treatment. Furthermore, these conditions often affect the type and programming of the pacing system used.

COMPONENTS AND TYPES OF PACING SYSTEMS

- A permanent artificial cardiac pacing system consists of a pulse generator (pacemaker) and a pacing lead. The pulse generator contains electronic circuitry and a lithium-iodide power cell (battery) sealed within a metal case with a connector block into which the lead is inserted. The pacing lead consists of an insulated wire or set of wires to conduct electrical impulses from the generator to the myocardium, but the lead also enables the generator to detect or sense native (endogenous) cardiac electrical activity.
- Modern cardiac pacemakers have sophisticated electronic circuitry capable of discharging pacing impulses of varying duration and voltage, sensing intracardiac signals, filtering signals, providing rate response functions, and storing rhythm data. Data retrieval and generator programming are done via telemetry using a pacemaker programmer. The programmer is also used to display real-time ECG and intracardiac electrograms and to test battery life, lead impedance, retrograde ventriculoatrial conduction, and pacing thresholds.
- The heart can be paced by an epicardial lead placed surgically (or thoracoscopically) or by a permanent endocardial pacing lead placed transvenously. Permanent transvenous pacing has largely replaced epicardial pacing because of its ease and safety; however, epicardial leads remain available and may be preferred when venous access is limited or when there is an associated condition that would increase likelihood of bacteremia or embolism with a permanent transvenous lead (e.g., a focus of sepsis or a hypercoaguable state). Epicardial leads are often used in feline patients.
- Permanent transvenous pacing leads use either active or passive fixation for attachment of the lead tip to the endomyocardium. A passive fixation transvenous lead has a "collar" of tines encircling the distal tip which anchor the lead by becoming enmeshed in the right ventricular trabeculae (Figure 21-1). An active fixation lead has a small metal helix that exits the tip of the lead to penetrate the endomyocardium (see Figure 21-1). Although the type of fixation of a transvenous lead does not appear to affect the incidence of lead dislodgement, it is wise to avoid use of passive fixation in animals with significant right ventricular dilation.

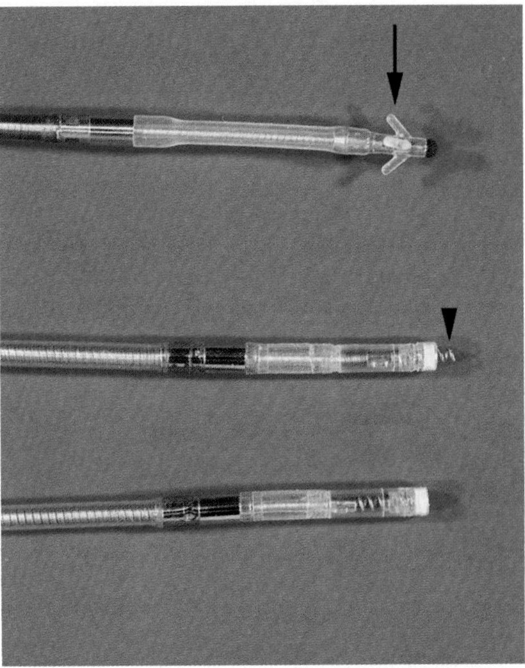

Figure 21-1. The distal ends of several transvenous (endocardial) pacing leads are shown. The lead at the top is a passive fixation lead. Note the collar of tines (arrow) which become trapped within trabeculae to anchor the tip of the lead to the right ventricular endocardium. At the bottom are two active fixation leads, one showing the helix retracted into the lead for placement and the other showing the helix extruded for as it would be for attachment into the endomyocardium (arrowhead).

- Another consideration for selection of the pacing system is whether a unipolar or bipolar system is desired. A unipolar pacing system uses the lead tip as the cathode (negative pole) of the electrical circuit and the metal case of the pulse generator as the anode (positive pole). The impulse travels from generator to myocardium via the lead and returns to the generator via the soft tissues. A major disadvantage of unipolar pacing is the proximity of the electrical circuit to skeletal muscle which may result in skeletal muscle twitching. Advantages of unipolar pacing include smaller diameter of the pacing lead, a single attachment site of the lead to the epicardium when epicardial pacing is used, and superior sensing of endogenous cardiac potentials. Bipolar pacing systems have two closely spaced electrodes located distally on a transvenous lead or closely adjacent at two ends of an epicardial lead (Figure 21-2). One electrode

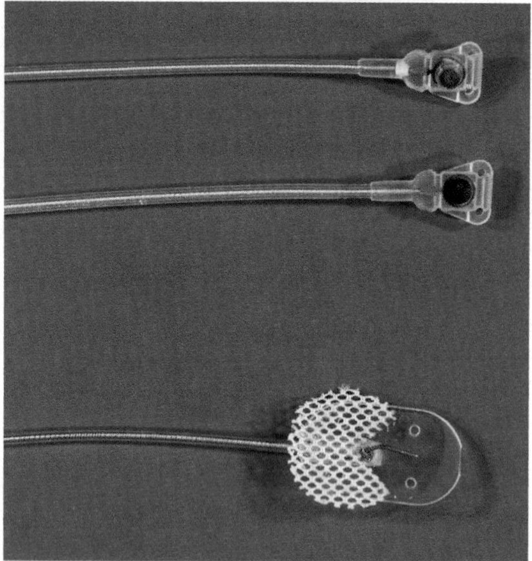

Figure 21-2. Shown are distal tips of two epicardial pacing leads. The lead at the bottom of the photo is a unipolar lead with a single electrode (cathode) which has an epicardial stab-in fixation mechanism. The lead at the top of the photo is a bipolar lead with two suture-on electrodes (cathode and anode).

(usually the distal electrode on a transvenous bipolar lead) is the cathode, and the other is the anode. Electrical impulses travel to the cathode from the pulse generator and return to the anode to complete the circuit. In the majority of cases a bipolar pacing system is preferred because there is less potential for electromagnetic interference (EMI) with bipolar pacing and because of absence of skeletal muscle stimulation.

- Although lead length should be given consideration prior to pacemaker implantation, length is often determined by availability. Most leads are longer than necessary, and excess length can be accommodated within the generator pocket; however, in large or giant breed dogs, adequate lead length may become an important factor.

KEY POINT

When selecting a permanent pacing lead, it is imperative that the lead be compatible with the pacing site selected (epicardial vs. endocardial, atrial vs. ventricular), that the lead and generator be of compatible size (typically IS-1), that the polarity of the lead matches polarity of the generator, and that the lead is of sufficient length.

Pacing with Chronotropic Competence (Rate Responsiveness)

- Initially, permanent cardiac pacing systems used in people and in dogs had a single lead that paced the ventricles at a constant rate. Later, rate responsive pacing generators became available, which allowed the paced rate to vary depending on the activity of the patient.
- Rate response is achieved through use of sensors in the pacemaker, often motion sensors or minute ventilation sensors, which adjust the paced rate between programmed upper and lower limits to match changing metabolic requirements. Thus, rate responsive pacing better mimics the normal physiologic response of the heart to exercise.

Single- vs. Dual-Chamber Pacing

- The original goal of permanent cardiac pacing was to alleviate hemodynamic instability resulting from an abnormally low ventricular rate, and this remains the primary goal of pacemaker therapy in most veterinary patients. However, it is now recognized that cardiac output is dependent, not solely on ventricular rate, but also on physiologic heart rate variation, synchrony between atrial and ventricular contraction, and the ventricular activation sequence. Modern cardiac pacing has evolved in people from single-chamber ventricular pacing to dual-chamber (atrial and ventricular sensing and pacing) primarily to provide pacing with AV synchrony.
- AV synchrony is attained either by pacing the atrium or by sensing intrinsic atrial activity and tracking this activity. Either a paced atrial depolarization or an endogenous atrial depolarization triggers an AV delay, programmable in length, after which the ventricle is paced (if intrinsic ventricular activity is not sensed). Atrial synchronous pacing provides not only AV synchrony but also physiologic heart rate variation (see Pacing Modes).
- Although AV synchrony may not be clinically important for many dogs and cats needing chronotropic support, pacing that provides AV synchrony will provide higher systemic pressure and lower ventricular filling pressures than single-chamber ventricular pacing. Therefore, dual-chamber pacing to provide AV synchrony is likely to be important in animals with underlying structural heart disease or in working animals such as military dogs and agility dogs.

Table 21-1 Pacemaker Nomenclature for Antibradycardia Pacing

Position	I	II	III	IV	V
	Chamber(s) paced	Chamber(s) sensed	Response to sensing	Rate modulation	Multisite pacing
	O = None	O = None	O = None	O = None	O = None
	A = Atrium	A = Atrium	T = Triggered	R = Rate responsive	A = Atrium
	V = Ventricle	V = Ventricle	I = Inhibited		V = Ventricle
	D = Dual (A + V)	D = Dual (A + V)	D = Dual (T + I)		D = Dual (A + V)

Manufacturers' designation only: *S* = Single (A or V).
From Bernstein AD et al: North American Society of Pacing and Electrophysiology/British Pacing and Electrophysiology Group: The revised NASPE/BPEG generic code for antibradycardia, adaptive-rate, and multisite pacing, Pacing Clin Electrophysiol 25: 260-264, 2002.

- Dual-chamber pacing is becoming increasingly used in veterinary medicine as a means of providing both heart rate response and AV synchrony. Disadvantages of dual-chamber pacing include its more complex programming, increased expense (when two leads are used), and the technical challenge of placing atrial sensing/pacing leads in small patients.
- Normalization of the left ventricular activation sequence may be achieved by means of site-specific pacing within the right atrium and right ventricle.

Pacemaker Nomenclature

- Pacing nomenclature was established in 1974 and updated in 2002 for use in human medicine. This nomenclature also applies to veterinary pacemaker therapy, and awareness of the nomenclature is important for understanding cardiac pacing. Pacing nomenclature classifies pacing based on the site and mode of both pacing and sensing using a series of three to five letters (Table 21-1).
- The first letter (position I) indicates the cardiac chamber or chambers in which pacing occurs: A = atrium, V = ventricle, D = dual chamber (both A and V), and O = none.
- The second letter (position II) indicates the chamber or chambers in which sensing of electrical activity occurs. The letters are the same as those for the first position. (Some pacemaker manufacturers use the letter *S* in both the first and the second positions to indicate that a generator is capable of pacing or sensing only a single cardiac chamber.)
- The third letter (position III) refers to the mode of response to sensed electrical activity. In this position the letter *I* indicates that a sensed electrical event inhibits the output pulse and causes the generator to recycle for one or more timing cycles. The letter *T* indicates that an output pulse is triggered in response to a sensed electrical event. A letter *D* in this position indicates that both *I* and *T* responses can occur, and this designation is limited to dual-chamber systems.
- The fourth letter (position IV) of the pacemaker nomenclature code refers to presence or absence of rate modulation. A letter *R* in this position designates that the generator has one or more sensors (such as a motion sensor or a minute ventilation sensor) to adjust the paced heart rate independently of intrinsic cardiac activity.
- The fifth letter (position V) of the code is used to indicate whether multisite pacing is present in: A = one or both atria, V = one or both ventricles, D = any combination of the atria and ventricles, or O = none of the cardiac chambers. For example, a patient with a dual-chamber rate-responsive pacemaker with biventricular stimulation would be designated having a DDDRV pacing system. Currently, the fifth letter is often omitted when describing pacing of veterinary patients because multisite pacing within the atria and ventricles is rarely done.

Pacing Modes

- At the present time, the most commonly used pacing mode in veterinary patients and in human patients worldwide is single-chamber, ventricular inhibited synchronous pacing either with (VVIR) or without (VVI) rate response. In this mode the artificial pacing stimulus is delivered to the

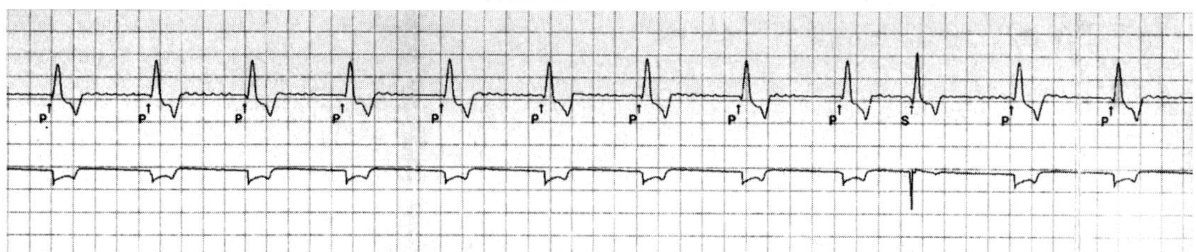

Figure 21-3. This figure shows a lead II ECG rhythm strip (top) and a simultaneous intracardiac electrogram (bottom) recorded from the pacing lead of a canine patient with complete AV block and a bipolar VVIR pacemaker. Small arrows labeled P indicate pacing stimuli, and each small pacing stimulus artifact results in a paced QRS complex. The tenth QRS complex is an endogenous ventricular depolarization that is sensed by the generator resulting in brief interruption of the paced rhythm. The sensed intrinsic activity resets the timing of the next paced beat (25 mm/s).

ventricle (the right ventricle if transvenous) and ventricular sensing allows sensed endogenous ventricular events to inhibit the pacemaker output. Inhibition of the output in response to endogenous ventricular activity is an important feature that prevents competitive rhythms and potentially fatal consequences of an electrical stimulus delivered during the vulnerable period of the cardiac cycle. A VVI (or VVIR) pacemaker is refractory for a specified, programmable interval after either a paced or sensed ventricular depolarization. This interval is the ventricular refractory period, and ventricular events occurring within the ventricular refractory period will not reset the ventricular timing. However, an endogenous ventricular depolarization occurring after the ventricular refractory period will be sensed, the generator output inhibited, and the timing cycle restarted from the intrinsic QRS complex. Thus, the cardiac rhythm may be irregular on auscultation in patients with VVI or VVIR pacing and RR intervals may vary on the ECG if there is intrinsic ventricular activity (Figure 21-3).

- Single-chamber, atrial inhibited pacing (AAI or AAIR) is identical to VVI pacing with the obvious difference that pacing and sensing occur from the atrium and pacemaker output is inhibited by sensed atrial events. Although this pacing mode is appropriate for patients with sinus node dysfunction (sick sinus syndrome) and normal AV conduction, its obvious disadvantage is lack of ventricular depolarization should AV block occur. Because most dogs with sinus node dysfunction have coexisting dysfunction of the AV node and/or bundle branches, AAI pacing is not widely used.
- Atrial synchronous pacing (VDD) is becoming increasingly popular for use in dogs with AV block. With this mode pacing occurs only in the ventricle, sensing occurs in both chambers, and ventricular output is inhibited by intrinsic ventricular activity but stimulated by ventricular tracking of sensed atrial activity. In other words, there is ventricular pacing in response to endogenous P waves. A single pacing lead with a pair of sensing electrodes located on the intraatrial portion of the lead is typically used (Figure 21-4). However, VDD pacing can also be accomplished using separate atrial and ventricular leads. In the VDD pacing mode sensed atrial events initiate an AV delay. If an endogenous ventricular depolarization occurs during the AV delay, ventricular stimulation is inhibited, and the timing cycle is reset. If no endogenous ventricular activity occurs, then a paced ventricular beat occurs at the end of the AV delay resetting the timing cycle. If no atrial event occurs, the pacemaker escapes with a paced ventricular depolarization at the lower rate. In other words, with VDD pacing the patient will be paced VVI in absence of sensed atrial activity. VDD pacing is appropriate only for animals

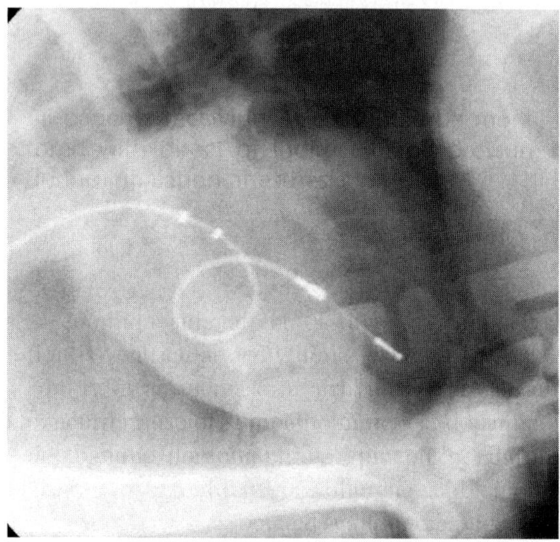

Figure 21-4. Lateral radiograph obtained from a canine with a transvenous VDD pacing system. The ventricular electrodes are within the right ventricle with the cathode at the ventricular apex. The atrial sensing electrodes, located more proximally on the lead, are within the right atrium.

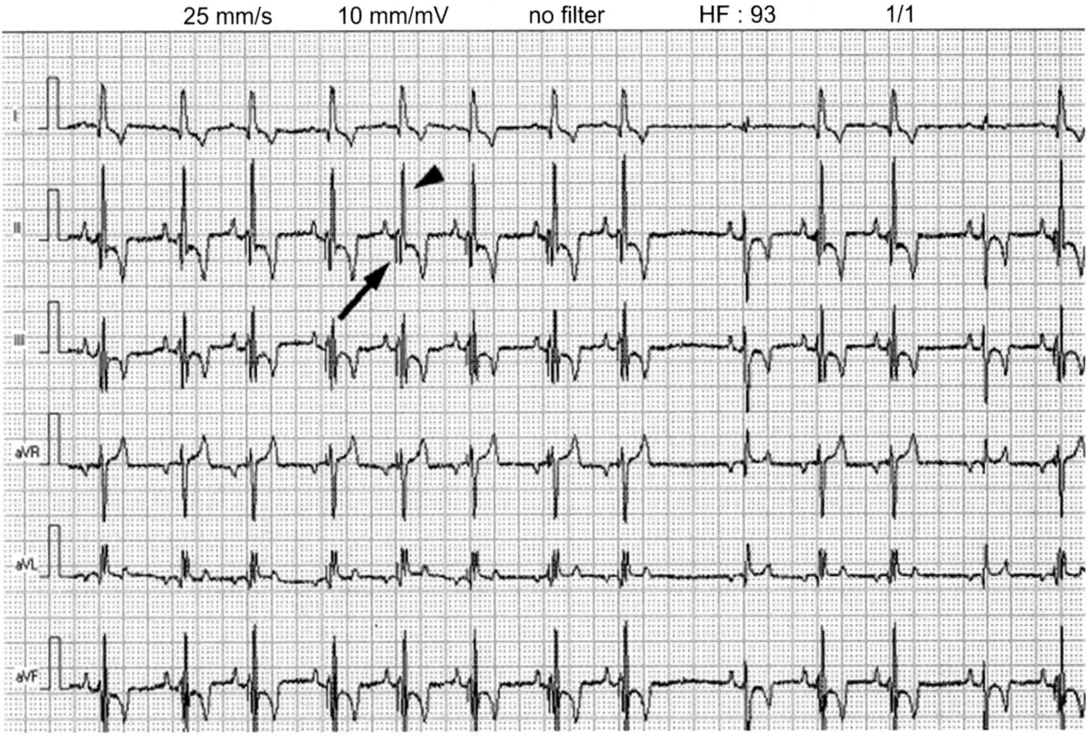

Figure 21-5. This six-lead II ECG was recorded from a dog with a transvenous VDD pacing system implanted because of high-grade second-degree AV block. The dog has normal sinus node function resulting in normal-appearing P waves with sinus-arrhythmia. The P waves are sensed by the generator and after a delay of 120 ms, there are pacing stimulus artifacts (arrow) followed immediately by paced QRS complexes, which have left bundle branch block morphology (arrowhead). The ninth and twelfth complexes are endogenous QRS complexes resulting from conduction of the P waves through the AV node. These QRS complexes have right bundle branch block morphology (25 mm/s).

with AV block and normal sinus node function. If a single VDD pacing lead is to be used, the patient must be large enough for the atrial sensing electrodes (located 11.5, 13.5, or 15.5 cm from the ventricular electrodes) to be placed in a stable position within or closely adjacent to the right atrium. Figure 21-5 shows an ECG recorded from a dog with a VDD pacing system.

- Dual-chamber pacing and sensing with inhibition and tracking (DDD) is a common mode of antibradycardia pacing in man. The primary difference between this mode and VDD mode is that in DDD mode when there is absence of sensed intrinsic atrial activity, the atrium is paced and the atrial paced beat is tracked by ventricular pacing. Thus, with exception of ectopic endogenous ventricular depolarizations AV synchrony is continuously present. This mode of pacing is important in human patients who frequently have both sinus node dysfunction and AV block; however, most dogs with complete AV block have a normal sinus node making atrial pacing unnecessary. Furthermore, DDD pacing alone does not provide rate response during AV sequential pacing (DDDR is required).

PACEMAKER IMPLANTATION

- The rate of complications associated with pacemaker implantation is inversely related to the experience of the implanter. Therefore, only highly experienced, well qualified veterinarians should attempt pacemaker implantation.
- Whereas transvenous pacemaker implantation is generally done with sedation and local anesthesia in human patients, general anesthesia is used for nearly all veterinary patients to maintain aseptic technique during the implantation.
- Application of a temporary external pacing system prior to induction of anesthesia is strongly recommended because a rapid and profound decrease in heart rate may occur unpredictably at any time after induction of anesthesia.
- Regardless of the type of pacing lead used, specific measurements of lead impedance, amplitude and slew rate of intrinsic cardiac electrical events (measured through the lead), and pacing threshold(s) should be obtained using a pacemaker system analyzer at the time of implantation. These measurements assure optimal placement of the lead for pacing and sensing.

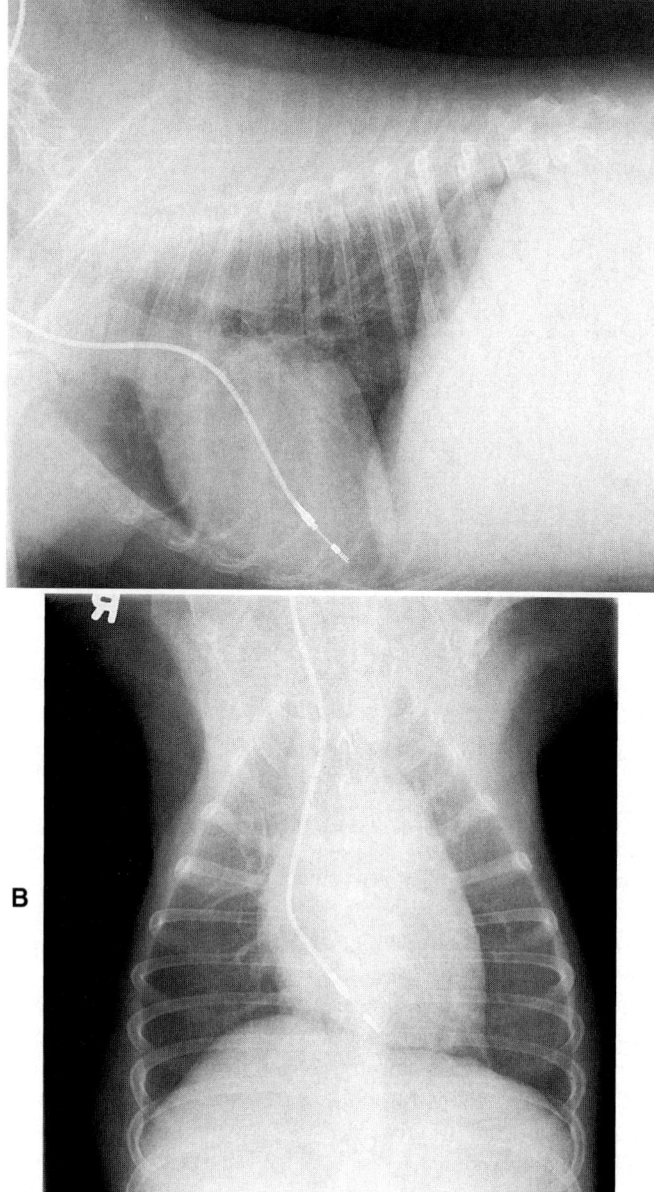

Figure 21-6. Lateral **(A)** and ventrodorsal **(B)** thoracic radiographs showing typical placement of a transvenous pacing lead in a dog. The lead tip is at the right ventricular apex.

- Radiographs should be obtained immediately after implantation to document final lead position(s).
- Permanent transvenous pacing leads are typically inserted into the right external jugular vein and advanced fluoroscopically into the ventricle leaving the lead tip in the most apical portion of the right ventricle angled toward the diaphragm (Figure 21-6). The rare exception would be site specific placement of a transvenous ventricular lead in the right ventricular outflow tract done in attempt to reduce mitral regurgitation and remodeling in patients with valvular disease or dilated cardiomyopathy.
- Right jugular venipuncture should not be attempted after implantation, and a halter or gentle leader should be used instead of a neck lead to avoid damaging transvenous pacing wires.
- When a transvenous pacing system is used, the generator is usually placed into a subcutaneous pocket made on the dorsolateral region of the neck. If a unipolar system has been used, skeletal muscle twitching may occur with each paced beat in the area of the generator pocket.
- Perioperative antibiotics are generally administered intravenously at the time of implantation and 8 hours following implantation.

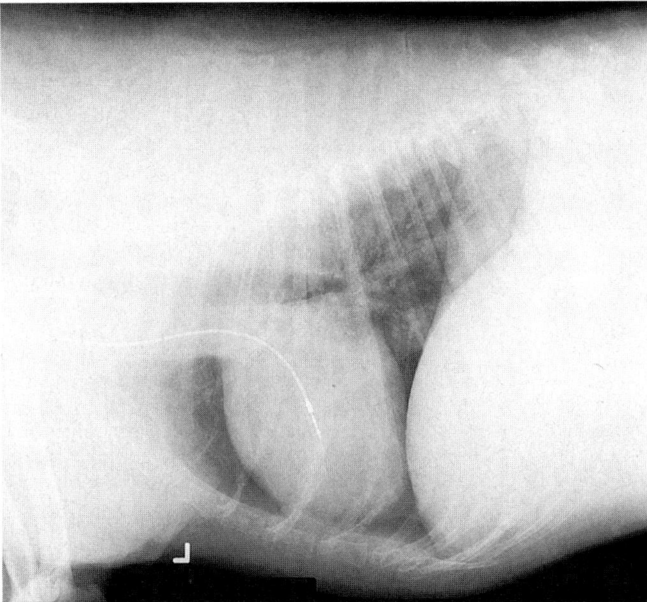

Figure 21-7. Lateral thoracic radiograph obtained from the same dog as in Figure 21-6 after dislodgement of the lead. Note that the distal tip of the lead is now located at the level of the tricuspid valve rather than at the apex. This radiograph was taken after reoccurrence of bradycardia caused by lack of contact between the cathode and the myocardium.

PACEMAKER COMPLICATIONS

- Permanent artificial cardiac pacing, whether endocardial or epicardial, is relatively safe but not completely innocuous. A 5-year retrospective study of 154 dogs receiving permanent cardiac pacemakers showed that 84 dogs (55%) had complications. Furthermore, the complications were life threatening in 51 dogs (33%). There was no significant difference in the rate of major complications between epicardial and endocardial pacing systems.
- The most frequent major complication in dogs with artificial cardiac pacemakers is lead malfunction due to lead dislodgement. Lead dislodgement occurs more often with transvenous leads than with epicardial leads, but is equally likely to occur with either active or passive fixation leads. Surprisingly, this complication does not appear to be affected by the experience of the implanter, and may be either acute or chronic (hours to months after implantation). Lead dislodgement may be radiographically apparent (macrodislogement) or not radiographically apparent (microdislodgement), and radiographs showing lead position should be compared to radiographs taken at the time of implantation (Figures 21-6 and 21-7). Lead dislodgement often necessitates a second procedure to reposition the lead. Occasionally, the generator can be programmed to higher output to reestablish effective pacing without repositioning of the lead.
- Another potential cause of lead malfunction is intermittent or complete failure of pacing due to a loose connection at the interface of the lead and the connector block of the generator. This problem is usually the result of inadequate securing of the lead at the time of implantation. When connection of the lead to the generator is loose, manipulation of the generator or generator pocket may induce the pacing malfunction. The poor connection may also be apparent radiographically (Figure 21-8). A second operative procedure to secure the lead pin into the generator connector block is needed to restore reliable pacemaker function.
- Lead fracture or lead insulation breaks are causes of pacemaker malfunction occasionally encountered in veterinary patients. Fractures or insulation breaks may cause impaired sensing, impaired pacing, or both. These complications may result from biting injuries, venipuncture, excessive repetitive lead motion, or traction with a neck leash. Lead fracture or lead insulation breaks are often identified by unacceptably high or low lead impedance measurements. Lead fractures may also be identified radiographically (Figure 21-9).
- Exit block refers to failure of the pacing stimulus to depolarize the myocardium (failure to capture), a complication most often due to development of fibrous tissue at the electrode cardiac interface (Figure 21-10). Fibrosis is frequently secondary to inflammation incited at the time of implantation, and use of leads with steroid eluting tips may minimize

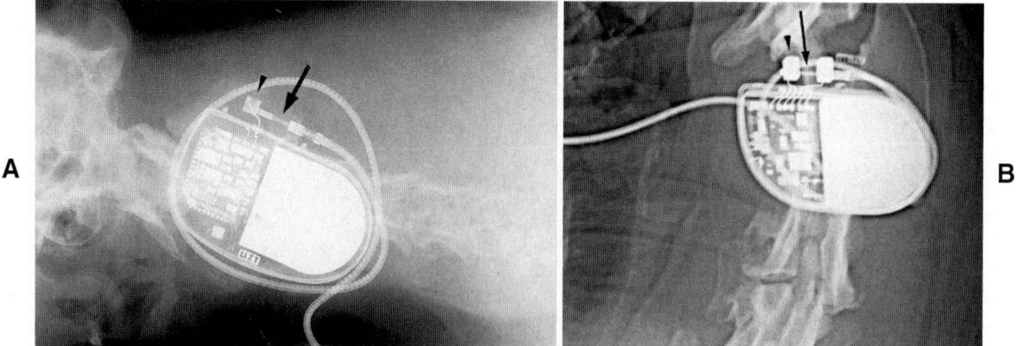

Figure 21-8. **A,** This radiograph was obtained from a dog with intermittent failure to pace caused by a loose connection at the interface of the unipolar lead and the connector block. The loose connection occurred because the lead pin was not adequately secured at the time of pacemaker implantation. Note that the connector pin (arrow) has withdrawn from the block (arrowhead) and is not passing all of the way through the block screw. **B,** For comparison, this radiograph shows an appropriately engaged connector pin from a patient with a bipolar pacing lead. The connector pin (arrow) is visible beyond the connection block screw (arrowhead).

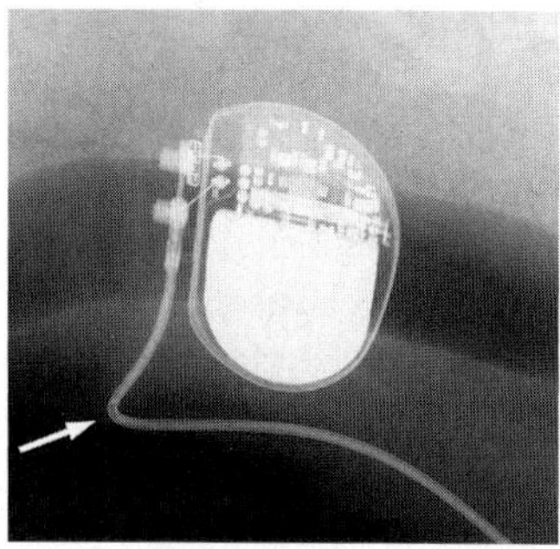

Figure 21-9. This radiograph was taken from a dog that experienced failure of a pacemaker system because of lead fracture. The fracture is visible at the tip of the arrow.

or prevent this problem. However, exit block may also occur from progression of underlying myocardial disease.

- Perforation of the right ventricular wall by a transvenous pacing lead is a rare complication that may occur at implantation or chronically. This complication may result in acute, fatal hemorrhage or loss of effective cardiac pacing caused by failure to capture.
- Pacemaker infections may involve the pocket, lead, or both and may cause fatal septicemia or endocarditis. In dogs most pacemaker infections occur within 3 months following implantation. With very few exceptions treatment of an infected pacemaker or lead requires removal and replacement of the entire system.
- Other potentially lethal pacemaker complications reported in dogs and cats include generator failure; significant arrhythmias such as ventricular asystole, atrial fibrillation, ventricular tachycardia and ventricular fibrillation; infection; development of congestive heart failure; and chylothorax. Extensive thrombosis and thromboembolism may also occur.
- Minor complications associated with pacemaker implantation include formation of hematomas and seromas at the generator or cervical lead site, skeletal muscle twitching at the generator site, transient or minor arrhythmias, and suture line dehiscence. To avoid contamination or lead damage, needle aspiration or other forms of mechanical drainage of seromas or hematomas should be avoided; conservative management with pressure, warm compresses, and prophylactic antibiotics are the recommended management.
- EMI is a pacemaker complication that occurs when any signal, biologic or nonbiologic, originating outside of the heart is detected by the sensing circuitry of the pacemaker. EMI can result in inappropriate inhibition of pacing, asynchronous pacing, damage to the generator or myocardium, or reprogramming of the pacing parameters. Sources of EMI include electrocautery, electrical cardioversion or defibrillation, magnetic resonance imaging, and electroshock therapy.

PACEMAKER PROGRAMMING AND FOLLOW-UP

- State of the art pacemakers have programmable parameters that can be evaluated and altered to optimize and monitor function of the pacing system. Although there is some variation between generators, typical data obtained during a pacemaker programming and evaluating session would include output current, output voltage, lead impedance, battery status, sensitivity (sensing parameters), event records, ECG monitoring, pacing histogram, and pacing thresholds. A real time intracardiac electrogram can be displayed with a simultaneous

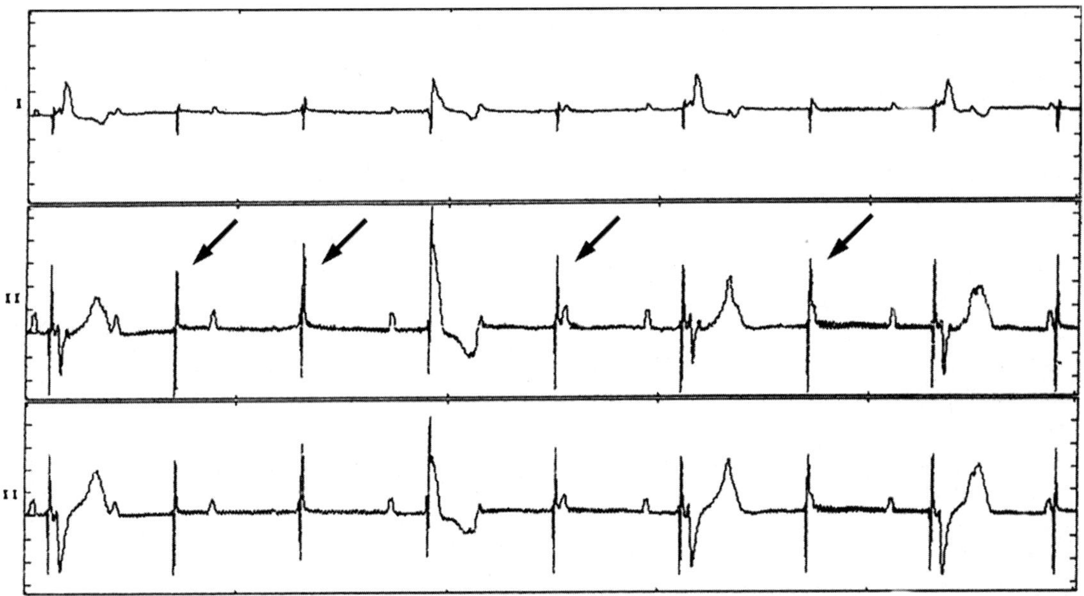

Figure 21-10. A simultaneous lead I, II, and III ECG recorded from a dog with a malfunctioning unipolar pacemaker. The ECG shows numerous pacing stimuli that do not depolarize the myocardium (intermittent failure to capture) (arrows).

surface ECG to show timing of pacing and sensing on the monitor, and a hard copy tracing may also be obtained (see Figure 21-3).

- Output programming, referring to programming of the pulse width and voltage amplitude of the pacing signals, is the most important aspect of programming that should be done routinely. Output should be high enough to provide an adequate pacing margin of safety while also maintaining output as low as possible to maximize battery longevity. Although there is no consensus regarding the best way to program output parameters, acceptable methods include doubling the threshold voltage amplitude, tripling the pulse width at threshold, and plotting strength duration curves. Because capture threshold usually increases immediately after pacemaker implantation as healing occurs, energy output should be set relatively high at implant and then reprogrammed after healing (approximately 8 weeks after implant).
- Sensing parameters also need to be programmed and checked. Appropriate sensing of intrinsic cardiac activity is extremely important for proper pacemaker function whether the patient has a single- or dual-chamber pacing system. A common programming error is over sensing of T waves in canine patients. This problem can usually be corrected by increasing the sensing threshold.
- Appropriate programming of the refractory period is also essential for correct pacemaker function. If the refractory period is too long, intrinsic QRS complexes may cause multiple restarting of the refractory period causing the generator to switch to asynchronous pacing. The recommended method for programming of the refractory period is that the refractory period should include the T wave and be slightly longer than the QT interval; however, dogs and cats with concurrent tachyarrhthmias may require programming with a slightly shorter refractory period to prevent noise reversion.
- Although a pacemaker programmer is often necessary for trouble shooting and thoroughly evaluating pacemaker function, standard ECG recording may also be helpful. The ECG appearance of paced beats differs from that of endogenous beats. A paced beat includes a pacing stimulus artifact, a depolarization wave, and a repolarization wave. The pacing stimulus artifact is typically small with bipolar pacing and relatively large with unipolar pacing (see Figures 21-5 and 21-10). The QRS morphology of a paced beat will depend on location of the ventricular pacing lead; transvenous pacing from the right ventricular apex usually produces QRS complexes with a left bundle branch block configuration in the frontal plane leads (see Figure 21-5). If the pacing mode is VVI or VVIR the paced beats are inhibited by sensed spontaneous beats, and the basic pacing cycle is reset.
- ECG abnormalities in patients with pacemakers may be broadly classified as failure to capture,

failure to output, and abnormal sensing. Failure to capture is recognized as a pacing stimulus artifact without ventricular depolarization (see Figure 21-10). Causes of failure to capture include lead dislodgement, high thresholds with inadequately programmed output, partial lead fracture, insulation defect, impending battery depletion, poor or incompatible connection of the lead to the generator, and functional noncapture (pacing stimulus during the refractory period of a spontaneous beat).

- Failure to pace is recognized as failure of the generator to deliver an appropriately timed stimulus. This problem is often caused by oversensing, but it may be due to true failure of the generator or to circuit interruption (the electrical signal does not reach the heart). Reasons for true failure to output include circuit failure, complete or intermittent lead wire fracture, intermittent or permanent loose screw set, incompatible lead, battery depletion, internal insulation fracture (bipolar lead), and lack of anodal contact (unipolar lead). When a pacemaker battery reaches the end state of depletion, either failure to capture because of reduced voltage output or failure to pace because of total battery depletion may occur.
- Sensing abnormalities, both under sensing and oversensing, may also be recognized on a surface ECG in many patients. Causes of sensing abnormalities include lead dislodgement or poor lead positioning, lead insulation failure, circuit failure, magnet application, malfunction of the generator (reed switch), EMI, and battery depletion.

Frequently Asked Questions

When and why should dual-chamber pacing be done?
Dual-chamber pacing provides AV synchrony whereas single-chamber ventricular pacing does not. Pacing with AV synchrony reduces ventricular filling pressures and mitral regurgitation compared to VVI (or VVIR) pacing. Therefore, dual-chamber pacing is preferable in patients with chronic valvular disease or myocardial disease. AV synchrony is also essential for high level athletic activity, and, therefore, dual-chamber pacing should be considered in athletic dogs and working dogs. Placement of a VDD lead or two conventional transvenous leads is technically difficult, however, in animals weighing less than 10 kg.

What are the major advantages of atrial synchronous pacing (VDD pacing) compared to ventricular inhibited synchronous pacing (VVI)?
Advantages of VDD pacing include chronotropic competence based on intrinsic sinus rate and restoration of AV synchrony. A disadvantage of this pacing mode is that it is appropriate only for treatment of patients with bradycardia caused by AV block. Therefore, this method of pacing cannot be used in patients with atrial fibrillation, atrial standstill, or sinus node dysfunction. Furthermore, VDD pacing is limited to patients large enough to accommodate two leads or a special VDD lead.

What is an appropriate diagnostic approach for a patient with an implanted pacemaker that has reoccurrence of clinical signs suggestive of bradyarrhythmia?
A physical examination and standard ECG should be done. The physical examination will confirm bradycardia if the pacemaker dysfunction is continuous. Occasionally, event recording or Holter monitoring is needed to confirm bradycardia that is episodic as a result of intermittent pacemaker dysfunction. Physical exam may occasionally reveal a cause of pacemaker dysfunction such as significant generator migration causing traction on a pacing lead. Standard ECG is used to identify underlying rhythm which, in turn, may confirm sustained pacemaker malfunction. In addition, standard ECG may help identify a specific cause of pacemaker malfunction. For example, regular pacing stimuli that occur at a rate below the lower programmed rate suggest battery depletion. Pacing stimuli with appropriate timing but without capture may indicate lead dislodgement, lead fracture, lead insulation defect, or inadequate capture threshold. Survey radiographs may confirm fractures or macrodislodgements of pacing leads. Use of a pacemaker programmer to evaluate output and sensing, to test lead impedance, and to determine capture thresholds is often necessary for definitive diagnosis of the cause of pacemaker dysfunction.

SUGGESTED READINGS

Bernstein AD, Daubert JC, Fletcher RD, et al: North American Society of Pacing and Electrophysiology/British Pacing and Electrophysiology Group: The revised NASPE/BPEG generic code for antibradycardia, adaptive-rate, and multisite pacing, Pacing Clin Electrophysiol 25:260-264, 2002.

Bonagura JD, Helphrey ML, Muir WW: Complications associated with permanent pacemaker implantation in the dog. J Am Vet Med Assoc 182:149-155, 1983.

Bulmer BJ, Oyama MA, Lamont LA, et al: Implantation of a single-lead atrioventricular synchronous (VDD) pacemaker in a dog with naturally occurring 3rd-degree atrioventricular block, J Vet Intern Med 16:197-200, 2002.

Bulmer BJ, Oyama MA, Sisson DD: Acute hemodynamic consequences of physiologic VDD pacing in dogs with naturally occurring third degree atrioventricular block, J Vet Intern Med 16(abstract):341, 2002.

Gammage M, Lieberman RA: Selective site pacing. Medtonic Technical Concept Paper, Minneapolis, 2004, Medtronic Inc.

Moise NS, Estrada A: Noise reversion in paced dogs, J Vet Card 4:13-21, 2002.

Oyama MA, Sisson DD, Lehmkuhl LB: Practices and outcome of artificial cardiac pacing in 154 dogs, J Vet Intern Med 15:229-239, 2001.

Petrie J-P: Permanent transvenous cardiac pacing, Clin Tech Small Anim Pract 20:164-172, 2005.

Phibbs B, Marriott HJL: Complications of permanent transvenous pacing, N Engl J Med 312:1428-1432, 1985.

Prosek R, Sisson DD, Oyama MA: Runaway pacemaker in a dog, J Vet Inter Med 18:242-244, 2004.

Sisson D, Thomas WP, Woodfield J, et al: Permanent transvenous pacemaker implantation in forty dogs, J Vet Intern Med 5:322-331, 1991.

APPENDIX 1

Canine Breed Predilections for Heart Disease

Kathleen E. Cavanagh and Francis W. K. Smith, Jr.

Breed	Disease
Afghan Hound	DCM
Airedale	PS
Akita	VSD
Basset Hound	PS VSD
Beagle	PS VSD
Bichon Frise	PDA Degenerative valve disease
Bloodhound	SAS
Boston Terrier	Degenerative valve disease DCM Chemodectoma (± pericardial effusion)
Bouvier des Flandres	SAS
Boxer	SAS PS ASD DCM Arrhythmogenic right ventricular cardiomyopathy (Boxer cardiomyopathy) Chemodectoma (± pericardial effusion)
Boykin Spaniel	PS Degenerative valve disease
Brittany Spaniel	Persistent right aortic arch
Bullmastiff	PS DCM
Bull Terrier	Mitral valve dysplasia Mitral valve stenosis SAS
Cavalier King Charles Spaniel	Inherited ventricular arrhythmias Right atrial hemangiosarcoma (± pericardial effusion) PDA Degenerative valve disease
Chihuahua	PDA PS Degenerative valve disease
Chow Chow	PS VSD
Cocker Spaniel	PDA PS Degenerative valve disease DCM Sick sinus syndrome
Collie	PDA
Dachshund	Degenerative valve disease Mitral valve prolapse Sick sinus syndrome PDA
Dalmatian	DCM Mitral valve dysplasia
Doberman Pinscher	ASD DCM Bundle of His degeneration
English Bulldog (Bulldog)	PS Tetralogy of Fallot VSD SAS Chemodectoma (± pericardial effusion) Mitral valve dysplasia Persistent right aortic arch
English Sheepdog	DCM
English Springer Spaniel	PDA VSD Persistent atrial standstill
Fox Terrier	Degenerative valve disease PS Tetralogy of Fallot (wirehaired)
German Shepherd	SAS Mitral valve dysplasia Tricuspid valve dysplasia Persistent right aortic arch Inherited ventricular arrhythmias Right atrial hemangiosarcoma (± pericardial effusion) Infective endocarditis DCM PDA

DCM, Dilated cardiomyopathy; *PS,* pulmonic stenosis; *VSD,* ventricular septal defect; *PDA,* patent ductus arteriosus; *SAS,* subaortic stenosis; *ASD,* atrial septal defect.

Continued

Breed	Disease
German Shorthair Pointer	SAS
Golden Retriever	SAS Mitral valve dysplasia Tricuspid valve dysplasia Taurine deficient familial DCM Canine X-linked muscular dystrophy Pericardial effusion, idiopathic Right atrial hemangiosarcoma (± pericardial effusion)
Great Dane	Mitral valve dysplasia Tricuspid valve dysplasia SAS PS Persistent right aortic arch DCM Lone atrial fibrillation
Great Pyrenees	Tricuspid valve dysplasia
Greyhound	Persistent right aortic arch
Husky	VSD
Irish Setter	Persistent right aortic arch DCM Right atrial hemangiosarcoma (± pericardial effusion)
Irish Wolfhound	DCM Lone atrial fibrillation
Keeshond (Keeshonden)	Conotruncal Defects (CTD)—A series of genetically related congenital cardiac malformations that include conal septum, conal VSD, Tetralogy of Fallot, and persistent truncus arteriosus PDA PS Mitral valve dysplasia
Kerry Blue Terrier	PDA
Labrador Retriever	Tricuspid valve dysplasia PDA PS DCM Pericardial effusion, idiopathic Right atrial hemangiosarcoma (± pericardial effusion)

DCM, Dilated cardiomyopathy; *PS,* pulmonic stenosis; *VSD,* ventricular septal defect; *PDA,* patent ductus arteriosus; *SAS,* subaortic stenosis; *ASD,* atrial septal defect.

Breed	Disease
Lakeland Terrier	VSD
Lhasa Apso	Degenerative valve disease
Maltese	PDA
Mastiff	Mitral valve dysplasia PS
Miniature Pinscher	Degenerative valve disease
Newfoundland	SAS Mitral valve dysplasia Mitral valve stenosis PDA PS DCM ASD
Old English Sheepdog	Tricuspid valve dysplasia Persistent atrial standstill DCM
Pekingese	Degenerative valve disease
Poodle	PDA (toy and miniature poodle) Degenerative valve disease (toy and miniature poodle) VSD ASD (standard poodle)
Pomeranian	PDA Degenerative valve disease Sick sinus syndrome
Portuguese Water Dog	Inherited juvenile DCM
Pug	Atrioventricular block
Rottweiler	SAS DCM
St. Bernard	DCM
Samoyed	PS SAS ASD
Schnauzer, Miniature	PS PDA Degenerative valve disease Sick sinus syndrome
Scottish Deerhound	DCM
Scottish Terrier	PS
Shetland Sheepdog	PDA Degenerative valve disease
Shih Tzu	VSD Degenerative valve disease
Springer Spaniel	DCM
Terriers (e.g., Fox Terrier, Mixed Terriers)	PS Degenerative valve disease

Continued

Breed	Disease
Weimaraner	Tricuspid valve dysplasia Peritoneopericardial diaphragmatic hernia
West Highland White Terrier	PS VSD Tetralogy of Fallot Degenerative valve disease
Whippet	Degenerative valve disease
Yorkshire Terrier	PDA Degenerative valve disease

DCM, Dilated cardiomyopathy; *PS,* pulmonic stenosis; *VSD,* ventricular septal defect; *PDA,* patent ductus arteriosus; *SAS,* subaortic stenosis; *ASD,* atrial septal defect.

RESOURCES

Alroy J, Rush JE, Freeman L, et al: Inherited infantile dilated cardiomyopathy in dogs: genetic, clinical, biochemical, and morphologic findings. Am J Med Genet 95(1):57-66, 2000.

Basso C, Fox PR, Meurs KM, et al: Arrhythmogenic right ventricular cardiomyopathy causing sudden cardiac death in boxer dogs: a new animal model of human disease. Circulation 109(9):1180-1185, 2004. e-pub: March 1, 2004.

Bélanger MC, Ouellet M, Queney G, et al: Taurine-deficient dilated cardiomyopathy in a family of Golden Retrievers. JAAHA 41:284-291, 2005.

Chetboul V, Charles V, et al: Retrospective study of 156 atrial septal defects in dogs and cats. J Vet Med A Physiol Pathol Clin Med 53(4):179-184, 2006.

Chetboul V, Trolle JM, et al: Congenital heart diseases in the boxer dog: a retrospective study of 105 cases (1998-2005). J Vet Med A Physiol Pathol Clin Med 53(7):346-351, 2006.

Dambach DM, Lannon A, Sleeper MM, et al: Familial dilated cardiomyopathy of young Portuguese water dogs. J Vet Intern Med 13(1):65-71, 1999.

Fox PR, Sisson D, Moïse NS, eds: Textbook of canine and feline cardiology, ed 2, Philadelphia 1999, WB Saunders.

Gordon SG, Saunders AB, et al: Atrial septal defects in an extended family of standard poodles. In *Proceedings,* The Annual ACVIM Forum, p 730, 2006.

Gunby JM, Hardie RJ, Bjorling DE: Investigation of the potential heritability of persistent right aortic arch in Greyhounds. J Am Vet Med Assoc 224(7):1120-1122, 2004.

Hyun C, Lavulo L: Congenital heart diseases in small animals. I. Genetic pathways and potential candidate genes. Vet J 171(2):245-255, 2006. Comment in Vet J 171(2):195-197, 2006.

Hyun C, Park IC: Congenital heart diseases in small animals. II. Potential genetic aetiologies based on human genetic studies. Vet J 171(2):256-262, 2006. Comment in Vet J 171(2):195-197, 2006.

Kittleson MD, Kienle RD, eds: Small animal cardiovascular medicine. Philadelphia, 1998, Mosby.

MacDonald KA: Congenital heart diseases of puppies and kittens. Vet Clin North Am Small Anim Pract 36(3):503-531, 2006.

Meurs KM: Inherited heart disease in the dog. In *Proceedings,* 2003 Tufts Genetics Symposium, 2003.

Meurs KM: Update on Boxer arrhythmogenic right ventricular cardiomyopathy (ARVC). In *Proceedings,* The Annual ACVIM Forum, p 106, 2005.

Meurs KM, Fox PR, Nogard M, et al: A prospective genetic evaluation of familial dilated cardiomyopathy in the Doberman Pinscher. J Vet Intern Med 21:1016-1020, 2007.

Meurs KM, Spier AW, Miller MW, et al: Familial ventricular arrhythmias in boxers. J Vet Intern Med 13(5):437-439, 1999.

Meurs KM, Spier AW, Wright NA, et al: Comparison of the effects of four antiarrhythmic treatments for familial ventricular arrhythmias in Boxers. J Am Vet Med Assoc 221(4):522-527, 2002.

Moïse NS: Update on inherited arrhythmias in German Shepherds. In *Proceedings,* The Annual ACVIM Forum, pp 67-68, 2005.

Olsen LH, Fredholm M, Pedersen HD: Epidemiology and inheritance of mitral valve prolapse in Dachshunds. J Vet Intern Med 13(5):448-56, 1999.

Parker HG, Meurs KM, Ostrander EA: Finding cardiovascular disease genes in the dog. J Vet Cardiol 8: 115-127, 2006.

Schober KE, Baade H: Doppler echocardiographic prediction of pulmonary hypertension in West Highland white terriers with chronic pulmonary disease. J Vet Intern Med 20:912-920, 2006.

Spier AW, Meurs KM, Muir WW, et al: Correlation of QT dispersion with indices used to evaluate the severity of familial ventricular arrhythmias in Boxers. Am J Vet Res 62(9):1481-1485, 2001.

Tidholm A: Retrospective study of congenital heart defects in 151 dogs. J Small Anim Pract 38(3):94-98, 2006.

Vollmar AC, Fox PR: Assessment of cardiovascular diseases in 527 Boxers. In *Proceedings,* The Annual ACVIM Forum, p 65, 2005.

Vollmar AC, Trötschel C: Cardiomyopathy in Irish Wolfhounds. In *Proceedings,* The Annual ACVIM Forum, p 66, 2005.

Werner P, Raducha MG, Prociuk U, et al: The Keeshond defect in cardiac conotruncal development is oligogenic. Human Genet 116(5):368-377, 2005. e-pub: Feb 12, 2005.

APPENDIX 2

Common Cardiovascular Drugs

Francis W. K. Smith, Jr., Larry P. Tilley, Mark A. Oyama, and Meg M. Sleeper

Advancing technology has provided clinicians with ever more powerful and effective drugs for treating diseases. As more drugs become available, it becomes progressively more difficult for practitioners to make rational choices between similar drugs. It is also difficult to be aware of the numerous side effects, contraindications, and drug interactions of the many cardiopulmonary drugs available. The following tables and charts have been designed and provided in the hope of facilitating rational drug selections for the treatment of cardiopulmonary disease.

An attempt has been made to make these tables as complete as possible, while focusing on the more common or serious side effects and drug interactions. For a more exhaustive review of individual drugs, the reader should refer to the package insert and drug chapters in this book. The reader should also follow the current veterinary literature, as new dosing recommendations may become available as a result of clinical use and scientific research. This advice is especially appropriate for new or infrequently used drugs.

DISCLOSURE

Medicine is a science that is constantly changing. Changes in treatment and drug therapy are required with new research and clinical experiences. The author, editor, and publisher of this book have made every effort to ensure that the drug dosage schedules are accurate. The drug dosages are based on the standards accepted at the time of publication. The product information sheet included in the package of each drug should be checked before the drug is administered to be certain that changes have not been made in the recommended dose of or in the contraindications for administration. Primary responsibility for decisions regarding treatment of patients remains with the attending clinician. All patients should be carefully monitored for desired efficacious and undesired toxic effects while instituting, titrating, and maintaining therapy.

Drugs are listed in alphabetical order by generic name. The order of presentation in no way reflects the preference for use. General recommendations for therapy may be found in the main body of this document.

KEY TO FORMULARY ABBREVIATIONS

ACE	Angiotensin-converting enzyme
ACT	Activated clotting time
ADP	Adenosine diphosphate
APTT	Activated partial thromboplastin time
BP	Blood pressure
Cap	Capsule
CHF	Congestive heart failure
COPD	Chronic obstructive pulmonary disease
CRI	Constant-rate infusion
CV	Cardiovascular
D5W	5% dextrose in water
ECG	Electrocardiogram
g	Gram
GFR	Glomerular filtration rate
GI	Gastrointestinal
IM	Intramuscular
Inj	Injectable
INR	International normalization ratio
IO	Intraosseous
IT	Intratracheal
IV	Intravenous
LRS	Lacated Ringer's solution
mcg	Microgram
mg	Milligram
mL	Milliliter
P0	Per os (oral)
PT	Prothrombin time
q	Every, as in q 8 h = every 8 hours
SC	Subcutaneous
Tab	Tablet
U	Units
WPW	Wolff-Parkinson-White syndrome

Cardiopulmonary Drugs—Formulations, Indications, Dosages

Drug Trade Name	Formulation	Indications	Dog Dose (D) Cat Dose (C)	Comments
Acetylsalicylic acid (Aspirin)	Tab: 81, 325 mg	Prevention of thromboembolism	D: 5-10 mg/kg PO q 24-48 h C: 25 mg/kg PO q 3 days (81 mg/cat q 72 h PO)	Platelet inhibitor Nonsteroidal antiinflammatory drug Not 100% effective in preventing emboli May decrease efficacy of ACE inhibitors
Albuterol (Proventil, Ventolin)	Tab: 2, 4 mg Syrup: 0.4 mg/mL	Bronchodilation in patients with reversible obstructive lung disease and asthma Symptomatic bradycardia	D: 0.02-0.05 mg/kg PO q 8 h C: Same	Beta-2 agonist bronchodilator Reduce dose by 50% first 4 days to prevent anxiety side effect Decrease dose with renal disease
Aminophylline (Aminophyllin)	Tab: 100, 200 mg Ampules: 25 mg/mL Oral solution: 21 mg/mL	Asthma, COPD Symptomatic bradycardia	D: 11 mg/kg q 6-8 h, PO, IV, IM (slowly IV) C: 5 mg/kg q 8-12 h; PO)	Methylxanthine bronchodilator Reduce dose with CHF, liver disease
Amiloride (Midamor)	Tab: 5 mg	See Triamterene	D: 1.25 mg/10 kg PO q 12-24 h with food	See Triamterene
Amiodarone (Cordarone)	Tab: 200 mg	Severe refractory atrial and ventricular arrhythmias	D: Loading dose of 10 mg/kg PO q 12 h for 1 week, thereafter 5 mg/kg PO q 12-24 h C: None	Class III antiarrhythmic Use as last resort for recurrent unstable ventricular tachycardia; takes weeks to achieve therapeutic levels
Amlodipine besylate (Norvasc)	Tab: 2.5, 5, 10 mg	Systemic hypertension	D: 0.05-0.20 mg/kg PO q 12-24 h C: 0.18 mg/kg PO q 24 h (0.625-1.25 mg/cat q 24 h)	Dihydropyridine calcium channel blocker Monitor for hypotension
Amrinone lactate (Inocor)	Ampule: 5 mg/mL	Short-term management of severe myocardial failure	D: 1-3 mg/kg bolus, then 30-100 mcg/kg/min CRI (titrate up to effect) C: Same	Phosphodiesterase inhibitor Can use with digoxin and catecholamines Positive inotrope with arterial vasodilating properties Do not administer in solutions with dextrose Pretreat with digitalis in patients with atrial fibrillation
Atenolol (Tenormin)	Tab: 25, 50, 100 mg Oral suspension: 25 mg/mL	Atrial and ventricular arrhythmias, hypertrophic cardiomyopathy, hypertension, aortic stenosis	D: 0.25-1.5 mg/kg PO q 12-24 h C: 6.25-12.5 mg PO q 12-24 h	Beta-1 selective beta-blocker Less bronchoconstriction and vasoconstriction than nonselective beta-blockers Taper dose when discontinue therapy

Continued

Cardiopulmonary Drugs—Formulations, Indications, Dosages—cont'd

Drug Trade Name	Formulation	Indications	Dog Dose (D) Cat Dose (C)	Comments
Atropine sulfate	Inj: 0.05, 0.1, 0.3, 0.4, 0.5, 0.8, 1.0 mg/mL	Sinus bradycardia, atrioventricular block, sick sinus syndrome, cardiac arrest	D: 0.01-0.04 mg/kg IV, IM, IO 0.02-0.04 mg/kg SC q 6-8 h (IT: double dose) C: Same	Anticholinergic May transiently worsen bradyarrhythmia More potent chronotropic effects than glycopyrrolate
Benazepril (Fortekor-Canada), Lotensin	Tab: 5, 20 mg	Balanced vasodilation in CHF, hypertension Renal disease in cats	D: 0.25-0.50 mg/kg PO q24h C: 0.25-0.5 mg/kg q24h (2.5 mg/cat/day)	ACE inhibitor Monitor electrolytes and renal function Excreted in bile and urine
Butorphanol tartrate (Torbutrol, Stadol)	Inj: 0.5, 1, 2 mg/mL Tab: 1, 5, 10 mg (Torbutrol)	Nonproductive cough (COPD, tracheal collapse)	D: 0.055-0.11 mg/kg SC q 6-12 h; 0.55 mg/kg q 6-12 h PO C: None	Narcotic cough suppressant More potent than dextromethorphan
Carnitine (Carnitor)	Tab: 330 mg Can be purchased in bulk as powder	Canine dilated cardiomyopathy accompanied by taurine or carnitine deficiency	D: 50-100 mg/kg PO q 8 h C: None	Amino acid L isomer is active form Not effective in all cases
Carvedilol (Coreg)	Tab: 3.125, 6.25, 12.5 mg	Myocardial failure	D: 0.1-0.5 mg/kg q 12 h (based on pharmacokinetic studies, may be able to titrate to 1.5 mg/kg PO q 12 h if tolerated) Start slowly at 0.05-0.1 mg/kg PO q 12 h for 2 weeks; up-titrate the dose every 2-4 weeks C: Not established	Alpha and nonselective beta blocker Do not use with atrioventricular block Monitor closely for worsening of heart failure Absorption highly variable in dogs
Chlorothiazide (Diuril)	Tab: 250, 500 mg Oral suspension: 50 mg/mL	Diseases associated with fluid retention (CHF, hepatic disease, nephrotic syndrome), hypertension	D: 20-40 mg/kg PO q 12 h C: Same	Thiazide diuretic Less potent than loop diuretics Not effective with low GFR (renal failure) Can use with loop diuretics for increased diuresis, but reduce initial thiazide dose by 50% May precipitate hepatic encephalopathy in patients with severe liver disease

Clopidogrel (Plavix)	Tab: 75 mg	Prevention of thromboembolism in cats that have already had a thrombembolic event or are at high risk for thromboembolism	D: 10 mg/kg loading dose followed by 2-4 mg/kg PO q 24 h C: 18.75 mg PO q 24 h	Platelet inhibitor (ADP receptor blocker) Can be used in combination with aspirin or heparin Be aware of possibility of hemorrhage when using combinations of platelet inhibitors and anticoagulants
Dalteparin (Fragmin)	Inj: 16 mg (2500 U)/0.2 mL; 32 mg (5000 U/0.02 mL) prefilled syringes; 64 mg (10,000 U)/mL multidose vials	Antithrombotic	D: 100-150 U/kg SC q 8 h C: 180 U/kg SC q 6 h	Low-molecular-weight heparin Dose extrapolated from humans and pharmacokinetic studies in animals; optimal dose in dogs and cats unknown Less likely to cause bleeding complications than warfarin Expensive
Dextromethorphan	In many OTC cough formulas	Nonproductive cough (COPD, tracheal collapse)	D: 2 mg/kg PO q 6-8 h C: Same	Nonnarcotic cough suppressant Only cough suppressant safe for use in cats
Digoxin (Lanoxin)	Tab: 0.125, 0.25, 0.5 mg Inj: 0.25 mg/mL Elixir: 0.05 mg/mL Cap: 0.05, 0.1, 0.2 mg	Supraventricular arrhythmias, myocardial failure	D: *Maintenance dose*: 0.22 mg/m^2 PO q12 h, 0.0055-0.01 mg/kg PO q12 h *Oral loading dose*: Twice the maintenance dose for the first 24-48 h C: 0.01 mg/kg PO q 48 h (Tab preferred), 0.007 mg/kg PO q 48 h (w/Lasix and aspirin)	Digitalis glycoside Toxicity potentiated by hypokalemia, hyponatremia, hypercalcemia, hypothyroidism, hypoxia Dose on lean body weight, reduce dose 10%-15% with elixirs Therapeutic range 0.5-2 ng/mL; 8 hours after a dose. Studies in humans show longer survival with range of 0.5-1 ng/ml than with 1-2 ng/ml.

Continued

Cardiopulmonary Drugs—Formulations, Indications, Dosages—cont'd

Drug Trade Name	Formulation	Indications	Dog Dose (D) Cat Dose (C)	Comments
Diltiazem (Cardizem, Dilacor)	Tab: 30, 60, 90, 120 mg Inj: 5 mg/mL Cardizem CD: 120, 180, 300 mg Dilacor XR: 120, 180, 240 mg	Supraventricular arrhythmias, hypertrophic cardiomyopathy, hypertension	D: 0.5-2 mg/kg PO q 8 h (consider higher dose of 5 mg/kg based on recent studies), 0.1-0.2 mg/kg IV bolus, then 2-6 mcg/kg/min IV CRI Dilacor XR: 1.5-6 mg/kg PO q 24 h C: 1.0-2.5 mg/kg PO q 8 h, 0.1-0.2 mg/kg IV bolus, then 2-6 mcg/kg/min IV CRI, Dilacor XR: 30-60 mg PO q 24 h	Calcium channel blocker Less myocardial depression than verapamil Dilacor XR capsules contain 60-mg tablets that are used for dosing cats
Dobutamine HCl (Dobutrex)	Inj: 12.5 mg/mL	Short-term management of severe myocardial failure	D: 2.5-20 mcg/kg/min (titrate up to effect). Administer in D5W C: 2-10 mcg/kg/min (titrate up to effect). Administer in D5W	Beta-adrenergic agonist Monitor ECG, BP, and pulse quality Preferable to dopamine in CHF but more expensive Inotropic effect is dose dependent Less arrhythmogenic than most other catecholamines Use with caution in cats
Dopamine HCl (Intropin, Dopastat)	Inj: 40, 80, or 160 mg/mL	Shock, short-term management of severe myocardial failure Anuric or oliguric renal failure	D: 2-10 mcg/kg/min (titrate up to effect). Administer in D5W, saline, or LRS C: Same	Dopaminergic agonist Monitor ECG, BP, and pulse quality May cause tissue necrosis if extravasation occurs Can administer intraosseously
Enalapril maleate (Enacard)	Tab: 1, 2.5, 5, 10, 20 mg	Balanced vasodilation in CHF, hypertension	D: 0.5 mg/kg PO q 12-24 h (titrate up to effect) C: 0.25-0.5 mg/kg PO q 24-48 h (titrate up to effect)	ACE inhibitor Monitor renal function and electrolytes Increased survival in heart failure patients Decrease dose with renal disease

Enoxaparin (Lovenox)	Inj: 30mg/0.3 mL	Antithrombotic	D: 0.8 mg/kg SC q 12 h C: 1.25 mg/kg SC q 12 h	Low-molecular-weight heparin Dose-extrapolated from humans and pharmacokinetic studies in animals. Optimal dose in dogs and cats unknown Less likely to cause bleeding complications than warfarin Expensive
Epinephrine (Adrenalin)	Inj: 1:1000 conc (1 mg/mL) 1:10000 conc (0.1 mg/mL)	Cardiac arrest	D: 0.2 mg/kg IV, IO q 3-5 min. Double dose for IT administration C: Same	Beta-adrenergic agonist Monitor with ECG Previously recommended dose of 0.02 mg/kg may be a safer starting dose if a defibrillator is not available
Esmolol (Brevibloc)	Inj: 100, 250 mg/mL	Short-term management of supraventricular tachyarrhythmias, ventricular tachycardia, and systemic hypertension	D: 50-500 (usually 50-100) mcg/kg IV bolus every 5 min (up to 500 mcg/kg max), 50-200 mcg/kg/min CRI C: Same	Ultra-short-acting beta-selective beta adrenergic blocker
Furosemide (Lasix)	Tab: 12.5, 20, 40, 50, 80 mg Inj: 10 and 50 mg/mL Oral solution: 10 mg/mL	Diseases associated with fluid retention (CHF, hepatic disease, nephrotic syndrome), hypertension	D: 2-6 mg/kg PO, IM, IV q 8-48 h, 2-8 mg/kg IV q 1-2 h for severe pulmonary edema CRI: 0.66 mg/kg IV bolus followed by 0.66 mg/kg/h IV C: 1-4 mg/kg PO, IM, IV q 12-48 h. Titrate to lowest effective dose for maintenance	Loop diuretic Decreased oral absorption in decompensated CHF Monitor hydration and electrolytes Hypokalemia uncommon in dogs unless anorexic or high dose May precipitate hepatic encephalopathy in patients with severe liver disease Bioavailability reduced with food
Glycopyrrolate (Robinul)	Inj: 0.2 mg/mL	Sinus bradycardia, atrioventricular block, sick sinus syndrome	D: 0.005-0.01 mg/kg IV, IM, 0.01-0.02 mg/kg SC C: Same	Anticholinergic Longer duration of action with less of a chronotropic effect than atropine
Heparin (Calciparine, Liquaemin)	Inj: 1000, 5000, 10,000 U/mL	Short-term prevention of thromboembolism	D: Loading dose: 100-500 U/kg SC q 8 h Chronic dose: 10-50 μ/kg q 6-8 h C: Loading dose: 100-300 U/kg SC q 8 h	Anticoagulant Antidote: Protamine sulfate Maintain APTT or ACT at 2-2.5 times the pretreatment values

Continued

Cardiopulmonary Drugs—Formulations, Indications, Dosages—cont'd

Drug Trade Name	Formulation	Indications	Dog Dose (D) Cat Dose (C)	Comments
Hydralazine HCl (Apresoline)	Tab: 10, 25, 50, 100 mg Inj: 20 mg/mL	Arterial dilation in CHF, hypertension	D: 1-3 mg/kg PO q12h (titrate up to effect) C: 0.5-0.8 mg/kg PO q 12 h	Direct-acting arterial vasodilator Causes sodium retention, requiring increased diuretic doses Reflex tachycardia can be controlled with digitalis Decreasing dose 50%-75% for 1-2 weeks and then titrating upward may reduce risk of vomiting Can use injectable formulation orally for more accurate dosing in small patients
Hydrochlorothiazide (HydroDIURIL)	Tab: 25, 50, 100 mg Oral solution: 10, 100 mg/ml	Diseases associated with fluid retention (CHF, hepatic disease, nephritic syndrome), hypertension	D: 2-4 mg/kg PO q 12 h C: Same	Thiazide diuretic Less potent than loop diuretics Not effective with low GFR (renal failure) Can use with loop diuretics for increased diuresis, but reduce inital thiazide dose by 50% May precipitate hepatic encephalopathy in patients with severe liver disease
Hydrocodone bitartrate (Hycodan)	Tab: 5 mg Syrup: 1 mg/mL	Nonproductive cough (COPD, tracheal collapse)	D: 0.22 mg/kg PO q 6-12 h C: Do not use	Narcotic antagonist More potent than dextromethorphan
Hyoscyamine sulfate (Levsin, Anaspaz, Cystospaz, Donnamar)	0.125 mg tab 0.375 mg tab (Extended release) 0.125 mg/5 cc	Sinus bradycardia, atrioventricular block, sick sinus syndrome	D: 0.003-0.006 mg/kg q 8 h	Anticholinergic Similar to atropine
Isoproterenol (Isuprel)	Inj: 1:5000 (0.2 mg/mL)	Short-term management of sinus bradycardia, atrioventricular block, sick sinus syndrome	D: 0.04-0.09 mcg/kg/min IV (titrate up to effect), 10 mcg/kg/min IM, SC q 6 h C: Same	Sympathomimetic agent Used as an emergency treatment until artificial pacing can be accomplished
Isosorbide dinitrate (Isordil, Sorbitrate)	Tab: 5, 10, 20, 30, 40 mg	Venodilation in CHF	D:0.2-1.0 mg/kg PO q 12 h C: Same	Nitrate venodilator Can combine with hydralazine for balanced vasodilation Schedule 12-hour drug-free period to try and avoid tolerance

Lidocaine (Xylocaine)	Inj: 5, 10, 15, 20 mg/mL (without epinephrine)	Ventricular arrhythmias	D: 2-8 mg/kg slowly IV or IO (double the dose IT) in 2 mg/kg boluses followed by IV drip at 25-75 (occasionally up to 100) mcg/kg/min CRI C: 0.25-0.75 mg/kg IV over 5 min CRI: 10-40 mcg/kg/min	Class I antiarrhythmic Use with caution in cats as may cause seizures Drug of choice for initial control of ventricular tachycardia Effects increased by high potassium and decreased by low potassium Seizures controlled with diazepam
Lisinopril (Prinivil, Zestril)	Prinivil unscored tablets, 2.5, 5, 10, 20, 40 mg	Balanced vasodilation in CHF, hypertension	D: 0.25-0.5 mg/kg PO q 12-24 h	ACE inhibitor Monitor renal function and electrolytes Decrease dose with renal disease
Magnesium	20% $MgCl_2$ solution for injection (contains 1.97 mEq of Mg^{++} per mL)	Ventricular arrhythmias-hypomagnesemia can potentiate ventricular tachycardia	D: 0.75-1 mEq/kg/24 h IV infusion (50% of total dose can be given in 2-4 hours if necessary); for ventricular fibrillation: 0.15-0.30 mEq/kg IV over 5-10 min.	Electrolyte For treating refractory arrhythmias
Melarsomine (Immiticide)	Inj: 25 mg/mL	Heartworm disease	D: 2.5 mg/kg/day IM give a single injection of 2.5 mg/kg and then in 1 month give two additional doses 24 hours apart C: None	Heartworm adulticide Administer via deep IM injection Divided protocol is now recommended in all infected dogs by the American Heartworm Society
Metoprolol (Lopressor)	Tab: 25, 50, 100 mg Inj: 1 mg/mL	Atrial and ventricular arrhythmias, hypertrophic cardiomyopathy, hypertension, myocardial failure	D: 0.25-1.0 mg/kg PO q 8 h C: Same	Beta-1 selective beta blocker Less bronchoconstriction, and interference with insulin therapy than with nonselective beta blockers Taper dose when stopping Dose should be slowly titrated over several weeks in dogs with myocardial failure Less expensive than carvedilol
Mexiletine (Mexitil)	Cap: 150, 200, 250 mg Inj: 1 mg/mL Mexitil, 250 mg for injection	Ventricular arrhythmias	D: 5-8 mg/kg PO q 8-12 h; 2.5 mg/kg bolus IV given over 10 min, followed by 30 mcg/kg/min for 3 hours CRI, followed by 5-8 mcg/kg/min CRI for 24-48 hours IV (currently available in Europe) C: None	Class I antiarrhythmic Reduce dose with liver disease Take with food to reduce gastrointestinal side effects

Continued

Cardiopulmonary Drugs—Formulations, Indications, Dosages—cont'd

Drug Trade Name	Formulation	Indications	Dog Dose (D) Cat Dose (C)	Comments
Nitroglycerin (Nitro-BID, Nitrol, Nitrostat) Minitran transderm patches 2.5, 5, 10, 15 mg/24h	2% ointment (1 inch = 15 mg)	Venodilation in CHF	D: 0.25 inch/5 kg cutaneously q 6-8 h; Patch: 2.5-10 mg (small-giant dog) C: ⅛-¼ inch cutaneously q 6-8 h	Nitrate venodilator Can combine with hydralazine for balanced vasodilation Apply to ears if warm to touch, otherwise use shaved area in inguinal or axillary region (use gloves when applying) Schedule 12-hour drug-free period to try and avoid tolerance
Nitroprusside sodium (Nipride, Nitropress)	Inj: 50 mg/vial	Short-term balanced vasodilation in severe CHF	D: 1-10 mcg/kg/min in D5W C: Unknown	Nitrate vasodilator Protect solution from light Adjust drip rate to maintain mean arterial pressure of ~70 mm Hg Discontinue if metabolic acidosis develops Large dose or prolonged use may cause cyanide toxicity
Omega-3 fatty acids (ALA, EPA and/or DHA)		Heart failure (to counter cachexia); renal hypertension; ventricular arrhythmias	D: C: 50-250 mg/kg/24 h PO	Fatty acid Side effects rare
Pimobendan (Vetmedin)	Chewable tablets: 1.25 mg, 5 mg (USA) Capsules: 1.25 mg, 2.5 mg, 5 mg (Canada, Europe, and Australia)	Licensed for treating dogs with signs of mild, moderate, or severe CHF (modified NYHA Class II, III, or IV) due to dilated cardiomyopathy or valvular insufficiency.	D: 0.25 mg/kg q 12 h PO C:1.25 mg/cat q 12 h PO (anecdotal)	Phosphodiesterase III inhibitor and a calcium sensitizer that acts as an inotropic vasodilator Do not use in aortic stenosis, hypertrophic cardiomyopathy, or other conditions in which an augmentation of cardiac output is inappropriate
Prazosin HCl (Minipress)	Cap: 1, 2, 5 mg	Balanced vasodilation in CHF, hypertension	D: 1 mg/15 kg PO q 8 h. Titrate to effect C: None	Direct acting vasodilator Tolerance develops

Procainamide (Pronestyl, generic)	Cap: 250, 375, 500 mg Tab: 250, 375, 500 mg Tab: CR, SR: 250, 500, 750, 1000 mg Inj: 100, 500 mg/mL	Ventricular and supraventricular arrhythmias, WPW	D: 10-30 mg/kg IM, PO q 6 h; 2 mg/kg IV over 3-5 min up to total dose of 20 mg/kg; 20-50 mcg/kg/min CRI C: 3-8 mg/kg PO, IM, q 6-8 h	Class 1 antiarrhythmic agent Beware hypotension with IV administration Effects increased by high potassium and decreased by low potassium Monitor ECG: 25% prolongation of QRS is sign of toxicity Fewer gastrointestinal and cardiovascular side effects than quinidine Use with caution in cats Reduce dose with severe renal and liver disease Use largely replaced by mexiletine and sotalol
Propranolol (Inderal)	Tab: 10, 20, 40, 60, 80, 90 mg Inj: 1 mg/mL Solution: 4, 8, 80 mg/mL	Atrial and ventricular arrhythmias, hypertrophic cardiomyopathy, hypertension, thyrotoxicosis	D: 0.2-1.0 mg/kg PO q 8 h; 0.02-0.06 mg/kg IV over 5-10 minutes C: < 4.5 kg: 2.5-5 mg PO q 8-12 h; > 4.5 kg: 5 mg PO 8-12 h; 0.02-0.06 mg/kg IV over 5-10 minutes	Nonselective beta blocker Start with low dose and titrate to effect Taper dose when discontinue therapy Reduce dose with liver disease Beware of possible bronchoconstriction
Quinidine gluconate (Quinaglute Dura-Tabs) Quinidine polygalacturonate (Cardioquin) Quinidine sulfate (Quinidex)	Tab: 324 mg Inj: 80 mg/mL Tab: 275 mg Tab: 100, 200, 300 mg Tab SR: 300 mg Cap: 200, 300 mg Inj: 200 mg/mL	Ventricular and supraventricular arrhythmias, WPW, conversion of atrial fibrillation	D: 6-20 mg/kg PO, IM q 6 h; 6-20 mg/kg PO q 8 h with sustained release products; 5-10 mg/kg IV (very slowly) C: None Note: Dose calculated for quinidine base equivalent, which varies with each quinidine salt. See Comments.	Class 1 antiarrhythmic Decrease digoxin dose 50% when using quinidine Effects increased by high potassium and decreased by low potassium Monitor ECG: 25% prolongation of QRS is sign of toxicity Has vagolytic, negative inotropic, and vasodilating properties Reduce dose in CHF, hepatic disease, and hypoalbuminemia Quinidine base (%) in each quinidine salt: quinidine gluconate (62%): 324 mg tab = 200 mg quinidine Quinidine polygalacturonate (60%); 275 mg tab = 166 mg quinidine Quinidine sulfate (83%); 200 mg tab = 166 mg quinidine Use largely replaced by mexiletine and sotalol
Sildenafil (Viagra)	Tab: 25, 50, 100 mg	Pulmonary hypertension	D: 0.5-1 mg/kg q 12 h (higher dose of 2-3 mg/kg q 8 h may be tolerated and needed C: Same	Phosphodiesterase 5 inhibiting vasodilator Expensive May be effective for pulmonary hypertension*

Continued

Cardiopulmonary Drugs—Formulations, Indications, Dosages—cont'd

Drug Trade Name	Formulation	Indications	Dog Dose (D) Cat Dose (C)	Comments
Sotalol (Betapace)	Tab: 80, 160, 240 mg	Ventricular arrhythmias	D: 1-2 mg/kg PO q 12 h C: ⅛ of 80 mg tab PO q 12 h	Antiarrhythmic agent with class II (beta-blocking) and class III effects
Spironolactone (Aldactone)	Tab: 25, 50, 100 mg	Diseases associated with fluid retention (CHF, hepatic disease, nephrotic syndrome), hypertension, hypokalemia	D: 1-2 mg/kg PO q 12 h C: Same D,C: 0.5-1.0 mg/kg/day (possible cardiac anti-remodeling)	Potassium-sparing diuretic 2-3 days to achieve peak effect Weak diuretic Usually combines with a loop diuretic Ulcerative facial dermatitis in third of cats
Taurine (Taurine V)	Tab: 250 mg Cap: 500 mg as a generic	Dilated cardiomyopathy (cats) and selective cases in dogs (especially the American Cocker Spaniel)	D: 500 mg PO q 12 h C: 250 mg PO q12 h	Amino acid Clinical improvements noted in 4-10 days Echo improvement usually by 6 weeks Continue supplement for 12-16 weeks while correcting diet
Terbutaline (Brethine, Bricanyl)	Tablet: 2.5, 5 mg Inj: 1 mg/mL	Asthma, COPD	D: 1.25-5 mg/dog PO q 8-12 h C: 0.1 mg/kg PO q 12 h; 0.05 mg/kg SC, IM, IV	Beta-2 agonist bronchodilator Reduce dose by 50% first 4 days to prevent restless behavior. Decrease dose with renal disease
Theophylline (Extended Release)	Tab: 100, 200, 300, 450 mg Cap: 50, 75, 125, 200 mg	Asthma, COPD, sick sinus syndrome	D: 9 mg/kg PO q 8-12 h; Extended release: 10 mg/kg PO q 12 h C: 4 mg/kg PO q 12 h; Extended release tab: 15 mg/kg PO q 24 h at night; Extended release cap: 19 mg/kg PO q 24 h at night	Methylxanthine bronchodilator Extended release dose based on Inwood Laboratories formulation Reduce dose with CHF, liver disease, cimetidine, orbifloxacin, enrofloxacin Reduce dose by 50% first 4 days to prevent anxiety side effect Therapeutic range: 10-20 mcg/mL Dose on lean body weight
Tocainide (Tonocard)	Tab: 400, 600 mg	Ventricular arrhythmias	D: 10-20 mg/kg PO q 8-12 h C: None	Class I Antiarrhythmic Oral analog of lidocaine Giving with food may decrease gastrointestinal upset

Drug Trade Name	Formulation	Indications	Dog Dose (D) Cat Dose (C)	Comments
Triamterene (Dyrenium)	Cap: 50, 100 mg	Diseases associated with fluid retention (CHF, hepatic disease, nephrotic syndrome), hypertension, hypokalemia	D: 1-2 mg/kg PO q 12 h C: Same	Potassium-sparing diuretic Weak diuretic Usually combined with loop diuretic Does not block aldosterone
Verapamil (Calan, Isoptin)	Tab: 80, 120, 240 mg Inj: 2.5 mg/mL	Supraventricular arrhythmias, hypertrophic cardiomyopathy	D: 0.05-0.2 mg/kg slow IV (1-2 min) in boluses of 0.05 mg/kg given at 10-30 minute intervals (to effect) to a maximum cumulative dose of 0.2 mg/kg C: None	Calcium channel blocker Diltiazem is a safer alternative in heart failure Potent vasodilator and negative inotrope
Warfarin (Coumadin)	Tab: 2, 2.5, 5, 7.5, 10 mg	Prevention of thromboembolism	D: 0.1-0.2 mg/kg PO q 24 h C: Same	Anticoagulant Initiate therapy with 4 days of heparin to prevent initial hypercoagulable state Control animal's lifestyle and environment to minimize risk of trauma Adjust dose to maintain PT at 1.5-2 times baseline value or INR of 2-3

*Bach et al. JVIM 20(5).

CALCULATING A CONSTANT-RATE INFUSION FOR LIDOCAINE

A CRI dosage of 25 to 75 mcg/kg/min of lidocaine can be used in dogs with an intravenous loading dose of 1-2 mg/kg. In cats, various sources support a CRI dosage of 10-40 mcg/kg/min of lidocaine with an intravenous loading dose of 0.25 to 0.75 mg/kg. Use with caution in cats because it may cause seizures.

Lidocaine solution is made up by replacing 75 ml of fluid from a liter bag with 75 ml of 2% lidocaine (half the amount if 500 ml bag). Using the appropriate body weight and corresponding fluid rate in the table below will achieve a CRI dosage of 50 mcg/kg/min.

BW (kg)	ml/hr
5	10
10	20
20	40
30	60
40	80
50	100
60	120
70	140

REFERENCES

Tilley LP, Smith FWK, eds: The five minute veterinary consult, ed 4. Ames, Iowa, 2008, Blackwell Publishing.

Kittleson MD, Kienle, RD: Small animal cardiovascular medicine. Philadelphia, 1998, Mosby.

Papich MG: Saunders handbook of veterinary drugs, ed 2. St Louis, 2007, WB Sanunders.

APPENDIX 3

Echocardiographic Normals

Normal Canine Echocardiographic Values*

	Weight (kg)										
Parameter	**3**	**5**	**7**	**10**	**15**	**20**	**25**	**30**	**35**	**40**	**50**
LVID$_d$	24.6	27.4	30.0	32.7	37.1	41.4	44.8	48.3	51.7	54.8	60.7
(mm)	(6.2)	(5.2)	(4.5)	(3.5)	(2.4)	(2.2)	(2.9)	(3.9)	(5.0)	(6.1)	(8.3)
LVID$_s$	13.6	16.0	17.9	20.6	24.3	28.0	31.0	33.9	36.9	39.6	44.6
(mm)	(5.5)	(4.7)	(4.0)	(3.1)	(2.1)	(2.0)	(2.5)	(3.4)	(4.5)	(5.4)	(7.4)
LVPW$_d$	5.0	5.4	5.7	6.2	6.8	7.4	7.9	8.4	8.9	9.3	10.2
(mm)	(2.1)	(1.7)	(1.5)	(1.2)	(0.8)	(0.7)	(1.0)	(1.3)	(1.7)	(2.0)	(2.8)
LVPW$_s$	7.2	7.9	8.4	9.2	10.2	11.3	12.1	13.0	13.8	14.5	16.0
(mm)	(1.7)	(1.6)	(1.4)	(1.3)	(1.1)	(1.1)	(1.2)	(1.3)	(1.5)	(1.7)	(2.2)
IVS$_d$	5.8	6.2	6.5	7.0	7.6	8.2	8.7	9.2	9.7	10.2	11.0
(mm)	(2.1)	(1.7)	(1.5)	(1.2)	(0.8)	(0.7)	(0.9)	(1.3)	(1.7)	(2.0)	(2.7)
IVS$_s$	9.8	10.2	10.4	10.9	11.5	12.3	13.0	13.9	14.6	15.4	—
(mm)	(2.6)	(2.2)	(2.0)	(1.7)	(1.2)	(1.1)	(1.5)	(2.3)	(2.6)	(3.5)	
LA	12.7	14.0	15.0	16.3	18.3	20.2	21.8	23.3	24.8	26.2	28.8
(mm)	(5.3)	(4.5)	(3.8)	(3.0)	(2.0)	(1.9)	(2.4)	(3.3)	(4.3)	(5.2)	(7.1)
Ao	13.8	15.3	16.4	18.1	20.4	22.8	24.6	26.4	28.3	30.0	33.1
(mm)	(3.6)	(3.0)	(2.6)	(2.0)	(1.4)	(1.3)	(1.6)	(2.2)	(2.9)	(3.5)	(4.8)

From Ware WA: Diagnostic tests for the cardiovascular system. In Nelson RW, Couto CG (eds): Essentials of small animal internal medicine. St. Louis, 1992, Mosby. Data from Bonagura JD, O'Grady MR, Herring DS: Echocardiography: principles of interpretation. Vet Clin North Am Small Anim Pract 15:1177, 1985.

LVID$_d$, Left ventricular internal dimension at end diastole; *LVID$_s$,* left ventricular internal dimension at end systole; *LVPW$_d$,* left ventricular posterior wall at end diastole; *LVPW$_s$,* left ventricular posterior wall at end systole; *IVS$_d$,* interventricular septum at end diastole; *IVS$_s$,* interventricular septum at end systole; *LA,* left atrium (systole); *Ao,* aortic root (diastole).

*Fractional shortening: 28% to 40%; mitral valve E point to septal separation: <5 to 6 mm. Mean value given, ±SD in parentheses below.

Normal Feline Echocardiographic Values

Parameter	Range (Unsedated)* (n = 30)	Range (Sedated With Ketamine)† (n = 30)
$RVID_d$ (mm)	2.7–9.4	1.2–7.5
$LVID_d$ (mm)	12.0–19.8	10.7–17.3
$LVID_s$ (mm)	5.2–10.8	4.9–11.6
SF (%)	39.0–61.0	30–60
$LVPW_d$ (mm)	2.2–4.4	2.1–4.5
$LVPW_s$ (mm)	5.4–8.1	—
IVS_d (mm)	2.2–4.0	2.2–4.9
IVS_s (mm)	4.7–7.0	—
LA (mm)	9.3–15.1	7.2–13.3
Ao (mm)	7.2–11.9	7.1–11.5
LA/Ao	.95–1.65	.73–1.64
EPSS (mm)	.17–.21	—
PEP (s)	—	.024–.058
LVET (s)	.10–.18	.093–0.176
PEP/LVET	—	.228–.513
Vcf (circumf/s)	2.35–4.95	2.27–5.17

$RVID_d$, Right ventricular internal dimension at end diastole; *$LVID_d$*, left ventricular internal dimension at end diastole; *$LVID_s$*, left ventricular internal dimension at end systole; *SF*, shortening fraction; *$LVPW_d$*, left ventricular posterior wall at end diastole; *$LVPW_s$*, left ventricular posterior wall at end systole; *IVS_d*, interventricular septum at end diastole; *IVS_s*, interventricular septum at end systole; *LA*, left atrium (systole); *Ao*, aortic root (end diastole); *EPSS*, E point to septal separation; *PEP (s)*, pre-ejection period (seconds); *LVET (s)*, left ventricular ejection time (seconds); *Vcf (circumf/s)*, velocity of circumferential fiber shortening.

*Data from Jacobs G, Knight DH: M-Mode echocardiographic measurements in nonanesthetized healthy cats: effects of body weight, heart rate, and other variables. Am J Vet Res 46:1705, 1985.

†Data from Fox PR, Bond BR, Peterson ME: Echocardiographic reference values in healthy cats sedated with ketamine hydrochloride. Am J Vet Res 46:1479, 1985.

Median and Range of Observed Heart Rate and Echocardiographic Measurements of Dogs of Four Different Breeds (Differing Somatotypes)

Measurement	Miniature Poodle (n=20)	Pembroke Welsh Corgie (n=20)	Afghan Hound (n=20)	Golden Retriever (n=20)
Weight (kg)	3* (1.4–9)†	15 (8–19)	23 (17–36)	32 (23–41)
Heart rate (bpm)	150 (100–200)	120 (80–160)	120 (80–140)	100 (80–140)
LVWD (mm)	5 (4–6)	8 (6–10)	9 (7–11)	10 (8–12)
LVWS (mm)	8 (6–10)	12 (8–13)	12 (9–18)	15 (10–19)
LVCD (mm)	20 (16–28)	32 (28–40)	42 (33–52)	45 (37–51)
LVCS (mm)	10 (8–16)	19 (12–23)	28 (20–37)	27 (18–35)
FS (%)	47 (35–57)	44 (33–57)	33 (24–48)	39 (27–55)
EPSS (mm)	0 (0–2)	2 (0–5)	4 (0–10)	5 (1–10)
RVCD (mm)	4 (2–9)	10 (6–14)	10 (5–20)	13 (7–27)
IVSD (mm)	5 (4–6)	8 (6–9)	10 (8–12)	10 (8–13)
IVSS (mm)	8 (6–10)	12 (10–14)	13 (8–18)	14 (10–17)
AO (mm)	10 (8–13)	18 (15–22)	26 (20–34)	24 (14–27)
LA (mm)	12 (8–18)	21 (12–24)	26 (18–35)	27 (16–32)

From Morrison, S.A., et al: Effect of breed and body weight on echocardiographic values in four breeds of dogs of differing somatotypes, J Vet Intern Med, 6:223, 1992.

LVWD, Left ventricular wall thickness at end-diastole; *LVWS,* left ventricular wall thickness at systole; *LVCD,* left ventricular chamber dimension at end-diastole; *LVCS,* left ventricular chamber dimension at systole; *FS,* percent fractional shortening; *EPSS,* E-point septal separation; *RVCD,* right ventricular chamber dimension at end-diastole; *IVSD,* interventricular septal thickness at end-diastole; *IVSS,* interventricular septal thickness at systole; *AO,* aortic root; *LA,* left atrium.

*Median.

†Range.

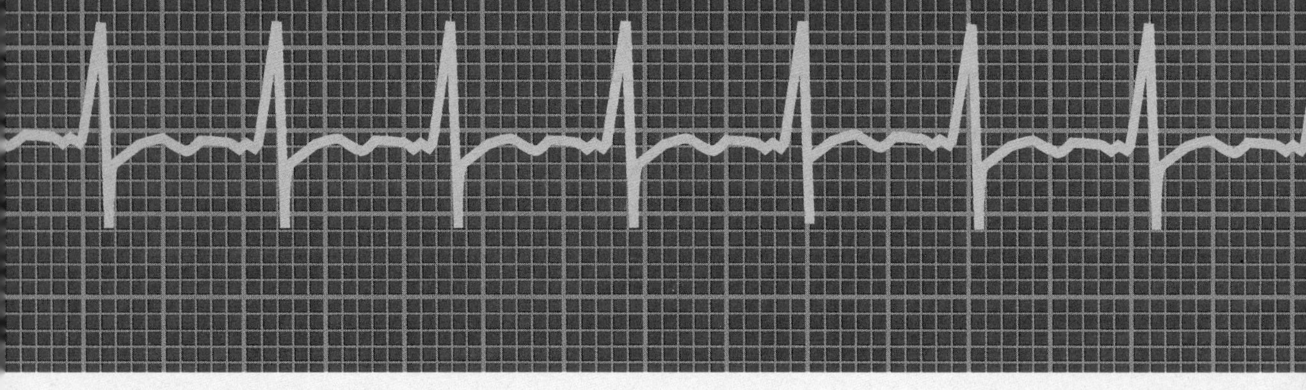

Index

Note: Page numbers followed by *b*, *f*, or *t* indicate boxes, figures, or tables.

B

C

D

E

M

U

V

W

X

Z